TEXTBOOK OF
EAR, NOSE AND THROAT WITH HEAD AND NECK SURGERY FOR MEDICAL STUDENTS

Gabriel Duarte

ALLIED
HEALTH
PRESS

Textbook of Ear, Nose and Throat with Head and Neck Surgery for Medical Students

Author: **Gabriel Duarte**

Allied Health Press
4164 Lakeshore Road
Burlington ON L7L 1A4
Canada
www.alliedhealthpress.com
Email: orders@arclereducation.com

ISBN: 978-1-77956-837-3

ABOUT THE AUTHOR

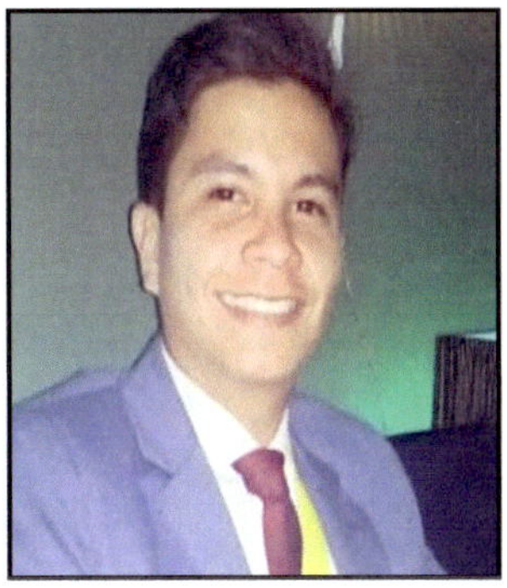

Gabriel is a doctor passionate about writing, clinical practice, diagnostic imaging, surgery, and teaching. His training is solid, having completed medical studies at the University of Los Andes, Venezuela, and subsequently received refresher courses in imaging, ultrasound, and educational consulting. He has also worked as a surgical assistant, providing high-quality medical care. His passion for writing and scientific research has led him to create content and author numerous publications, making him a highly regarded professional.

Brief Table of Contents

1. Introduction to ENT and Head and Neck Surgery	1
2. Anatomy and Physiology of the Ear	35
3. Diseases of the External Ear	65
4. Middle Ear Disorders	93
5. Inner Ear and Vestibular Disorders	123
6. Hearing Assessment and Rehabilitation	153
7. Anatomy and Physiology of the Nose and Paranasal Sinuses	185
8. Nasal and Sinus Disorders	215
9. Disorders of the Nasopharynx	243
10. Anatomy and Physiology ofthe Throat and Larynx	275
11. Tonsillar and Pharyngeal Diseases	305
12. Trauma Reconstruction in Facial Cosmetic	337
13. Congenital and Developmental Deformities in Facial Cosmetic	369
14. Oncologic and Post-Tumor Reconstruction in Facial Cosmetic	401
15. Advances, Technologies, and Practice Management in Facial Cosmetic	433
Index	467

Getting Started with This Book

Chapter Openers

A list of Chapter Outline is presented providing a brief Introduction to what will be covered in the chapter.

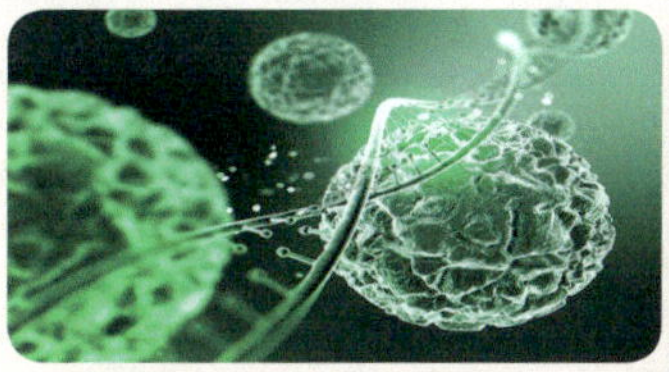

LEARNING OBJECTIVES

After studying this chapter, you will be able to:

1. Discuss the scientific method in biology;
2. Explain the cell theory;
3. Discuss the genetics and heredity;
4. Evolution and natural selection;
5. Focus on ecology and ecosystems;
6. Learn about human biology;
7. Evaluate the plant biology;
8. Explain the microbiology;
9. Focus on current trends in biology.

Introduction

Often referred to as the science of life, biology is a broad field of study aimed at comprehending the several kinds of life on Earth, from tiny creatures to sophisticated multicellular entities. Comprising several subfields, including molecular biology, ecology, and evolutionary biology, each of which advances our knowledge of living systems, this field clarifies the mechanisms controlling life events, including development, reproduction, and interaction with the surroundings, which is the central goal of biology. Moreover, biology fills in the void between the natural sciences and medicine by offering a necessary understanding of health, illness, and the interactions between organisms and their environments. Dealing with urgent global issues such as climate change, biodiversity loss, and new diseases depends on an awareness of these complex biological interactions, therefore highlighting the critical part biology plays in modern civilization. Fundamentally, biology explores and tests ideas about the living world using the scientific method. Through methodical observation and experimentation,

1.1. The Scientific Method in Biology

Learning Outcome

1. Describe the steps of the scientific method;
2. Focus on hypothesis formation;
3. Learn about experimental design.

Learning Outcomes

The beginning of each section of every chapter contains a set of Learning Outcomes that inform students of concepts they should understand. These outcomes help students understand what they should be able to do if they have mastered the material in that section.

Test Your Knowledge

Throughout each chapter, Test Your Knowledge cues you to note which topics have been covered and to self-test your understanding of the material presented.

Test Your Knowledge

1. Explain why correlation does not imply causation in scientific experiments.
2. How does the scientific method help reduce the influence of personal opinions in research?

Chapter Summary

The Summary Section appear at the end of each chapter and summarize main concepts covered throughout the chapter. These points provide key concepts in an engaging and meaningful way.

Summary

The investigation of biological principles highlights the importance of a comprehensive view of life by reflecting the intricate interactions that occur within living systems. The complexity of biology goes beyond individual species or systems, as this essay highlights; it also includes the interactions that mold ecosystems and affect biodiversity. Researchers can conduct in-depth analyses of metabolomic data using sophisticated technologies like MetaboAnalyst, which offer insights into the molecular mechanisms underlying these interactions. As demonstrated by the developments in MetaboAnalyst, for example, the integration of diverse omics data promotes a thorough understanding of metabolic pathways and helps identify important biological markers necessary for research on development and disease (Chong et al., 2018). Additionally, the phenomenon of ecological invasions is a key component of biological research and a vital field of study. The introduction of non-native species into unfamiliar habitats has significant ramifications and calls for multidisciplinary management strategies. Examining the origins and effects of these biological incursions, invasion science has become a crucial field that highlights the need to comprehend ecological dynamics and community interactions. As interest in biological invasions increases, new findings are emerging that put conventional ecological theories and practices to the test. The importance of incorporating various scientific viewpoints is shown by this developing discipline, which also highlights how invasive species shape ecosystems and advances our knowledge of ecological resilience (David et al., 2013). When taken as a whole, these discoveries from invasion science and metabolomics highlight the value of multidisciplinary biology research. Fostering cross-disciplinary collaboration and utilizing technological breakthroughs to improve our comprehension of intricate biological interactions are crucial as we look to the future of biological research. In addition to deepening our understanding of the complexities of life, this method lays the groundwork for tackling urgent environmental issues. Future studies can ensure the continued relevance of biology in a world that is constantly changing by acknowledging the interconnection of biological systems and opening the door to creative solutions that support sustainability and biodiversity conservation. We might imagine a thorough comprehension of life that serves both academia and society at large through ongoing investigation and integration of scientific knowledge.

Knowledge Assessment

The chapter includes material designed to review and reinforce each content. It includes Critical Thinking Questions to help test of your understanding of information presented in the chapter and Short answer Questions to review your understanding of the key concepts presented in the chapter.

Critical Thinking Questions

1. **Who is known as the "Father of Modern Biology"?**
   a. Aristotle
   b. Charles Darwin
   c. Gregor Mendel
   d. Louis Pasteur
2. **What is the basic unit of life?**
   a. Atom
   b. Molecule
   c. Cell
   d. Organism
3. **Which branch of biology studies the interaction of organisms with their environment?**
   a. Genetics
   b. Ecology
   c. Physiology
   d. Botany
4. **Which macromolecule is the main source of energy for living organisms?**
   a. Proteins
   b. Lipids
   c. Carbohydrates
   d. Nucleic acids
5. **DNA is primarily responsible for which function in living organisms?**
   a. Energy production
   b. Protein synthesis
   c. Storing genetic information
   d. Regulating body temperature

Short Answer Questions

1. What is biology, and why is it important to study biology?
2. What are the three main domains of life, and how are they different from one another?
3. Define homeostasis and give an example of how it works in living organisms.
4. What is the cell theory, and why is it fundamental to biology?
5. How do autotrophs and heterotrophs differ in the way they obtain energy?
6. What is the scientific method, and how is it applied in biological research?
7. Discuss how biology helps address global challenges such as climate change, disease, and food security.
8. Explain the levels of biological organization from the smallest unit to the largest. Provide examples at each level.
9. Describe the relationship between structure and function in biology, giving specific examples from cells or organs.
10. How has the discovery of genetics shaped our understanding of inheritance and variation among organisms?

Supplementary Materials

Key Terms: A list of key terms is given for quick reference

KEY TERMS FROM THIS CHAPTER

Annotation enrichment analysis	Biological structure	Cell
Cell theory	Cellular structure	Ecology
Ecosystems	Genetics	Human biology
Microbiology	Natural selection	Organism
Plant biology		

Further Resources: Recommendations for additional readings, websites, and multimedia resources.

References

1. Argelaguet, R., Velten, B., Arnol, D., Dietrich, S., Zenz, T., Marioni, J. C., Buettner, F., et al. (2018). Multi-omics factor analysis—A framework for unsupervised integration of multi-omics data sets. *Molecular Systems Biology, 14*. https://doi.org/10.15252/msb.20178124.
2. Bacher, S., Blackburn, T. M., Essl, F., & Genovesi, P. (2017). *Socio-Economic Impact Classification of Alien Taxa (SEICAT)*. https://core.ac.uk/download/286567949.pdf (accessed on 8th March 2025).
3. Barnett, R., Brace, S., Cucchi, T., & Dobney, K. (2013). *Divergent Evolutionary Processes Associated with Colonization of Offshore Islands*. https://core.ac.uk/download/20664364.pdf (accessed on 8th March 2025).

Detailed Table of Contents

List of Figures *xvii*
Preface *xxv*

CHAPTER 1

Introduction to ENT and Head and Neck Surgery 1

Introduction 1
1.1. Anatomy Relevant to ENT and Head and Neck Surgery 4
1.1.1. Structure and Function of the Ear 5
1.1.2. Anatomy of the Nasal Cavity and Sinuses 6
1.1.3. Overview of the Throat and Neck Structures 7
1.2. Common Conditions Treated in ENT 9
1.2.1. Otitis Media and Other Ear Disorders 9
1.2.2. Sinusitis and Nasal Obstruction 11
1.2.3. Throat Conditions, Including Tonsillitis and Laryngitis 11
1.3. Surgical Techniques in Head and Neck Surgery 12
1.3.1. Endoscopic Procedures in ENT 13
1.3.2. Open Surgical Techniques for Head and Neck Conditions 14
1.3.3. Innovations in Minimally Invasive Surgery 15
1.4. Diagnostic Tools and Technologies 16
1.4.1. Role of Imaging in ENT Diagnosis 17
1.4.2. Use of Endoscopy in Examination 18
1.4.3. Audiological Assessments and Their Importance 19
1.5. Patient Management and Care 20
1.5.1. Preoperative Assessment and Preparation 20
1.5.2. Postoperative Care and Recovery 21
1.5.3. Multidisciplinary Approach to Patient Management 22
1.6. Challenges and Future Directions in ENT 22
1.6.1. Addressing the Rise of Antibiotic Resistance 23
1.6.2. Advances in Technology and Their Impact on Surgery 24
1.6.3. The Importance of Research and Education in ENT 25
Summary 27
References 30

CHAPTER 2

Anatomy and Physiology of the Ear 35

Introduction 35
2.1. Anatomy of the Outer Ear 39
2.1.1. Structure and Function of the Pinna 40
2.1.2. The Auditory Canal and Its Role 40
2.1.3. The Tympanic Membrane (Eardrum) 42
2.2. Anatomy of the Middle Ear 43
2.2.1. The Ossicles: Malleus, Incus, and Stapes 44
2.2.2. The Eustachian Tube and Its Function 45
2.2.3. The Role of the Middle Ear in Sound Amplification 46
2.3. Anatomy of the Inner Ear 47
2.3.1. The Cochlea and Its Structure 48
2.3.2. The Vestibular System and Balance 49

2.3.3. The Auditory Nerve and Signal Transmission 50
2.4. Physiology of Hearing **51**
2.4.1. Sound Wave Transmission Through the Ear 53
2.4.2. Mechanotransduction in Hair Cells 53
2.4.3. Neural Processing of Auditory Information 54
2.5. Physiology of Balance **55**
2.5.1. The Role of the Vestibular System in Equilibrium 56
2.5.2. Interaction Between the Inner Ear and the Brain 57
Summary **59**
References **62**

CHAPTER 3

Diseases of the External Ear 65

Introduction **65**
3.1 Common Diseases of the External Ear **68**
3.1.1. Otitis Externa (Swimmer's Ear) 69
3.1.2. Earwax Impaction 70
3.1.3. Perichondritis 71
3.2. Symptoms and Diagnosis **72**
3.2.1. Common Symptoms Associated with External Ear Diseases 73
3.2.2. Diagnostic Methods Used by Healthcare Professionals 74
3.2.3. Importance of Early Diagnosis 75
3.3. Treatment Options **76**
3.3.1. Medical Treatments for External Ear Diseases 76
3.3.2. Surgical Interventions When Necessary 77
3.3.3. Home Remedies and Preventive Measures 78
3.4. Risk Factors **79**
3.4.1. Environmental Factors Contributing to Ear Diseases 80
3.4.2. Personal Hygiene and Its Impact on Ear Health 80
3.4.3. Genetic Predispositions to Ear Conditions 81
3.5. Prevention Strategies **82**
3.5.1. Proper Ear Care Practices 83
3.5.2. Importance of Regular Check-Ups 84
3.5.3. Education on Ear Health Awareness 84
Summary **86**
References **89**

CHAPTER 4

Middle Ear Disorders 93

Introduction **93**
4.1. Common Middle Ear Disorders **97**
4.1.1. Otitis Media 98
4.1.2. Eustachian Tube Dysfunction 99
4.1.3. Cholesteatoma 99
4.2. Causes of Middle Ear Disorders **101**
4.2.1. Infections and Inflammation 102
4.2.2. Allergies and Environmental Factors 103
4.2.3. Anatomical Abnormalities 104
4.3. Symptoms of Middle Ear Disorders **105**
4.3.1. Hearing Loss 106
4.3.2. Ear Pain and Discomfort 107
4.3.3. Fluid Drainage from the Ear 108
4.4. Diagnosis of Middle Ear Disorders **109**
4.4.1. Physical Examination Techniques 110
4.4.2. Audiological Assessments 111
4.4.3. Imaging Studies 112
4.5. Treatment Options for Middle Ear Disorders **113**
4.5.1. Medical Management 113
4.5.2. Surgical Interventions 114
4.5.3. Home Care and Preventive Measures 115
Summary **116**
References **119**

CHAPTER 5

Inner Ear and Vestibular Disorders 123

Introduction **123**
5.1. Common Inner Ear Disorders **126**
5.1.1. Meniere's Disease 127
5.1.2. Vestibular Neuritis 128
5.1.3. Benign Paroxysmal Positional Vertigo (BPPV) 129
5.2. Symptoms of Vestibular Disorders **130**

5.2.1. Dizziness and Vertigo 131
5.2.2. Balance Issues 132
5.2.3. Nausea and Vomiting 133
5.3. Diagnosis of Inner Ear Disorders 134
5.3.1. Clinical History and Physical Examination 135
5.3.2. Audiometric Testing 136
5.3.3. Imaging Studies (e.g., MRI, CT Scans) 136
5.4. Treatment Options 138
5.4.1. Medications for Symptom Relief 139
5.4.2. Vestibular Rehabilitation Therapy 140
5.4.3. Surgical Interventions 140
5.5. Impact on Quality of Life 142
5.5.1. Psychological Effects of Vestibular Disorders 143
5.5.2. Social Implications and Isolation 143
5.5.3. Coping Strategies for Patients 144
Summary 146
References 149

CHAPTER 6

Hearing Assessment and Rehabilitation 153

Introduction 153
6.1. Anatomy Relevant to ENT and Head and Neck Surgery 156
6.1.1. Anatomy of the Nasal Cavity and Paranasal Sinuses 156
6.1.2. Overview of the Throat and Laryngeal Structures 157
6.2. Common Conditions Treated in ENT 158
6.2.1. Otitis Media and Its Implications 159
6.2.2. Sinusitis and Its Treatment Options 160
6.2.3. Disorders of the Larynx, Including Vocal Cord Nodules 161
6.3. Surgical Techniques in Head and Neck Surgery 162
6.3.1. Endoscopic Procedures and Their Applications 162
6.3.2. Open Surgical Techniques for Tumor Removal 163
6.3.3. Reconstructive Surgery in Head and Neck Cases 164
6.4. Diagnostic Tools in ENT and Head and Neck Surgery 165
6.4.1. Role of Imaging Techniques (CT, MRI) 166
6.4.2. Importance of Endoscopy in Diagnosis 167
6.4.3. Audiological Assessments and Their Relevance 168
6.5. Patient Management and Care 169
6.5.1. Preoperative Assessment and Preparation 170
6.5.2. Postoperative Care and Recovery 171
6.5.3. Multidisciplinary Approach to Patient Management 171
6.6. Advances and Innovations in ENT and Head and Neck Surgery 173
6.6.1. Technological Advancements in Surgical Tools 174
6.6.2. Emerging Treatments and Therapies 175
6.6.3. Research Trends and Future Directions in the Field 176
Summary 177
References 180

CHAPTER 7

Anatomy and Physiology of the Nose and Paranasal Sinuses 185

Introduction 185
7.1. Anatomy of the Nose 188
7.1.1. External Structures of the Nose 189
7.1.2. Internal Nasal Cavity and Its Components 190
7.1.3. Nasal Septum and Its Significance 191
7.2. Physiology of the Nose 192
7.2.1. Functions of the Nose in Respiration 193
7.2.2. Role of the Nose in Olfaction 193
7.2.3. Mechanisms of Filtration and Humidification of Air 194
7.3. Anatomy of the Paranasal Sinuses 195
7.3.1. Types of Paranasal Sinuses and Their Locations 196
7.3.2. Structure and Lining of the Sinuses 197
7.3.3. Relationship Between Sinuses and Nasal Cavity 198
7.4. Physiology of the Paranasal Sinuses 199

7.4.1. Functions of the Paranasal Sinuses in the Respiratory System 200
7.4.2. Role in Voice Resonance and Sound Production 201
7.4.3. Contribution to the Immune Defense System 202
7.5. Common Disorders of the Nose and Sinuses 203
7.5.1. Rhinitis and Its Types 204
7.5.2. Sinusitis: Causes and Symptoms 205
7.5.3. Nasal Polyps and Their Implications 206
7.6. Diagnostic Techniques 207
7.6.1. Physical Examination of the Nose and Sinuses 208
7.6.2. Imaging Techniques: CT and MRI 208
7.6.3. Endoscopic Evaluation of Nasal Passages 209
Summary 211
References 214

CHAPTER 8

Nasal and Sinus Disorders 215

Introduction 215
8.1. Common Nasal Disorders 218
8.1.1. Allergic Rhinitis 218
8.1.2. Nasal Polyps 219
8.1.3. Deviated Septum 220
8.2. Common Sinus Disorders 221
8.2.1. Sinusitis (Acute and Chronic) 222
8.2.2. Fungal Sinus Infections 222
8.2.3. Barometric Sinusitis 223
8.3. Symptoms and Diagnosis 224
8.3.1. Common Symptoms of Nasal and Sinus Disorders 225
8.3.2. Diagnostic Methods (e.g., Imaging, Endoscopy) 226
8.3.3. Importance of Accurate Diagnosis 227
8.4. Treatment Options 228
8.4.1. Medications (e.g., Antihistamines, Decongestants) 229
8.4.2. Surgical Interventions (e.g., Endoscopic Sinus Surgery) 230
8.4.3. Home Remedies and Lifestyle Changes 231
8.5. Prevention Strategies 232
8.5.1. Avoiding Allergens and Irritants 232
8.5.2. Maintaining Nasal Hygiene 233
8.5.3. Importance of Regular Medical Check-Ups 234
Summary 236
References 239

CHAPTER 9

Disorders of the Nasopharynx 243

Introduction 243
9.1. Anatomy and Physiology of the Nasopharynx 247
9.1.1. Structure and Location of the Nasopharynx 247
9.1.2. Functions of the Nasopharynx in the Respiratory System 248
9.1.3. Relationship Between the Nasopharynx and Other Anatomical Structures 249
9.2. Common Disorders of the Nasopharynx 251
9.2.1. Allergic Rhinitis 251
9.2.2. Nasopharyngeal Carcinoma 252
9.2.3. Adenoid Hypertrophy 253
9.3. Symptoms and Diagnosis 254
9.3.1. Common Symptoms Associated with Nasopharyngeal Disorders 255
9.3.2. Diagnostic Techniques Used in Evaluating Nasopharyngeal Conditions 256
9.3.3. Importance of Early Diagnosis in Treatment Outcomes 257
9.4. Treatment Options of the Nasopharynx 258
9.4.1. Medical Management of Nasopharyngeal Disorders 259
9.4.2. Surgical Interventions for Severe Cases 260
9.4.3. Role of Lifestyle Changes in Managing Symptoms 260
9.5. Complications of Nasopharyngeal Disorders 262
9.5.1. Potential for Airway Obstruction 263
9.5.2. Impact on Hearing and Speech 264
9.5.3. Risk of Systemic Infections 265
9.6. Preventive Measures of the Nasopharynx 266
9.6.1. Importance of Regular Medical Check-Ups 267
9.6.2. Strategies for Reducing Exposure to Allergens 268

9.6.3. Vaccination and Its Role in Preventing Infections 269
Summary 270
References 273

CHAPTER 10

Anatomy and Physiology of the Throat and Larynx 275

Introduction 275
10.1. Anatomy of the Throat 278
10.1.1. Description of the Pharynx 279
10.1.2. Structure of the Esophagus 280
10.1.3. Relationship Between the Throat and Surrounding Structures 281
10.2. Anatomy of the Larynx 282
10.2.1. Components of the Larynx 282
10.2.2. Location and Function of the Vocal Cords 283
10.2.3. Role of the Larynx in Respiration 284
10.3. Physiology of the Throat 285
10.3.1. Mechanisms of Swallowing 286
10.3.2. Role in Speech Production 287
10.3.3. Interaction with the Respiratory System 288
10.4. Physiology of the Larynx 289
10.4.1. Sound Production and Modulation 290
10.4.2. Protective Functions During Swallowing 291
10.4.3. Role in Regulating Airflow 292
10.5. Common Disorders of the Throat 293
10.5.1. Pharyngitis and Its Causes 293
10.5.2. Tonsillitis and Its Implications 294
10.5.3. Impact of Allergies on Throat Health 295
10.6. Common Disorders of the Larynx 296
10.6.1. Laryngitis and Its Symptoms 297
10.6.2. Vocal Cord Nodules and Their Effects 298
10.6.3. Cancer of the Larynx and Treatment Options 298
Summary 300
References 303

CHAPTER 11

Tonsillar and Pharyngeal Diseases 305

Introduction 305
11.1. Anatomy of the Tonsils and Pharynx 308
11.1.1. Description of the Tonsils and Their Functions 309
11.1.2. Overview of the Pharynx and Its Role in the Respiratory System 310
11.1.3. Relationship Between Tonsils and Pharyngeal Health 311
11.2. Common Tonsillar Diseases 312
11.2.1. Acute Tonsillitis: Causes and Symptoms 313
11.2.2. Chronic Tonsillitis: Diagnosis and Treatment Options 314
11.2.3. Peritonsillar Abscess: Complications and Management 315
11.3. Common Pharyngeal Diseases 316
11.3.1. Pharyngitis: Viral vs. Bacterial Causes 317
11.3.2. Allergic Pharyngitis: Triggers and Symptoms 318
11.3.3. Pharyngeal Cancer: Risk Factors and Early Signs 318
11.4. Diagnostic Methods 320
11.4.1. Physical Examination Techniques 320
11.4.2. Laboratory Tests and Imaging Studies 321
11.4.3. Differential Diagnosis of Tonsillar and Pharyngeal Diseases 322
11.5. Treatment Options 323
11.5.1. Pharmacological Treatments: Antibiotics and Analgesics 324
11.5.2. Surgical Interventions: Tonsillectomy and Adenoidectomy 325
11.5.3. Home Remedies and Lifestyle Modifications 325
11.6. Prevention Strategies 326
11.6.1. Vaccination and Its Role in Prevention 327
11.6.2. Hygiene Practices to Reduce Infection Risk 328
11.6.3. Dietary Considerations for Maintaining Throat Health 329
Summary 330
References 333

CHAPTER 12

Trauma Reconstruction in Facial Cosmetic 337

Introduction 337

12.1. Types of Facial Trauma 340

12.1.1. Common Causes of Facial Injuries 341

12.1.2. Classification of Facial Trauma 342

12.1.3. Impact of Trauma on Facial Structure 343

12.2. Psychological Effects of Facial Trauma 344

12.2.1. Emotional and Mental Health Implications 344

12.2.2. Social Stigma and Its Effects on Recovery 345

12.2.3. Role of Self-image in Psychological Healing 346

12.3. Surgical Techniques in Facial Reconstruction 347

12.3.1. Overview of Surgical Options Available 348

12.3.2. Innovations in Surgical Technology 349

12.3.3. Importance of Personalized Treatment Plans 350

12.4. Role of Cosmetic Procedures in Reconstruction 351

12.4.1. Integration of Cosmetic Techniques in Trauma Recovery 352

12.4.2. Non-Surgical Options for Facial Enhancement 353

12.4.3. Patient Satisfaction and Quality of Life Improvements 354

12.5. Multidisciplinary Approach to Treatment 355

12.5.1. Collaboration Between Surgeons, Psychologists, and Therapists 356

12.5.2. Importance of a Holistic Treatment Plan 357

12.5.3. Case Studies Demonstrating Successful Multidisciplinary Outcomes 357

12.6. Ethical Considerations in Facial Reconstruction 358

12.6.1. Informed Consent and Patient Autonomy 359

12.6.2. Balancing Aesthetic Desires with Medical Needs 360

12.6.3. Addressing Disparities in Access to Care 361

Summary 362

References 365

CHAPTER 13

Congenital and Developmental Deformities in Facial Cosmetic 369

Introduction 369

13.1. Types of Congenital Deformities 372

13.1.1. Cleft Lip and Palate 373

13.1.2. Craniosynostosis 374

13.1.3. Hemifacial Microsomia (HFM) 375

13.2. Types of Developmental Deformities 376

13.2.1. Facial Asymmetry 377

13.2.2. Acquired Deformities Due to Trauma 378

13.2.3. Deformities Resulting from Medical Conditions 379

13.3. Causes of Congenital Deformities 380

13.3.1. Genetic Factors 381

13.3.2. Environmental Influences 381

13.3.3. Maternal Health During Pregnancy 382

13.4. Psychological Impact of Facial Deformities 383

13.4.1. Self-esteem and Body Image Issues 384

13.4.2. Social Stigma and Discrimination 385

13.4.3. Mental Health Implications 386

13.5. Treatment Options for Facial Deformities 387

13.5.1. Surgical Interventions 388

13.5.2. Orthodontic Treatments 389

13.5.3. Psychological Support and Counseling 390

13.6. Advances in Facial Aesthetic Procedures 391

13.6.1. Innovations in Surgical Techniques 392

13.6.2. Role of 3D Imaging and Modeling 393

13.6.3. Non-Surgical Aesthetic Enhancements 393

Summary 395

References 398

CHAPTER 14

Oncologic and Post-Tumor Reconstruction in Facial Cosmetic 401

Introduction **401**

14.1. Understanding Oncologic Surgery **405**

14.1.1. Types of Cancers Affecting the Facial Region 406

14.1.2. Surgical Techniques Used in Oncologic Procedures 407

14.1.3. Goals of Oncologic Surgery in Facial Aesthetics 408

14.2. The Role of Reconstruction in Facial Cosmetic Surgery **410**

14.2.1. Definition and Purpose of Reconstructive Surgery 411

14.2.2. Techniques Used in Facial Reconstruction 411

14.2.3. Psychological Impact of Facial Reconstruction on Patients 412

14.3. Preoperative Considerations **414**

14.3.1. Patient Assessment and Evaluation 414

14.3.2. Importance of Multidisciplinary Teams 415

14.3.3. Planning for Aesthetic Outcomes 416

14.4. Surgical Techniques in Reconstruction **418**

14.4.1. Flap Techniques and Their Applications 419

14.4.2. Grafting Methods in Facial Reconstruction 419

14.4.3. Innovations in Surgical Technology 420

14.5. Postoperative Care and Recovery **421**

14.5.1. Importance of Follow-up Care 422

14.5.2. Managing Complications and Risks 423

14.5.3. Rehabilitation And Support For Patients 423

14.6. Ethical Considerations in Oncologic and Reconstructive Surgery **424**

14.6.1. Informed Consent and Patient Autonomy 425

14.6.2. Balancing Aesthetics with Medical Necessity 426

14.6.3. Addressing Disparities in Access to Care 427

Summary **428**

References **431**

CHAPTER 15

Advances, Technologies, and Practice Management in Facial Cosmetic 433

Introduction **433**

15.1. Historical Context of Facial Cosmetics **437**

15.1.1. Evolution of Cosmetic Practices 438

15.1.2. Key Milestones in Cosmetic Technology 439

15.1.3. Cultural Influences on Cosmetic Use 440

15.2. Current Technologies in Facial Cosmetics **441**

15.2.1. Innovations in Cosmetic Formulations 442

15.2.2. Advances in Application Techniques 443

15.2.3. Role of Digital Technology in Cosmetic Design 444

15.3. Non-Surgical Cosmetic Procedures **445**

15.3.1. Overview of Popular Non-Surgical Treatments 446

15.3.2. Safety and Efficacy of Non-Surgical Options 447

15.3.3. Patient Satisfaction and Outcomes 448

15.4. Surgical Advances in Facial Cosmetics **449**

15.4.1. Latest Techniques in Facial Surgery 450

15.4.2. Minimally Invasive Surgical Options 451

15.4.3. Ethical Considerations in Surgical Practices 452

15.5. Practice Management in Cosmetic Clinics **453**

15.5.1. Importance of Effective Management Strategies 454

15.5.2. Staff Training and Development 454

15.5.3. Patient Relationship Management 455

15.6. Regulatory and Ethical Considerations **456**

15.6.1. Overview of Regulations Governing Cosmetic Practices 457

15.6.2. Ethical Dilemmas in Cosmetic Procedures 458

15.6.3. Impact of Regulations on Practice Management 458

Summary **460**

References **463**

Index 467

LIST OF FIGURES

Figure 1.1. The field of ear, nose, and throat (ENT)
Figure 1.2. Importance of head and neck surgery in medical practice
Figure 1.3. The historical development of ENT (ear, nose, and throat) and head and neck surgery
Figure 1.4. Anatomy plays a crucial role in the practice of ENT and head and neck surgery
Figure 1.5. The human ear is an intricate organ that plays a vital role in the processes
Figure 1.6. The anatomy of the nasal cavity and sinuses
Figure 1.7. An overview of the throat and neck structures
Figure 1.8. The landscape of ear disorders
Figure 1.9. Sinusitis and nasal obstruction
Figure 1.10. In the context of head and neck surgery, surgical techniques
Figure 1.11. Endoscopic procedures in ENT
Figure 1.12. Innovations in minimally invasive surgery
Figure 1.13. Use of endoscopy in examination
Figure 1.14. Patient management and care
Figure 1.15. Addressing the rise of antibiotic resistance
Figure 2.1. The ear serves a multifaceted role in human anatomy and physiology
Figure 2.2. Anatomy of the outer ear
Figure 2.3. Structure and function of the pinna
Figure 2.4. The auditory canal and its role
Figure 2.5. The tympanic membrane (eardrum)
Figure 2.6. The anatomy of the middle ear plays a crucial role in the auditory function
Figure 2.7. The ossicles: malleus, incus, and stapes
Figure 2.8. Anatomy of the inner ear
Figure 2.9. The cochlea is a spiral-shaped, fluid-filled structure located within the inner ear
Figure 2.10. The auditory nerve and signal transmission
Figure 2.11. Physiology of hearing

Figure 2.12. The role of the vestibular system in equilibrium
Figure 2.13. Interaction between the inner ear and the brain
Figure 3.1. Ear examination of a child
Figure 3.2. Common diseases of the external ear
Figure 3.3. Otitis externa (swimmer's ear)
Figure 3.4. Earwax impaction
Figure 3.5. Comparison of an inflamed ear and a normal ear
Figure 3.6. Checking for signs of an ear infection in a child
Figure 3.7. Otoscopic examination of the ear
Figure 3.8. Medical treatments for external ear diseases
Figure 3.9. Personal hygiene and its impact on ear health
Figure 3.10. Proper ear care practices
Figure 3.11. Education on ear health awareness
Figure 4.1. Anatomy of the middle ear
Figure 4.2. Common middle ear disorders
Figure 4.3. Otitis media
Figure 4.4. Eustachian tube dysfunction
Figure 4.5. Development of cholesteatoma in the middle ear
Figure 4.6. Causes of middle ear disorders
Figure 4.7. Common symptoms of middle and outer ear infections, including pain, discharge, and swelling
Figure 4.8. Symptoms of middle ear disorders
Figure 4.9. Hearing loss
Figure 4.10. Ear pain and discomfort
Figure 4.11. Fluid drainage from the ear
Figure 4.12. Diagnosis of middle ear disorders
Figure 5.1. The vestibular system
Figure 5.2. Vestibular neuritis is an inner ear disorder
Figure 5.3. The symptoms of vestibular disorders
Figure 5.4. Balance issues are a significant consequence of inner ear and vestibular disorders
Figure 5.5. The diagnosis of inner ear disorders
Figure 5.6. Imaging studies, particularly MRI and CT scans
Figure 5.7. Medications for symptom relief
Figure 5.8. Surgical interventions for inner ear disorders

Figure 5.9. The impact of inner ear and vestibular disorders on an individual's quality of life
Figure 5.10. The experience of inner ear and vestibular disorders significantly affects an individual's social interactions and community engagement
Figure 6.1. The historical development of Ear, Nose, and Throat (ENT) and head and neck surgery has roots that trace back to ancient civilizations
Figure 6.2. Common conditions treated in ENT
Figure 6.3. Sinusitis and its treatment options
Figure 6.4. Endoscopic procedures have significantly advanced the field of auditory assessment and treatment
Figure 6.5. The reconstructive surgery for head and neck cases plays a pivotal role in restoring both functionality and aesthetic integrity
Figure 6.6. Role of imaging techniques (CT, MRI)
Figure 6.7. Audiological assessments serve as critical elements in the understanding and management of hearing health
Figure 6.8. The preoperative assessment and preparation for cochlear implantation play a crucial role in determining the likelihood of successful auditory rehabilitation outcomes
Figure 6.9. Multidisciplinary approach to patient management
Figure 6.10. Advances and innovations in ENT and head and neck surgery
Figure 6.11. The field of hearing assessment and rehabilitation is evolving rapidly, with emerging treatments and therapies being developed to address various auditory impairments
Figure 7.1. The nose and paranasal sinuses in the respiratory system
Figure 7.2. The anatomy of the nose is both complex and functional
Figure 7.3. The internal nasal cavity serves as a fundamental anatomical structure in the respiratory system
Figure 7.4. The physiology of the nose
Figure 7.5. Role of the nose in olfaction
Figure 7.6. Anatomy of the paranasal sinuses
Figure 7.7. Structure and lining of the sinuses
Figure 7.8. The physiology of the paranasal sinuses
Figure 7.9. Role in voice resonance and sound production
Figure 7.10. Common disorders of the nose and sinuses
Figure 7.11. Sinusitis: causes and symptoms
Figure 7.12. The otorhinolaryngology
Figure 7.13. The application of imaging techniques, particularly Computed Tomography

(CT) and Magnetic Resonance Imaging (MRI)
Figure 8.1. The nasal and sinus disorders
Figure 8.2. Nasal disorders represent a diverse range of conditions
Figure 8.3. While nasal polyps are a common manifestation in various nasal and sinus disorders
Figure 8.4. Common sinus disorders
Figure 8.5. Fungal sinus infections, classified under the broader spectrum of sinusitis
Figure 8.6. The symptoms associated with nasal and sinus disorders
Figure 8.7. Diagnostic methods play a crucial role in the assessment and management of nasal and sinus disorders
Figure 8.8. The management of nasal and sinus disorders encompasses a variety of treatment options
Figure 8.9. Surgical interventions (e.g., endoscopic sinus surgery)
Figure 8.10. The prevention strategies for nasal and sinus disorders
Figure 8.11. Maintaining nasal hygiene is essential in preventing various nasal and sinus disorders
Figure 9.1. The nasopharynx
Figure 9.2. The common disorders affecting the nasopharynx
Figure 9.3. The nasopharynx serves a crucial structural and functional
Figure 9.4. Relationship between the nasopharynx and other anatomical structures
Figure 9.5. Allergic rhinitis emerges as a significant clinical concern within the spectrum of nasopharyngeal disorders
Figure 9.6. Adenoid hypertrophy represents a significant pathological condition
Figure 9.7. Common symptoms associated with nasopharyngeal disorders
Figure 9.8. Importance of early diagnosis in treatment outcomes
Figure 9.9. Medical management of nasopharyngeal disorders
Figure 9.10. Role of lifestyle changes in managing symptoms
Figure 9.11. The potential for airway obstruction
Figure 9.12. The disorders of the nasopharynx, particularly otitis media, pose a significant risk for systemic infections
Figure 9.13. Importance of regular medical check-ups
Figure 10.1. The throat and larynx
Figure 10.2. The anatomy of the throat
Figure 10.3. Structure of the esophagus

Figure 10.4. The larynx is predominantly constituted of several vital components
Figure 10.5. Role of the larynx in respiration
Figure 10.6. The mechanisms of swallowing
Figure 10.7. The intricate relationship between the throat and larynx and the respiratory system
Figure 10.8. The intricate mechanisms of sound production and modulation in the throat and larynx
Figure 10.9. The throat and larynx play a pivotal role in regulating airflow
Figure 10.10. Pharyngitis, an inflammatory condition of the pharynx
Figure 10.11. Allergies can significantly impact throat health
Figure 10.12. Laryngitis and its symptoms
Figure 11.1. Tonsillar and pharyngeal diseases
Figure 11.2. Studying tonsillar
Figure 11.3. Anatomy of the tonsils and pharynx
Figure 11.4. Description of the tonsils and their functions
Figure 11.5. Common tonsillar diseases
Figure 11.6. Chronic tonsillitis: diagnosis and treatment options
Figure 11.7. Common pharyngeal diseases
Figure 11.8. Pharyngitis: viral vs. bacterial causes
Figure 11.9. Pharyngeal cancer
Figure 11.10. Physical examination techniques for pharyngeal cancer
Figure 11.11. Treatment options for tonsillar and pharyngeal diseases
Figure 11.12. Prevention strategies for tonsillar and pharyngeal diseases
Figure 12.1. Laryngeal and voice disorders
Figure 12.2. Laryngeal disorders
Figure 12.3. Role of vocal cords in sound production
Figure 12.4. Types of laryngeal disorders
Figure 12.5. Neurological voice disorders
Figure 12.6. Causes of voice disorders
Figure 12.7. Symptoms of voice disorders
Figure 12.8. Difficulty in pitch control in voice disorders
Figure 12.9. Diagnosis of laryngeal disorders
Figure 13.1. Head and neck infections and emergencies

Figure 13.2. Diagnosis of head and neck infections
Figure 13.3 Lymphatic system
Figure 13.4. Common head and neck infections

Figure 13.5. Sinusitis (sinus infection)
Figure 13.6. Pharyngitis and tonsillitis
Figure 13.7. Signs and symptoms of head and neck infections
Figure 13.8. Systemic symptoms indicating the severity of head and neck infections
Figure 13.9. Neck pain red flags
Figure 13.10. Taking a patient history
Figure 13.11. CT neck with annotated scrollable images
Figure 13.12. Treatment options of head and neck infections
Figure 13.13. Antibiotic therapy of head and neck infections
Figure 13.14. Surgical interventions for abscesses
Figure 13.15. Spread of infection to adjacent structures
Figure 14.1. Head and neck cancers or tumors
Figure 14.2. Studying head and neck tumors
Figure 14.3. Types of head and neck tumors
Figure 14.4. Benign tumors
Figure 14.5. Malignant tumors
Figure 14.6. Risk factors in the head and neck
Figure 14.7. HPV throat cancer
Figure 14.8. Symptoms and diagnosis in the head and neck
Figure 14.9. Diagnostic imaging techniques in the head and neck
Figure 14.10. Biopsy and histopathological examination of the head and neck
Figure 14.11. Head and neck cancer treatment options
Figure 14.12. Radiation therapy in the treatment of head and neck tumors
Figure 14.13. Chemotherapy options for head and neck tumors
Figure 14.14. Prognosis and Survival Rates of head and neck tumors
Figure 15.1. ENT clinical skills
Figure 15.2. Surgical procedures and investigations in ENT
Figure 15.3. Clinical skills in ENT
Figure 15.4. Otoscopic examination

Figure 15.5. Communication skills with patients in ENT
Figure 15.6. Common investigations in ENT
Figure 15.7. Audiometry and hearing tests
Figure 15.8. Nasal endoscopy
Figure 15.9. Surgical procedures in ENT
Figure 15.10. Tonsillectomy and adenoidectomy
Figure 15.11. Functional endoscopic sinus surgery
Figure 15.12. Cochlear implantation
Figure 15.13. Role of technology in ENT
Figure 15.14. Telemedicine in ENT consultations
Figure 15.15. Managing patient expectations in ENT practice

PREFACE

The human head and neck area is a remarkable convergence of structures that allow us to perceive the world around us, express our ideas, and carry out essential functions. Ranging from the fragile organs that facilitate hearing and equilibrium to the intricate channels that permit breathing, swallowing, and speech, the area calls for meticulous investigation and exact intervention. Advances in the operative skills, allied to advances in diagnostic and rehabilitative techniques, have transformed patient management in ear, nose, and throat (ENT) practice. But here too, success will continue to depend upon a strong grasp of basic principles, diligent clinical assessment, and judicious application of surgical skills.

Students entering the specialty of ENT and head and neck surgery will encounter a broad spectrum of conditions—ranging from routine infections to esoteric neoplasms—that require analytical skill and technical competence to manage. Successful treatment of disorders of hearing, breathing, speech, and facial appearance hinges on the integration of anatomical data, physiologic understanding, and surgical skill. In order to achieve knowledge in this field, one not only learns the process of how procedures are performed but also why they need to be performed and how they improve the patient's outcome.

This text, *Textbook to Ear, Nose, and Throat with Head and Neck Surgery for Medical Students*, is designed to lead students through the basics of ENT practice. Between its covers, readers will find brief descriptions of anatomy and physiology, systematic descriptions of disease mechanisms, step-by-step descriptions of diagnostic tests, and functional outlines of both routine and advanced surgical procedures. Clinical pearls and case examples are woven throughout to instruct the reader in how theoretical principles are translated into practice in patient care.

Chapter 1 presents a synopsis of the history and development of ENT practice, following significant milestones that have shaped modern surgical practice. It delineates the current scope of the specialty, charting the diversity of conditions managed by ENT surgeons, and introducing the major instruments and examination techniques that form the basis of each clinical consultation.

Chapter 2 covers the anatomy and physiology of the ear, including the functions of the external, middle, and inner ear, guiding students through the anatomy of these structures. Vestibular and auditory glandular physiology is supplemented with explanations of standard audiological tests so that students are able to interpret results of tests and understand their clinical implications.

Chapter 3 covers outer ear disorders, including causes, presentations, and treatment for otitis externa, traumatic injury, congenital malformations, and benign or malignant neoplasms. Special care is taken to address when surgery is indicated and how to perform simple tasks safely.

Chapter 4 covers middle ear pathology such as acute and chronic otitis media, Eustachian tube dysfunction, and complications of perforations of the tympanic membrane and cholesteatoma. Principles of repair and reconstructive surgery are introduced to prepare students for advanced study.

Chapter 5 deals with sensorineural hearing loss and vestibular disorders. The subjects are inner ear trauma mechanisms, tinnitus clinical evaluation, diagnosis, and treatment of Meniere's disease and other causes of vertigo. Practical guidance on the management of chronic symptoms completes this section.

Chapter 6 includes hearing testing and rehabilitative options. Pure tone and speech audiometry techniques are addressed along with tympanometry and brainstem evoked response audiometry (BERA). The chapter concludes with a review of equipment such as hearing aids and cochlear implants, including candidacy specifications and postoperative management.

Chapter 7 summarizes the anatomy and physiology of the nasal cavity and paranasal sinuses. The mucociliary clearance mechanisms, olfactory apparatus, and the vascular supply relevant to both medical and surgical treatment will be taught to the student.

Chapter 8 explains prevalent nasal and sinus disease. Allergic and non-allergic rhinitis is explained in great detail, followed by acute, chronic, and fungal sinusitis. Nasal polyp treatment and management of epistaxis control are also explained.

Chapter 9 addresses nasopharyngeal illness, including adenoid hypertrophy and congenital choanal atresia. Presentation and staging of nasopharyngeal carcinoma and the uses of surgery and adjunctive therapy in habitual snoring and sleep apnea are also addressed in the chapter.

Chapter 10 addresses the anatomy and function of the pharynx and larynx. The chapter defines the biomechanics of swallowing and phonation and sets the stage for the associated pathologies.

Chapter 11 discusses tonsillar and pharyngeal illness. Acute and chronic tonsillitis is contrasted, and treatment of peritonsillar abscess is presented. Pharyngitis types and treatments, including surgical procedures for obstructive sleep apnea, are discussed.

Chapter 12 discusses laryngeal and voice disorders. Explanations are provided for the diagnosis and treatment of acute and chronic laryngitis, the treatment of vocal cord paralysis, and the examination and treatment of hoarseness and stridor.

Chapter 13 discusses head and neck infection and emergency. Careful case scenarios illustrate recognition and management of deep neck space infections, Ludwig's angina, and airway obstruction. Tracheostomy in the acute setting is discussed, along with instructions on how to perform it.

Chapter 14 discusses benign and malignant head and neck tumors. The chapter includes discussion of thyroid and salivary gland neoplasms, oncologic principles in surgery, and neck dissection. Particular emphasis is placed on disease control, with minimal functional impairment.

Chapter 15 concludes with a handy manual of clinical skills, investigations, and surgical procedures in ENT. This chapter introduces common instruments and endoscopic surgery, outlines the use of imaging modalities such as X-ray, CT, and MRI, and provides a step-by-step guide to procedures like tonsillectomy, septoplasty, and mastoidectomy.

Aimed at medical students and early trainees, this book has a direct progression from basic science through clinical application to surgical technique. Through completing each chapter, the reader will acquire the knowledge and skills needed to perform effective examinations, interpret investigations, and participate in surgical management under supervision.

INTRODUCTION TO ENT AND HEAD AND NECK SURGERY

1

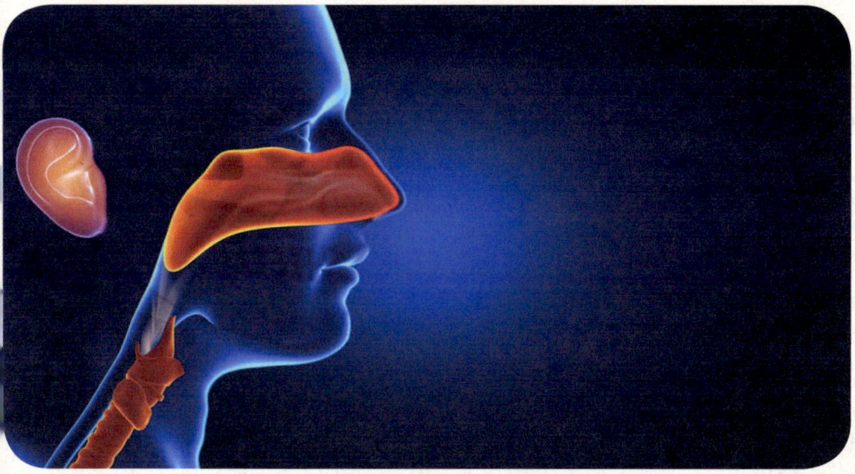

LEARNING OBJECTIVES

After studying this chapter, you will be able to:

1. Anatomy relevant to ENT and head and neck surgery.
2. Common conditions treated in ENT.
3. Surgical techniques in head and neck surgery.
4. Diagnostic tools and technologies.
5. Patient management and care.
6. Challenges and future directions in ENT.

Introduction

ENT and Head and Neck Surgery encompasses a wide spectrum of medical and surgical specialties that treat conditions of the upper airway, hearing, balance, and head and neck anatomy. ENT physicians often address common ailments, such as otitis media, sinusitis, and tonsillitis, besides managing complex conditions like neoplasms of the head and neck. Underlying ENT practice is an in-depth understanding of the anatomy and physiology of the area in question so that one can accurately diagnose and efficiently treat. The integration of medical, surgical, and rehabilitative techniques reflects the sophistication of this specialty and its utility in both pediatric and adult populations. Furthermore, advanced surgical techniques, such as minimally invasive surgery, improve patient outcomes and safety in this rapidly evolving field. Children's ENT conditions warrant special attention because of differences in their anatomy and physiology. Obstructive sleep apnea syndrome (OSAS), say, is a serious condition with an estimated incidence rate of roughly 2% in children aged two to eight years. It is usually caused by enlarged adenoid tissue in the upper airway and can manifest as a range of symptoms, including sleep disturbances, behavioral issues, and growth retardation. The diagnosis and management challenges of OSAS are typical of pediatric ENT, where risk factors differ from those in adults. Practitioners must navigate through these issues with respect to the impact of interventions on a childs total growth. An understanding of the factors is imperative for effective treatment planning, which does not merely address immediate symptoms but also supports long-term health outcomes (Bellini et al., 2019). Surgeons often collaborate with oncologists, speech therapists, and audiologists, particularly when treating head and neck malignancies or associated functional impairments. Multidisciplinary care offers greater efficacy to treatments and the patient journey as a whole. For example, in the management of head and neck cancers, teamwork among specialists enables the maximization of operations, such as reconstructive surgery, to preserve function and beauty. Additionally, research and development into the specialty, as seen through institutional initiatives such as those presented by TJUHs Quality and Safety Group, further highlight the importance of improving patient safety and care processes. Such collaborative frameworks are critical to addressing the challenges of ENT disorders and delivering excellent patient-centered care (N/A, 2018).

Definition and Scope of ENT (Ear, Nose, and Throat)

ENT primarily concerns itself with the medical and surgical management of ear, nasal passages, sinuses, and throat ailments, as well as voice disorders. ENT is a comprehensive specialty, encompassing patients with hearing loss and chronic sinusitis, as well as those with sleep apnea and allergies. This variety is reflective of the varied nature of the specialty that requires practitioners to possess a sophisticated understanding of varied medical conditions and their relation to one another. As scientific research and technological advancements continue to evolve, so does the scope of conditions addressed in otolaryngology, firmly establishing ENT as an important branch of modern medicine and working to enhance both the quality of life and the health of patients. Ongoing expansion into its line of work, ENT professionals also extend to critical areas such as head and neck surgical procedures, addressing conditions like tumors and congenital deformities. This operative aspect encompasses interventions ranging from minimally invasive endoscopy to major surgeries that may involve the salivary glands or the thyroid gland. Further, complications in the treatment of head and neck disease call for a multidisciplinary approach, where otolaryngologists work in concert with other specialists, such as oncologists and radiologists, to develop comprehensive treatment plans.

The term and scope of ENT are extended to incorporate patient education and preventive care with the prime emphasis placed on awareness and early diagnosis in the treatment of ear, nose, and throat conditions. Preventive care includes regular screenings for hearing loss, chronic diseases and schemes of child vaccination to prevent dominant infections. Patient education programs equip patients with the knowledge to take charge of risk factors and symptoms of ENT conditions, promoting active health management. Moreover, with the expansion of telehealth, ENT care is now more accessible, and patients can receive consultations and follow-up visits remotely. Not only does this technology minimize barriers to care, particularly for disadvantaged groups, but it also enhances patient participation and treatment adherence, highlighting the ENT specialty's responsiveness and flexibility in meeting the demands of the contemporary healthcare landscape (Akyol et al., 2019) (Figure 1.1).

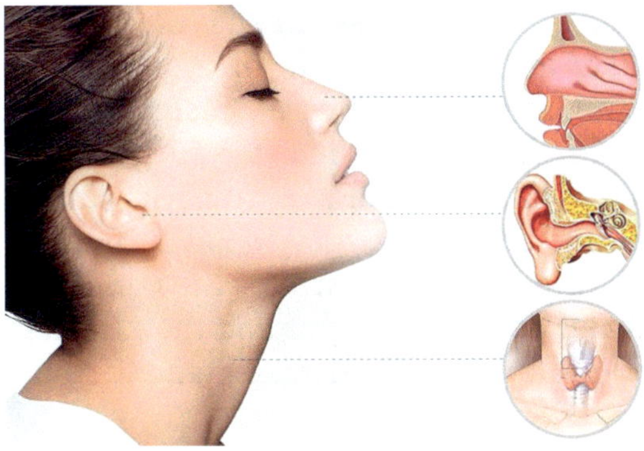

Figure 1.1. The field of ear, nose, and throat (ENT).

Source: https://globehealthcare.org/wp-content/uploads/2025/01/ent-surgery-about.jpg.

Importance of Head and Neck Surgery in Medical Practice

The head and neck surgery specialty is of great importance in medical practice, particularly because it offers a comprehensive approach to the diagnosis and management of a wide spectrum of disorders affecting this critical anatomical region. Surgeons who practice this specialty are trained to manage disorders ranging from benign neoplasms to malignancies, underscoring the importance of timely and accurate diagnosis. By developing operation methods sensitive to specific disorders, head and neck surgeons not only enhance patient outcomes but also address quality-of-life concerns.

For instance, the management of oral cancer requires a carefully planned surgical approach to preserve function and aesthetic potential, highlighting the delicate interplay between operative skill and patient care. Moreover, the specialized expertise required for head and neck surgery ensures that head and neck surgeons excel at overcoming the complexity posed by structures such as nerves, blood vessels, and lymphatics, underscoring their pivotal role in medical practice. Moreover, the essential role of head and neck surgery has been underscored by the COVID-19 pandemic, which revealed new challenges for medical practitioners. Lastly, the education and training of medical professionals in conducting head and neck examinations are important in facilitating the overall success of this medical practice. The results of a study evaluating comfort levels among medical students performing head and neck physical examinations demonstrate the long-lasting impact of targeted educational interventions. Following educational sessions, students reported greater confidence in conducting these critical assessments, which can lead to earlier detection of pathological states. This health initiative introduces a new cohort of health practitioners who are trained to recognize signs and understand the multifactorial nature of head and neck disorders. This comprehensive training ultimately serves the specialty's ultimate goals, establishing the necessity of head and neck surgery as both a medical subspecialty and an integral component of well-rounded patient care (Armstrong et al., 2015) (Figure 1.2).

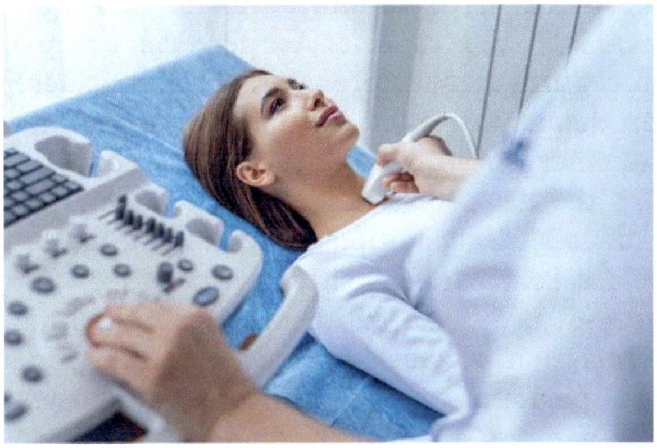

Figure 1.2. Importance of head and neck surgery in medical practice.

Source: https://www.drpaulgoonan.com.au/static/uploads/images/2head-and-neck-istock-1189207524-wfokezjmvogr.jpg?autorotate=true&mode=max&upscale=true&width=602.

Historical Development of ENT and Head and Neck Surgery

The history of ENT (ear, nose, and throat) and head and neck surgery is deeply linked to medical knowledge and surgical ingenuity. Ancient evidence shows that early practitioners used rudimentary methods to treat neck and head-related diseases. Surprisingly enough, Egyptians were observed administering crude trepanation for the control of cranial trauma, while Hippocratic texts documented knowledge of sinusitis and pharyngitis. The Renaissance was a milestone; anatomists such as Andreas Vesalius needed a more detailed understanding of human anatomy, on which surgical practice was founded. By the 19th century, increased attention to ear, nose, and throat anatomy led to the establishment of ENT as a specialty in its own right, facilitated by advances in both technique and instruments that greatly improved patient outcomes. The development of surgical methods for managing head and neck disorders accelerated in the 20th century, especially with the advent of specialized training for otolaryngologists. The introduction of anesthetic methods and advances in surgery increased the capacity to perform complex procedures that had previously been considered too dangerous. This era did not just witness the emergence of evidence-based practice but also the dawn of a new era of epidemiologic knowledge of conditions often treated in these fields. For instance, intensive research into sleep-disordered breathing brought to light the association between obstructive sleep apnea and perioperative complications, showing that patients had higher complications during perioperative periods due to undiagnosed upper airway conditions (Doghramji et al., 2012). These developments marked the turning point at which the integration of surgical expertise and comprehensive patient care began to take shape. Furthermore, contemporary approaches in ENT and head and neck surgery have increasingly followed a multidisciplinary paradigm, recognizing the diverse needs of patients. Specialists are now capable of managing not only traumatic injury but also chronic pain syndromes that can occur after surgery, such as post-sternotomy pain syndrome in patients undergoing cardiac surgery (Bordoni et al., 2017). This evolution illustrates the complexity of head and neck pathologies and their need for ongoing study and novel treatment methods. (Figure 1.3).

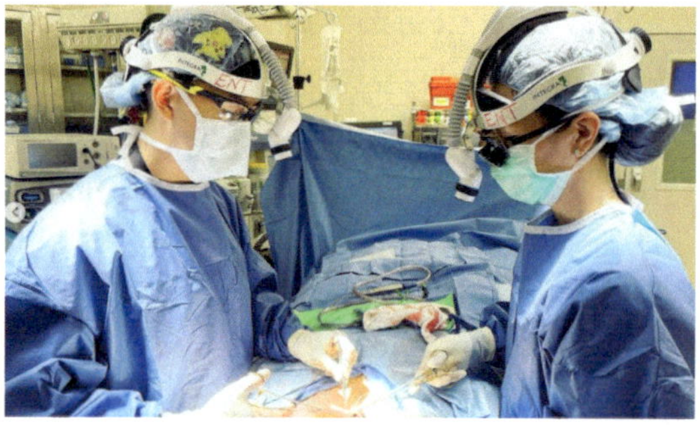

Figure 1.3. The historical development of ENT (ear, nose, and throat) and head and neck surgery.

Source: https://cdn.bcm.edu/sites/default/files/styles/two_thirds_width_component_image/public/2022-12/head-and-neck-surgery-education-.png?h=5267cd90&itok=g5uQL80c.

1.1. Anatomy Relevant to ENT and Head and Neck Surgery

Learning Outcome

1. Structure and Function of the Ear
2. Anatomy of the Nasal Cavity and Sinuses
3. Overview of the Throat and Neck Structures

Anatomy plays a crucial role in the practice of head and neck and ENT surgery since it acts as the foundation upon which the sophisticated structures involved in these procedures are comprehended. The head and neck region comprises a diversified set of organs that constitute the nasal cavities, the pharynx, the larynx, the salivary glands, and the cranial nerves. For instance, the vagus nerve, an important component of the nervous system, innervates many structures involved in swallowing and voice production. Knowledge of the spatial relationship and anatomical variations of these structures helps surgeons avoid complications during surgery, such as damage to adjacent nerves or arteries. Good knowledge of anatomy not only promotes surgical precision but also improves preoperative planning and postoperative management, which are critical to optimal patient outcomes in ENT and head and neck surgery (N/A, 2018). Facial anatomy, like the mandible and maxilla, governs the surgical complexities of all the conditions, ranging from traumatic injuries to congenital deformities. The facial skeleton serves not only a structural role but also includes critical sensory and motor functions. Important anatomical landmarks, such as the facial nerve and its branches, must be worked around by surgeons in an attempt to minimize the risk of postoperative complications such as facial paralysis. On top of this, the facial anatomy itself, for example, the musculature of tongues and the floor of the mouth, comes to form a focal point of procedures such as tonsillectomy and cleft lip repair. A detailed understanding of facial anatomy ensures that surgeons are best positioned to manage functional impairments while maximizing aesthetic outcomes, thereby responding to both the physiological and psychological requirements of patient care in head and neck surgery (N/A, 1997). Additionally, the relationship of anatomy to pathology is a vital component of ENT and head and neck surgery. Tumors, infections, and congenital abnormalities frequently occur in this anatomical region and require a profound knowledge of the anatomical structures beneath it to be diagnosed and treated adequately. For example, the proximity of the thyroid gland to the recurrent laryngeal nerve requires thoughtful vigilance on the part of surgeons so they do not accidentally damage the nerve during thyroidectomies. This intersection of anatomy and clinical presentations informs surgical practice and intraoperative care. (Figure 1.4).

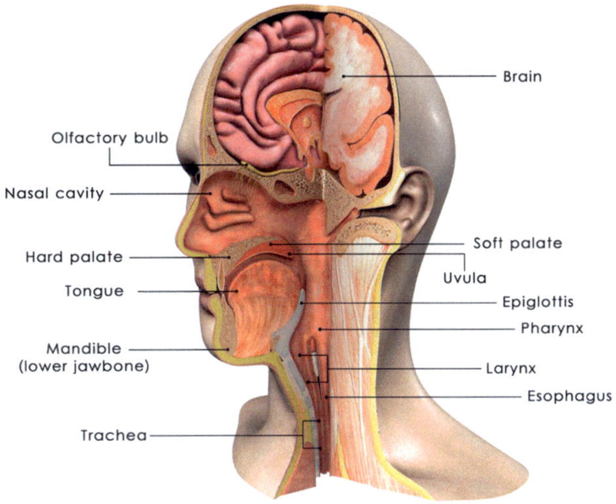

Figure 1.4. Anatomy plays a crucial role in the practice of ENT and head and neck surgery.

Source: https://external-content.duckduckgo.com/iu/?u=https%3A%2F%2Fwww.entkidsadults.com%2Fwp-content%2Fuploads%2F2015%2F12%2Fhead-anatomy-3D.jpg&f=1&nofb=1&ipt=3e14927a201b339ca90097d0ba0e6f2ba33e6c398b4697a87f653b3eff5359cc.

1.1.1. Structure and Function of the Ear

The human ear is a sophisticated organ that plays an essential role in the processes of hearing and balance, both of which are ever so important in everyday life. The anatomy of the ear divides it into three large sections: the outer ear, middle ear, and inner ear. The outer ear is composed of the pinna and the auditory canal and is utilized to receive sound waves and project them towards the eardrum. This vibration of the sound wave causes the eardrum to oscillate, which sets the stage for further sound processing. In the middle ear, the tympanic membrane transmits these vibrations to the ossicles, three small bones known as the malleus, incus, and stapes. This mechanical amplification is crucial for the effective transmission of sound energy into the fluid-filled inner ear, where more complex transduction occurs. The inner ear, or the labyrinthine structure, contains the cochlea, which does the job of converting the mechanical vibrations into neural signals. It is a spiral-shaped organ containing specialized hair cells that respond to fluid movement caused by sound waves, which in turn carry electrical impulses via the auditory nerve to the brain for interpretation.

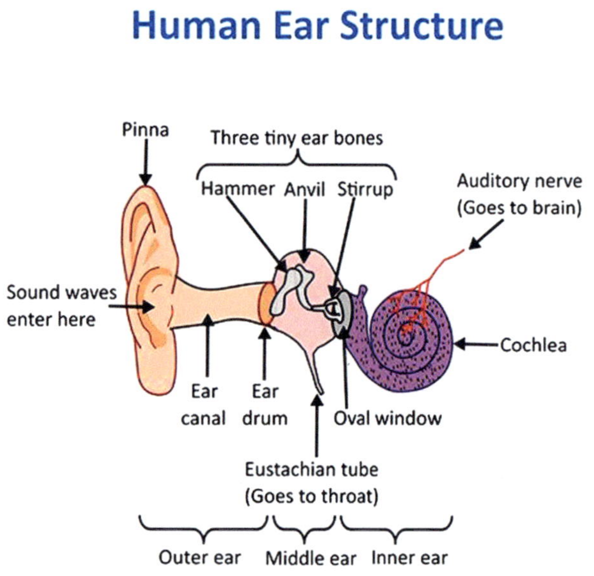

Figure 1.5. The human ear is an intricate organ that plays a vital role in the processes.

Source: https://external-content.duckduckgo.com/iu/?u=https%3A%2F%2Ftse1.mm.bing.net%2Fth%2Fid%2FOIP.9fWiJCXwNGkJMLYtMWtD_AHaHt%3Fr%3D0%26pid%3DApi&f=1&ipt=76197db047713f52e46076811425fe23b385ec6e610fd2e2ba833df0362f7842.

The vestibular system in the inner ear consists of semicircular canals and otolith organs that help maintain balance. It detects head movement and position and sends this information to the central nervous system to coordinate posture and balance. Understanding the specific functions of both the vestibular system and the cochlea is not only necessary in otolaryngology but also in treating conditions involving hearing and balance, such as vestibular disorders and hearing loss (Dimitriadis et al., 2017).

The similarity between the structural and functional components of the ears is reflective of the complexity of the auditory and balance functions. Furthermore, pathologies in any component of the ear can cause serious impairments in the quality of life. For instance, obstructive sleep apnea syndrome (OSAS) can complicate auditory processing and is often associated with intrinsic structural abnormalities of the upper respiratory tract that can extend to the ear (Bellini et al., 2019). Recognizing these interrelationships is significant in ENT and head and neck surgery, where an interdisciplinary approach to diagnosis and treatment can lead to improved outcomes for patients with ear disorders. It is the basis upon which successful intervention strategies in the ever-changing discipline of otolaryngology are built (Figure 1.5).

1.1.2. Anatomy of the Nasal Cavity and Sinuses

Nasal cavity and sinus anatomy is a highly complex and delicate structure needed for multiple physiological functions, especially in the context of ENT and head and neck surgery. The nasal cavity, from the nostrils to the choanae, performs multiple critical functions, including filtration, humidification, and warming of inspired air. It is divided into two asymmetrical halves by the nasal septum, which is made up of a combination of cartilage and bone. The lateral walls house three turbinates, or nasal conchae, that give it a greater surface area for air contact, enabling proper airflow and enhanced olfactory function. In addition, the nasal cavity connects to the paranasal sinuses, that is, the frontal, maxillary, ethmoidal, and sphenoidal sinuses, thereby playing a very significant role in resonance during the production of sounds and in protecting the upper respiratory tract from infection. The paranasal sinuses are air-filled spaces that empty directly into the nasal cavity. They are lined by mucous membranes that produce mucus, which protects the airway from pathogens and debris.

Each sinus coexists in a specific anatomical location and drainage pathway that is important to sinus health. For instance, frontal sinuses are located superior to the orbit and drain to the middle meatus through the frontal recess. Their unique position makes them susceptible to blockage and complication-inducing conditions such as chronic rhinosinusitis. Endoscopic techniques have been widely embraced as the standard for tackling these issues, since direct visualization and intervention within the sinuses and nasal passages are allowed. Surgical techniques such as balloon catheter dilatation and stent placement have emerged as the best options improve sinus ventilation (Azimonti et al., 2018). Recent studies present highly effective advanced surgical interventions for the treatment of nasal cavity and sinus diseases. The modified endoscopic Lothrop procedure (MELP) is used primarily to manage complex frontal mucoceles, which pose significant challenges due to their anatomical location. Research has shown that MELP not only improves drainage but also minimizes complications of sinus surgery and enhances patient outcomes. The research findings indicate that the efficacy and safety of endoscopic procedures are evident in both straightforward and complex sinus cases. These advances emphasize the importance of understanding complex nasal passage and sinus anatomy in the context of surgical procedures, informing clinical practice, and improving the quality of care for patients with upper respiratory disorders (Khong et al., 2004) (Figure 1.6).

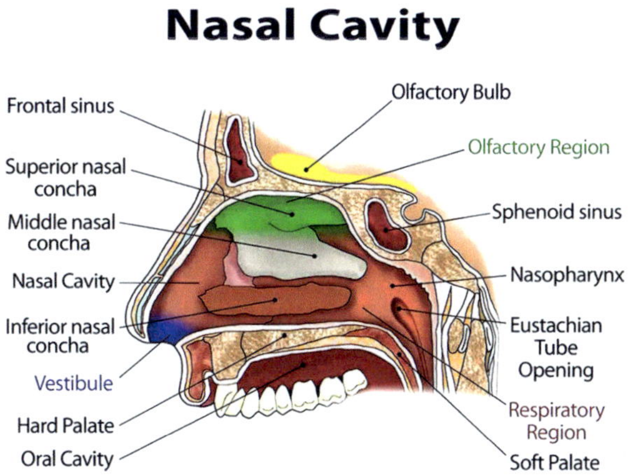

Figure 1.6. The anatomy of the nasal cavity and sinuses.

Source: https://external-content.duckduckgo.com/iu/?u=https%3A%2F%2Fwww.therespiratorysystem.com%2Fwp-content%2Fuploads%2F2017%2F07%2FNasal-Cavity.jpg&f=1&nofb=1&ipt=a712154d2ac18c0da35c9857dc1117ef64194759d08502cb9f61039c36eeaab8.

1.1.3. Overview of the Throat and Neck Structures

The throat and neck are advanced anatomical regions that perform critical roles in numerous physiological processes, including respiration, digestion, and speech. The throat, or pharynx, consists of three distinct segments: the nasopharynx, oropharynx, and laryngopharynx. Each of these segments serves a specific function, with the nasopharynx providing a passage for air from the nasal cavities and the oropharynx serving as a conduit for air and food. The laryngopharynx opens into the esophagus and larynx, dividing the gastrointestinal and respiratory tracts.

The structures are lined with mucosal tissues that provide defense and sensory functions, creating an effective barrier against infection. Such intricate arrangements underscore the importance of understanding the anatomical and functional nuances of the neck and throat when considering various otolaryngological conditions and their attendant interventions. One of the major features of the throat is its relationship to other structures in the neck, such as the larynx and numerous important blood vessels and nerves that traverse the neck. The larynx, or voice box, is involved in phonation, as well as functioning as a protective device when swallowing by preventing food from entering the trachea.

The neck also houses important vascular structures, including the carotid arteries and jugular veins, which supply oxygenated blood to the brain and drain deoxygenated blood, respectively. These vascular structures are home to numerous lymph nodes that are important to the immune system. These elements are interlinked to ensure that the throat and neck function optimally, enabling vital interaction between the circulatory and respiratory systems that is essential to maintaining overall well-being. Appreciation of the complexity of the throat and neck structures is also highly relevant to pathology diagnosis and management. Pathologies such as obstructive sleep apnea syndrome (OSAS) and other sleep respiratory disorders can be caused by anatomical pathologies or by variation in these areas, particularly in children, with the prevalence being approximately 2% among certain age groups, often related to adenoid tissue size (Bellini et al., 2019). Additionally, a thorough examination of patients' symptoms can improve diagnosis, leading to the best treatment options for ENT condition-impacting conditions (Harthi et al., 2018). Hence, a solid grasp of neck and throat anatomical relationships is crucial for specialists in ENT and head and neck surgery to facilitate accurate recognition and management of a wide variety of disorders (Figure 1.7).

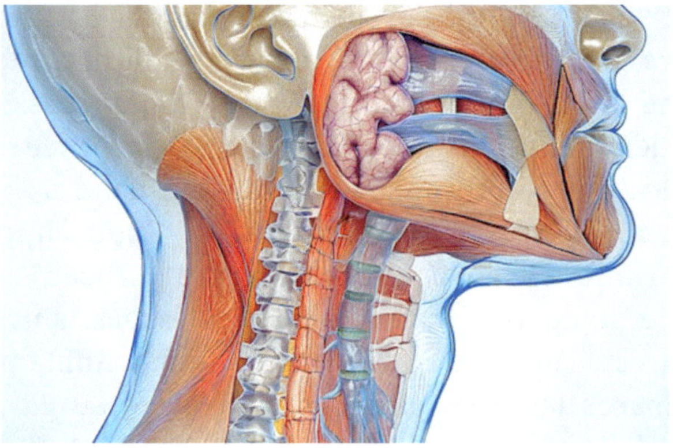

Figure 1.7. An overview of the throat and neck structures.

Source: https://external-content.duckduckgo.com/iu/?u=https%3A%2F%2Fimg.freepik.com%2Fpremium-photo%2Fanatomical-diagram-human-neck-throat-structures-clean-white-background_994764-173535.jpg&f=1&nofb=1&ipt=eb363f14e2380642a8fc2767895be995016e70c984a8457d544a5438a6f41dc1.

Test Your Knowledge

1. Temporal Bone and Middle Ear Anatomy
2. Neck Spaces and Fascial Planes

1.2. Common Conditions Treated in ENT

Learning Outcome

1. Otitis Media and Other Ear Disorders
2. Sinusitis and Nasal Obstruction
3. Throat Conditions, Including Tonsillitis and Laryngitis

ENT is a specialty involving a wide range of conditions affecting the upper aerodigestive tract.

Tinnitus is one of the most frequent conditions, characterized by the perception of sound in the absence of any external stimulus, most often associated with hearing loss. The effect of tinnitus is more than an individual's quality of life, and it leads to severe psychological distress. A literature review finds that approximately 7% of tinnitus patients initiate medical visits; thus, it is important to provide early intervention for those presenting with acute cases. Given the existence of psychiatric comorbidity among tinnitus conditions, developing robust diagnostic and therapeutic strategies is essential to avoid exacerbated risks such as increased morbidity related to distress and even suicidal ideation, as noted by Altissimi et al. (2016).. In addition to tinnitus, another cross-cutting disorder managed in ENT is vertigo, which is most commonly caused by vestibular system disease. A major cause of vertigo is conditions such as Meniere's disease or benign paroxysmal positional vertigo, which present with episodes of dizziness and imbalance. Management can include a complete assessment of symptoms through detailed audiological investigations and imaging techniques to identify the underlying etiology. For instance, the diagnosis of Enlarged Vestibular Aqueduct (EVA) syndrome, which is associated with sensorineural hearing loss and vestibular problems, requires appropriate diagnostic methods. Intratympanic corticosteroid therapy success has shown effective outcomes in responding to hearing improvement and diminishing symptoms of vertigo, as indicated in Nola et al. (2017). Psychological effects are also worthy of note, as persistent vertigo can lead to anxiety and affect daily life, requiring a multidisciplinary treatment pathway.

Chronic sinusitis is also a prevalent condition in ENT practice. It refers to inflammation of the nasal sinuses lasting over 12 weeks; in most cases, pressure, congestion, and facial pain ensue, severely affecting patients' lives. Chronic sinusitis is treated both medically and surgically with the aim of reducing inflammation and easing drainage of the sinuses. There is growing evidence in favor of using endoscopic sinus surgery to achieve relief in patients resistant to standard therapies. As diagnostic-therapeutic protocols are developed by ENT specialists, it is necessary to consider the patient's overall condition, potential comorbidities, and lifestyle factors that may complicate treatment. By combining medical advancements with age-old practices, ENT practices aim to enhance the patient experience and address the complex nature of chronic sinusitis.

1.2.1. Otitis Media and Other Ear Disorders

The spectrum of ear disorders is vast, and among them, ***otitis media*** is among the most common. The inflammatory process in the middle ear typically develops as a sequel to infection, resulting in fluid accumulation behind the eardrum. What is particularly striking about otitis media is that it exists in several varieties, ranging from acute to chronic, each with its own clinical presentation and patient care implications. Acute otitis media (AOM) most often presents with an abrupt onset of disease, that is, pain and fever, while chronic otitis media is characterized by recurrent fluid accumulation and potential impairment of hearing. The impact of otitis media is most significant in children, where recurrent infections may lead to delayed development and learning disabilities, underscoring the need for strict clinical management (Bailey et al., 2007). Along with otitis media, numerous other ear disorders can disrupt auditory function and lead to far-reaching health problems.

Eustachian tube dysfunction, which disrupts the normal pressure equilibration of the middle ear, may also increase otological issues through increased susceptibility to infection and formation of a collection of fluid, and thus necessitate multi-problem diagnosis and treatment in ENT practice. Management of ear disorders such as otitis media and tinnitus must be personalized to the patient's unique needs and clinical presentation. Medical or surgical management, or both, is usually effective in controlling these disorders. For instance, management of otitis media can include antibiotics for a bacterial infection or tympanostomy tubes for drainage for chronic otitis media. Conversely, tinnitus treatment may include sound therapies, counseling, and cognitive-behavioral strategies to reduce distress. Such a diverse strategy is particularly noteworthy given the interconnectedness of physical and psychological factors that accompany ear disorders. Early detection and intervention are important because the earlier one gets treated, the better outcomes will result, as well as reduce long-term effects typically associated with such disorders (Bailey et al., 2007; Altissimi et al., 2016) (Figure 1.8).

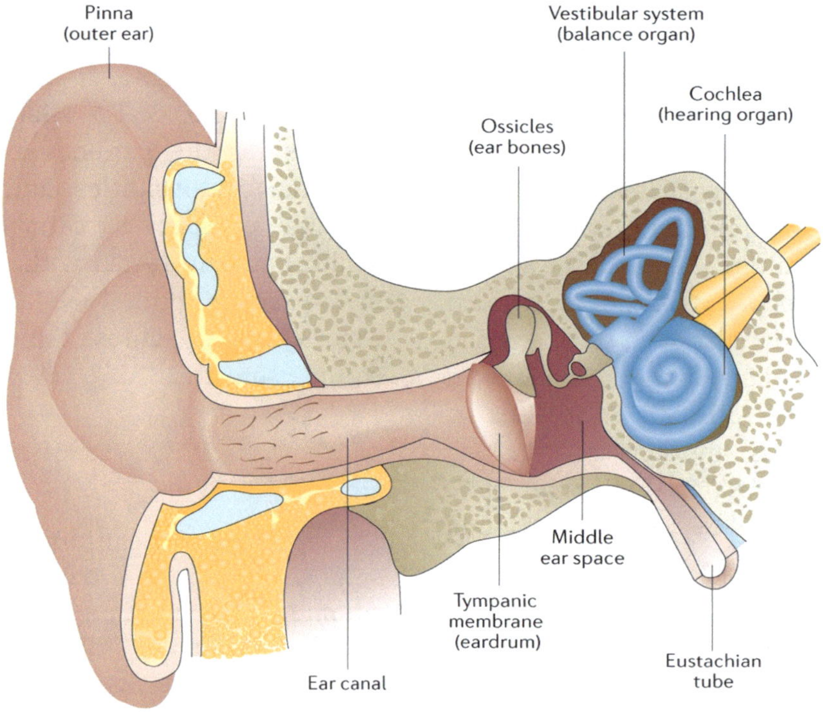

Figure 1.8. The landscape of ear disorders.

Source: https://media.springernature.com/full/springer-static/image/art%3A10.1038%2Fnrdp.2016.63/MediaObjects/41572_2016_Article_BFnrdp201663_Fig1_HTML.jpg

1.2.2. Sinusitis and Nasal Obstruction

In fact, the following are three exhaustive and well-spun paragraphs solely dedicated to Sinusitis and nasal obstruction that fit the requirements of the chapter Introduction to ENT and Head and Neck Surgery. Sinusitis, a highly prevalent condition encountered in practice in ENT, typically ensues due to inflammation of sinus cavities and may be associated with numerous symptoms that may significantly influence patients' quality of life. The illness is characterized by nasal obstruction, facial pain, and nasal purulent secretions. The most significant sequela of sinusitis is its ability to disrupt normal nasal airflow and drainage, leading to a cycle of chronic infection and inflammation. Furthermore, the worsening of nasal blockage can lead to complications such as chronic sinusitis, which can require surgical intervention. Diagnosis of sinusitis is typically based on clinical history, physical examination, and imaging studies, which allow otolaryngologists to tailor an effective treatment regimen for the patient. Nasal obstruction is typically a complicating condition in most respiratory diseases, including allergic rhinitis, which has been shown to play an important role in the general well-being of patients. Among children, in particular, nasal obstruction can have indirect consequences, such as sleep disturbances, caused by adenoid hypertrophy and other related diseases (Hardjojo et al., 2012). In allergic rhinitis, nasal blockage is more than a mere blockage; it can lead to sinus infections that aggravate the condition and increase the risk of more serious ENT diseases, making treatment for the patient even more complicated. When treating sinusitis and nasal blockage, ENT professionals must also consider a multidisciplinary approach that combines medical and surgical interventions. Effective treatment often includes corticosteroids to reduce inflammation, antihistamines for allergies, and, in advanced cases, surgery to address sinus drainage and alleviate nasal blockage (Basnyat et al., 2016). This surgery may be in the form of endoscopic sinus surgery or adenoidectomy, primarily among children, where obstructive symptoms lead to recurrent respiratory issues. Furthermore, patients are also generally required to have ongoing follow-up to observe recurrence and manage any co-morbidities. By combining comprehensive care strategies, otolaryngologists can optimize patient outcomes and significantly reduce the burden of chronic sinusitis and related nasal obstruction (Figure 1.9).

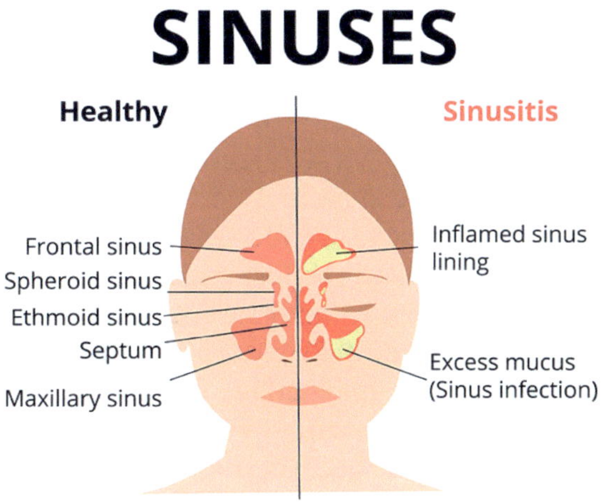

Figure 1.9. Sinusitis and nasal obstruction.

Source: https://external-content.duckduckgo.com/iu/?u=http%3A%2F%2Fceenta.com%2Fstorage%2Fwysiwyg%2Fchronicsinsutisweb_1.jpg&f=1&nofb=1&ipt=a3f7f699e928ddca595348c15d22e88d1743a8217ab476987fd58ef2d7be5fa4.

1.2.3. Throat Conditions, Including Tonsillitis and Laryngitis

Throat infections, particularly tonsillitis and laryngitis, are prevalent conditions within the field of otolaryngology and significantly impact patients' quality of life in those who experience these conditions. Tonsillitis, in which the tonsils become inflamed, is often caused by viral or bacterial infection and typically presents with fever, dysphagia, and a sore throat. Among children, tonsillitis is a leading cause of illness visits, underscoring the need for prompt diagnosis and treatment. In addition, recurrent tonsillitis, if left untreated, may lead to serious complications like peritonsillar abscesses, necessitating surgery, and therefore highlights the necessity for early medical intervention (Moran et al., 2025). Given these effects, healthcare systems are forced to prioritize effective treatment regimens to manage this widespread disorder and improve patient outcomes. Another extremely common throat disorder is laryngitis, which involves inflammation of the larynx and is most often characterized by hoarseness or loss of voice. This is caused by several etiological factors, including viral infections, overuse of the voice, and exposure to irritants such as smoke or allergens. While often self-limited, chronic laryngitis can reflect underlying disease requiring further management. The effects of chronic laryngitis extend beyond voice dysfunction and may affect communication, social interactions, and overall psychosocial adaptation. The heterogeneous nature of laryngitis necessitates a treatment approach that ranges from lifestyle changes to medical interventions that reduce inflammation and restore the voice to normal. By understanding the subtleties of laryngitis, clinicians are well placed to deliver targeted interventions tailored to individual patient needs (Moran et al., 2025). The epidemiologic burden of throat illnesses such as tonsillitis and laryngitis warrants significant attention in the health sector. The research identifies the nature of such illnesses, especially in regions with limited access to specialized ENT services. Studies show that disorders such as chronic tonsillitis account for a significant share of hospital discharges, underscoring the need for effective health planning and resource management (Imad et al., 2025). Moreover, public health interventions, such as public education on throat health, can reduce the prevalence and severity of such disorders. Awareness can help patients seek early medical consultation and prevent throat illnesses from becoming more serious health problems. Lastly, addressing tonsillitis and laryngitis improves patient outcomes and enhances the overall success of ENT and head and neck surgery clinics.

Test Your Knowledge

1. A 35-year-old man presents with a sudden onset of severe vertigo, nausea, and hearing loss in his right ear. On examination, he has nystagmus and tinnitus. Which of the following is the most likely diagnosis?
2. A 7-year-old child has recurrent sore throat, difficulty swallowing, and enlarged tonsils with white exudates. What is the most common causative organism?

1.3. Surgical Techniques in Head and Neck Surgery

Learning Outcome

1. Endoscopic Procedures in ENT
2. Open Surgical Techniques for Head and Neck Conditions
3. Innovations in Minimally Invasive Surgery

In head and neck surgery, surgery is very important in the treatment of most conditions, ranging from benign lesions to malignancy. A key approach is careful planning of the operation to minimize complications and achieve the best functional and aesthetic outcome. The delicate anatomy of the head and neck region requires thorough knowledge of surgical anatomy and techniques to perform interventions. Surgeons apply contemporary techniques such as endoscopic surgery, which is associated with less morbidity and quicker recovery, and traditional open surgery. The union of these two approaches facilitates increased customization of patient management protocols according to the specific pathology and individual anatomical considerations in each case. Surgical management of infection in the head and neck region, such as deep neck infection, requires a method that combines clinical experience and surgical dexterity. For instance, treatment of an abscess, such as a peritonsillar or retropharyngeal abscess, is usually by surgical drainage through incisions that leave extensive scarring. A good understanding of pathophysiology is crucial to prevent procedure-related complications, including mediastinitis and septicemia. The requirement of more than one incision for proper drainage not only highlights the technical difficulty of the procedure but also reflects on the psychological distress patients may experience due to potential scarring and a change in appearance. The literature indicates that effective preoperative communication is required to ensure patients provide informed consent when they know the life-threatening nature of these diseases (Bălălău et al., 2018). Another critical aspect of head and neck surgical techniques is how necrotizing fasciitis, aggressive infection with high morbidity and mortality rates, and rapid progression, is treated. This condition most often requires early and aggressive surgical intervention to debride dead tissue and control spread of infection. Specifically, the operation could vary depending on the affected compartments, underscoring the importance of proper imaging studies to guide the operation effectively. Early diagnosis and early surgery are integral to maximizing outcomes, particularly in high-risk populations such as the immunocompromised. By curing the infection in a holistic way with both medical and surgical treatment, good outcomes can be achieved, which reduce long-term complications, ultimately advancing the multispectral character of head and neck surgery (Abramo et al., 2012) (Figure 1.10).

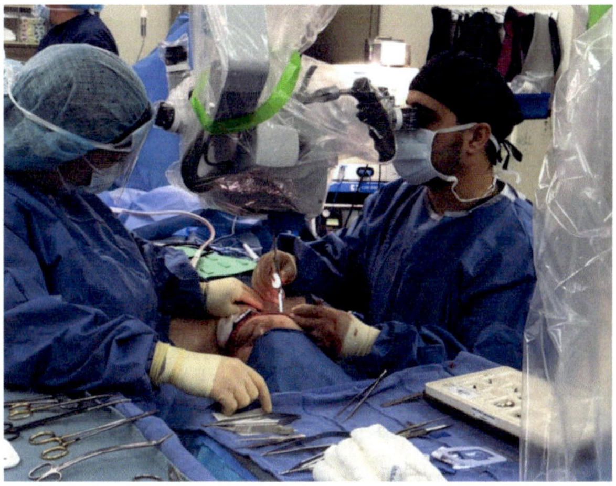

Figure 1.10. Surgical techniques in the context of head and neck surgery .

Source: https://external-content.duckduckgo.com/iu/?u=https%3A%2F%2Fwww.nextgenoms.com%2Fwp-content%2Fuploads%2F2020%2F11%2Fhead-and-neck-surgery-doctor-1024x797-1.jpg&f=1&nofb=1&ipt=4733125f8fa47d6b8ccb8141098f574db3f27103746725ff92488b5690a6d161.

1.3.1. Endoscopic Procedures in ENT

The evolution of endoscopic surgery has completely transformed the practice of otolaryngology, providing new methods in both diagnosis and treatment in ENT. Endoscopy uses flexible or rigid scopes with cameras, enabling physicians to examine the ear, nose, and throat without performing open surgery. This minimally invasive technique not only reduces recovery time and pain but also enhances the accuracy of interventions. In conditions such as chronic sinusitis and nasal polyps, endoscopic methods offer immediate access to sinusal anatomy, facilitating site-specific treatment and maximizing the efficacy of surgical intervention. As the need for minimal invasive options becomes more pressing, endoscopic treatments are progressively in the forefront of ENT disease management, underscoring their relevance in contemporary head and neck surgery. But with the advantages of endoscopic procedures come some inherent risks, specifically regarding surgical site infection (SSI). Appreciation of microbiological factors during these procedures is pivotal to achieving maximal patient benefit. ENT procedures, which are frequently performed on colonized areas with rich bacterial flora, are more susceptible to SSIs than other surgical sites. For example, guidelines for antimicrobial surgical prophylaxis apply directly to procedures such as endoscopic paranasal sinus surgery and tonsillectomy (Bianchini et al., 2022). These results highlight the need for individualized antibiotic regimens, especially in children, where differences in microbiota profiles can confound surgical outcomes (Bianchini et al., 2022).

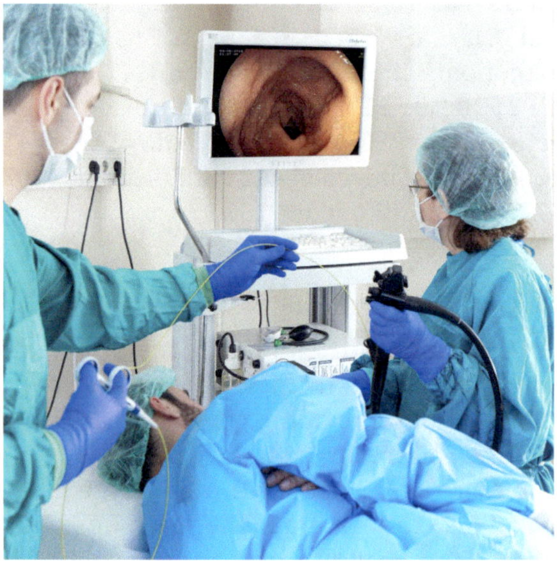

Figure 1.11. Endoscopic procedures in ENT.

Source: https://external-content.duckduckgo.com/iu/?u=https%3A%2F%2Fgastro-md.com%2Fwp-content%2Fuploads%2F2020%2F01%2FUGIE-Graphics3-min-2048x2048.jpg&f=1&nofb=1&ipt=f298cbd808f1a7c4cd29b19886c58ef1aea4d2c00b980dbd66107cefed6638a2.

Resolution of these concerns is necessary to ensure the success of endoscopic interventions and prevent complications with these new technologies. Future advances in endoscopic technology could further hone ENT surgeons' skills. Emerging technologies such as high-definition imaging, narrow-band imaging, and robotic-assisted endoscopic systems are elevating surgical precision and visualization. As these technologies become routine practice, they should improve diagnostic accuracy and extend the range of conditions that can be treated minimally invasively. ENT surgeon training and skill acquisition must shift in tandem to equip them to perform these new treatments. Also, ongoing research is important to determine the long-term efficacy and safety of these procedures, ensuring that endoscopic techniques continue to meet complex patient needs in head and neck surgery (Figure 1.11).

1.3.2. Open Surgical Techniques for Head and Neck Conditions

Open surgical approaches for head and neck disease are vital to managing advanced disease in this highly anatomically complex region. Surgical intervention is often required to treat malignancies, congenital and acquired anatomical malformations, and inflammatory lesions of the head and neck. In recurrent head and neck carcinoma, in particular, open surgical resection is an initial treatment of choice, with potential for complete tumor extirpation followed by reconstruction. Techniques such as permanent interstitial brachytherapy, in this instance using isotopes like Cesium-131, represent an advancement in this field. Radiation postoperatively delivered by this method reaches residual cancer cells without harming adjacent healthy tissues, suggesting potential for use in recurrent cases in patients previously irradiated (Bar-Ad et al., 2019). The application of advanced surgical techniques has been extended to the treatment of chronic rhinosinusitis (CRS) of the frontal sinuses, where restenosis is prevalent. Open surgery techniques for sinus surgery, although efficient, occasionally present complications, necessitating steps for improvement in outcomes. Techniques such as balloon catheter dilation (BCD) and stent or spacer implantation are recent advances designed to enhance sinus ventilation. These techniques aim at reducing inflammation and scarring during surgery, thus providing better healing and surgical outcome duration. Research on various methods indicates that while BCD has been shown to be effective, stenting also warrants further investigation to determine additional benefits in both mild and severe CRS (Azimonti et al., 2018). The integration of open surgery methods into the broader categorization of ENT and head and neck surgery indicates the need for continued shifts in surgical practice. Surgeons must remain competent in applying a variety of techniques to tailor interventions to individual patients' needs while balancing the risks and benefits of each approach. As surgical techniques expand to include minimally invasive strategies and advanced tools, the field is moving toward faster patient recoveries and improved surgical outcomes. This constantly evolving atmosphere necessitates ongoing education and communication within the surgical community to share ideas and develop better techniques, ultimately with the aim of delivering patients the optimal and safest care available for their head and neck pathology.

1.3.3. Innovations in Minimally Invasive Surgery

The landscape of minimally invasive ENT and head and neck surgery has been significantly transformed by surgical innovations and technological advances. The evolution of robotic surgery and endoscopic techniques has increased precision and reduced recovery times for patients. These modalities facilitate reduced incisions, diminished tissue trauma, and enhanced visualization, with the ultimate aim of optimizing surgical outcomes without causing unnecessary postoperative complications. The minimally invasive trend is also particularly relevant in the management of head and neck cancers, where traditionally it involves extensive surgical resection and significant morbidity. As documented in recent literature, a multidisciplinary approach is critical, with innovations aimed at improving not only cancer management but also the preservation of key functions such as speech and swallowing, which are most important to patient quality of life (Andry et al., 2012). Among notable advancements in minimally invasive surgery are the use of gasless transaxillary endoscopic thyroidectomy (GTET) and minimally invasive video-assisted thyroidectomy (VAT). Both techniques have been debated for their potential to minimize postoperative complications and improve aesthetic outcomes. Comparison of GTET and VAT revealed subtle implications in operating time, pain, and incidence of nerve injury. While GTET is a technically demanding procedure associated with longer operating times and higher immediate pain scores, findings indicate no difference in patient satisfaction with the scars' cosmetic appearance between the two procedures (Lang, B. H. H., & Wong, K. P., 2012). This reiterates the ongoing quest in surgical practice to advance techniques that optimize patient-oriented outcomes while reducing invasiveness, further symbolizing the progress of surgical technologies in the ENT domain. The focus on the innovations in minimally invasive surgery has necessitated a paradigm shift in training in ENT and head and neck surgery residency programs. Surgeons today must learn to become more skilled with advanced technologies such as robotic systems and novel endoscopic instruments. As more residency programs integrate these minimally invasive techniques, their inclusion in surgical curricula is required to prepare the next generation of surgeons. Simulation training and mentorship programs are starting to become a necessary component of education, ensuring that the trainees do not only learn the technical details but a whole concept about the associated risks and benefits of such complex procedures. The continuous development of surgical techniques promises not only better clinical outcomes but also a climate of innovation that disrupts established practice in the field, with the ultimate goal of enhancing the quality of care provided to patients undergoing ENT and head and neck operations (Figure 1.12).

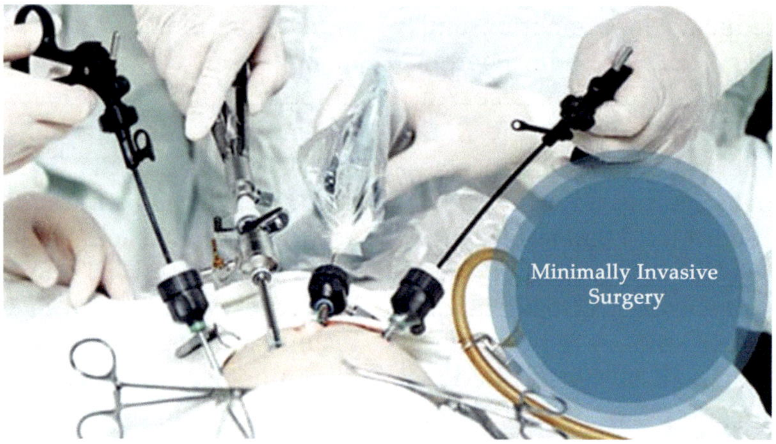

Figure 1.12. Innovations in minimally invasive surgery.

Source: https://external-content.duckduckgo.com/iu/?u=https%3A%2F%2Fs3-ap-south-1.amazonaws.com%2Fimages.hospals.com%2Fuploads%2Fblogs%2Fimg_60c4cb6670d2b1623509862.png&f=1&nofb=1&ipt=1de619061432953f366e2c88012528d12a002fc37b498ad58968eaca905704bd.

Test Your Knowledge

1. Describe the surgical approaches to the thyroid gland. Discuss indications, key anatomical landmarks, and potential complications.
2. Discuss the principles and techniques of neck dissection in the management of head and neck malignancies.

1.4. Diagnostic Tools and Technologies

Learning Outcome

1. Role of Imaging in ENT Diagnosis
2. Use of Endoscopy in Examination
3. Audiological Assessments and Their Importance

The field of diagnostic technology and equipment in ENT and head and neck surgery is of greatest significance in the appropriate assessment and care of disease. Advanced technologies such as endoscopy have totally revolutionized the process of observing inner structures. This least invasive technique provides real-time imaging of the nasal passages, sinuses, and pharynx, which is very important for diagnosing diseases such as chronic sinusitis and vocal cord lesions. In addition, advances in imaging modalities such as computed tomography (CT) and magnetic resonance imaging (MRI) provide cross-sectional imaging of complex anatomical structures, thereby aiding precise tumor localization and the identification of anatomical defects. Integration of these technologies not only improves diagnostic precision but also guides surgical planning, ultimately facilitating better patient outcomes in ENT and head and neck clinics. In addition to visual inspection, identifying hearing disorders is important through audiometric tests. Audiometers and tympanometers are just a few of the instruments used by practitioners to quantify hearing sensitivity and middle-ear function, respectively. This information is vital for diagnosing conditions such as conductive hearing loss and sensorineural hearing impairment and helps practitioners make informed decisions about interventions. Such as the results from tympanometry, which can reveal the presence of middle ear or eustachian tube dysfunction, both of which necessitate specific treatment modalities. Additionally, the evolving discipline of telemedicine has enabled remote audiological testing, increasing access to specialized ENT care. Using these diagnostic tools, healthcare providers can ensure timely and effective management of hearing conditions, particularly given the potential for long-lasting consequences for communication and quality of life. Emerging diagnostic technologies, including new molecular techniques, are also continuing to expand the boundaries of ENT and head and neck surgery. Techniques such as DNA sequencing and biomarker profiling are proving significant for early diagnosis and stratification of head and neck malignancies. These molecular diagnoses assist in delivering a more personalized treatment by facilitating the identification of patients at higher risk for disease and informing therapy based on tumor genetic content. Additionally, technologies such as fluorescence-guided surgery are being explored to improve tumor resection rates while preserving crucial adjacent structures. With such developments still underway, they hold the promise of radically improving diagnostic accuracy and therapeutic outcomes in ENT and transforming patient care. The integration of multifaceted diagnostic technologies will eventually provide broader insight into head and neck pathologies, enabling customized and effective interventions in patient care.

1.4.1. Role of Imaging in ENT Diagnosis

Imaging is a critical component of diagnosing ear, nose, and throat (ENT) conditions, providing deeper insight into pathology that may not be evident on clinical examination. Imaging modalities such as X-rays, computed tomography (CT) scans, and magnetic resonance imaging (MRI) provide valuable information about anatomical structures, lesions, and potential complications. For instance, CT scanning is better at imaging the intricate bony architecture of the skull and sinuses, which is required to diagnose sinusitis, fractures, or tumors. MRI, with its superior contrast in soft tissues, is particularly helpful for evaluating neurologic structures and soft-tissue tumors in the head and neck. By using these imaging methods side by side, the ENT specialist can render a full diagnosis, tailor treatments, and manage patient care accordingly. In cases of infection, particularly those that compromise major anatomical structures around the neck, imaging is essential for early recognition and proper management. Conditions like necrotizing fasciitis can rapidly advance, and such cases require urgent surgical intervention to avoid major morbidity and mortality. Imaging helps determine the spread of infection and inform surgical methods. For example, a CT scan will delineate the spread of infection from superficial to deeper fascial planes, so the ENT surgeon can evaluate whether drainage or decompression is required. Moreover, the difficulty of head and neck infections necessitates a multidisciplinary case and underscores the important role of imaging. Deep neck space infections can complicate quickly, with severe consequences such as mediastinitis or airway compromise, potentially leading to fatality. Imaging assists in defining the nature of infection, such as peritonsillar or retropharyngeal abscess, and informs the decision to operate. Awareness of anatomical relationships on imaging can also guide the placement of feeding tubes or tracheostomies when necessary, significantly impacting patient management and outcomes. With ENT surgeons navigating through the intricate landscape of head and neck surgery, integration of novel imaging techniques is a cornerstone in diagnosis, management, and ultimately better quality of life in managing patients with complex infections and pathologies (Bălălău et al., 2018).

1.4.2. Use of Endoscopy in Examination

Endoscopy is an important tool for examining the head and neck, particularly in otolaryngology. This technique of minimally invasive visual investigation allows clinicians and surgeons to observe structures within the body without making an incision. With the aid of flexible and rigid endoscopes, doctors can assess pathologies that occur in the nasal cavity, sinuses, larynx, and pharynx. As technology advances, endoscopic surgery has evolved to include digital imaging and video recording, which provide real-time visual feedback and enable detailed post-procedural analysis. All of these are absolutely crucial for precise diagnosis and treatment planning in ENT and head and neck surgery, underscoring the significance of endoscopy as an essential instrument in modern medical practice.

The use of endoscopic techniques allows careful examination of anatomical regions that are traditionally hard to access. For instance, during laryngoscopy, visualization of the larynx and hypopharynx is classically compromised by the physical limitations of the examination. Endoscopes may, however, be maneuvered to provide a full view of these regions, allowing precise assessment of pathology. Technologies such as panoramic imaging, made feasible by stitching video sequences, open up a new approach to archiving and documenting laryngoscopy results. A trial of post-processing video sequences recorded with a rigid laryngoscope demonstrates how the technology improves both visual inspection and documentation, thereby enhancing ENT experts' diagnostic capability (Bergen et al., 2012). Aside from evaluating structural pathology, endoscopy also has an important function in the diagnosis of obstructive sleep apnea syndrome (OSAS), particularly in children. With a prevalence rate estimated at 2% among children between the ages of 2 and 8, an effective method of diagnosis is required. Endoscopic evaluation can identify adenoid hypertrophy, which is typically one of the underlying causes of the condition. With accurate assessment of the condition and size of the upper airway tissues through endoscopy, medical practitioners can formulate appropriate management strategies tailored to individual patients' needs. Through this targeted intervention, screening and treatment of children's respiratory sleep disorders are significantly enhanced, highlighting the decisive role of endoscopy in facilitating ENT and head and neck management (Bellini et al., 2019) (Figure 1.13).

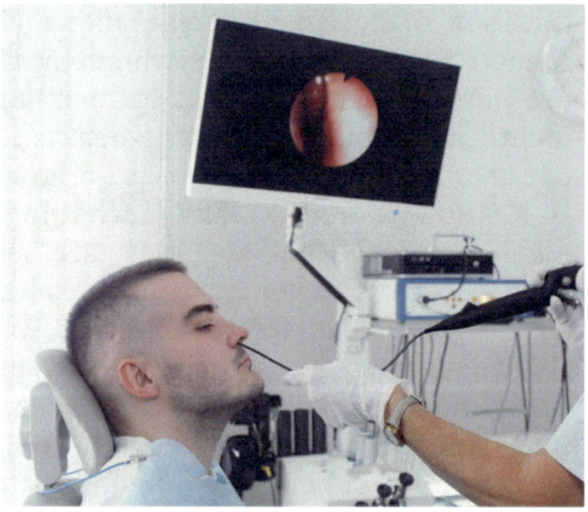

Figure 1.13. Use of endoscopy in examination.

Source: https://otorrinoclinicalperu.com/wp-content/uploads/2023/02/nasofibrolaringoscopia.png.

1.4.3. Audiological Assessments and Their Importance

Audiological testing is a core role of ENT and Head and Neck Surgery, namely the diagnosis and management of various hearing disorders. Audiological tests are conducted by applying various techniques, including pure-tone audiometry, speech reception tests, and auditory steady-state responses (ASSR), which provide essential information regarding a person's ability to hear. Implementing appropriate stopping criteria for ASSR testing, as emphasized in recent literature, improves the efficiency of obtaining accurate thresholds without necessarily affecting outcome quality. The objective nature of such tests not only aids the earlier identification of hearing disorders but also helps clinicians individualize treatment regimens. Because hearing impairment can have an immense impact on quality of life, early audiological evaluation is an integral aspect of ensuring patients receive proper interventions tailored to their needs, thereby ensuring improved healthcare outcomes. Outcomes of audiological evaluation extend beyond mere diagnosis, enhancing general knowledge of factors that may lead to hearing impairment. For example, the incidence of sensorineural hearing loss among recovered patients with bacterial meningitis underscores the importance of conducting routine auditory tests in vulnerable populations. Reports indicate that approximately 28% of those with this disease also develop hearing loss, underscoring the importance of conducting audiometric tests after recovery to monitor auditory status. Furthermore, studies have shown that while some patients have consistent hearing levels, others may require ongoing assessment to determine the need for treatment. This validates the role of audiology in ENT clinics, showing how early and ongoing audiological assessment can help prevent permanent auditory impairment and enable prompt referral for specialist review when needed. Apart from their diagnostic value, audiological testing is also needed to enable holistic care and coordination of medical professionals. The treatment of hearing-impaired patients must be multidisciplinary; therefore, audiologists often collaborate with otolaryngologists, speech-language pathologists, and educators to provide a range of rehabilitation services. Effective communication between these experts will help ensure that the care plans are patient-centered and holistic. The results gained from audiological testing also allow for public health activities aimed at preventing hearing loss through events and educational outreach and screening campaigns. In total, the contribution of audiological testing to ENT and Head and Neck Surgery is not just determined by its diagnostic role but also by its multiple contributions towards enhancing patient treatment, reducing the prevalence of hearing impairments, and promoting interdisciplinary communication.

Test Your Knowledge

1. How do imaging technologies such as X-rays, CT scans, and MRI differ in their principles of operation and clinical applications?
2. What role do laboratory diagnostic tools (e.g., blood tests, PCR, and biopsy) play in early disease detection and treatment planning?

1.5. Patient Management and Care

Learning Outcome

1. Preoperative Assessment and Preparation
2. Postoperative Care and Recovery
3. Multidisciplinary Approach to Patient Management

Adequate patient care and management in ENT and Head and Neck Surgery are of utmost priority for optimal outcomes and to avoid risks associated with various procedures and diseases. Understanding the particular challenges posed by the anatomy and functions of these regions is the basis for patient assessment. In addition to infectious complications, conditions such as necrotizing fasciitis illustrate the subtlety of caring for patients within this surgical subspecialty.

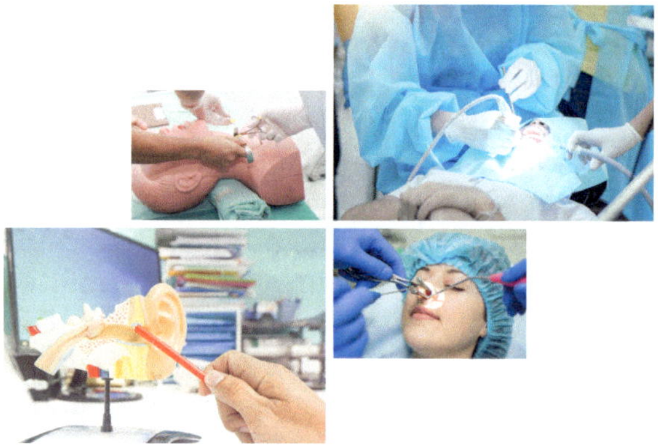

Figure 1.14. Patient management and care.

Source: https://external-content.duckduckgo.com/iu/?u=https%3A%2F%2Fviswanathanhospital.com%2Fwp-content%2Fuploads%2F2021%2F10%2FENT-1.png&f=1&nofb=1&ipt=6bac6bcc0b7e9f095d4fd83c8179d4f9ece4d1cff867f832921c143af56d2dad.

This rapidly spreading infection, particularly in immunocompromised hosts, requires prompt diagnosis and treatment. Finally, multidisciplinary patient care. The requirement for ongoing evaluation and adaptation to evolving clinical scenarios is fundamental to enhanced patient outcomes. Systematic training and strict adherence to standard guidelines enable clinicians to address the complexities of multiple medical conditions, particularly amid new public health challenges. By fostering a safety culture and ongoing learning, healthcare teams can ensure they not only provide effective therapies but also manage patient care and support systems in an integrated way. This integrated approach is necessary to establish trust between patients and medical professionals and, therefore, enhance the overall health care experience (Figure 1.14).

1.5.1. Preoperative Assessment and Preparation

Preoperative assessment and preparation are essential components of ENT and head and neck surgery, as they directly affect surgical outcomes and reduce complications. The full preoperative assessment involves evaluating the patients' general health, any potential risks they may face, and familiarizing oneself with comorbidities that may affect recovery. This is followed by a thorough medical history, physical examination, and relevant laboratory tests. For instance, evaluating factors such as age, smoking habits, and past medical histories, including respiratory illnesses or diabetes, can provide patient risk profiles. Ultimately, effective preoperative assessment helps avoid complications, such as pharyngocutaneous fistula, which remains a frequent complication after total laryngectomy (Sabri, 2010). The preparation process also includes educating patients about the surgical procedure and establishing clear lines of communication about postoperative care. Educating the patient as to what they can expect before, during, and after surgery will decrease anxiety and increase compliance with preoperative regulations, vital for optimal surgical success. The education may involve descriptions of the surgical technique employed, potential postoperative complications, and rehabilitative strategies that may be necessary. Furthermore, involving multidisciplinary personnel, such as anesthesiologists and nutritionists, helps ensure that various areas of patient management are covered, providing a more comprehensive preparation plan. Incorporating the elements of advanced technology, such as 3D printing, can also be helpful, enabling customized surgical guides and models tailored to patients' anatomy, thus enhancing surgical efficacy and accuracy (Annemans et al., 2016). Effective preoperative preparation extends beyond mere evaluations; it also involves making patients as optimal as possible before surgery. This may involve preoperative optimization steps, such as smoking cessation programs, nutritional interventions, or the management of comorbid medical conditions. For example, chronic diseases like obstructive pulmonary disease or diabetes must be controlled so as to reduce postoperative complications. Also, the use of formal preoperative protocols can significantly improve patients' readiness for surgery. This forward-looking approach not only improves the quality of surgical care overall. By focusing on improving patient outcomes through thoughtful assessments and tailored preparation strategies, ENT and head and neck surgery practice can enhance procedural success and quality of life after treatment (Sabri, 2010).

1.5.2. Postoperative Care and Recovery

Successful postoperative care and recovery are critical components in the patient care continuum for individuals who have undergone ENT and head and neck surgeries. The nature of these surgeries might demand a holistic method of postoperative care, including pain control, vigilance for complications, and enabling the best healing environment. For instance, surgeries such as endoscopic tympanomastoidectomy have shed light on how normal mucosa should be preserved during operation, which in turn promotes quicker recovery and better hearing results. By prioritizing individualized postoperative regimens, practitioners can help prevent complications and improve patient comfort, thereby reducing hospital stays and improving overall satisfaction with surgical outcomes, underscoring the importance of meticulous postoperative care in ENT surgery (Kumar et al., 2012). In postoperative convalescence, some risk factors for the complication of healing are taken into account, particularly in patients with obstructive sleep apnea syndrome (OSAS). The prevalence in surgical candidates is much higher than in the general population, posing serious risks to anesthetic management and postoperative monitoring. Sedation and anesthesia are known to increase upper airway collapsibility, a risk factor for postoperative respiratory complications. Hence, preoperative identification of OSAS and the use of appropriate perioperative management measures—such as specialized monitoring and adjusted anesthetic techniques—are important to reduce patient risk and optimize recovery outcomes. The perioperative team must work together to minimize these risks and identify high-risk patients early in the surgery process (Doghramji et al., 2012). Furthermore, postoperative rehabilitation and education are integral to the process after ENT and head and neck surgery. The patients must be instructed on how things will work out during the recovery phase, what symptoms could signal complications, and lifestyle modifications that can make the recovery easier. Speech therapy for patients undergoing surgery on the voice box or swallowing pathways is possible through rehabilitation. This aspect of care is crucial because it can significantly affect functional recovery and quality of life after surgery. Patient involvement in the recovery process can encourage compliance with rehabilitation programs and help patients take control of their care. When healthcare workers are informed about the various elements of postoperative care, including education and rehabilitation, they can better optimize recovery and help patients achieve the best possible results from surgery.

1.5.3. Multidisciplinary Approach to Patient Management

The surgical intricacy of head and neck operations generally requires a multidisciplinary treatment plan, involving different specialists to ensure proper care. This treatment plan is compulsory in the management of complex conditions that might arise as a result of trauma, infections, or congenital anomalies of the head and neck region. With interdisciplinary coordination among otolaryngologists, reconstructive surgeons, radiologists, and anesthesiologists, treatment protocols can be optimally tailored to patient needs. This partnership not only enhances surgical outcomes but also minimizes complications by offering a comprehensive analysis of the patient's medical history and pre-existing health conditions. This partnership is symptomatic of the growing recognition that combined care improves patient safety and satisfaction, and of the necessity of a robust support system in the complex setting of ENT and head and neck surgery. In the treatment of complex injuries such as those that accompany trauma, the multidisciplinary process is the key to the ideal result. An otolaryngologist may coordinate with emergency medicine physicians, intensivists, and surgeons to plan and carry out a lengthy course of treatment. The coordinated effort ensures proper drainage of abscesses and maintains the patient's overall stability. The psychological impact on the patients who undergo these procedures cannot be overlooked either; effective counseling about surgical outcomes prevents their anxiety and stress about the functional and aesthetic repercussions of treatment. Thus, the multidisciplinary approach is essential in addressing both the physical and psychological aspects of patient care (Bălălău et al., 2018).

Test Your Knowledge

1. How does effective communication between healthcare providers and patients improve patient outcomes and overall quality of care?
2. What are the key steps involved in developing and implementing an individualized patient care plan?

1.6. Challenges and Future Directions in ENT

Learning Outcome

1. Addressing the Rise of Antibiotic Resistance
2. Advances in Technology and Their Impact on Surgery
3. The Importance of Research and Education in ENT

The field of ENT surgery is faced with a number of challenges that greatly impact patient outcomes as well as treatment efficacy. Among the challenges is the heterogeneity of head and neck cancers, particularly the locally advanced squamous cell carcinoma (LA SCCHN). The biology of these cancers is complex, necessitating complex treatment interventions such as induction chemotherapy (ICT) protocols. Recent advances, particularly the performance of TPF (docetaxel, cisplatin, and fluorouracil) as a superior regimen compared with traditional chemotherapy options, highlight the need for ongoing research in this area. Regardless, the administration of TPF needs to be carefully managed by an interdisciplinary team, underscoring the need for coordination among medical professionals. As the specialty advances, maintaining the safe and effective use of new treatments is critical to further improving patient care in ENT surgery (Cohen et al., 2018). Another critical issue for ENT is the need for comprehensive guidelines that guide treatment decisions, taking into account patients' quality of life. For instance, the management of diseases such as Mucopolysaccharidosis VI (MPS VI) illustrates the importance of a multidisciplinary team in delivering optimal care to patients.

The relentless nature of MPS VI, coupled with the heterogeneity of manifestations ranging from respiratory to hearing impairments, underscores the importance of evidence-based guidelines and standardized monitoring protocols. Heterogeneity of such patients' needs can make treatment modalities, such as enzyme replacement therapies to surgery, challenging. Ensuring that all physicians involved on a case are oriented by consensus statements not only improves treatment outcome but also meets the patient's overall needs (Akyol et al., 2019). In overcoming inherent challenges in the field, ENT surgery has no choice but to prioritize innovative methods to improve treatment accuracy and the delivery of care to patients. One such direction is the meeting of personalized medicine and advanced technologies, such as genomics and targeted therapy, that have the potential to revolutionize treatment for head and neck disease. Tumor profiling and biomarker investigation could lead to more tailored, potent therapy, especially for highly aggressive cancer subtypes. Additionally, fostering collaboration among schools, clinicians, and industry partners will be instrumental in advancing ENT practice. By providing both clinical and research solutions, the specialty can turn challenges into opportunities, thereby improving clinical outcomes and defining the future of ENT and head and neck surgery.

1.6.1. Addressing the Rise of Antibiotic Resistance

The emergence of antibiotic resistance is a significant challenge in ENT and head and neck surgery, especially in managing diseases such as chronic suppurative otitis media (CSOM). The treatment of CSOM commonly involves topical antibiotics, but there is considerable uncertainty about their effectiveness and safety in clinical practice. Studies have shown that the small body of existing literature is of low quality and, therefore, when comparing topical antibiotics and systemic therapy, creates uncertainty about outcomes (Hashmi et al., 2022). For instance, evidence shows that applying topical antibiotics improves the clearance of ear discharge but also indicates that many potential side effects are underreported, casting doubt on the selection of effective treatment modalities (Hashmi et al., 2022). This underscores the need for careful scrutiny of antibiotic stewardship plans to counter the growing tide of resistance. Appropriate management of antibiotic resistance also requires harmonizing clinical guidelines with the latest information and practice trends. The European Position Paper on Rhinosinusitis and Nasal Polyps (EPOS2020) provides updated guidelines for managing acute and chronic rhinosinusitis, emphasizing the escalating problems of antibiotic misuse. This full guide emphasizes evidence-based interventions that utilize multidisciplinary teams, including patients and pharmacists, to optimize condition management. Through redefined definitions and classes, EPOS2020 ensures that effective intervention is possible only with ongoing education and collaboration from all healthcare providers to maximize prescribed therapy and avoid unnecessary antibiotic use (Alobid et al., 2020). By applying these dynamic guidelines, practitioners are better equipped to respond to and manage the threat of antibiotic resistance in relevant ENT diseases. Therefore, management of antibiotic resistance in ENT and head and neck surgery involves an all-encompassing approach that integrates clinical vigilance with public health interventions. Physicians must remain steadfast in advocating for antibiotic stewardship, not merely responsible prescribing, but also research into alternative therapies and better diagnostic methods. In this context, the rise of pharmacological resistance requires that physicians adopt practices emphasizing delayed antibiotic prescribing or the use of adjunctive therapies that can bolster the body's defense mechanism. Simultaneously, public education campaigns to enlighten about appropriate antibiotic use can reduce overprescription and misuse considerably. By fostering a cultural shift toward judicious use of antibiotics, the medical community can help prevent the catastrophic consequences of antibiotic resistance, ensuring that effective therapy remains available to future ENT and head and neck disease patients (Figure 1.15).

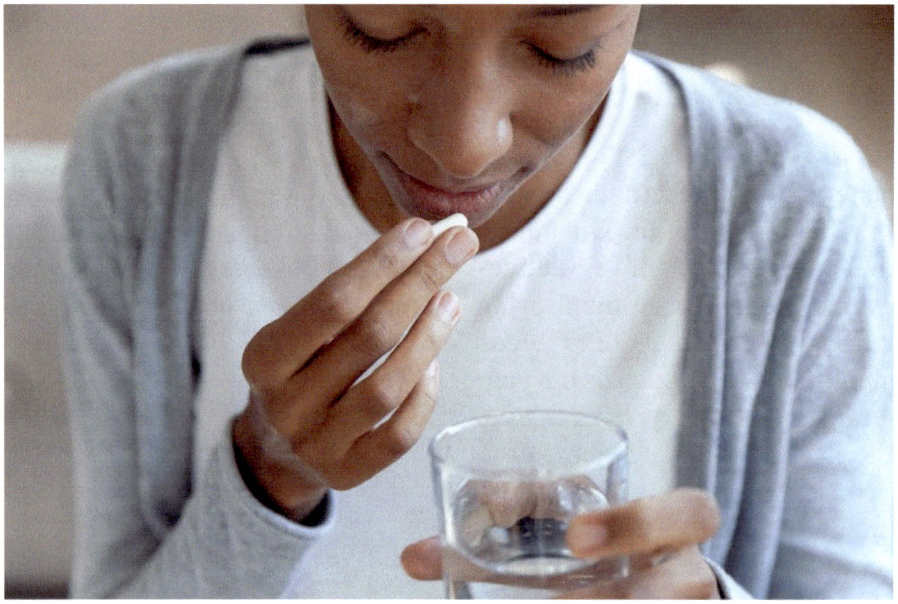

Figure 1.15. Addressing the rise of antibiotic resistance.

Source: https://external-content.duckduckgo.com/iu/?u=https%3A%2F%2Fhealth.umms.org%2Fwp-content%2Fuploads%2F2024%2F10%2FAntibiotic-Resistance_1200.jpg&f=1&nofb=1&ipt=d7ac3a84ba6e95bceece3ddc104186192be9178c7b580bdc6035414d138948e7.

1.6.2. Advances in Technology and Their Impact on Surgery

Advancements in technology have significantly changed surgical procedures, particularly in ENT and head and neck surgery. A major advancement is the use of virtual surgical planning, which employs three-dimensional imaging to enhance the precision and success of surgery. It can be used by surgeons to rehearse complex procedures, streamline their strategy to adapt to patient anatomy, and visualize major structures before incision. Such a preoperative plan is particularly helpful in oncologic surgery, as it enables surgeons to achieve optimal safety margins in tumor resections while minimizing damage to adjacent normal tissues. It has been established through research that virtual planning not only maximizes functional outcomes but also generates higher degrees of patient satisfaction concerning facial aesthetics postoperatively, which underscores its multiple benefits (Battiston et al., 2024). Simultaneously with advances in virtual planning, the development of specialty surgical packs demonstrates the technology's ability to streamline operating room protocols. Specialty packs, which consolidate all the necessary medical disposable elements into a single sterile bundle, have become valuable tools for optimizing workflow efficiency in the operating room. Traditional arrangements typically require additional preparation time and can cause delays or problems during a procedure. Through reducing points of contact, or physical contact between equipment and staff, these packs promote faster setups while also decreasing the possibility of contamination. Research has indicated that hospitals using optimized custom packs can significantly streamline operations and ensure surgical teams' rapid access to all necessary instruments and equipment, thereby enhancing patient safety and outcomes (Belien et al., 2015). Furthermore, the introduction of robotic-assisted surgery is revolutionizing minimally invasive surgery in the head and neck as well as ENT. Robotic systems enhance visualization and instrumentation beyond the human hand, allowing surgeons to perform intricate maneuvers with greater accuracy. Robotic systems provide surgeons with a three-dimensional view of the operating field, making it easier to manipulate complicated anatomical structures. This technology has been particularly revolutionary in procedures such as endoscopic sinus surgery and thyroidectomy, where surgical accuracy is of the highest priority. Reducing patient recovery times through robot-assisted surgery underscores the growing adoption of this technology in modern surgical practice and signals a clear shift toward incorporating sophisticated technology to improve patient care and surgical outcomes. The implications of these advances are profound, as they not only enhance the effectiveness of surgery but also improve overall patient outcomes in ENT and head and neck surgery (Belien et al., 2015; Battiston B et al., 2024).

1.6.3. The Importance of Research and Education in ENT

Education and research are essential parts of progress in the discipline of otolaryngology, especially in the field of head and neck surgery. As medical information continues to grow exponentially, a solid research foundation enables practitioners to implement evidence-based interventions that improve patient outcomes. Research into different conditions, including head and neck cancers, guides clinical decisions through determining incidence, symptomatology, and intervention. Moreover, curriculum programming aimed at residents and medical students is critical to building a wide foundation of knowledge of complex procedures, such as the head and neck physical examination (NPE). Research confirms that formally organized teaching interventions significantly enhance students' confidence in performing these procedures, thereby leading to a new era of efficient practitioners committed to excellence in care (Armstrong et al., 2015). The value of research in otolaryngology lies in its capacity to treat head and neck diseases with multiple causative factors. Cancerous cases analysis, which recent studies are focusing on, indicates correlations of disease formation and habits such as smoking and alcohol consumption (Gopalakrishnan, S., & Kumar, P., 2013). Such understanding not only identifies populations at risk but also underscores the importance of education-based preventive programs. Educational coursesfor healthcare providers and the general public are adequately geared toward providing information about risk factors and symptoms of head and neck cancers. Incorporation of such knowledge into curricula, therefore, prepares future clinicians and optimizes public health education, advocating for a culture where preventive care is prioritized in addition to therapeutic advances. In addition to enhancing clinical competence and expertise, ongoing research in ENT is important for advancing therapeutic techniques. As head and neck ailments evolve, so do the treatments applied to treat them. Advanced research drives new surgical innovations, advances in targeted therapy, and the development of diagnostic equipment. Research fosters a culture of investigation among otolaryngologists, who are motivated to stay current in their profession. Such synergy between research and education empowers practitioners not only to address current health issues effectively but also to prepare for future demands, ultimately advancing the body of knowledge for patients and the medical community at large. By prioritizing research and education in ENT, we position ourselves to make significant advances in patient care and outcomes.

Test Your Knowledge

1. What are the major challenges currently faced in ENT practice, and how do they impact patient outcomes?
2. Discuss the future directions and innovations that are shaping the field of ENT.

SUMMARY

For ENT and Head and Neck Surgery, closing comments emphasize the utmost importance of developing surgical techniques and outcomes for patients. This specialty's nature requires a multidisciplinary approach to treating patients, particularly for severe deep neck space infections. These infections are not only a clinical challenge but require extensive management strategies to avoid mediastinitis and septic shock. Given the potential for significant aesthetic and psychological influence from surgical interventions, it is imperative that patients are properly educated preoperatively about the nature of the procedures and what to expect. Informed patientness helps set realistic expectations and, in the long term, helps build a trusting rapport between the medical professional and the client (Bălălău et al., 2018).

In short, ENT and Head and Neck Surgery is an essential specialty of medicine with subtleties that demand a solid understanding of both surgical and medical management. The intricate interplay among pathophysiology, surgical technique, and patient management underscores the need for continuing education for healthcare workers. While advancing with advances in medical technology and changes in demographic profiles of health, practitioners need to give patient-centered care approaches precedence that emphasize informed consent and psychological support. The destiny of this surgical specialty lies in an alliance dedicated to maximizing patient outcomes through innovative research, interprofessional practice, and sustained efforts to combat the ongoing challenges of ENT and Head and Neck Surgery.

The field of ENT and Head and Neck Surgery encompasses a wide array of surgical procedures and complex factors that affect patient outcomes. Among them, obstetric-free surgery during pregnancy is a key point of discussion in this context. The new research reveals the association between such procedures and adverse delivery outcomes like spontaneous abortion and preterm delivery. This study emphasized that 1-2% of pregnancies involve non-obstetric surgery, but the risk factors and outcomes remain poorly delineated in current NHS guidelines.

Overall, recognition of a more accurate definition of these risks can influence surgical decision-making and enhance patient consultations, obtaining critical information on how to balance surgical treatment with likely maternal and fetal health outcomes (Aylin et al., 2016). Secondly, the unique problem of management of head and neck cancer, that is, head and neck squamous cell carcinomas (HNSCC), has significant treatment and patient implications. One of the significant issues, as contended, is the poor overall survival of 40-60%, and therefore, there is an urgent need for new treatment interventions.

The most recent developments in preserving tumor biopsies in microfluidic tissue culture systems enable researchers to study tumors' responses to various therapies in a laboratory setting. Not only does this preserve tissue viability and morphology, but it also allows for investigating personalized medicine that can lead to tailored regimens that maximize efficacy and improve patient outcomes (Bower et al., 2017). Finally, ENT and Head and Neck Surgery complexities vary from the delicate balance of performing surgery on vulnerable groups, such as pregnant women, to the novel techniques applied in cancer treatment. Parallel to this, research on treatment modalities in HNSCC is increasingly focused on personalized medicine and patient-based treatment. Together, these two significant discussions provide key insights into the evolving nature of ENT and Head and Neck Surgery, underscoring the need for ongoing research and debate among physicians to ensure that treatment maximizes patient care and surgical outcomes (Aylin et al., 2016; Bower et al., 2017).

KEY TERMS FROM THIS CHAPTER

Otorhinolaryngology	Otology
Rhinology	Laryngology
Audiology	Pharyngology
Vestibular System	Eustachian Tube
Tympanic Membrane	Ossicles
Cochlea	Semicircular Canals
Nasal Septum	Turbinates
Paranasal Sinuses	Adenoids
Tonsils	Epiglottis

CRITICAL THINKING QUESTIONS

1. **The most common cause of epistaxis in adults is:**
   a. Juvenile nasopharyngeal angiofibroma
   b. Hypertension
   c. Trauma to Little's area
   d. Bleeding disorder
2. **The nerve most commonly injured during parotid gland surgery is:**
   a. Hypoglossal nerve
   b. Glossopharyngeal nerve
   c. Facial nerve
   d. Accessory nerve
3. **The most common malignant tumor of the larynx is:**
   a. Adenocarcinoma
   b. Squamous cell carcinoma
   c. Small cell carcinoma
   d. Lymphoma
4. **The most common cause of conductive hearing loss in young adults is:**
   a. Otosclerosis
   b. Acoustic neuroma
   c. Presbycusis
   d. Meniere's disease
5. **The first lymph node involved in carcinoma of the tongue is usually:**
   a. Submental
   b. Submandibular
   c. Jugulodigastric
   d. Preauricular

Short Answer Questions

1. Describe the blood supply of the nasal septum.
2. Enumerate the boundaries of the tonsillar bed.
3. List the complications of otitis media.
4. What are the indications for tracheostomy?
5. What are the parts of the ear?
6. What is the most common cause of conductive hearing loss?
7. What are the common causes of epistaxis?
8. What are the symptoms of acute tonsillitis?
9. What are the indications for tonsillectomy?

Answers to Critical Thinking Questions

1. (c) 2. (c) 3. (b) 4. (a) 5. (c)

REFERENCES

1. Abramo, A., Ferri, E., Spinato, G., Tirelli, G., et al. (2012). *Necrotizing fasciitis of the posterior cervical compartment: An atypical case due to Streptococcus agalactiae.* https://core.ac.uk/download/pdf/9634056.pdf (accessed on 7th August 2025).

2. Akyol, M. U., Co-Chairs, M. C. P., Alden, T. D., Amartino, H., Ashworth, J., Belani, K., Berger, K. I., Borgo, A., Braunlin, E., Eto, Y., Gold, J. I., Jester, A., Jones, S. A., Karsli, C., Mackenzie, W., Marinho, D. R., McFadyen, A., McGill, J., Mitchell, J. J., . . . Scarpa, M. (2019b). Recommendations for the management of MPS IVA: systematic evidence- and consensus-based guidance. *Orphanet Journal of Rare Diseases, 14*(1), 137. https://doi.org/10.1186/s13023-019-1074-9Al Harthi, T. S., Al-Jehani, A. M., Alahmar, A. F., Alharbi, R. A., et al. (2018). *Head and Neck Surgery: A Differential Diagnosis in Otolaryngology.* https://core.ac.uk/download/234692535.pdf (accessed on 7th August 2025).

3. Alobid, I., Anselmo-Lima, W. T., Bachert, C., Baroody, F. M., et al. (2020). *European Position Paper on Rhinosinusitis and Nasal Polyps 2020.* https://core.ac.uk/download/288799867.pdf (accessed on 7th August 2025).

4. Altissimi, G., Cianfrone, G., Ciofalo, A., Greco, A., et al. (2016). *When Alarm Bells Ring: Emergency Tinnitus.* https://core.ac.uk/download/54538689.pdf (accessed on 7th August 2025).

5. Andry, J., Bernier, A., Bonner, R., Boudreaux, M., Bova, S., Buckley, T., Caglar, M., et al. (2012). *Current trends in initial management of hypopharyngeal cancer: The declining use of open surgery.* https://deepblue.lib.umich.edu/bitstream/2027.42/90087/1/21613_ftp.pdf (accessed on 7th August 2025).

6. Annemans, L., Gemmel, P., Tack, P., Victor, J., et al. (2016). *3D-Printing Techniques in a Medical Setting: A Systematic Literature Review.* https://core.ac.uk/download/84043719.pdf (accessed on 7th August 2025).

7. Armstrong, W. B., Badran, K. W., Kuan, E. C., Passy, V., et al. (2015). *Medical students' comfort levels with performing the basic head and neck examination in practice: Follow-up during the core clerkship year.* https://core.ac.uk/download/305124560.pdf (accessed on 7th August 2025).

8. Aylin, P., Balinskaite, V., Bennett, P., Bottle, A., et al. (2016). *Estimating the risk of adverse birth outcomes in pregnant women undergoing non-obstetric surgery using routinely collected NHS data: An observational study.* https://core.ac.uk/download/77021205.pdf (accessed on 7th August 2025).

9. Azimonti, D., Cavaliere, C., De Vincentiis, M., Dragonetti, A., et al. (2018). *Use of balloon catheter dilation and steroid-eluting stent in light and severe rhinosinusitis of frontal sinus: A multicenter retrospective randomized study.* https://core.ac.uk/download/188823049.pdf (accessed on 7th August 2025).

10. Bailey, C. M., Brain, C., Dillon, M. J., Richards, H., et al. (2007). *Craniometaphyseal and craniodiaphyseal dysplasia, head and neck manifestations, and management.* https://core.ac.uk/download/1703492.pdf (accessed on 7th August 2025).

11. Bălălău, C., Domuța, M., Egor, S., Sargarovschi, M., Mărginean, C., et al. (2018). *Management of Deep Space Infections of the Neck.* https://core.ac.uk/download/216808113.pdf (accessed on 7th August 2025).

12. Bar-Ad, V., Cognetti, D., Curry, J., Doyle, M., et al. (2019). *Single institution implementation of permanent 131Cs interstitial brachytherapy for previously irradiated patients with resectable recurrent head and neck carcinoma.* https://core.ac.uk/download/228068157.pdf (accessed on 7th August 2025).

13. Basnyat, S., Goldfarb, J. M., Nyquist, G. G., Rabinowitz, M. R., et al. (2016). *Head and neck manifestations of eosinophilic granulomatosis with polyangiitis: A systematic review.* https://core.ac.uk/download/83049399.pdf (accessed on 7th August 2025).

14. Battiston, B., Crosetti, E., Succo, G., Arrigoni, G., Berrone, M., & Tos, P. (2024). *Long-term follow-up of computer-assisted microvascular mandibular reconstruction: A retrospective study.* https://core.ac.uk/download/639899024.pdf (accessed on 7th August 2025).

15. Belien, J., Cardoen, B., & Vanhoucke, M. (2015). *On the Design of Custom Packs: Grouping of Medical Disposable Items for Surgeries.* https://core.ac.uk/download/55847234.pdf (accessed on 7th August 2025).

16. Bellini, C., Cammaroto, G., Colizza, A., De Vincentiis, M., et al. (2019). *Risk Factors for Obstructive Sleep Apnea Syndrome in Children: State of the Art.* https://core.ac.uk/download/231747914.pdf (accessed on 7th August 2025).

17. Bergen, T., Friedl, S., Muenzenmayer, C., Reiter, A., et al. (2012). *Laryngoscopic image stitching for view enhancement and documentation – First experiences.* https://core.ac.uk/download/19418344.pdf (accessed on 7th August 2025).

18. Bianchini, S., Caminiti, C., Carrara, E., Donà, D., Esposito, S., Giuffrè, M., Inserra, A., et al. (2022). *Antimicrobial prophylaxis in neonates and children undergoing dental, maxillo-facial or ear-nose-throat (ENT) surgery: A RAND/UCLA appropriateness method consensus study.* https://core.ac.uk/download/512044745.pdf (accessed on 7th August 2025).

19. Bišof, V., Brajković, L., Curić Radivojević, R., Prgomet, D., et al. (2022). *Multidisciplinarni tim u liječenju karcinoma glave i vrata – iskustvo KBC-a Zagreb.* https://core.ac.uk/download/553606766.pdf (accessed on 7th August 2025).

20. Bordoni, B., Marelli, F., Morabito, B., Sacconi, B., et al. (2017). *Post-Sternotomy Pain Syndrome Following Cardiac Surgery: Case Report.* https://core.ac.uk/download/127587320.pdf (accessed on 7th August 2025).

21. Bower, R., Crank, S. T., Green, V. L., Greenman, J., et al. (2017). *Maintenance of head and neck tumor on-chip: Gateway to personalized treatment?* https://core.ac.uk/download/151161858.pdf (accessed on 7th August 2025).

22. Chinn, S. B., Clayburgh, D., Davies, L., Givi, B., et al. (2020). *Safety recommendations for evaluation and surgery of the head and neck during the COVID-19 pandemic.* https://core.ac.uk/download/322846968.pdf (accessed on 7th August 2025).

23. Cohen, E. E. W., Haddad, R. I., Hitt, R., Lefebvre, J. L., et al. (2018). *Induction chemotherapy in locally advanced squamous cell carcinoma of the head and neck: Role, controversy, and future directions.* https://core.ac.uk/download/323065529.pdf (accessed on 7th August 2025).

24. D'Haenens, W., Dhooge, I., & Vinck, B. (2009). *Determination and evaluation of clinically efficient stopping criteria for the multiple auditory steady-state response technique.* https://core.ac.uk/download/55824629.pdf (accessed on 7th August 2025).

25. Dimitriadis, P., Dunn, M., & Ray, J. (2017). *The role of non-invasive camera technology for*

gait analysis in patients with vestibular disorders. https://core.ac.uk/download/84340284.pdf (accessed on 7th August 2025).

26. Doghramji, K., Grewal, R. G., Vasu, R., et al. (2012). *Obstructive sleep apnea syndrome and perioperative complications: A systematic review of the literature*. https://core.ac.uk/download/83049558.pdf (accessed on 7th August 2025).
27. Domuţa, M., Mărginean, E., Pantiş, A., Popescu, R., et al. (2017). *Necrotizing Fasciitis of the Neck: Case Presentation*. https://core.ac.uk/download/144553906.pdf (accessed on 7th August 2025).
28. Gopalakrishnan, S., & Kumar, P. (2013). *Epidemiological study on head and neck malignancies: A study of 150 cases*. https://core.ac.uk/download/pdf/9634081.pdf (accessed on 7th August 2025).
29. Hardjojo, A., Shedden, A., Stuck, B., Cruz, A. A., Stevenson, A. N., Chauhan, B., Engel-Yeger, B., et al. (2012). *Allergic rhinitis and its associated co-morbidities at Bugando Medical Centre in Northwestern Tanzania: A prospective review of 190 cases*. https://core.ac.uk/download/pdf/11307799.pdf (accessed on 7th August 2025).
30. Hashmi, S. S., Hussain, S. Z. M., & Qayyum, A. (2022). *Ototoxicity of topical antibiotic ear drops in chronic suppurative otitis media in humans: A review of the literature*. https://core.ac.uk/download/619410926.pdf (accessed on 7th August 2025).
31. Hoff, H. J., Lehmann, M., & Sudhoff, H. (2011). *Skull Repair After Major Crush Injury*. https://core.ac.uk/download/193425091.pdf (accessed on 7th August 2025).
32. Imad, N. K., Ullah, S., Shah, S. M., Zaman, H., Jan, M. U., Ahmad, M., et al. (2025). *Frequency of ear, nose, and throat conditions leading to hospital admissions in Mardan Medical Complex, Mardan: A cross-sectional study*. https://core.ac.uk/download/647976427.pdf (accessed on 7th August 2025).
33. Khong, J., Malhotra, R., Selva-Nayagam, D., Wormald, P. J., et al. (2004). *Efficacy of endoscopic sinus surgery for paranasal sinus mucocele, including modified endoscopic Lothrop procedure for frontal sinus mucocele*. https://core.ac.uk/download/12734664.pdf (accessed on 7th August 2025).
34. Kumar, S., Ramamoorthy, M., & Thiagarajan, B. (2012). *Endoscopic Typmpanomastoid Exploration [Functional Endoscopic ear Surgery–FEES]*. https://core.ac.uk/download/pdf/9634108.pdf (accessed on 7th August 2025).
35. Lang, B. H. H., & Wong, K. P. (2012). *A comparison of surgical morbidity and scar appearance between gasless, transaxillary endoscopic thyroidectomy (GTET) and minimally invasive video-assisted thyroidectomy (VAT)*. https://core.ac.uk/download/37994273.pdf (accessed on 7th August 2025).
36. Moran, N., Sangma, R., & Yasmin, S. I. (2025). *A study on the pediatric cases admitted to the otorhinolaryngology department in a tertiary care center*. https://core.ac.uk/download/655504272.pdf (accessed on 7th August 2025).
37. N/A. (1997). *Focal Spot, Summer 1997*. https://core.ac.uk/download/129069308.pdf (accessed on 7th August 2025).
38. N/A. (2001). *Focal Spot, Summer 2001*. https://core.ac.uk/download/129069321.pdf (accessed on 7th August 2025).

39. N/A. (2004). *Focal Spot, Summer/Fall 2004.* https://core.ac.uk/download/129069330.pdf (accessed on 7th August 2025).

40. N/A. (2005). *Focal Spot, Winter 2004/2005.* https://core.ac.uk/download/129069331.pdf (accessed on 7th August 2025).

41. N/A. (2018). *Download Entire Issue: Gibbon Surgical Review,* 1 (1), 2018. https://core.ac.uk/download/155271707.pdf (accessed on 7th August 2025).

42. Nola, G., Ralli, G., Ralli, M., Sparvoli, L., et al. (2017). *Unilateral enlarged vestibular aqueduct syndrome and bilateral endolymphatic hydrops.* https://core.ac.uk/download/98349074.pdf (accessed on 7th August 2025).

43. Oostenbrink, R., Rodenburg-Vlot, M. B. A., Ruytjens, L., Schroeff, M. P., et al. (2018). *Repeated audiometry after bacterial meningitis: Consequences for future management.* https://core.ac.uk/download/158596627.pdf (accessed on 7th August 2025).

44. Sabri, I. F. (2010). *8 years of study of pharyngocutaneous fistula following total laryngectomy at C. H. Baragwanath Hospital.* https://core.ac.uk/download/39667763.pdf (accessed on 7th August 2025).

ANATOMY AND PHYSIOLOGY OF THE EAR

2

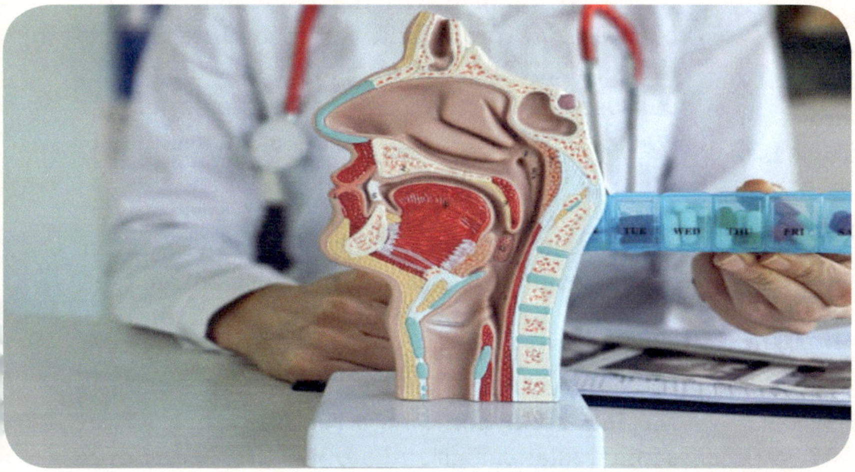

LEARNING OBJECTIVES

After studying this chapter, you will be able to:

1. Anatomy of the outer ear.
2. Anatomy of the middle ear.
3. Anatomy of the inner ear.
4. Physiology of hearing.
5. Physiology of balance.
6. Common ear disorders.

Introduction

The ear, a complex organ used for hearing and balance, contains intricate structures that work in harmony to detect sound. From the external ear, responsible for collecting sound waves, right through the middle ear ossicular chain utilized to amplify vibrations, to the inner ear's cochlea, where transduction occurs, all components play an integral role in hearing. An understanding of the ear's anatomy and physiology is crucial not only to comprehend basic auditory function but also to appreciate the pathologies that interfere with such function. While scientists investigate the evolution and adaptations of hearing mechanisms via interspecific comparison, what comparative anatomy provides about the specialized mechanism of human hearing sheds light. The diversity and complexity of vertebrate ear morphology confirm the evolutionary significance of auditory processes through a direct relationship of form to function and adaptation. Furthermore, research into the versatility of the tympanic middle ear has important physiological implications. Variability in tympanic structure, as found in comparative studies, demonstrates how these adaptations confer functional advantages across species. For instance, the mobility of the ossicles allows movement, perhaps to facilitate better sound transmission under certain conditions. More flexibility, as suggested by models, would tend to reduce sound energy transmission, but certain configurations may enhance hearing performance. The protective functions of such flexible units are also significant, as they help cushion the inner ear against excessive vibrations or displacements that could cause damage.

Emerging this dynamic capability underscores the need for continued studies of the middle ear's function in health and disease, and more particularly on inter-ossicular joint dysfunction and its clinical implications in humans, thereby illustrating the congruence of structure and functional integrity. Scanning through recent findings, advances in imaging technology in the form of micro-computed tomography come in handy with valuable inputs on the evolutionary background of the ears as well as the structure-function correlations. Extinct avian species, such as Prophaethon shrubsolei, provide important evidence of the evolution of auditory features over millions of years. The study of these fossilized samples provides evidence of inner-ear cochlear duct development, which reveals auditory sensitivities equal to those of modern birds. The marked expansion of brain areas involved in sensory functions, such as the eminentia sagittalis, suggests highly developed auditory and visual systems during the Mesozoic. These findings not only add to our understanding of the evolution of ear anatomy but also validate the correlation between auditory anatomy and overall sensory abilities in vertebrates, thereby opening opportunities for future work on the complexity of ear physiology and its evolutionary pathway.

Definition of the Ear and Its Importance

The ear serves a multifaceted role in human anatomy and physiology, functioning as both a hearing and a balance organ. The three divisions of the ear—the outer ear, middle ear, and inner ear—possess specialized anatomy for the purpose of sound wave detection, processing sound information, and controlling equilibrium. The outer ear receives sound vibrations and transmits them down the ear canal into the eardrum. As the sound waves bounce against the eardrum, they are transmitted via the middle ear ossicles to the cochlea in the inner ear, where they are transferred into electric impulses for the brain to interpret. This elaborate process illustrates the ear's role not only in the transmission of communication via speech and listening experiences but also in humans' capacity to respond to their environment effectively. In addition to hearing, the ears' role in balance is critical. The vestibular system in the inner ear contains structures such as the semicircular canals and otoliths that detect head movement and changes in position. This sensory information is helpful in coordinating movement and posture, and it has an important role in the activities of daily life, from walking to sports. Vestibular interference can lead to vertigo, illustrating the ear is central role in overall physical equilibrium and spatial orientation. The ear's importance extends far beyond mere hearing; it's a full appreciation of how the ear helps integrate higher-order human experience, folding together sensory information into an integral grasp of the world. The significance of the ear also extends to broader social and health concerns. For instance, effective communication relies heavily on hearing processing, which may shape how one interacts socially and relates to others. Hearing impairments or disorders may lead one to withdraw from society and impact mental health, hence requiring early detection and treatment. Furthermore, increased awareness of the sensory city life indicates the need for sound-sensitive designs that recognize how our sense of place is enhanced by all senses, including hearing (Lucas et al., 2008). This complex, rich meaning of the ear extends well beyond a brief anatomical account; it influences how we find our way and comprehend our world (Figure 2.1).

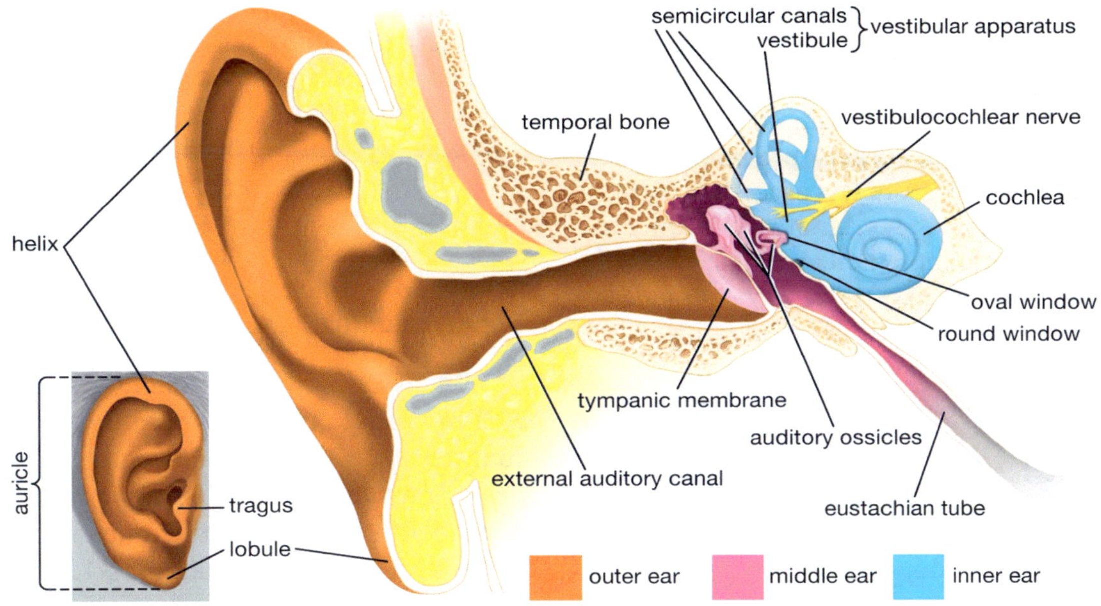

Figure 2.1. The ear serves a multifaceted role in human anatomy and physiology.

Source: https://cdn.britannica.com/04/14304-050-1A5E3289/structures-outer-ear.jpg

Overview of the Ear's Role in Hearing and Balance

The intricate structure of the ear is critical to hearing and balance, coordinating mechanical and neural functions to enable hearing and spatial localization. Essentially, sound waves enter the ear canal and strike the tympanic membrane, which vibrates. These vibrations are transmitted by a series of small bones referred to as the ossicles (malleus, incus, and stapes) that amplify sound before it reaches the cochlea in the inner ear. The cochlea is a sensory structure that translates mechanical energy into nerve impulses through hair cells that respond to different frequencies, enabling the brain to differentiate different sounds. This remarkable process of transduction is indicative of the ear's role not only in hearing but in compounding complex perceptions from external acoustics, thus signifying the profound interactivity between anatomical structure and auditive function. Balance, a significant human physiological activity, is regulated primarily by the vestibular system, which is located in the inner ear alongside the cochlea. This system detects head movement and space orientation through specialized structures: the semicircular canals and otolith organs. Rotational movement is detected by the semicircular canals, and linear acceleration and gravity are detected by the otolith organs. Sensory hair cells in these structures generate action potentials that are sent to the brain along the vestibular nerve. Therefore, the brain processes this information to maintain equilibrium, combining balance with visual and proprioceptive input from the body. This intricate interrelation of auditory and vestibular components is the ear's dual role and emphasizes its importance in complete sensory integration, serving to hear as well as balance. Refinement of surgical techniques, such as endoscopic tympanomastoidectomy, has improved diagnosis and treatment of ear disease, enhancing hearing outcomes and hearing preservation of ear anatomy and function. Endoscopic surgery provides greater illumination and access to less accessible regions of the middle ear and promotes clearance of pathologies, including cholesteatoma, without disrupting the integrity of overlying mucosal structures. By facilitating early re-aeration of the mastoid cavity, these methods allow for maximal postoperative recovery and improvement in auditory function. The benefits of adopting endoscopic methods resonate throughout the medical community, mirroring the tide of a paradigm shift toward more functional and reconstructive ear surgery methods. These advances emphasize ongoing research and understanding of the ears' function in hearing and balance, as evidenced by technologies such as Functional Endoscopic Ear Surgery (FEES) intended to restore physiological states critical to the maintenance of auditory and vestibular function.

Purpose and Scope of the Chapter

The purpose of this chapter is to provide an in-depth examination of the ear's anatomy and physiology, a highly advanced organ responsible for the perception of sound and balance. By dissecting the structural components—from the outer ear to the inner ear systems—this chapter explains how each role contributes to hearing. In addition, the discussion will examine how the ear's structure enables it to convert sound waves into neural impulses, the foundation of communication and interaction with the world. Anatomical knowledge of the ears provides a foundation for comprehension of the physiological mechanisms underlying hearing and balance, and is thus significant for academic and clinical endeavors in audiology and otology, as the auditory system itself, being healthy, directly affects overall quality of life. Further, the chapter will discuss the physiological mechanisms by which the ear operates, including how it transduces sound and how hair cells transduce signals. The sophisticated nature of the cochlea and the vestibular system will be elucidated, illustrating the way they work together to enable balance and orientation. Also discussed are issues such as frequency discrimination and sound localization, which show how the ear reacts to complex auditory stimuli.

By situating these physiological processes within the language of their anatomical counterparts, the chapter seeks to highlight the auditory system's reliance on the mutual dependence of structure and function. All of this is required because, in addition to explaining simple ear physiology more clearly, it lays the groundwork for the study of frequent pathologies of hearing loss and balance disorders, which are capable of inflicting great hardship on individuals. Finally, the scope of this chapter extends beyond basic anatomical and physiological explanations, aiming to bring these biological facts to practical use in medicine and education. In this regard, various education approaches will be assessed, focusing on visual aids and drawing methods that facilitate understanding of abstract ideas and enhance learning outcomes. In examining the educational value of ear anatomy, the chapter will reference established frameworks that encourage the incorporation of visual model-based argumentation in biology education. By equating pedagogy with scientific content, this discussion aims to promote greater integration of learning in the anatomy and physiology of the ear. This comprehensive review will not only inform future studies but also enable the development of effective teaching strategies and patient education programs in audiology and hearing sciences, ultimately improving learning and health outcomes (Quillin, K., & Thomas, S., 2015; Foster, 2017).

2.1. Anatomy of the Outer Ear

Learning Outcome

1. Structure and Function of the Pinna
2. The Auditory Canal and Its Role
3. The Tympanic Membrane (Eardrum)

The outer ear, one of the parts of the auditory system, consists of the pinna or auricle and the external auditory canal, which terminates at the eardrum. The shape of the auricle collects sound waves and directs them into the ear canal, which amplifies the sensory input of hearing. The auricle, in terms of anatomy, consists of a majority of cartilage and skin with ridges and grooves which aid in the localization of sound. This structure not only increases sound intensity but also aids in distinguishing auditory direction, an important factor in spatial perception and communication. The outer auditory canal, with an average length of around 2.5 centimeters, serves as a conduit for sound, allowing it to be conveyed to the tympanic membrane. These outer ear design elements highlight the intricacy of hearing and demonstrate how it is a key component of the body's sound system. Inside the external auditory canal is a specialized environment that plays an important role in ear health and hearing function. The canal is lined with skin containing ceruminous and sebaceous glands, which produce earwax, or cerumen. The waxy substance provides protection by trapping dust, debris, and pathogens, preventing them from invading the more delicate middle and inner ear structures. The canal's minimal curvature also facilitates the transmission of sound in addition to safeguarding the tympanic membrane from direct harm. Significantly, the outer ear serves not only as a sound collector but also as a filter that changes the acoustic quality of the hearing system, increasing certain frequency components and attenuating others. This activity illustrates the complexity of the interaction between physiological function and anatomical structure in hearing. Examination of various ear structures, such as the outer ear, is significant for understanding auditory diseases and therapeutic methods. For instance, anatomical and physiological studies of the ears provide critical data on disorders such as outer ear infections and the impact of structural defects on hearing.

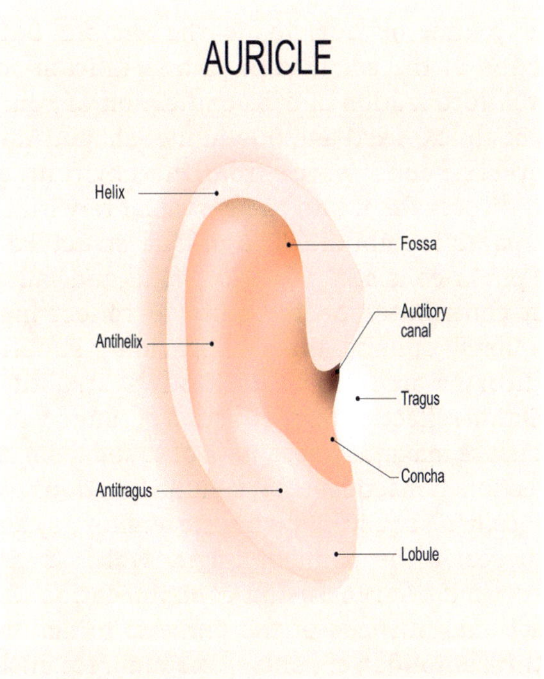

Figure 2.2. Anatomy of the outer ear.

Source: https://www.verywellhealth.com/thmb/lQOZkaj2fMXLdLRWy2v1IiXzZQk=/1500x0/filters:no_upscale():max_bytes(150000):strip_icc()/GettyImages-1071689464-a1bbf7541f9f41f1bd42c99f91f3d03b.jpg.

The function of the outer ears in hearing can also be analyzed using specific models, such as those relating to auditory neurons and their tuning properties, as reported in insect research. These comparative analyses demonstrate how anatomical features across species can shed light on human auditory function. As research into these dimensions continues, advances in our understanding of the ear's anatomy—particularly the external ear—will not only deepen our understanding of hearing but also aid in compensating for various types of hearing impairment and enhancing measures of auditory health (Figure 2.2).

2.1.1. Structure and Function of the Pinna

The pinna, or auricle, is the visible outer portion of the ear that plays a significant role in the localization and magnification of sound. Its complex, cartilaginous funnel-shaped form captures sound waves from the environment and directs them into the ear canal toward the tympanic membrane. The unique structure of the pinna, consisting of various folds and valleys, that contributes to its ability to collect high-frequency sounds, thereby providing superior auditory perception. The body's structures facilitate reflection and refraction of sound waves to ensure maximum reception of sound from any direction. Consequently, the pinna functions well in localizing sound, allowing the auditory system to perceive the point of origin, which is vital for spatial awareness and communication. One functional purpose of the pinna is to act as a natural amplifier, enhancing certain frequencies through its anatomy. Resonance from the shape of the outer ears will amplify sounds within the range of frequencies vital for human perception, between 1,000 and 4,000 Hz. This amplification is required for speech and environmental sound perception, as numerous studies indicate a relationship between the pinna's shape and auditory acuity. The interaction between the pinna and the auditory canal influences the quality and clarity of sounds reaching the inner ear. In addition, its intricate relationship with the surrounding musculature allows minor modifications when auditory stimuli are received, attesting to the auricle's dynamic capacity to respond to changes in environmental sound. Aside from its role in hearing, the pinna also provides overall protection and helps maintain ear health. By deflecting sound waves into the inner ear, it prevents foreign particles and dirt from entering the ear canal and thereby safeguards the delicate middle and inner ear structures. The pinna is also highly vascular and therefore has the potential to respond rapidly to changes in temperature or infection, and these two parameters can impair hearing function. In addition, studies have shown that there are some pathologies that can influence the shape and function of the pinna and hence impact the ability to perceive sound as well as their ability to localize sound. As shown in cochlear mechanical studies, optimizing these ear-structure interactions, including the function of the pinna, could benefit understanding of hearing function and related disorders (Cooper et al., 2018; N/A, 2018) (Figure 2.3).

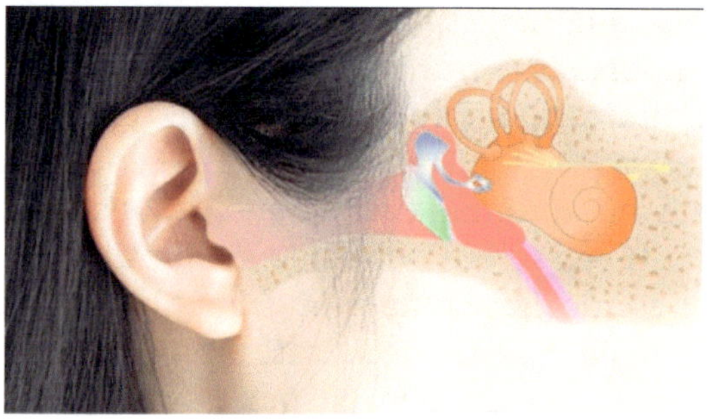

Figure 2.3. Structure and function of the pinna.

Source: https://www.shutterstock.com/image-photo/human-ear-anatomy-outer-middle-260nw-2244675129.jpg.

2.1.2. The Auditory Canal and Its Role

The auditory canal, or the external auditory meatus, is a critical pathway for introducing sound waves into the ear. Approximately 2.5

centimeters in length, the canal is covered with skin that contains ceruminous glands and hair follicles. The hair follicles ensnare dust and foreign particles, while the wax produced by the ceruminous gland, known as cerumen, is a natural barrier to the invasion of bacteria and additional debris. This placement is in the best-suited environment for sound transmission, highlighting the canals' protective nature and their function in processing sound. Therefore, not only is the auditory canal necessary for the transmission of sound directly, but also for the well-being of the ear based on its physiological and anatomical characteristics. In addition to transmitting sound and protecting the ear, the auditory canal plays a vital role in amplifying sound. The auditory canal vibrates sound at a particular frequency, thus enhancing the perception of particular auditory stimuli. This is particularly true in human speech perception, where the communication frequency range overlaps heavily with the canal's natural resonances. Research indicates that the shape and length of the canal can affect these resonant features and, consequently, auditory sensitivity. Comprehending this function can lead to significant advances in hearing aids and auditory prosthetics, underscoring the importance of understanding the anatomy of the auditory canals and their physiological role. This intricate function underscores the canal's importance within the auditory system and its contribution to successful auditory perception. The auditory canal is an adaptive structure that undergoes various changes in response to external influences. Cerumen production, and hence the acoustic impedance of the canals, may be affected by changes in temperature and humidity. Excess cerumen, for example, may cause occlusion and hence resulting defects in hearing. The health of the auditory canal, therefore, plays an important role in the total perception of sound and audiological health. The integration of proper care, including regular check-ups from medical professionals, becomes important in keeping the canals' integrity for maximum auditory performance. Continued research into the function of the auditory canal examines its complex relationship with the external environment and the internal ear tissues, as documented in extensive studies of ear anatomy. The significance of the auditory canal to auditory physiology cannot be overstated, as it not only serves functional but also protective roles in the auditory system (Figure 2.4).

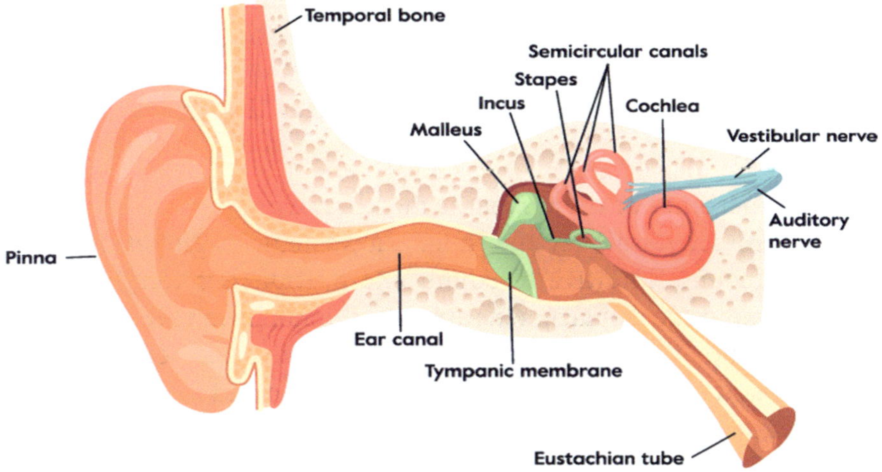

Figure 2.4. The auditory canal and its role.

Source: https://www.amplifonusa.com/content/dam/ahhc/content-factory/misc--health-images/Ear%20Anatomy-01.png/jcr:content/renditions/cq5dam.web.1280.1280.png.

2.1.3. The Tympanic Membrane (Eardrum)

The eardrum, or tympanic membrane, is a critical barrier to the external world and the middle ear and a key component of the auditory system. This thin, cone-shaped membrane vibrates upon exposure to sound waves and thereby converts acoustic energy into mechanical energy. Its composition is anatomically divided into three layers: the outer epithelial, the middle fibrous, and the inner mucosal layer. The compliance provided by these layers allows the tympanic membrane to respond effectively to changes in sound frequency, ultimately transmitting vibrations to the ossicular chain in the middle ear. Of particular significance is its ability to adjust to varying sound pressure, which allows sound conduction to be optimal without compromising the integrity of the inner ear, which can lead to hearing loss or auditory deficiency.

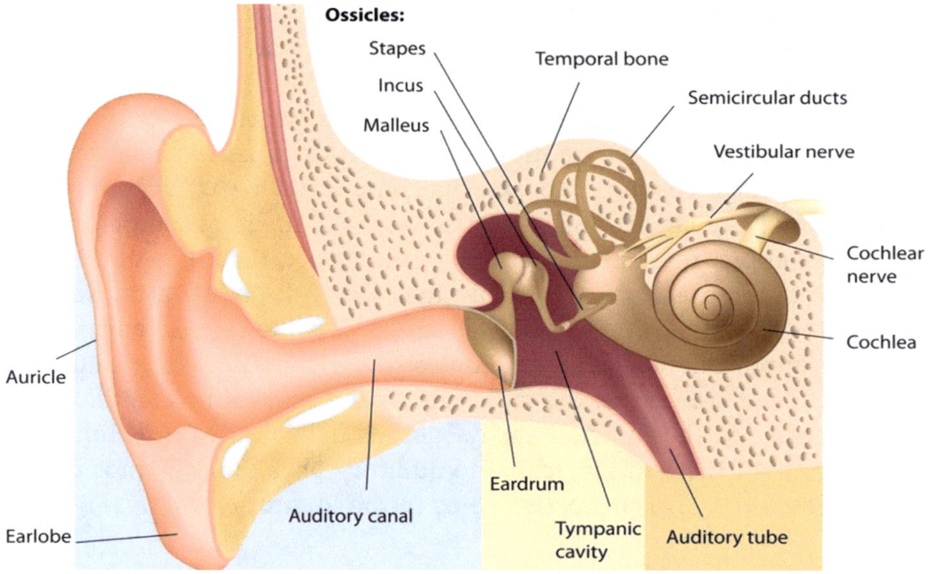

Figure 2.5. The tympanic membrane (eardrum).

Source: https://entkidsadults.com/wp-content/uploads/2013/10/ear-anatomy-.-copy1-1024x629.jpg.

The physiological importance of the tympanic membrane goes beyond the mere conduction of sound; it also serves a protective role for the inner ear structures. The elasticity of the eardrums may at first seem to be counterintuitive to sound energy transmission; however, it serves as a protection against high-amplitude displacement and destruction from severe sound stimuli. Both the ossicular chain and the tympanic membrane are greatly resilient, as demonstrated by Baird et al. (2012), and this is important in both the preservation of hearing and in shielding the sensitive inner ear from damaging vibrations. The tympanic membrane can also withstand and dissipate excessive acoustic energy, thereby acting as a resonator that amplifies sound across various frequencies. Thus, its structural integrity is vital to its proper sound function. Additionally, the anatomy of the tympanic membrane plays an important role in clinical practice, particularly in the diagnosis and treatment of ear pathology. Otitis media, for instance, can cause fluid buildup in the middle ear, preventing the eardrums from vibrating properly. It is very important to understand the mechanical characteristics of the tympanic membrane to develop effective interventions, such as surgery to treat tympanic membrane perforation or tympanostomy tube insertion. More recent studies suggest the need for improved prosthesis design that incorporates flexible components to mimic the physiological function of the natural tympanic membrane, as highlighted by investigations into the effects of ossicular joint dysfunction on hearing. To this end, the tympanic membrane emerges not just as a passive structure of the ear apparatus, but as a pivotal component that contributes to roles in the perception of sound, as well as ear health at large, reflective of its importance in anatomy within the greater physiological framework of the ear (Mason, 2015) (Figure 2.5).

Test Your Knowledge

1. List and describe the main anatomical parts of the outer ear, including the auricle (pinna) and the external auditory canal, and explain their roles in sound conduction and protection of the middle ear.
2. Describe the structural features, blood supply, and nerve supply of the outer ear and discuss their clinical importance in conditions such as otitis externa and trauma.

2.2. Anatomy of the Middle Ear

Learning Outcome

1. The Ossicles: Malleus, Incus, and Stapes
2. The Eustachian Tube and Its Function
3. The Role of the Middle Ear in Sound Amplification

Middle ear anatomy is crucial to the ear's functioning, and it is the transitional area that is required between the outer and inner ear. The middle ear includes the tympanic membrane and ossicular chain and is responsible for the amplification of sound waves and transmission to the cochlea. The eardrum, or tympanic membrane, oscillates when sound waves travel through and generates the mechanical process of hearing. This oscillation is carried over to three small bones known as the ossicles—the malleus, incus, and stapes—whose function is to amplify the sound further. Their arrangement allows efficient energy transmission while preventing excessive sound pressure, thereby maintaining delicate structures in the inner ear intact—a function especially important in preventing hearing loss from acoustic trauma. Perhaps the most fascinating feature of middle ear anatomy is the variation observed among species, which may have some effect upon hearing sensitivity. Comparative ear anatomy of the middle and inner ear structures reveals that, while most mammals share a similar configuration, minute anatomical differences can significantly affect hearing. A case in point is research on red fox *Vulpes* that demonstrates how its middle ear is quite similar to that of domestic dogs but possesses some distinguishing features, such as the absence of a fully developed bony septum in the bulla tympanica. This indicates how adaptive evolution affects ear structure and function across species, an adaptive requirement in different environments. Furthermore, studies show anatomical features such as the ossicular mass and bulla volume increase with age and may shape auditory capacity over a lifetime, thus highlighting the dynamic feature of the middle ear's anatomy (Burda et al., 2020). The physiological influence of the middle ear anatomy is not just mere sound conduction; there is a delicate interaction affecting overall hearing efficiency. Middle ear structure compliance, particularly the ossicular chain, allows for a delicate response to sound stimulation while, at the same time, providing some degree of protection against inrushing sound pressure. Research indicates that this flexibility may improve transmission in certain situations, making it a beneficial evolutionary trait. Dysfunction of the interossicular joints can, however, cause various pathologies of the auditory system, which warrants clinical consideration when planning prosthetic devices. Developments involving flexible components in prostheses aim to replicate natural flexibility and, therefore, improve auditory rehabilitation outcomes. The intricate interplay between middle-ear anatomy and physiology is essential for understanding hearing health and informing medical interventions in otology (Baird et al., 2012) (Figure 2.6).

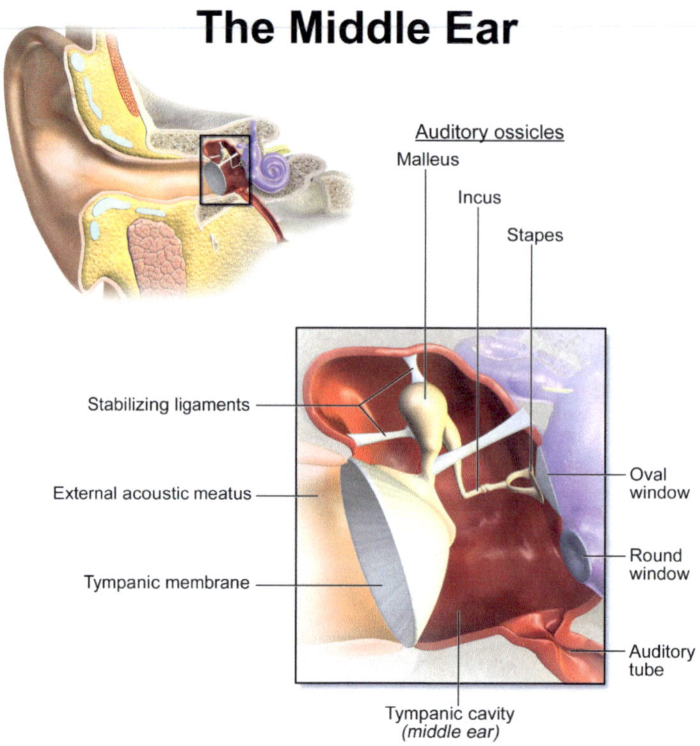

Figure 2.6. The anatomy of the middle ear plays a crucial role in the auditory function.

Source: https://upload.wikimedia.org/wikipedia/commons/8/81/Blausen_0330_EarAnatomy_MiddleEar.png.

2.2.1. The Ossicles: Malleus, Incus, and Stapes

Ossicles, which consist of the malleus, incus, and stapes, have very important functions within the hearing system by aiding sound conduction from the external ear to the internal ear. The tiny bones function in a lever-like manner by amplifying sound waves entering the ear canal. The malleus is the largest of the three bones and is fixed on the tympanic membrane (eardrum), where sound waves first hit. The incus, found in between the malleus and the stapes, assists in energy transfer of vibrational form, whereas the smallest bone within the human skeleton, the stapes, comes into contact with the oval window of the cochlea. Such hearing perception. One of the attractive qualities of ossicles is their flexibility in anatomy, which has a considerable impact on the protection and conduction of sound. It has been established in research that the series of conduction structures of the middle ear demonstrates an amount of flexibility that facilitates adaptive adjustment to different frequencies and amplitudes of sound. Even though flexibility seems to reduce the efficiency of sound transmission, it can help protect against excessive sound pressure that would otherwise damage the inner ear structures. In this respect, the ossicles not only transmit sound but also protect against potentially destructive acoustic stimulation, once again highlighting their dual role in auditory physiology (Baird et al., 2012).

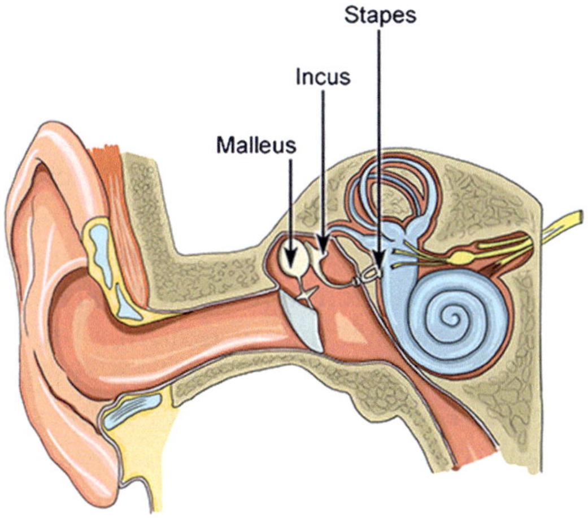

Figure 2.7. The ossicles: malleus, incus, and stapes.

Source: https://mammothmemory.net/images/user/base/uncategorised/1.32.59%20Diagram%20of%20the%20ear.jpg.

The dynamic balance between flexibility and rigidity of the ossicular chain is crucial for sustaining hearing integrity across varied sound environments. Structural properties of ossicles, although minute, play important roles in hearing sensitivity and overall hearing health. The ossicles' mass and shape can vary across species and influence their hearing capacity. For instance, anatomical studies have shown that although the middle ear anatomy of animals such as red foxes, dogs, and cats is similar, differences in ossicle size can affect sound performance. The link between ossicular anatomy and hearing sensitivity, which helps appreciate how small changes in anatomy affect subtle differences in hearing across mammals (Burda et al., 2020), is key. Here, the ossicles illustrate how intricate anatomical structures play important roles in the physiological process of hearing and why they are central to evolutionary biology and clinical audiology (Figure 2.7).

2.2.2. The Eustachian Tube and Its Function

The eustachian tube plays a crucial role in maintaining the physiological balance of the middle ear by equalizing pressure between the external environment and the inner ear. This thin tube connects the nasopharynx with the middle ear in order to drain off the fluids and also to ventilate the tympanic cavity. Normal tube function is vital for healthy auditory function because it allows the sound waves to reach the inner ear without any interference. Tubal abnormality can cause a range of complications, such as otitis media, where there is fluid buildup in the middle ear, most often as a consequence of allergies or infection, leading to congestion and blockade of the tube. The relevance of knowledge about these mechanisms extends beyond the anatomical sphere, as they have significant implications for treatment and prevention in clinical settings (Wilson, 2016). are that obstruction of the Eustachian tube, caused by factors ranging from allergic responses to infection, can be fatal. It may be deactivated by obstruction, creating a negative pressure that might suck fluid into the middle ear space. This is particularly prevalent in children, whose Eustachian tubes are typically shorter and more horizontal, making them more susceptible to collapse. In fact, anatomical findings associated with Eustachian tube function have been correlated with the high incidence of otitis media in children (Wilson,

2016). An understanding of these anatomical correlations allows for specific therapy. For instance, recent studies have explored the therapeutic role of H3 receptor blockade in alleviating middle ear congestion and hence improving Eustachian tube function, positing that drug treatments offer novel opportunities for management (Wilson, 2016). Understanding the dynamic interaction between anatomy, physiology, and surgical technique is the key to future advancements in ear health and improved quality of life in patients.

2.2.3. The Role of the Middle Ear in Sound Amplification

The middle ear is also a critical interface between the external auditory environment and the inner ear and amplifies sound through its unique anatomical structures. Three small bones referred to as ossicles—malleus, incus, and stapes—are located in this region, which function on a lever system to magnify the vibrations of the sound. When the sound waves hit the eardrum, or tympanic membrane, it oscillates. These vibrations are passed on to the ossicles, which amplify the sound energy before passing it on to the oval window of the cochlea. Through effective pressure increase in airborne sound waves, the middle ear guarantees that such vibrations are effectively transduced into fluid motions in the inner ear, which is essential in the process of transducing sound waves into neural signals necessary for the sense of hearing. The degree of effectiveness of sound amplification through the middle ear depends on several factors, including the flexibility of the osseous chain. It is noted that while stiffness in the ossicular system would appear to be better in the transduction of sound, flexibility can also be a beneficial factor in some conditions. For instance, the connections between the ossicles provide for restricted movement among the bones, which can help with the accommodation of various sound frequencies and defense against excessive sound wave intensity. Moreover, the same flexibility is essential for protecting the inner ear against potentially uncomfortable or injurious high-amplitude displacements, thereby illustrating an adaptive mechanism that reconciles the functions of amplification and protection. Therefore, the middle ear is an advanced adaptation that enables the complex processing of mammalian sounds (Baird et al., 2012). In addition to its amplification mechanism, the middle ear is crucial for pressure equalization between the external and internal ear, which supports overall auditory health. The Eustachian tube connects the middle ear to the nasopharynx, utilized for pressure equilibrium on both sides of the tympanic membrane. Pressure equilibrium is necessary to maximize the ossicular vibration efficiency and, consequently, the efficient transmission of sound. The Eustachian tube's role in middle ear function also influences hearing and the risk of diseases that may lead to auditory impairments, such as infections or blockages. Ultimately, the middle ear's intricate composition—involved with amplification by the ossicular chain and pressure regulation via the Eustachian tube—underscores its non-replaceable character in ear structure and function (Montealegre-Z, F., & Robert, D, 2014).

Test Your Knowledge

1. Describe the anatomy of the middle ear, including the tympanic cavity, auditory ossicles, and their articulations. Explain their role in sound transmission.
2. Explain the boundaries (walls), blood supply, and nerve supply of the middle ear. Discuss their clinical significance in conditions such as otitis media and during ear surgery.

2.3. Anatomy of the Inner Ear

Learning Outcome

1. The Cochlea and Its Structure
2. The Vestibular System and Balance
3. The Auditory Nerve and Signal Transmission

The inner ear, an essential component of the hearing mechanism, is designed to mediate hearing and balance. It consists of two important structures: the cochlea and the vestibular system. The cochlea, a spiral-shaped organ, transforms the sound waves into electrical impulses so that the brain may decode sounds. Within the cochlea, sensory hair cells are stimulated by fluid motion induced by sound vibration, which ultimately leads to neural impulses being transmitted to the auditory cortex. The vestibular system, comprising the semicircular canals and otolith organs, also plays a significant role in balance by detecting head position and changes in movement. This interaction of structures illustrates the complexity of inner-ear anatomy and reveals its dual function in hearing and vestibular processing.

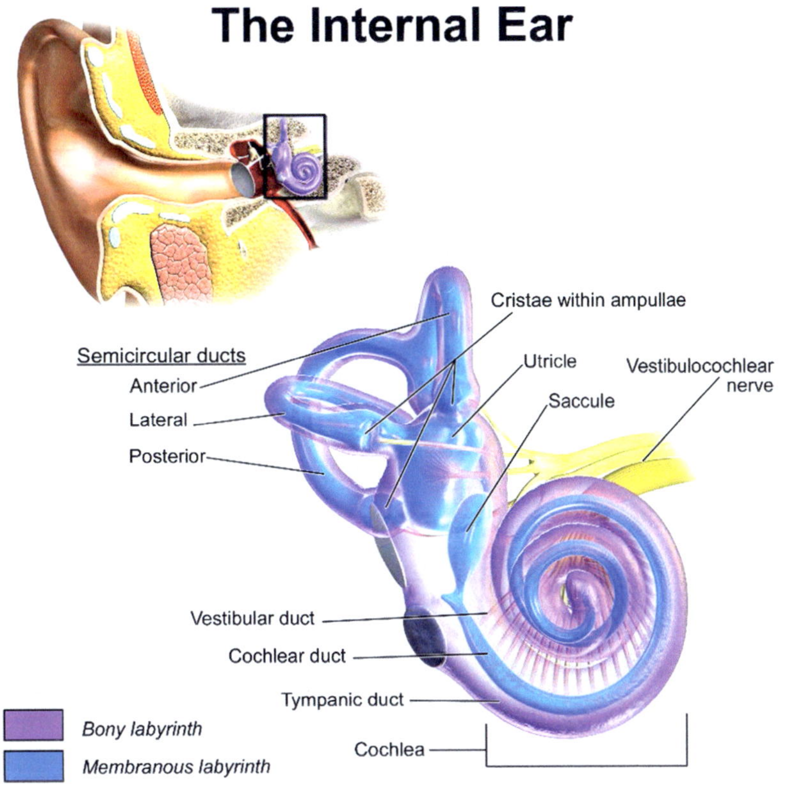

Figure 2.8. Anatomy of the inner ear.

Source: https://upload.wikimedia.org/wikipedia/commons/1/14/Blausen_0329_EarAnatomy_InternalEar.png.

Because of the significance of the internal ear's architecture, the advancement of medical technology has been met with further understanding and practice with respect to its anatomy. One notable development is the creation of realistic anatomical models from patient CT scans, employed for educational purposes by medical trainees. For example, the fabrication of a multi-material model of the ear canal allows surgeons and students to handle a tactile replica of inner ear structures, enhancing understanding of their anatomical correlations and physiological behaviors (Ali et al., 2017). These models provide pre-surgical training in a highly useful manner, particularly for procedures involving common conditions such as otitis media with effusion.

This exposure to teaching techniques not only hones surgical skill but also fosters a close appreciation for the subtleties of the inner ear. With the development of surgical techniques, particularly the increasing popularity of endoscopic ear surgery (EES), our understanding of inner-ear anatomy is expanding. EES facilitates less invasive treatment of ear disease without compromising essential anatomical structures. The use of endoscopes has not only improved visibility of the middle ear but also led to greater awareness of the complex anatomy of the inner ear (Marchioni et al., 2014).

This has also led to the identification of new anatomical landmarks and to the development of optimal treatment methods. Besides, ongoing practice and research with endoscopic techniques point toward the shift towards more accurate surgical procedures, highlighting the importance of extensive knowledge about the inner ear's structure and function. These advances underscore the need for ongoing education and new surgical training protocols to deliver optimal patient outcomes and to further research on ear physiology (Figure 2.8).

2.3.1. The Cochlea and Its Structure

The cochlea is a spiral, fluid-filled structure within the inner ear and is the focal point of the auditory system. The cochlea contains three large chambers: the scala vestibuli, the scala media, and the scala tympani, which are filled with endolymph and perilymph fluids. Scala media, often simply referred to as the cochlear duct, houses the organ of Corti, the sound-transducing sensory organ. This unique institution facilitates the conversion of sound waves into mechanical vibrations transmitted through the fluid, ultimately stimulating the hair cells lining the organ of Corti. When traveling through the cochlea, sound vibrations generate a traveling wave on the basilar membrane, whose amplitude varies with sound frequency. This intricate design underscores the cochlea's prominence in hearing, highlighting its complexity and the sophisticated mechanisms that enable hearing. General anatomical similarities among various mammals identify the structure of the cochlea's involvement in anticipating sensitivities in hearing among species. Research into the red fox cochlea, for example, has similarities with domestic dogs and cats, implying that these differences will have minimal effect on general auditory function. Of special interest is that middle ear morphology in such canids is unexpectedly conserved, though differing at specific cochlear structures. In particular, increasing age adds mass to the middle ear ossicles and bulla in red foxes, potentially expressing developmental compensation. These findings contradict the notion that large differences in hearing ability arise from small variations in anatomy and suggest that, although structure and function tend to be related, interactions among cochlear components remain complex and strongly influenced by evolutionary events (Burda et al., 2020). Intercellular communication within the cochlea also plays a significant role in cochlear function, particularly through connexins such as connexin 26 (Cx26) and connexin 30 (Cx30). These proteins assemble gap junction channels through which cochlear cells communicate, a feature crucial for ensuring the proper functioning of hair cells. The action of opening these channels allows the diffusion of calcium ions, a necessity in signaling pathways that guarantee cochlear homeostasis. Research establishes that G-protein coupled receptors are stimulated by the released ATP from supporting cells, generating calcium signals that propagate in the cochlear tissues. This cascading mechanism is important, especially in the postnatal formation of hearing, illustrating how impaired gap junction coupling can lead to hearing loss. Therefore, exploring connexin gene therapy emerges as a treatment strategy for auditory disease, emphasizing the interconnection between cochlear anatomy, cell communication, and hearing function (Hernandez et al., 2013) (Figure 2.9).

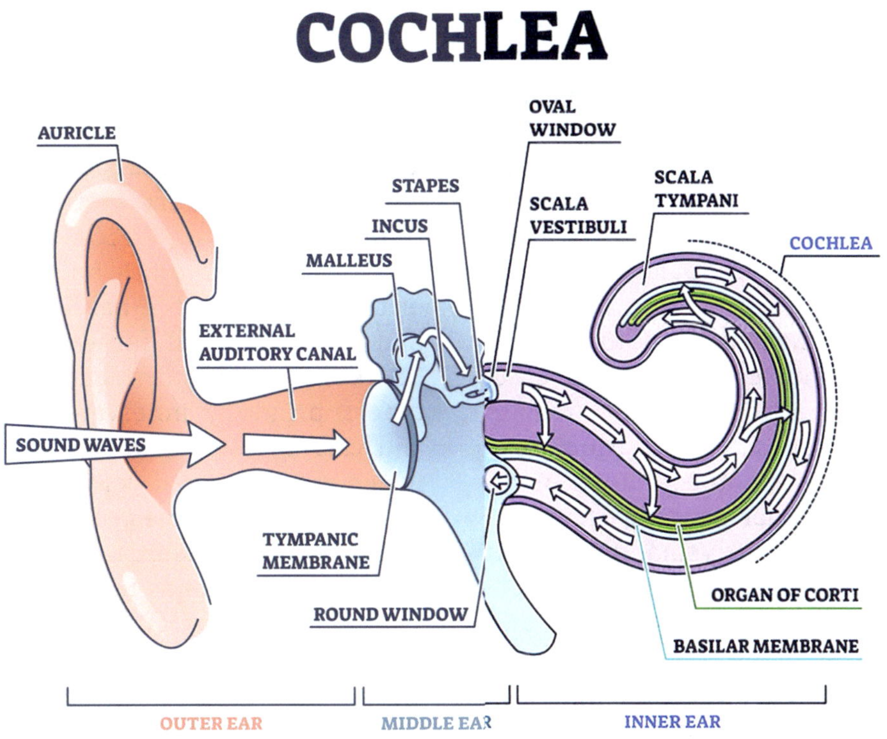

Figure 2.9. The cochlea is a spiral-shaped, fluid-filled structure located within the inner ear.

Source: https://media.istockphoto.com/id/1327025693/vector/cochlea-ear-anatomical-structure-with-organ-parts-description-outline-diagram.jpg?s=612x612&w=0&k=20&c=6EYvQrWDBqYxuZlOxET67lm8K1hKnogcY2qn9L1xM_g=.

2.3.2. The Vestibular System and Balance

The vestibular apparatus, as an aspect of ear anatomy and physiology, is responsible for maintaining the individual upright and oriented in space. It exists primarily in the inner ear and consists of the semicircular canals, the utricle, and the saccule. The semicircular canals, located in three-dimensional planes, are filled with fluid and detect head rotation. When the head rotates, fluid in these canals shifts, bending hair cells that induce neural impulses sent to the brain. These signals are vital for maintaining a sense of balance, as they inform the central nervous system of the head's position and motion. This mechanism is vital to daily life, from simple movements such as walking to more complex physiological functions, thereby making us generally more stable and coordinated in dynamic settings. The utricle and saccule complement the function of the semicircular canals by detecting linear accelerations and the force of gravity. These organs contain sensory hair cells embedded in a gelatinous membrane that is heavily calcified with calcium carbonate crystals. When the head moves or tilts, displacement of the seated hair cells by the movement of the gelatinous matrix creates signals that convey the change in position. This is critical information for maintaining balance in the brain. It is only by way of concomitant signals from the utricle and saccule and those from the semicircular canals that one can possess a complete response to varying postural requirements. Hence, the vestibular system not only assists with balance but also facilitates proprioception, enabling individuals to navigate their environment with confidence and ease. Malfunction in the vestibular system results in severe balance issues and proprioceptive impairment that impacts the quality of an individual's life. Vestibular neuritis, Meniere's disease, and benign paroxysmal positional vertigo (BPPV) are examples in which inner-ear dysfunction leads to dizziness, vertigo, and instability. An understanding of the anatomy and physiology of the vestibular system is essential not only for its identification but also for the formulation of effective remedial interventions. Rehabilitation interventions, such as vestibular rehabilitation therapy, aim to reeducate the brain to process vestibular information accurately. Therefore, research on the vestibular system is vital to the broader context of ear anatomy and physiology, as it facilitates balance and movement in a dynamic environment (N/A).

2.3.3. The Auditory Nerve and Signal Transmission

The auditory nerve plays a significant role in transmitting sound signals from the inner ear to the brain. Once the sound waves are converted into mechanical vibrations within the cochlea's fluid-filled chambers, hair cells, which are along the organ of Corti, become activated. These mechanosensitive hair cells generate electrical impulses by converting mechanical energy into neural signaling. The nerve of hearing collects these impulses and transports them to the brain, as it were, translating physical sound waves into sound meaning. This intricate process of translation indicates the sensitivity and precision of the auditory system, enabling animals, including humans, to distinguish a wide range of frequencies and intensities, which are significant for communication and environmental experience, as seen in comparative auditory systems across species (Kampschulte et al., 2016). The activity of the auditory systems relies on the electric signal of the auditory nerve based on a coordinated pattern of neuronal pathways. Auditory nerve fibers are generally divided into two categories: type I, primarily innervating inner hair cells and carrying sound information, and type II, which are associated with outer hair cells and have regulatory roles. The structure of the auditory nerve ensures efficient transmission of information about intensity and frequency. This arrangement enables rapid processing, which is critical for sound identification in noisy environments. Various mechanisms have evolved across animals to enhance auditory sensitivity and involve differences in the auditory neural pathways. For example, while mammals employ cochlear amplification to enhance hearing signals, insects such as katydids have comparable mechanisms that enable effective signal transmission despite their distinct anatomy (Montealegre-Z, F., & Robert, D, 2014). It is through the operation of the auditory nerve and its signaling pathways that one comes to understand how hearing processing occurs within the brain. The auditory cortex interprets signals from the auditory nerve, integrates them with other sensory inputs, and synthesizes a cohesive perceptual experience. This involves complex neural networks that encode various sound qualities, such as pitch, loudness, and timbre. The ability of the brain to distinguish between discrete sources of sound also illustrates the complexity of hearing. Temporal processing and response patterns in the auditory nerve play an important role in activities such as sound localization and speech comprehension. The auditory nerve can lead to various types of hearing impairments if it gets disturbed, emphasizing the importance of unaltered signal transmission in daily life communication and interaction with the environment (Kampschulte et al., 2016) (Figure 2.10).

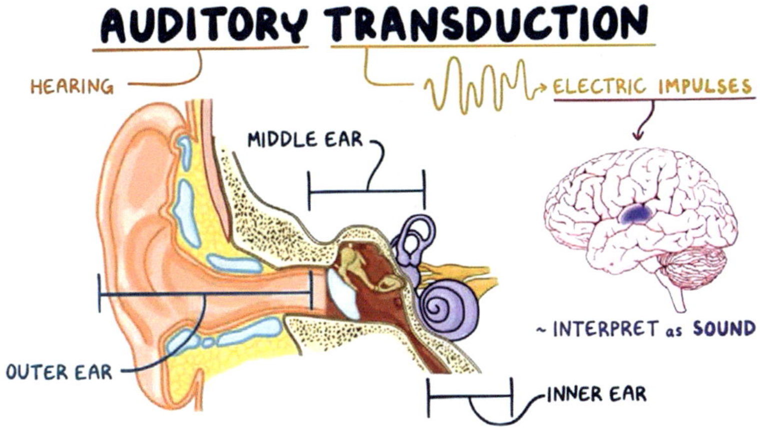

Figure 2.10. The auditory nerve and signal transmission.

Source: https://d16qt3wv6xm098.cloudfront.net/6do6_87kTrGlx1CiwWXXxNOVQBCJZHEQ/_.jpg.

Test Your Knowledge

1. Describe the anatomy of the inner ear, including the bony and membranous labyrinth, and explain the structure and function of the cochlea, vestibule, and semicircular canals.
2. Explain the nerve supply and blood supply of the inner ear and discuss their clinical importance in hearing loss and vestibular disorders.

2.4. Physiology of Hearing

Learning Outcome

1. Sound Wave Transmission Through the Ear
2. Mechanotransduction in Hair Cells
3. Neural Processing of Auditory Information

The hearing mechanism is a complex interplay of anatomical structures and physiological mechanisms that enable us to hear sound. The sound waves travel to the ear by entering the outer ear, traveling down the ear canal to the eardrum, or tympanic membrane. These vibrations are then passed on through the three little bones of the middle ear, incus, malleus, and stapes, which amplify the sound before it is allowed to pass into the cochlea, a spiral organ found in the inner ear. Within the cochlea, fluid movement is generated as vibrations from the sound move the basilar membrane, which leads to stimulation of hair cells found on the organ of Corti. This mechanical conversion converts sound waves into neural signals, which are subsequently relayed to the brain for interpretation and processing, thereby illustrating the role of anatomical structures in facilitating auditory function (Capra et al., 2023). Within the cochlea, mechanical energy is converted to electrical impulses by sensory hair cells. The stereocilia of hair cells are deflected by fluid motion induced by sound, thereby opening ion channels that allow calcium and potassium ions to enter. This leads to depolarization, generating action potentials that travel along auditory nerve fibers to the auditory cortex. Surprisingly, the process is not fixed; rather, it is highly responsive to sound intensity and frequency and represents a sophisticated system for frequency transduction from one location to another within the cochlea. In addition, the health and integrity of such hair cells are of utmost importance, as their damage can cause some degree of hearing impairment, underscoring the physiologic sophistication of the human hearing system (Steel, 2019). The physiology of hearing extends beyond the cochlea, with complex neural pathways that integrate hearing information. The signals of hearing are treated at several levels, including the brainstem and thalamus, before they get to the auditory cortex. At the center of this process is the capacity of the brain to distinguish and understand qualities of sound such as pitch, loudness, and direction. Moreover, genetics and the study of hearing have revealed the genetic basis of hearing, with numerous genes identified that contribute to auditory function and related disorders. Growing evidence suggests that multiple genes contribute to age-related or progressive hearing loss, indicating greater genetic complexity than previously recognized. The genetic factor is key to understanding multifaith hearing impairments, eventually resulting in improved diagnostic and treatment methods for subjects with hearing impairment (Capra et al., 2023) (Figure 2.11).

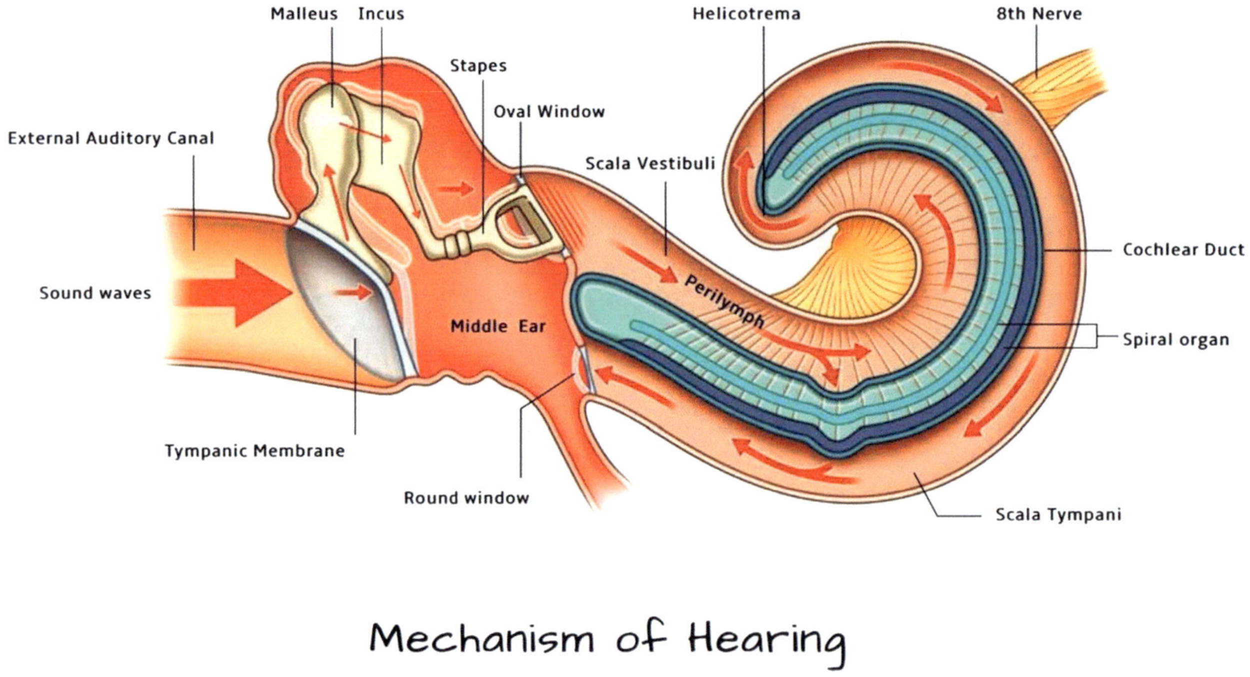

Figure 2.11. Physiology of hearing.

Source: https://www.entlecture.com/wp-content/uploads/2023/01/Dr-Rahul-Bagla-Mechanism-of-Hearing-2-2048x1319-1.jpg.

2.4.1. Sound Wave Transmission Through the Ear

Transmission of the sound wave to the ear is a complex process beginning in the outer ear, where sound waves are channeled through the auditory canal to the eardrum or tympanic membrane. When this membrane vibrates as a result of sound pressure waves, it converts acoustic energy into mechanical energy. The subsequent steps are those of the middle ear, which contains three tiny bones known as ossicles: malleus, incus, and stapes. They act as a system of levers, amplifying the vibrations of the eardrum and passing them on to the inner ear, the oval window. Here, mechanical vibrations are efficiently converted into sound waves in the fluid-filled cochlea, a critical transition point in hearing, thereby maximizing the transmission of sound energy from air to the liquid environment of the inner ear and facilitating effective perception. The cochlea is a sophisticated device that plays a central function in frequency analysis, a fundamental process of the transmission of sound waves. When the sound waves hit the cochlea, they create fluid motions that result in the basilar membrane vibrating. Certain frequencies activate specific locations along the membrane because the membrane is tonotopically organized. The most rapid frequencies shift the base of the cochlea, with slower frequencies shifting the apex. This spatial frequency sensitivity pattern enables the auditory system to decompose complex sounds into their component frequency components, allowing the brain to receive and interpret the signals appropriately. The mammals' complex cochlear mechanisms reflect evolutionarily advanced mechanisms that are significant for sound discrimination and localization, as documented in studies of various animal auditory systems (Montealegre-Z, F., & Robert, D., 2014). In addition to mammals, various other species have developed specialized hearing mechanisms adapted to their habitat requirements. For instance, certain insects possess a tympanate ear organ based on the tympanal membrane, unlike the mammalian system, yet it is functionally effective for hearing. Insects such as the sarcophagid fly possess a tympanic ear, which is ventrally placed and comprises a scolopidial sense organ and a tracheal air space connected to a larger tracheal system (Kampschulte et al., 2016). The adaptation enhances sensitivity to sound, particularly in vocal environments, representing an intriguing case of convergent evolution. The broad tuning and frequency-dependent sensitivity of such hearing systems illustrate the diversity of evolutionary strategies adopted by different taxa for the conduction of sound waves, ultimately illustrating the efficacy and complexity of auditory processing in all taxa.

2.4.2. Mechanotransduction in Hair Cells

Mechanotransduction in hair cells is the process responsible for hearing, converting mechanical stimuli into electrochemical signals. Hair cells are located within the cochlea and are overlaid with stereocilia that are sensitive to vibration caused by sound. When sound waves strike the ear, they cause fluid movement within the cochlea that results in the bending of stereocilia. This deflection opens ion channels, primarily allowing calcium and potassium ions to enter the hair cells, thereby causing depolarization. This process is significant because it establishes an electrical potential that is transmitted to auditory nerve fibers, ultimately relaying sound information to the brain. A genuine admiration for the intricate process illustrates how the neural network-like structure of the hair cell is specifically adapted for efficient signal transduction, thereby making the operation of mechanotransduction in hearing strictly essential. Intracellular signaling pathways in hair cells have been investigated in recent studies, focusing on the role of ATP in cochlear signaling. ATP from neighboring support and epithelial cells releases G-protein coupled receptors, which activate PLC-dependent signaling pathways. According to the research, citation of connexins (e.g., Cx26 and Cx30) forming gap junctions via which intercellular communication is realized through the diffusion of calcium-mobilizing second messengers like inositol trisphosphate (IP3) (Hernandez R et al., 2013). This signaling induces a regenerative spread of calcium signals via supporting cells, revealing that gap junction structure is essential to the cochlear environment in function. Mechanotransduction relies not only on the physical properties of hair cells but also on biochemical interactions between them, resulting in a complex interplay that enables robust sound perception.

The implications of such observations extend beyond the simple mechanics of hearing; they present possibilities for future therapeutic modalities for hearing loss. Gene delivery strategies, particularly with bovine adeno-associated viral vectors, have been shown to effectively restore connexin expression and enhance gap junction coupling of the cochlea. This new technique has been shown to directly increase mechanotransductive signaling in hair cells and is important for auditory function (Campioni et al., 2017). By manipulating connexin expression through targeted delivery of viral vectors, researchers are paving the way for the potential treatment of genetic deafness. This intersection of hearing physiology and molecular biology highlights the importance of advancing our knowledge of mechanotransduction mechanisms because it has the potential to give us new approaches for reversing hearing loss as well as improving auditory health.

2.4.3. Neural Processing of Auditory Information

Sound processing in the brain is a complex and vital process that begins in the inner ear and continues through the auditory cortex. As they enter the ear, the sound waves are changed into mechanical vibrations by the eardrum and transmitted through the ossicles to the cochlea. Within the cochlea, the motion of the fluid activates hair cells, and these convert the mechanical signals into electrical impulses. This transduction is essential to the interpretation of sound within the brain. The cochlear process is better at decomposing incoming sound waves into their spectral content and thereby measuring spectral quality, which is important for human and animal communication and survival, as evidenced by adaptive auditory processes across species such as katydids (Montealegre-Z, F., & Robert, D., 2014).

These skills highlight sophisticated evolutionary solutions to the problem of sound perception. The auditory nerve fibers perform the task of carrying these electrical impulses from the cochlea to the brainstem, where initial processing is done. Studies have shown that different fibers exhibit similar discharge responses to various acoustic stimuli. The precision of these patterns provides essential information about sound frequency and intensity, which is essential for sound discrimination and localization in hearing. For instance, studies of single-fiber discharge patterns in the cat auditory nerve illustrate the varied response patterns that enable fine hearing in loud environments (Clark et al., 2025). The signal from the auditory nerve is then passed to different areas of the brain, including the superior olivary complex and the inferior colliculus, which further process the auditory signal and integrate it with other sensory information. Ultimately, auditory processing ends in the auditory cortex, where the brain processes the nuances of sound. This processing in the brain enables individuals to listen to speech, distinguish musical tones, and appreciate ambient sounds. The auditory cortex comprises neurons that support auditory processing and memory, enhancing learning and adaptive behavior in response to sound stimuli. Moreover, the blending of auditory information with visual and spatial contexts occurs, enhancing overall sensory perception and environmental interaction. The intricate interaction among the cochlea, auditory pathways, and higher centers constitutes a highly sophisticated network essential for effective sound processing, underscoring the critical role of hearing in communication and mobility.

Test Your Knowledge

1. Describe the mechanism of hearing, starting from the entry of sound waves into the external ear up to the generation of nerve impulses in the cochlea.
2. Explain the role of the organ of Corti, basilar membrane, and hair cells in sound transduction and frequency discrimination.

2.5. Physiology of Balance

Learning Outcome

1. The Role of the Vestibular System in Equilibrium
2. Interaction Between the Inner Ear and the Brain
3. Common Disorders Affecting Balance

The physiology of balance is closely related to the anatomy and function of the inner ear, particularly in the vestibular system. The system consists of the semicircular canals, which are associated with the perception of rotational ; the otolith organs, which detect linear acceleration and position relative to gravity; and the otolith organs, which detect linear acceleration and position relative to motion. The integration of these structures enables the brain to be positioned and in balance, allowing one to perform ordinary functions such as walking and running. In addition, vestibular information is integrated with visual and proprioceptive information to create a consistent sense of body position in space. Dysfunction in any component of this complex system can result in balance disorders, emphasizing the importance of the ear's anatomy in enabling stable movement and locomotion. Research on the activity of the sympathetic nervous system offers balance physiology information, and particularly so through the lens of blood flow regulation. Significantly, sympathetic nerve activity influences circulation in peripheral and central regions of the body in response to cold, as shown by studies that used methods such as photoplethysmography to quantify changes in pulse transit time (PTT). During cold pressor tests, variations in PTT in the ear canal compared to the fingers demonstrated how varied sites respond to external stimuli (Ainslie et al., 2019). This shows that the vestibular system is not activated in isolation but is part of a larger physiological system that also controls vascular responses to maintain balance in a changing environment. Furthermore, integration of the balance mechanism is not restricted to the vestibular apparatus but involves intricate interactions among various brain regions, particularly the cerebellum and brainstem. These areas process information from the vestibular system, visual inputs, and proprioceptive feedback to coordinate muscle activity and maintain posture. The cerebellum, in particular, plays a significant role to fine-tune motor responses on the basis of sensory feedback in such a way that stability during movement is maintained. Experiments examining autonomic responses to environmental stressors, such as cold exposure, demonstrate the role of ear anatomy in these integrative processes (Ernst, C. H., & Ross, C. A., 1994). In the absence of optimal ear function and its connections with central nervous structures, subjects experience severe difficulty maintaining balance, underscoring the essential relationship between ear anatomy and balance physiology.

2.5.1. The Role of the Vestibular System in Equilibrium

The vestibular system is responsible for maintaining balance, enabling individuals to walk or navigate with stability and precision. Composed of interrelated inner-ear structures, primarily the semicircular canals and otolith organs, this system is particularly adapted to detect changes in head position and motion. The three semicircular canals in each ear are specifically designed to sense angular accelerations within different planes and therefore provide immediate feedback of rotation. These perceptions are transmitted via neural channels that coordinate muscular responses, enabling the body to respond accordingly. The impeccable coordination of these structures attests to the sophistication and efficiency of the vestibular apparatus in maintaining balance and spatial orientation, and thus to its significance in daily functioning, from the maintenance of posture to the execution of coordinated movement without conscious effort (Stewart et al., 2007). Other than the body structures, the operation of the vestibular system is supplemented by the intricate neural design. All the semicircular canals provide signals via an octahedrally symmetric neuronal network, whose integration is crucial for interpreting neck position and movement. With excitatory and inhibitory signals from the motoneurons linked to neck muscles, delicately controlled movements to balance are carried out. Experiments indicate that this organization is not merely mathematically elegant but also crucial for producing a large range of head movements in response to changes in orientation or applied force. By analyzing the outputs of these neuronal ensembles, researchers can infer how vestibular function accommodates difficulties of various types, thereby emphasizing its crucial role in human balance (Stewart I et al., 2007). the vestibular system can also significantly contribute to overall balance and stability. Pathological conditions such as Meniere's disease highlight the delicate balance preserved by the blood-labyrinthine barrier (BLB) of these organs. Observations of BLB cellular architecture in normal controls and subjects with vestibular disease yield pertinent insights into how microvascular changes can affect balance. In Meniere's disease, ultrastructural abnormalities in the vestibular end-organ can lead to impaired function and significant equilibrium difficulty. Recognition of such pathological changes underscores the importance of the vestibular system not only in the maintenance of balance but also in the preservation of robust auditory and vestibular function. From these studies, it is clear that the vestibular system is not merely an elementary component of the anatomy and physiology of the ear but also illustrates how sensory systems interact to achieve equilibrium (Figure 2.12).

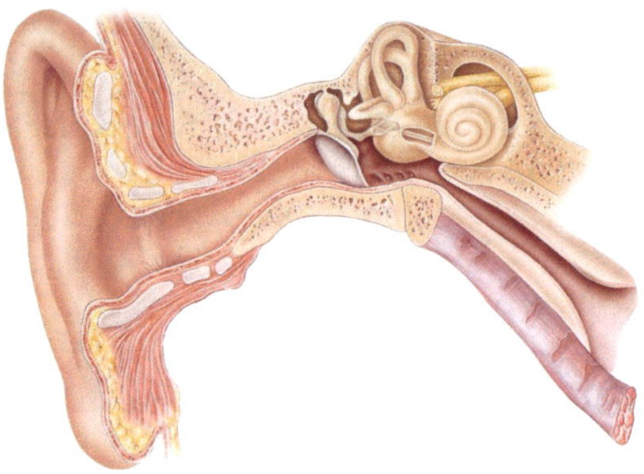

Figure 2.12. The role of the vestibular system in equilibrium.

Source: https://images.squarespace-cdn.com/content/v1/625e28e7e18f5966e5c14811/188164d3-dced-4cbb-8a66-5cc618e9e775/shutterstock_479354101+%28Custom%29.jpg.

2.5.2. Interaction Between the Inner Ear and the Brain

The intricate relationship between the brain and inner ear is key to appreciating auditory processing. The inner ear contains the cochlea that translates sound vibrations into neural impulses that are forwarded by the auditory pathway to the brain. The mechanism begins with sound waves passing through the ear canal, stimulating the tympanic membrane to vibrate. These vibrations are transmitted down through the ossicles to the cochlea, where they activate hair cells along the organ of Corti.

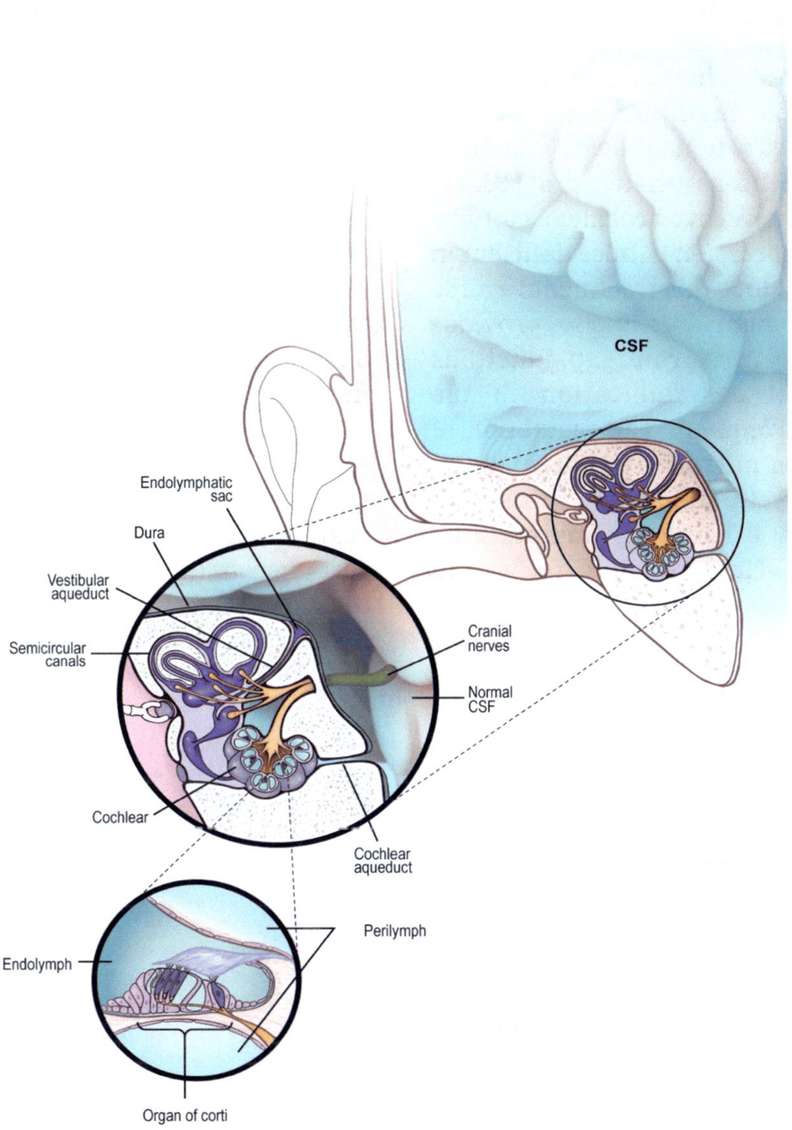

Figure 2.13. Interaction between the inner ear and the brain.

Source: https://pub.mdpi-res.com/brainsci/brainsci-14-00621/article_deploy/html/images/brainsci-14-00621-g001.png?1719219636.

The movement of these hair cells triggers electrical impulses, which are then transmitted through the auditory nerve to various regions of the brain to decode sound. Efficiency largely depends on the functional integrity of the cochlea and its underscoring the importance of neural communication in auditory physiology. Inner-ear and brain communication is again mediated by gap junctions, which facilitate cellular communication required for hearing. Recent studies have shown that connexin expression can be manipulated, thereby affecting the cochlea's function. For instance, the use of bovine adeno-associated viral (BAAV) vectors was found to recover cochlear culture-derived connexin expression in mice deficient in connexins. Not only does this treatment reverse the hearing impairment, but it also provides evidence for the central role gap junctions play in cell-to-cell communication in the cochlear microenvironment. The regulation of connexin expression mirrors how intercellular communication directly affects the mechanics of hearing and is critical for maintaining the tenuous equilibrium required for sound perception. Such findings underscore the need for further rigorous exploration of molecular interactions linking the inner ear to the central auditory pathways (Campioni et al., 2017). Moreover, the brain's capacity to process sound relies on feedforward and feedback pathways within the inner ear, indicating bidirectional interaction. This interaction ensures that not only auditory information is delivered to the brain, but also that the brain can modulate auditory processing according to contextual demands. Current research indicates that this interaction is impaired in patients with auditory processing disorders, reducing their ability to comprehend sound in noisy environments. The vulnerability of inner-ear structures to gene mutations—such as those affecting connexins—can further exacerbate these disorders. As such, an understanding of the relationships among the inner ear's physiology and the auditory cortex of the brain is vital for devising specific treatment options for hearing loss. These developments can lead to novel therapeutic approaches that restore hearing function by enhancing the resilience of inner ear structures or fine-tuning their coordination with the central nervous system (N/A) (Figure 2.13).

Test Your Knowledge

1. Explain the structure and function of the vestibular apparatus and describe how it helps maintain balance, posture, and spatial orientation.
2. Discuss the roles of the semicircular canals, utricle, and saccule in detecting angular and linear movements, and explain their contribution to equilibrium.

SUMMARY

The intricate anatomy and physiology of the ear exhibit a highly developed design that underscores the significance of these structures in sound processing. The ear is not only a sound-transmission device but also plays critical roles in balance and spatial orientation. Understanding of the different components, such as the outer, middle, and inner ear, is observed in how they work in concert to convert sound waves into electrical impulses perceived by the brain as sound. This cohesion indicates the importance of healthy ears since any malfunction in this system leads to impaired hearing or balance, underlining the ears' precise yet efficient design. The comparative morphological examination of the ear among various species reveals both the common characteristics and unique adaptations that define their hearing capabilities.

Research, such as studies of red fox anatomy compared with domestic dogs and cats, indicates that minute variations can influence hearing sensitivity and frequency response. It is clear that evolutionary pressures shape the anatomical form of the ear to improve hearing in varying environmental conditions. The findings reveal that, while there are common patterns in the structure of the ear, considerable variability can affect auditory perception, indicating that small anatomical variations can be highly functionally significant (Burda et al., 2020). In addition, tympanic middle-ear development in vertebrates highlights the adaptive significance of mutable auditory systems. Middle ear mechanics and the interaction of the ossicles with articulations demonstrate a compromise between the transmission of sound and the protection of the inner ear against potential damage. Understanding these mechanisms is important for informing clinical approaches to ear pathology management, particularly for designing prosthetic devices that can replicate such flexible forms (Baird et al., 2012). Thus, the anatomy and physiology of the ear not only shed light on the evolutionary biology of hearing but also open avenues for new medical interventions aimed at restoring hearing function in individuals with such problems.

When studying the anatomy and physiology of the ear, it is essential to understand the intricate structures that contribute to hearing. The ear has three major parts: the outer ear, the middle ear, and the inner ear, each with crucial functions in sound transmission and hearing. The outer ear collects sound waves and funnels them down the sound canal, where they make the eardrum in the middle ear vibrate. This section contains ossicles, small bones that pass these vibrations on before they arrive at the fluid-filled inner ear. The shared processes of these structures reveal the delicate yet coordinated efforts required for effective hearing, laying the groundwork for normal hearing functions and for potential disorders arising from physiological disturbances. Within the inner ear, the cochlea is a spiral organ that transduces sound-induced mechanical vibrations into neural impulses. Inside the cochlea, these vibrations are detected by specialized hair cells with varying sensitivities to varying frequencies, which ultimately transfer impulses through the auditory nerve to the brain.

Recent developments in neuro-electronic devices, particularly cochlear implants, are highly applicable clinical endeavors based on this anatomical information. The implants directly interface with the auditory nerve and enable hearing-impaired patients to hear. A critique of all these technologies is not only performed for their medicative intentions but also explores the social environment in which they are applied, much like literature today handles both medicinal and non-medicinal use in Ward (2000). The nerve itself plays a role in the delivery of sound information to the brain in terms of unique patterns of discharge in response to specific acoustic stimuli. Studies indicate that knowledge of fiber discharge patterns of the auditory nerve is critical to designing effective auditory prosthetics and appliances. These studies, such as single-fiber responses in the cat's auditory nerve, provide insight into how auditory signals are decoded and processed by the brain (Clark et al., 2025). Therefore, a coherent synthesis of ear anatomy and physiology must account for both the biological background and the technologies developed from these discoveries. An integrated perspective enables appreciation of the mechanisms of hearing and underscores the importance of continued research in this rich field of inquiry.

KEY TERMS FROM THIS CHAPTER

- Auricle
- Tympanic Cavity
- Malleus
- Stapes
- Eustachian Tube
- Round Window
- Cochlea
- Semicircular Canals
- Membranous Labyrinth
- External Auditory Meatus
- Tympanic Membrane
- Incus
- Ossicular Chain
- Oval Window
- Cochlear Duct
- Vestibule
- Bony Labyrinth
- Endolymph

CRITICAL THINKING QUESTIONS

1. **The external ear consists of:**
   a) Cochlea and vestibule
   b) Pinna and external auditory canal
   c) Tympanic cavity and ossicles
   d) Semicircular canals
2. **The ear is divided into how many parts?**
   a) Two
   b) Three
   c) Four
   d) Five
3. **The tympanic membrane separates:**
   a) External ear and middle ear
   b) Middle ear and inner ear
   c) External ear and inner ear
   d) Nose and ear
4. **Which of the following is NOT an ossicle?**
   a) Malleus
   b) Incus
   c) Stapes
   d) Cochlea
5. **The smallest bone in the human body is:**
   a) Malleus
   b) Incus
   c) Stapes
   d) Hyoid

Short Answer Questions

1. What are the three main parts of the ear, and what are their primary functions?
2. Describe the anatomy of the external ear, including the auricle and external auditory canal.
3. Explain the structure and function of the tympanic membrane (eardrum).
4. Discuss the anatomy of the middle ear cavity and its contents.
5. Describe the structure of the inner ear, including the cochlea, vestibule, and semicircular canals.
6. Explain the mechanism of hearing, tracing the pathway of sound waves from the external ear to the auditory cortex.
7. What is the role of the Eustachian (auditory) tube in ear function?
8. Explain the mechanism of balance and equilibrium in relation to the vestibular system.

Answers to Critical Thinking Questions

1. (b) 2. (b) 3. (a) 4. (d) 5. (c)

REFERENCES

1. Budidha, K., & Kyriacou, P. A. (2019). Photoplethysmography for quantitative assessment of sympathetic nerve activity (SNA) during cold stress. *Frontiers in Physiology, 9*, 1863. https://doi.org/10.3389/fphys.2018.01863Ali, A., Hairston, R., Locks, H., & Hunter, A. (2017). *3D Printed Ear Canal Model*. https://core.ac.uk/download/215483359.pdf (accessed on 7th August 2025).
2. Allison, P. A., Andrews, C. A., Milner, A., Cunningham, S., Dechaseaux, C., Harrison, C. J. O., et al. (2011). *Halcyornis toliapicus (Aves: Lower Eocene, England) indicates advanced neuromorphology in Mesozoic Neornithes*. https://core.ac.uk/download/pdf/1569383.pdf (accessed on 7th August 2025).
3. Altissimi, G., Cianfrone, G., Ciofalo, A., Greco, A., et al. (2016). *When Alarm Bells Ring: Emergency Tinnitus*. https://core.ac.uk/download/54538689.pdf (accessed on 7th August 2025).
4. Américo, R. dos R., Barauna Filho, I. S., Hermann, D. R., Nogueira Júnior, J. F., et al. (2007). *A Brief History of Otorhinolaryngology: Otology, Laryngology, and Rhinology*. https://core.ac.uk/download/37707315.pdf (accessed on 7th August 2025).
5. Baird, R. A., Bell, D. A., Burda, H., Dahmann, H., Feenstra, J., Fleischer, R. C., Goode, R. L., et al. (2012). *Flexibility within the Middle Ears of Vertebrates*. https://core.ac.uk/download/17030984.pdf (accessed on 7th August 2025).
6. Burda, H., Malkemper, E., & Mason, M. (2020). *Functional anatomy of the middle and inner ears of the red fox, in comparison to domestic dogs and cats*.
7. Campioni, M., Chiorini, J. A., Crispino, G., Di Pasquale, G., et al. (2017). *In vivo genetic manipulation of inner ear connexin expression by bovine adeno-associated viral vectors*. https://core.ac.uk/download/129592405.pdf (accessed on 7th August 2025).
8. Capra, D. R., DosSantos, M., Sanz, C., Gall Acosta Filha, L., Nunes, P., Heringer, M., Ximenes-da-Silva, A., et al. (2023). Pathophysiology and mechanisms of hearing impairment related to neonatal infection diseases. *Frontiers in Microbiology, 14*. https://www.semanticscholar.org/paper/b4a479a9680f204b0541cf2d05b537704a5c8838 (accessed on 7th August 2025).
9. Clark, L. F., Kiang, N. Y. S., & Takeshi, T. E. C. (2025). *Discharge Patterns of Single Fibers in the Cat's Auditory Nerve*. https://core.ac.uk/download/pdf/85249703.pdf (accessed on 7th August 2025).
10. Cooper, N. P., Vavakou, A., van der Heijden, M. (2018). Vibration hotspots reveal longitudinal funneling of sound-evoked motion in the mammalian cochlea. *Nature Communications, 9*. https://doi.org/10.1038/s41467-018-05483-z (accessed on 7th August 2025).
11. Eckert, S. A., Harms, C. A., Jones, T. T., Mann, D., et al. (2016). *Hearing in the juvenile green sea turtle (Chelonia mydas): A comparison of underwater and aerial hearing using auditory evoked potentials*. https://cupola.gettysburg.edu/cgi/viewcontent.cgi?article=1086&context=esfac (accessed on 7th August 2025).
12. Ernst, C. H., & Ross, C. A. (1994). *Alligator Mississippiensis*. https://core.ac.uk/download/211343484.pdf (accessed on 7th August 2025).
13. Foster, B. L. (2017). On the discovery of cementum. *Journal of Periodontal Research, 52*, 666–685. https://doi.org/10.1111/jre.12444 (accessed on 7th August 2025).

14. Ishiyama, A., Ishiyama, G., Ishiyama, P., Lopez, I., et al. (2017). *The blood-labyrinthine barrier in the human normal and Meniere's disease macula utricle*. https://core.ac.uk/download/323076450.pdf (accessed on 7th August 2025).

15. Jaafar, N. I. (2011). *Noise-Induced Hearing Loss Among Grass Trimming Workers*. https://core.ac.uk/download/141499431.pdf (accessed on 7th August 2025).

16. Kampschulte, M., Lakes-Harlan, R., Martels, G., Stumpner, A., et al. (2016). *The auditory system of the dipteran parasitoid Emblemasoma auditrix (Sarcophagidae)*. https://core.ac.uk/download/84117992.pdf (accessed on 7th August 2025).

17. Kumar, S., Ramamoorthy, M., & Thiagarajan, B. (2012). *Endoscopic Typmpanomastoid Exploration [Functional Endoscopic Ear Surgery–FEES]*. https://core.ac.uk/download/pdf/9634108.pdf (accessed on 7th August 2025).

18. Lee, J. (1999). *The utilization of transient evoked otoacoustic emissions and tympanometry in hearing screening of hearing-impaired children*. https://core.ac.uk/download/37885861.pdf (accessed on 7th August 2025).

19. Lucas, R., Mair, G., & Romice, O. (2008). *The Scale of Sense: Spatial Extent and Multimodal Urban Design*. https://core.ac.uk/download/9023652.pdf (accessed on 7th August 2025).

20. Lue, P.-Y., Oliver, M. H., Neeff, M., Thorne, P. R., Suzuki-Kerr, H. (2023). Sheep as a large animal model for hearing research: Comparison to common laboratory animals and humans. *Laboratory Animal Research, 39*. https://doi.org/10.1186/s42826-023-00182-3 (accessed on 7th August 2025).

21. Marchioni, D., Nogueira, J. F., Pothier, D. D., Presutti, L., et al. (2014). *Endoscopic Ear Surgery: Tips and Pearls*. https://core.ac.uk/download/217555463.pdf (accessed on 7th August 2025).

22. Mason, M. J. (2015). *Structure and Function of the Mammalian Middle Ear. II: INFERRING Function from Structure*. https://core.ac.uk/download/42338660.pdf (accessed on 7th August 2025).

23. Montealegre-Z, F., & Robert, D. (2014). *Biomechanics of Hearing in Katydids*. https://core.ac.uk/download/29176659.pdf (accessed on 7th August 2025).

24. N/A. (2025). *Aerospace medicine and biology: A continuing bibliography with indexes, supplement 130, July 1974*. https://core.ac.uk/download/pdf/42893215.pdf (accessed on 7th August 2025).

25. Pierpont, M. E., Brueckner, M., Chung, W. K., Garg, V., Lacro, R. V., McGuire, A. L., Mital, S., et al. (2018). Genetic basis for congenital heart disease revisited: A scientific statement from the American Heart Association. *Circulation, 138*. https://doi.org/10.1161/cir.0000000000000606 (accessed on 7th August 2025).

26. Quillin, K., & Thomas, S. (2015). Drawing-to-learn: A framework for using drawings to promote model-based reasoning in biology, *CBE—Life Sciences Education, 14*, es2–es2 https://doi.org/10.1187/cbe.14-08-0128 (accessed on 7th August 2025).

27. Rodriguez Hernandez, L. (2013). *Studies of intercellular Ca^{2+} signaling and gap-junction coupling in the developing cochlea of mouse models affected by congenital hearing loss*. https://core.ac.uk/download/17190110.pdf (accessed on 7th August 2025).

28. Steel, K. (2019). Lessons about hearing loss from mice. *The Hearing Journal*. https://www.semanticscholar.org/paper/afaf443e022ceaa4684cb9db63dff86f2b5b229a (accessed on 7th August 2025).

29. Stewart, I., Shiau, L., Golubitsky, M., Shinoda, Y., & Wilson, V. J. (2007). *Spatiotemporal symmetries in the disynaptic canal-neck projection*. https://core.ac.uk/download/49289.pdf (accessed on 7th August 2025).

30. Ward, J. A. (2000). *Neuro-Electronic Technology in Medicine and Beyond*. https://core.ac.uk/download/70097.pdf (accessed on 7th August 2025).

31. Wilson, J. D. (2016). *The Efficacy of Betahistine as Treatment for Eustachian Tube Dysfunction in an Allergic Rat Model*. https://open.bu.edu/bitstream/2144/16075/1/Wilson_bu_0017N_11091.pdf (accessed on 7th August 2025).

32. Zainun, Z. (2010). *Enhancing the Accuracy in Diagnosing Peripheral Vestibular Disorders*. https://core.ac.uk/download/132567102.pdf (accessed on 7th August 2025).

DISEASES OF THE EXTERNAL EAR

3

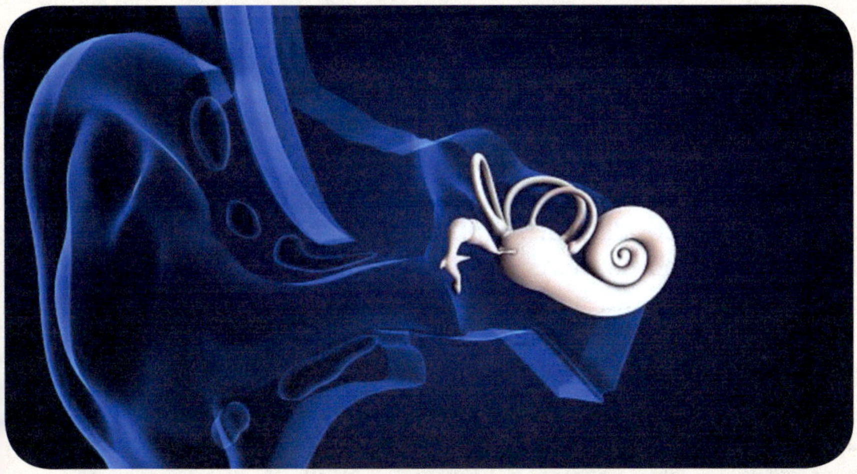

LEARNING OBJECTIVES

After studying this chapter, you will be able to:

1. Common diseases of the external ear.
2. Symptoms and diagnosis.
3. Treatment options.
4. Risk factors.
5. Prevention strategies.

Introduction

The outer ear, which consists of the auricle and external auditory canal, has a vital role to play in the ear system by capturing sound waves and channeling them to the inner and middle ear. The significance of identifying diseases affecting the outer ear cannot be overstated, as these conditions may cause pain, hearing loss, and even life-threatening complications if left untreated. A comprehensive overview of this topic must include the common disorders of the outer ear, such as otitis externa, cerumen impaction, and trauma. Because the outer ears are exposed to the external environment, including pathogens, allergens, and physical trauma, a deeper understanding of these diseases will enhance clinical diagnosis and prevention, ultimately improving outcomes for otology patients. With ongoing advances in medical technology, scientists have identified multiple etiological factors in external ear disease. For instance, microbial infection has been a leading cause of morbidity in conditions such as otitis externa, inflammation of the auricle or ear canal. The causative factors leading to increased susceptibility towards such infection are the occurrence of moisture, skin injury, and hypersecretion of earwax. Additionally, disorders such as craniofacial abnormalities can impair normal ear function and increase the risk of complications, including hearing impairment. By examining these associations, practitioners can establish a more apparent link between environmental extrinsic stimuli and the pathophysiology of external ear disease and thus ultimately guide targeted intervention and preventive strategies (Abita et al., 2019). In addition, it is important to assess the long-term impact of external ear diseases, above all, their impact on quality of life and emotional well-being. Affected patients may be ostracized due to embarrassment or pain, and the effects may extend to educational and occupational environments. The correlation between sensorineural impairment and psychosocial status underscores the importance of early diagnosis and management of external ear diseases. While medicine continues to seek to understand the underlying mechanisms of these illnesses, emerging research suggests that a multi-component approach, encompassing genetic, environmental, and developmental factors, may be the solution. This multi-approach strategy, taking into account areas such as craniofacial dysmorphology, may significantly contribute to understanding differences in the presentation of diseases of the external ear and to future therapeutic planning (Bowman et al., 2017).

Importance of Ear Health

The importance of ear health cannot be overemphasized, especially with reference to many diseases affecting the outer ear. An efficient auditory system plays an essential role in effective communication, socialization, and quality of life. Ear health is closely linked to academic success and career prospects. For instance, children with chronic ear disease, such as otitis media, will experience hearing loss that can impair their academic performance. The effects continue beyond childhood; if untreated, ear infections lead to long-term consequences such as increased unemployment and interactions with the criminal justice system later in life, particularly among historically marginalized groups. Therefore, prioritizing ear health can address these potential drawbacks, underscoring its importance not only for individual health but also for societal improvement (N/A). Understanding the root causes of ear diseases underscores the importance of preventive healthcare measures. Poverty, lack of good access to healthcare, and environmental issues are some of the underlying social determinants that support the prevalence of ear diseases, particularly among Indigenous populations. High rates of otitis media in these populations necessitate targeted interventions to address these causes. Although some interventions have attempted to address this, most have been unsuccessful due to insufficient planning and evidence-based practice, yielding little benefit. New health programs, such as the Stronger Futures policy in the Northern Territory, have shown promise in combating ear disease by significantly reducing the rates and severity of hearing loss. Ensuring adequate funding and support for such programs will be key to improving ear health outcomes among high-risk groups (Bell et al., 2017). Furthermore, routine follow-up and early intervention are essential for maintaining ear health, particularly among children and other high-risk groups. For example, monitoring ear temperature can be an effective tool for identifying infants predisposed to complications from underlying ear disease. Through the use of instruments like constant temperature probes, medical officers can diagnose fever and intervene promptly through certain treatments, which in the end prevent long-term conditions. Evidence in veterinary medicine research, though on calves, illustrates the significance of appropriate treatment techniques in time. It shows that treating with non-steroidal anti-inflammatory drugs (NSAIDs) alone can clear certain conditions without adverse effects, again emphasizing monitoring and effective intervention (Bell et al., 2017). Best practices in one area of work typically guide and optimize strategies for improving ear health across different populations (Figure 3.1).

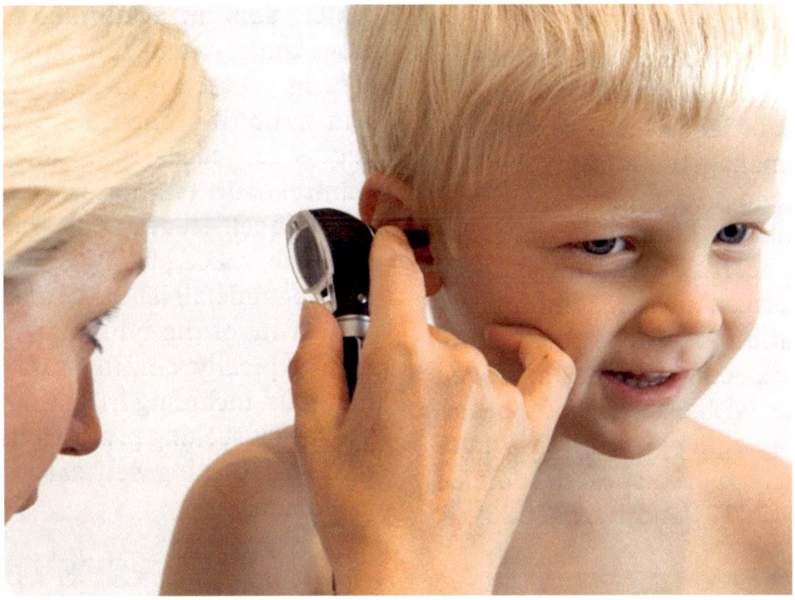

Figure 3.1. Ear examination of a child.

Source: https://external-content.duckduckgo.com/iu/?u=https%3A%2F%2Fwww.aljazeera.net%2Fwp-content%2Fuploads%2F2017%2F08%2F1bed4dbf-2dfe-4998-8b4d-3c13518a8743.jpeg&f=1&nofb=1&ipt=16fd9b45397e7d82697c7f7500e3f2fa1ff4e97ad3b6e57714448a1c398303c1.

Overview of Common Diseases Affecting the External Ear

The outer ear, comprising the auricle and the ear canal, is susceptible to a number of diseases that involve hearing and overall ear health. Otitis externa, or swimmers' ear, as it is popularly referred to, is a common condition of the outer ear. The infection involves inflammation of the ear canal caused by moisture accumulation, bacterial infection, or fungal infection. The most common symptoms are itching, redness, swelling, and discharge from the ear. The condition is prevalent in individuals who swim frequently and engage in other activities that involve exposing the ear to water. Prevention by keeping the ear dry and refraining from inserting foreign bodies is critical in reducing the incidence of otitis externa, highlighting the importance of ear hygiene and health awareness. A second frequent disease of the outer ear is cerumen impaction, or earwax occlusion. While cerumen has a protective function by keeping debris and bacteria out, overaccumulation may lead to a variety of symptoms from hearing loss to pain and even tinnitus. Impacted cerumen is due to prolonged use of earplugs or hearing aids, along with normal variations in earwax amount in people. Treatment is often professional ear cleaning, but some individuals attempt home remedies. However, improper technique can exacerbate the condition, as evidenced by the need for cautious, well-informed techniques in ear care. Successful removal of impacted cerumen can restore auditory function and alleviate distress, underscoring the benefits of regular ear health checks in clinical practice. A third common disease of the outer ear is dermatitis, an inflammatory cutaneous condition that may the ear canal. Dermatitis has multiple causes, ranging from metal allergy to jewelry to skin care cosmeceuticals and environmental allergens. Symptoms most commonly present as erythema, scaling, and pruritus, which may significantly impair quality of life and functioning. The intricate interaction between skin and external ear disease requires a multidisciplinary management approach that includes identifying and preventing irritants and allergens. Additionally, new studies examine the impact of systemic health alterations on skin disease, as characterized in recent literature. Therefore, information on the etiology and control of dermatitis can lead to improved outcomes for patients with external ear disease, particularly among an aging population, where skin sensitivity is likely to predispose, as posited by Majumder et al. (2017) and N/A (2018).

3.1 Common Diseases of the External Ear

Learning Outcome

1. Otitis Externa (Swimmer's Ear)
2. Earwax Impaction
3. Perichondritis

The outer ear, encompassing the auricle and the external ear canal, is prone to several recurring conditions, one of which is otitis externa, or swimmers' ear. Infection or inflammation of the ear canal is commonly associated with contact with water, which provides a conducive environment for bacterial and fungal growth. Redness, irritation, and discharge are symptoms that may provoke pain and hearing loss. Otitis externa most often can be treated by the application of topical corticosteroids and antibiotics to alleviate inflammation and eradicate infection. Further evaluation is warranted in severe or prolonged cases to rule out predisposed underlying conditions that predispose to chronic infection, necessitating a comprehensive treatment and preventive regimen. The second most prevalent issue of the external ear is cerumen impaction, in which earwax accumulates abnormally and clogs the ear canal. Cerumen plays an essential role in protecting the ear by entraping debris and inhibiting microbial growth; however, an excess can cause symptoms such as ear pain, tinnitus, and temporary hearing loss. Patients attempt self-treatment to remove the blockage; however, these attempts are more detrimental than beneficial, leading to adverse effects such as tearing of the tympanic membrane. Medical staff typically employ safe cerumen removal methods, including irrigation or aspiration, with a focus on seeking professional assistance rather than performing self-care to prevent further ear damage.

DISEASES OF THE EXTERNAL EAR

1. Boils

(furuncolosis or circumscribed otitis media)

Causes:

- Poor Hygiene
- Bacterial Infection

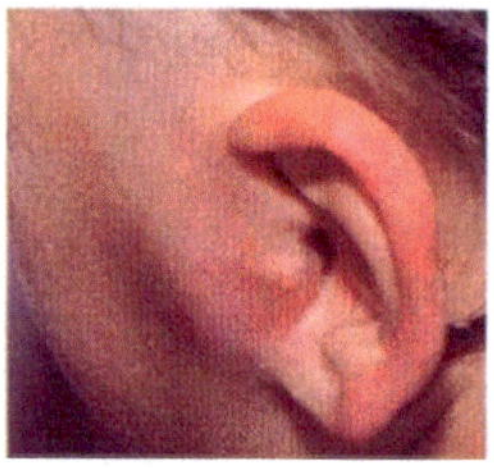

Figure 3.2. Common diseases of the external ear.

Source: https://external-content.duckduckgo.com/iu/?u=https%3A%2F%2Fimage.slidesharecdn.com%2Fsecondary20common20ear20diseases-110407105503-phpapp02%2F95%2Fcommon-ear-diseases-4-728.jpg%3Fcb%3D1333693874&f=1&nofb=1&ipt=3e6f64ae24fb0b4a6006fd5b462848808b7b8139362c14df5ef5abf09a703588.

Lastly, eczema and psoriasis may also manifest in the outer ear, causing inflammation and pain. These cutaneous conditions may be localized to the auricular skin and lining of the ear canal and present as scaling, redness, and itching. Psoriasis and eczema are both influenced by environmental and genetic factors and result in chronic skin conditions that require management. Treatment is primarily with topical corticosteroids and emollients to inhibit inflammation and hydrate the skin. It must be managed with care to prevent secondary infection from scratching or skin barrier compromise. Understanding the interaction between dermatological conditions and ear health is necessary, as it indicates that such individuals require comprehensive care strategies (Nola et al., 2017; Gall, L. S., & Riely, P. E., 2025) (Figure 3.2).

3.1.1. Otitis Externa (Swimmer's Ear)

Otitis externa, commonly referred to as swimmers' ear, is an infection of the external auditory canal that is primarily caused by contact with water, particularly swimming. It presents with a variety of symptoms, including ear pain, itching, and discharge, with or without odor. The etiology of acute otitis externa is typically mixed bacterial and fungal, necessitating confirmation of the infecting agent. University of Nigeria Teaching Hospital studies indicate that clinical diagnoses of otitis externa were confirmed by microbiological examinations, with most isolates from these conditions being bacterial (Ezeanolue et al., 2013). This information provides important insight into the microbiological background of this disease, underscoring the need for specific therapy against the responsible agents. The management of otitis externa in clinical practice usually involves topical antimicrobial agents, with analgesics used to relieve pain. The preferred treatment is largely determined by the etiologic agents, given evidence of high rates of bacterial and fungal infections among patients with the condition (Ezeanolue et al., 2013). In most cases, disease progression can be prevented through proper ear hygiene and preventive measures, particularly among individuals who engage in swimming and water sports. Education on how to prevent exposure to water and how to properly dry the ears following swimming can reduce the incidence of swimmers' ear considerably, bolstering the value of a comprehensive approach that involves both medical and preventive treatments. Epidemiologically, otitis externa is a common condition that manifests in various age groups without any gender predisposition as reflected by demographic outcomes among patients (Ezeanolue et al., 2013).

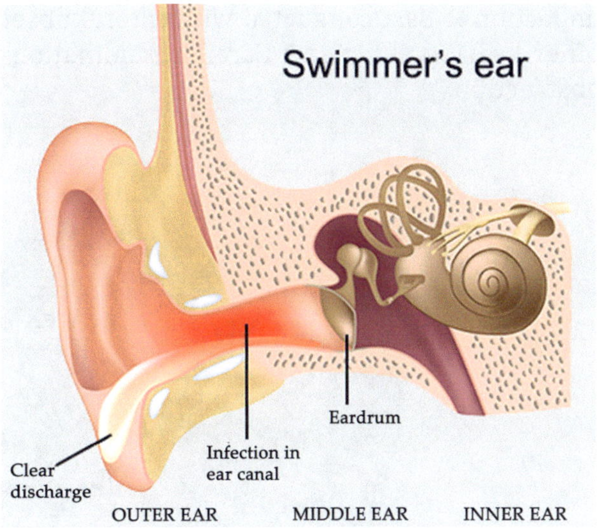

Figure 3.3. Otitis externa (swimmer's ear).

Source: https://external-content.duckduckgo.com/iu/?u=https%3A%2F%2Fmedia.healthdirect.org.au%2Fimages%2Finline%2Foriginal%2Fswimmers-ear-illustration-inline-29d4d4.jpg&f=1&nofb=1&ipt=8258146fa7171e7bc038a60562e814df36d44230bfdb597f30aa80bc53ae975d.

Awareness of the prevalence and clinical presentation in a given population may elucidate patterns to guide health practitioners in optimizing diagnostic and treatment approaches. While advances in otologic education—such as those described in materials submitted to otolaryngology students—can enhance knowledge of otitis externa, community education and prevention must also be prioritized. The two-way approach has the potential not only to improve individual outcomes but also to reduce the overall burden of this common external ear condition (Figure 3.3).

3.1.2. Earwax Impaction

Earwax impaction is a common condition in which cerumen accumulates in the ear canal, obstructing sound conduction and causing pain. Buildup comes from the shape of a person's ear canal, misuse of cotton swabs or other objects for cleaning, or certain skin issues that encourage overproduction of cerumen. In some cases, individuals with developmental disorders or auditory sensitivities, for instance, autism spectrum disorder, may experience challenges in the efficient handling of sensory inputs, which inadvertently lead to the perpetuation of earwax accumulation. In addition to temporarily affecting hearing, the condition may also cause tinnitus-like symptoms, itching, and ear fullness, thereby impairing communication and overall quality of life. Diagnosis of earwax impaction is best conducted with careful observation because it has diverse signs that also signify other hearing afflictions. Careful examination typically involves otoscopy to assess the degree of obstruction.

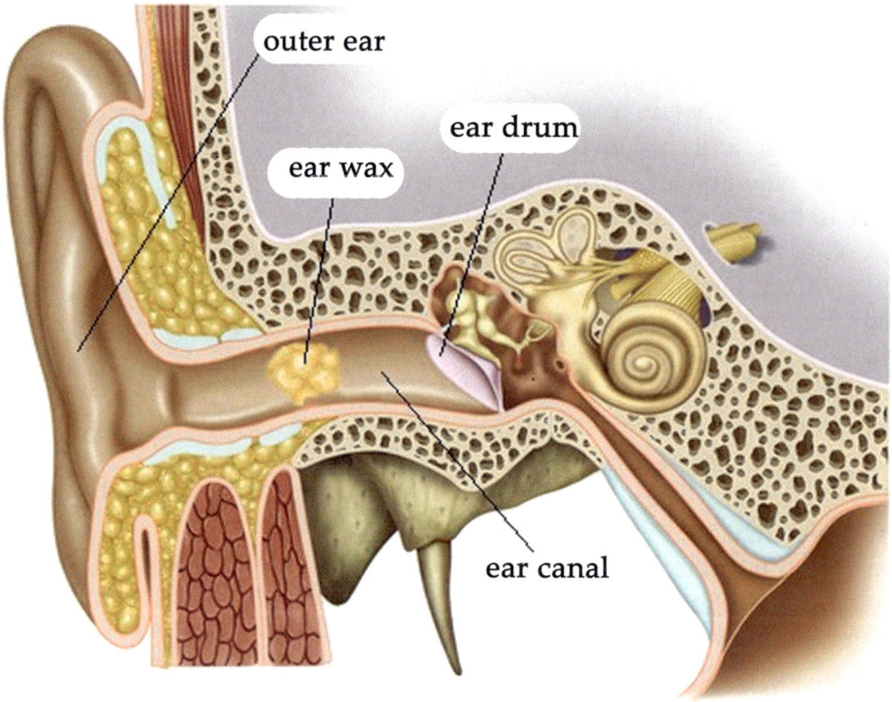

Figure 3.4. Earwax impaction.

Source: https://external-content.duckduckgo.com/iu/?u=https%3A%2F%2Fwww.earclean.com.au%2Fwp-content%2Fuploads%2F2015%2F03%2Fear.jpg&f=1&nofb=1&ipt=25462de9e186fe7f3dc881ada3e9acbb5a4790c0145e5bd1be55ee96e92933cf.

Moreover, the anatomy and physiology of the outer ear canals predominantly influence susceptibility to impaction. Temperature, humidity, and the ear's defense mechanisms also significantly contribute to maintaining a healthy microenvironment. The outer ear canal has been said to exhibit antimicrobial activity as per studies due to the antimicrobial substance cerumen, which bars excessive overgrowth of pathogenic microbes. However, when there is an imbalance due to allergic states or excessive cleansing behavior, the conditions may be conducive to impaction and microbial colonization, thereby exacerbating problems (Houtsaeger et al., 2024; Jamal et al., 2025). Management of earwax impaction is typically preventive and interventional. For individuals prone to excessive buildup, ongoing professional cleaning and avoidance of aggressive cleaning methods are recommended. In cases of obstruction, professionals can use methods such as irrigation, suction, or the application of softening agents to excavate impacted wax. Wherever there are recurrent infections or complications due to impaction, ongoing follow-up and specific treatment protocols are critical to avert detrimental effects on hearing and overall ear health. Lastly, recognizing the multifaceted nature of earwax impaction can help formulate effective steps that promote overall health and enhance patients' listening experience and social life (Houtsaeger et al., 2024; Jamal et al., 2025) (Figure 3.4).

3.1.3. Perichondritis

Perichondritis, or inflammation of the cartilage of the external ear, is the most important aspect of auricular diseases. The etiology often involves bacterial infection, usually secondary to trauma, that is, surgery or piercing. Infections may also result from microorganisms being introduced into the cartilage as a consequence of loss of integumentary continuity. The resulting inflammation manifests as localized swelling, redness, and pain in the surrounding tissue. Significantly, the immune response to such infections may lead to additional complications, making early medical attention imperative to prevent cartilage necrosis and potential disfigurement. Knowledge of perichondritis pathophysiology can inform treatment options and preventive interventions more effectively, thereby ensuring ear health. Diagnosis of perichondritis is made with careful clinical evaluation along with proper patient history, primarily ear surgery or trauma-related history. Techniques such as otoscopy and imaging can be employed for assessing the severity of infection and cartilage involvement. Recent advances in diagnostic modalities, such as culturing aspirated material from the affected area, also enhance diagnostic accuracy. Prompt identification is essential because the condition can deteriorate rapidly, leading to serious complications such as abscesses or systemic infection. The integration between ancient and contemporary clinical practices is crucial in successful management because what is derived from ancient texts, such as texts described in Shalakya Tantra, imbues a total sense into ear pathologies and their implication for contemporary treatment modalities (Narayanan, A., & Sarvabhouma, G. V. S. S. N., 2023; Ramadevi et al., 2024). Treatment of perichondritis is primarily antibiotic therapy, with surgical drainage of abscesses or necrotic tissue fragments required in more severe infections. Antibiotic selection is commonly guided by culture results to identify the most prevalent etiological pathogens. Aside from drug management, incorporation of therapeutic modalities as outlined in Ayurvedic treatment, including diet modification and lifestyle modification, may also enhance general healing reactions and functional rehabilitation of the ear. Emphasizing preventive measures—such as proper ear hygiene, caution with ear piercings, and protective measures against trauma—will significantly reduce the incidence of perichondritis. Because ear health is related to overall health, ongoing education and research are vital for minimizing disease-related risks, enabling patients to receive optimal care and achieve the best outcomes (Figure 3.5).

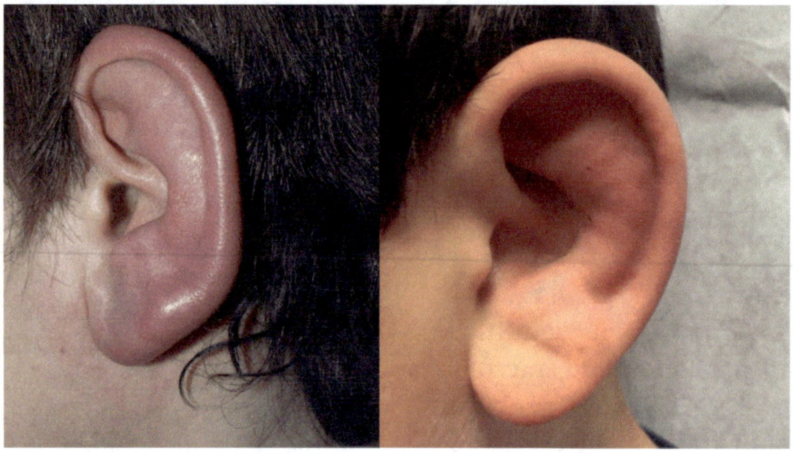

Figure 3.5. Comparison of an inflamed ear and a normal ear.

Source: https://external-content.duckduckgo.com/iu/?u=https%3A%2F%2Frebelem.com%2Fwp-content%2Fuploads%2F2022%2F11%2FScreenshot-2022-11-14-at-1.52.27-PM.png&f=1&nofb=1&ipt=1be02e740a03967bfcfa845aa671c6f012d6317571c020f40beff51fe4c5ed14.

Test Your Knowledge

1. Describe the common diseases of the external ear, including otitis externa, impacted cerumen, and perichondritis, highlighting their causes, clinical features, and management.
2. Explain the risk factors, symptoms, complications, and preventive measures of otitis externa.

3.2. Symptoms and Diagnosis

Learning Outcome

1. Common Symptoms Associated with External Ear Diseases
2. Diagnostic Methods Used by Healthcare Professionals
3. Importance of Early Diagnosis

For diseases of the external ear, it is crucial to recognize symptoms and their correct diagnosis so that they can be treated appropriately. Symptoms vary widely by disease, but common signs include hearing loss, tinnitus (ringing in the ears), and otalgia (ear pain). For instance, patients with enlarged vestibular aqueduct syndrome may have had various auditory complaints varying from mild hearing loss to severe deafness and vestibular complaints of vertigo or dizziness. These vestibular and auditory presentations require an appropriate diagnostic order, typically based on patient history and physical examination, followed by imaging studies, such as high-resolution CT or MRI, to identify any underlying anatomical pathology, thereby informing appropriate management interventions. Further, awareness of these symptoms, as well as imaging diagnosis, aids differentiation between mimicking clinical presentations of diseases. The diagnosis of external ear disease is often multifactorial, particularly when distinguishing among diseases with overlapping presentations. Cogan's syndrome, for example, can cause vestibular and auditory dysfunction, complicating the diagnosis because it also manifests with interstitial keratitis as well as potential systemic involvement. There must be careful observation and consideration of the possibility of underlying autoimmune processes. The use of serological tests for inner ear illness-associated antibodies could be extremely useful in diagnosis. Early diagnosis is essential because patients responding to Cogan's syndrome benefit from corticosteroid treatment. Timely diagnosis not only alleviates symptoms but also is highly effective in preventing further complications, such as hearing loss or worsening vestibular impairment, thereby making an integrated diagnostic approach necessary. Finally, early and accurate diagnosis of external ear diseases can significantly affect treatment outcomes and patients' quality of life. This is optimally achieved in conditions such as enlarged vestibular aqueduct syndrome, where therapeutic interventions, such as intratympanic corticosteroid injections, have been shown to be useful for hearing gain. However, the relationship between symptoms and pathologic processes should be well understood to avoid misdiagnosis and to enable proper management. For instance, Cogan's syndrome patients may first come in with nonspecific ear complaints that may be misleading for primary common middle or inner ear pathology. Therefore, an interdisciplinary team of audiologists, ENT specialists, and maybe rheumatologists is needed to enhance diagnostic practices and develop patient-tailored treatment plans, ultimately enhancing patient care and outcomes in the management of external ear disease.

3.2.1. Common Symptoms Associated with External Ear Diseases

The external ear is a conduit for sound waves and plays a crucial role in the functioning of the ear. External ear disease often presents with a broad spectrum of recurrent symptoms that obstruct normal hearing and cause significant discomfort. Ear pain (otalgia) is a common symptom and may be caused by otitis externa, an infection of the ear canal. This discomfort is frequently stabbing, dull, or aching and increases with jaw movement or on touching the ear. Pruritus (itching) is similarly reported, leading to ear rubbing by the patient, which can exacerbate the condition or precipitate a secondary infection. Clinicians would therefore be required to evaluate such symptoms not only in isolation but in the context of patient history, as they could be suggestive of underlying, more serious conditions of the external auditory system. Related and significant as well is discharge or otorrhea, which is frequent in conditions of otitis externa or tympanic membrane perforation. Discharge is either purulent, indicating bacterial infection, or serous, and it could suggest non-infectious pathology. This discharge is followed by other related symptoms such as hearing impairment and ear fullness. Otorrhea can be bothersome to patients and needs prompt medical evaluation to identify the cause and offer appropriate treatment. Additionally, hearing loss due to external ear disease can be either transient conductive loss or a more persistent type, depending on the nature of the condition and the extent and duration. This supports the importance of thorough assessments, as untreated hearing disturbances can lead to chronic conditions that affect quality of life (Chen et al., 2023). Lastly, swelling and redness of the outer ear, more frequently known as outer otitis or ear canal inflammation, is another feature that most diseases of the ear have in common. This condition typically presents as a response to allergy, infection, or irritant and can cause overt redness, warmth, and pain over the ear. The patient will have painful, localized areas on palpation, which will aid in diagnosis. Systemic manifestations, such as fever, may also be present alongside these local signs and symptoms, particularly in severe infection. Practitioners must be familiar with the differential diagnoses of external ear disease to accurately treat and reduce these signs and symptoms. Early diagnosis and treatment are not only capable of alleviating pain but can also prevent complications like chronic otitis or hearing loss and hence enhance patient outcomes (Johnson et al., 2020) (Figure 3.6).

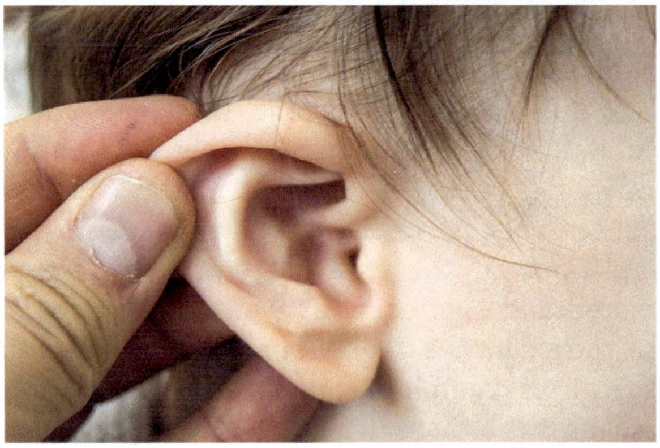

Figure 3.6. Checking for signs of ear infection in a child.

Source: https://external-content.duckduckgo.com/iu/?u=https%3A%2F%2Fwww.pedpartners.com%2Fwp-content%2Fuploads%2FSigns-of-ear-infection.jpg&f=1&nofb=1&ipt=e97d46c5e4bdad4e7b3dd1f850ee984f800744b1a3d838b45743feaa5433184b.

3.2.2. Diagnostic Methods Used by Healthcare Professionals

Diagnosis of diseases of the external ear is based on a blend of clinical examination and specialist diagnostic procedures. The first step is a detailed medical history and physical examination by healthcare providers, which serve as the basis for subsequent examinations. Through this study, a specialist can examine the outer ear and ear canal with an otoscope, enabling visualization of pathology such as redness, swelling, or discharge. Tuning fork tests are also used to assess conductive hearing, differentiating between conductive and sensorineural hearing loss. This initial assessment is crucial, as it provides a baseline understanding of the patient's condition before any diagnostic testing is performed to guide the diagnostic process and optimize treatment options. For more complex situations or when initial assessments are noninformative, consideration of audiometric testing can be indicated. This encompasses a complete evaluation of hearing ability, employing pure-tone audiometry and speech audiometry to define the degree and character of hearing impairment. These tests quantify hearing thresholds across different tones and frequencies, which in turn inform the treatment plan. On top of that, tympanometry can be used to measure middle ear function by ascertaining the mobility of the tympanic membrane and the conduction of sound via the ear. These tests play a crucial role in the diagnosis of specific ear pathology, namely otitis media or tympanic membrane perforation, thereby guiding healthcare professionals in prescribing a treatment plan to address the pathology. Sophisticated imaging modalities, such as magnetic resonance imaging (MRI) or computed tomography (CT) scans, are also critical for evaluating suspected external ear pathology. These modalities provide accurate cross-sectional images of anatomical structures and enable the identification of more refined defects that cannot be identified with standard examination methods. These images are particularly valuable in assessing the severity of infection, developmental defects, or neoplastic changes involving the outer ear and surrounding tissue. Additionally, the use of these diagnostic methods can enhance patient care by improving understanding of the condition, enabling timely intervention and preventing complications arising from delayed diagnosis. The combined use of these diagnostic methods reflects the complexity of healthcare practitioners' role in the successful management of external ear disease and in maximizing patient outcomes during the diagnostic process.

3.2.3. Importance of Early Diagnosis

Among the diseases of the external ear, the need for early detection cannot be overstressed. External ear conditions often present with symptoms that appear harmless or transitory, leading individuals to delay treatment. Early treatment is necessary, however, because most external ear conditions, such as otitis externa, have serious implications if left untreated. Early proper diagnosis allows early treatment, which not only dispels sudden pain but also prevents secondary complications, like chronic infection or structural damage. This aspect of early diagnosis is particularly significant, as it can ultimately decide the overall well-being of the auditory apparatus and prevent potential long-term hearing damage. Furthermore, establishing a definitive diagnosis of external ear conditions typically relies on clinical evaluation and advanced diagnostic imaging. According to recent articles, although an extensive neurologic examination can localize vestibular disturbances to specific sites, additional diagnostic studies are usually required before a final diagnosis can be made (LeCouteur et al., 1999). This is especially true in cases where the symptoms can be close to those of other illnesses, hence presenting a tricky clinical feature. Lack of proper, timely diagnosis may lead to inappropriate management or treatment, posing a risk to disease progression and further complicating the patient's health and well-being. Hence, implementing an active diagnostic strategy not only simplifies the treatment process but also improves patient outcomes. The implication of early diagnosis extends beyond the individual patient; it involves the general public health implications as well. Early detection of external ear disease can lead to improved management practices, reducing healthcare spending on chronic conditions and complications. For instance, in genetic conditions such as Townes-Brocks syndrome, where the initial presentation may be external ear malformations, early detection can enable genetic counseling and appropriate management measures to potentially prevent catastrophic outcomes, such as end-stage renal failure (Bian et al., 2016). Overall, the advantages of an early diagnosis of an individual's health resonate through improved treatment outcomes and efficient use of resources in healthcare, speaking to its central role in external ear disease management (Figure 3.7).

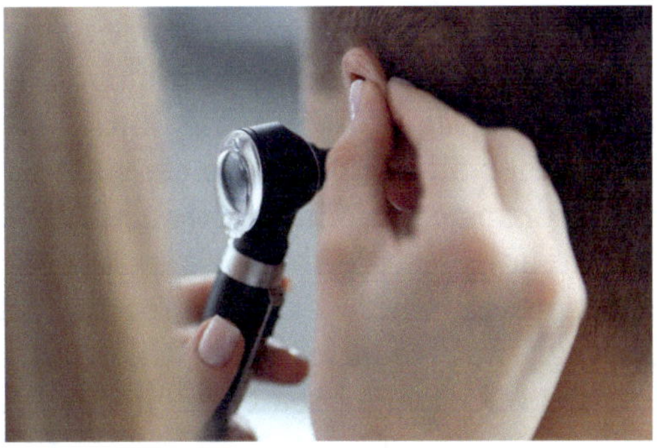

Figure 3.7. Otoscopic examination of the ear.

Source: https://external-content.duckduckgo.com/iu/?u=https%3A%2F%2Fimages.squarespace-cdn.com%2Fcontent%2Fv1%2F576aa49f03596e7bb34631de%2F1707325172159-5113V6Y8C2ZDCUZJXTNP%2FThe%2BImportance%2Bof%2BEarly%2BDiagnosis%2Bin%2BENT%2Band%2BAllergy%2BHealth.png&f=1&nofb=1&ipt=c8dcd03b279c48158cd4ef9c7f3a9b48fda7edbf1749e342fef52dcc49de2c7d.

Test Your Knowledge

1. What are the common symptoms of external and middle ear disorders? Describe how pain, discharge, hearing loss, itching, and swelling help in clinical diagnosis.
2. Explain the methods used in diagnosing ear diseases, including history taking, physical examination, otoscopy, audiological tests, and imaging studies.

3.3. Treatment Options

Learning Outcome

1. Medical Treatments for External Ear Diseases
2. Surgical Interventions When Necessary
3. Home Remedies and Preventive Measures

The therapy of outer ear disorders will involve a multifaceted approach, as varied as the symptomatic pathology. For instance, external otitis, which typically involves inflammation and infection of the canal, is usually treated with a course of topical antibiotics and corticosteroids aimed at reducing inflammation and eliminating pathogens. More advanced infections may require systemic antibiotics, particularly when evidence of spread beyond the initial site is present. Other adjuvant therapies, such as the use of ear drops containing acetic acid, can also be used to help restore the ear's natural acidic state and prevent microbial overgrowth, further enhancing the treatment regimen. Finally, success depends on accurate diagnosis and an individualized treatment regimen that addresses both symptomatic and underlying disease processes. In cases of sudden sensorineural hearing loss, particularly in diabetic patients, treatment should be approached cautiously, taking into account interactions between their chronic diseases and therapeutic modalities. Adjustment of treatment strategies for diabetic patients is paramount because the change in glycemia can aggravate the underlying microvascular disease of the inner ear. Therefore, researchers emphasize the need to adjust medication selection to prevent exacerbation of the patient's condition. Some of the adjustments include changes in classes and routes of drug administration in such a manner as to optimize the benefits for diabetic patients with sudden hearing loss. Such precise management is required to achieve optimal functional hearing outcomes, underscoring the importance of personalized treatment protocols in external ear diseases (Badiu et al., 2019). Cogans syndrome is yet another complex problem in ear disease treatment. The autoimmune disorder, with auditory and vestibular symptoms as well as ocular inflammation, requires an intense treatment protocol. Corticosteroids are the first choice of treatment, which effectively manage inflammation as well as hearing loss. Due to the autoimmune nature of the pathology of Cogan's syndrome, other immunosuppressive agents, such as tumor necrosis factor-alpha blockers, have been shown to be potential adjunct therapies with differential effectiveness. Surgical interventions, such as cochlear implantation, may also be planned for severely sensorineural hearing loss unresponsive to medical treatment. These decisions must be personalized, weighing the risks and benefits relative to each patient's disease severity and response to initial treatment (D'Aguanno et al., 2017). Understanding these diverse treatment trajectories enables clinicians to better manage complex cases of disease in the external ear.

3.3.1. Medical Treatments for External Ear Diseases

Management of external ear disease, specifically acute otitis externa (AOE), has advanced significantly, reflecting an improved understanding of the pathophysiology and microbial etiology of these conditions. AOE is typically characterized by inflammation of the external ear canal, most commonly precipitated by bacterial or fungal infection. Clinical studies, such as those conducted at the University of Nigeria Teaching Hospital, show that bacterial infections predominate over fungal infections in diagnosed cases. In particular, 71 ears had only bacterial isolates, underscoring the need for targeted antimicrobial treatment. Topical antibiotics such as fluoroquinolones and aminoglycosides are employed in classical therapy and exert instant action on the site of infection, facilitating an immediate relief of symptoms and restoration of the ear's barrier function (Ezeanolue et al., 2013). These drugs are typically supplemented by corticosteroids in order to reduce inflammation and improve patient comfort. Pharmacological therapy is not limited to antibiotics; treatment of outer-ear infections may involve anti-inflammatory drugs and analgesics. Non-steroidal anti-inflammatory agents are part of the drugs that can be prescribed for patients with evident pain or inflammation. NSAIDs work by inhibiting the cyclooxygenase enzymes, thus reducing the production of inflammatory mediators (Bell et al., 2017). While NSAIDs are prescribed to reduce pain, monitoring the response of the patient to therapy is also crucial, particularly when fever or generalized symptoms are present. When inflammation and fever do not subside despite NSAIDs, additional antimicrobial therapy may be warranted. Strategic use of such therapies ensures symptomatic relief and effective control of the root cause and the underlying infection. The management and complexity of external ear disease treatment mandate a careful diagnostic process. Clinicians should pay close attention to the clinical manifestations of the diseases, which are as diverse as the patients themselves. Early diagnosis is crucial, particularly for determining whether bacterial or fungal infections are present, as the choice of treatment depends on this. In addition, follow-up management is obligatory; patients may need to be seen more than once to evaluate treatment outcomes and make appropriate adjustments. For example, persistence of symptoms would imply inadequate initial treatment or the need for other drugs. The integration of antimicrobial stewardship principles into the management of external ear disease ensures the judicious use of antibiotics, thereby avoiding the emergence of resistance and improving patient outcomes. An integrated management plan with a plethora of medical treatments according to what the individual requires, therefore, represents the best available practice in the management of external ear diseases (Figure 3.8).

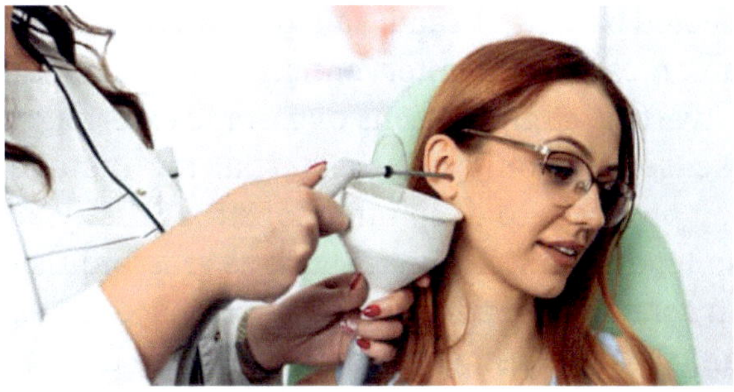

Figure 3.8. Medical treatments for external ear diseases.

Source: https://external-content.duckduckgo.com/iu/?u=https%3A%2F%2Fwww.hearingandaudiology.com.au%2Fwp-content%2Fuploads%2F2023%2F05%2FWhat-are-the-best-ear-wax-treatments-in-Perth_-768x345.jpg&f=1&nofb=1&ipt=5d5fb401ddab4fe67948723db1bda8eee3c461f5eb210331b319dff424067b08.

3.3.2. Surgical Interventions When Necessary

Surgical treatment plays a significant role in external ear disease, particularly when non-surgical steps cannot restore normal function or alleviate symptoms. Some conditions, such as chronic otitis externa, neoplasms, or trauma, can result in severe tissue destruction and infection, in which less aggressive treatment cannot be employed, and more aggressive treatment is necessary. Surgical treatment, like lateral ear canal ablation or total ear canal removal, is typically reserved following proper examination and imaging.

These procedures are designed to remove diseased tissue while preserving as much healthy tissue as possible in an effort to maintain ear function. The success of surgical treatment depends on accurate diagnosis, patient condition, and adequate postoperative management. By treating the causative factors of external ear disease, surgical treatment not only improves clinical outcomes but also the quality of life in infected patients. In addition to improving patient outcomes, surgical interventions could be pivotal in averting complications of chronic external ear diseases. Chronic otitis externa, for instance, may progress to deep infections that ossify and can lead to complications such as mastoiditis or intracranial infections. Surgery can avert these dangers by excising necrotic tissue and draining accumulated infections, thereby preventing fatal complications. Veterinary evidence indicates that surgical enlargements such as lateral ear canal ablation (LECA) have yielded encouraging clinical outcomes in animal models, with the majority of patients recovering well without evidence of recurrent disease (Willems et al., 2025). These procedures emphasize the benefits of early surgical intervention and may be lifesaving, reminding clinicians when surgical intervention is necessary in treating external ear disease. Lastly, whether to undertake surgical intervention should depend on an accurate understanding of the disease process and the patient's particular needs. Preoperative assessment, including imaging, diagnostic tests, and thorough physical examination, allows for the formulation of customized surgical planning. Postoperative care, including observation for complications and proper wound healing, is equally important for achieving favorable outcomes. Otoplasty or corrective surgery for external ear deformities in human medicine is another example that attests to the importance of surgical repair in addressing both cosmetic and functional problems. With the enhanced realization of the interplay between immune response and outer ear health, as now being foregrounded by current research into immunity's role in inner ear illness (Li et al., 2025), the potential for the future of surgery is certain to expand, thereby creating new and more innovative treatment possibilities in the treatment of external ear disease.

3.3.3. Home Remedies and Preventive Measures

Home remedies for the prevention and control of outer ear infections have gained popularity due to their ease of access and natural makeup. Simple measures such as applying garlic oil, which has antimicrobial and anti-inflammatory properties, can alleviate pain and prevent infection in the ear. The use of warm compresses has also been found to provide pain relief associated with ear infections. They are preferred by individuals seeking holistic alternatives to conventional medicine because they have fewer side effects and are readily available in most homes. Hence, the inclusion of these home remedies in one's health program can promote ear health and reduce the incidence of external ear diseases, making them a central component of preventive care within community health programs (Groot et al., 2011).

Preventive measures are fundamental to controlling the spread of external ear diseases, especially among those with limited access to healthcare. Educational campaigns on ear hygiene in the community can significantly reduce the risk of infection. Simple habits such as drying the ears, avoiding the insertion of foreign objects, and regularly wiping the outer ear with a cloth can be effective preventive measures. Where healthcare access is limited, as in Guatemala, informing individuals about these prevention practices is especially important (Gragnolati, M., & Marini, A., 2025). Moreover, these programs can facilitate community empowerment to actively engage in their health care, promoting an environment conducive to improved overall health outcomes. Moreover, the fusion of indigenous knowledge with modern approaches in health can enhance the effectiveness of prevention interventions. In some societies, awareness of local herbs and natural products for ear care can be beneficial for the treatment and prevention of external ear diseases. For instance, the use of chamomile tea as a rinse is not only a soothing treatment but also has anti-inflammatory properties, thereby contributing to ear health. This linkage of home remedies with scientific health programs can help develop a more comprehensive approach to ear disease prevention. By encouraging collaboration between contemporary physicians and traditional healers, communities can develop tailored programs that respect local culture while addressing contemporary health issues of the external ear (Groot et al., 2011).

Test Your Knowledge

1. Describe the medical management of common external ear diseases such as otitis externa, impacted cerumen, and furunculosis, including the use of topical and systemic medications.
2. Explain the role of antibiotics, antifungal agents, anti-inflammatory drugs, and analgesics in the treatment of external ear infections.

3.4. Risk Factors

Learning Outcome

1. Environmental Factors Contributing to Ear Diseases
2. Personal Hygiene and Its Impact on Ear Health
3. Genetic Predispositions to Ear Conditions

Understanding the risk factors that predispose individuals to external ear diseases is essential for prevention and early management. These risk factors can be broadly categorized as environmental, genetic, and medical factors. For instance, exposure to loud noise can lead to acoustic trauma, a well-known risk factor for conditions such as ear infection and transient threshold shift. In addition, genetics plays an important role: individuals with a family history of ear problems may be prone to developing the same. Underlying diseases such as asthma or allergies can also aggravate ear problems by causing inflammation and accumulation of fluid in the middle ear, eventually influencing the outer ear as well. Recognition of these risk factors enables medical personnel to develop individualized strategies to reduce risk and improve health outcomes in high-risk groups. Furthermore, certain demographic characteristics significantly influence the incidence of external ear diseases. The age of the individual, for example, is a significant risk factor; children and older adults are most susceptible to infection and to structural abnormalities. In infants and children, illnesses such as secondhand smoke exposure and chronic upper respiratory infection have been associated with higher rates of otitis media, a common outer ear disorder. Conversely, in older adults, declines in the physical components of the ear and long-term environmental noise exposure can increase the risk of disorders such as presbycusis, which impairs hearing function. The interaction among these demographic risk factors underscores the importance of prevention- and education oriented public health activities at age- and setting-specific levels. In addition, certain health care practices, particularly neonatal care, introduce specific risk factors for the development of external ear disease. Infants admitted to neonatology intensive care units (NICU), for instance, often have multiple risk factors such as prolonged mechanical ventilation and ototoxic agents. These interventions can lead to complications, including sensorineural hearing loss (SNHL). Studies have found that there is a significant correlation between the number of risk factors present and the incidence of SNHL in NICU infants, as increased exposure to these risk factors demonstrates an association with increased auditory impairment, as indicated in studies comparing hearing outcomes in terms of these conditions. Thus, identifying these clinical risk factors is important for developing strategies to reduce adverse outcomes and for effective monitoring and early intervention for vulnerable infants (Aylin et al., 2016; Abita et al., 2019).

3.4.1. Environmental Factors Contributing to Ear Diseases

Varying environmental conditions play significant roles in the prevalence and extent of ear diseases, particularly in vulnerable groups. Otitis media, for instance, is prevalent among children due to exposure to contaminated water sources. This is an issue, particularly in regions with limited access to clean water and sanitation, where bacteria and viruses proliferate. Where frequent pest infestations have led to the subsequent use of toxic pesticides, the effect also mediates further aggravation of ear diseases through direct exposure and secondary impacts. Traditional populations, as reported by the Australian Indigenous HealthInfoNet (2025), generally have a single environmental factor that explains health inequalities, including ear diseases. Thus, understanding the intricate interaction between environmental factors and public health is crucial for designing effective interventions to mitigate these risks and optimize outcomes for affected groups. Noise pollution is yet another critical environmental factor that contributes significantly to ear diseases, particularly in individuals with noisy occupations. Chronic exposure to high levels of noise is a well-established risk factor for sensory disorders such as noise-induced hearing loss (NIHL) and tinnitus. A recent study found that employees in hazardous jobs had poorer hearing thresholds, particularly in the left ear, confirming a direct correlation between noise exposure in the workplace and the development of hearing impairment (Altissimi et al., 2017). Notably, groups of affected patients reflect occupational hazards that disproportionately affect men, raising questions about the regulation of workplace safety. Mitigating these causes of noise pollution by enhancing workplace design and implementing comprehensive health education programs can prevent NIHL and reduce the prevalence of concomitant ear diseases. Climate change is a long-term environmental factor that indirectly influences ear diseases by altering ecosystems and increasing the prevalence of certain pathogens. With rising temperatures and climatic variations, mold and allergen growth increases, and allergy conditions such as allergic rhinitis worsen, thereby impacting ear health through Eustachian tube dysfunction. The rise in the incidence of natural disasters such as floods and hurricanes will likely increase the risk of waterborne infections, including otitis media and other ear infections. In regions that are in Australian Indigenous HealthInfoNet (2025), such climatic changes have long-lasting impacts on the health of populations, mounting present disparities. It will therefore be essential to address the intricate interactions among climate change, public health, and ear disease to develop more resilient health systems and reduce future morbidity from these diseases.

3.4.2. Personal Hygiene and Its Impact on Ear Health

Good personal hygiene is crucial for overall health, especially for the delicate mechanisms of the external ear. The external ear serves as the first line of defense against environmental pathogens, and poor hygiene can lead to the accumulation of wax, debris, and moisture. These conditions create a favorable environment for fungi and bacteria, resulting in external ear infection (otitis externa). Evidence indicates that unsound ear hygiene practices can lead to clogging, infection, and pain, and necessitate that appropriate cleansing methods be taken seriously. By paying attention to ear hygiene—such as avoiding cotton swabs, which can push wax deeper into the ear—individuals reduce their risk of infection and other ear issues that threaten ear health. Furthermore, personal hygiene is not limited to the cleaning of easily seen surfaces, but rather it includes the general health practices that support overall well-being. Careful washing of hands before and after handling the ears is a basic practice that avoids much of the transfer of pathogens. It is especially vital in the current era, given the widespread presence of infectious agents that can enter the ear canal via touch or water penetration. When bathing or swimming, one should also use earplugs or earplug-like devices to prevent water accumulation, which can be a causative factor in infection. Greater awareness in this regard directly reduces ear diseases. Prevention of ear diseases through hygiene indicates awareness of the delicate nature of ear health and the preventive measures available to maintain it.

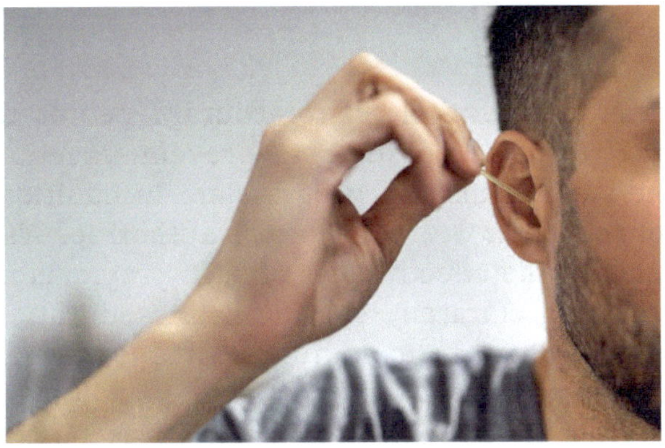

Figure 3.9. Personal hygiene and its impact on ear health.

Source: https://external-content.duckduckgo.com/iu/?u=https%3A%2F%2Fimg.freepik.com%2Fpremium-photo%2Fear-cleaning-health-hygiene_1016675-1989.jpg&f=1&nofb=1&ipt=d2f0470b838acd5a12aed424f3326b192041917ab56966a8fb395009685c1784.

Finally, hygiene is promoted as ear health through practices that appear unrelated yet play a direct role in ear health. Smoking, for instance, has been linked to a number of ear diseases due to its effect on mucosal coverings of the respiratory system and, in turn, the ear apparatus. These adverse effects may be compounded by poor hygiene habits. In addition, the recent upsurge in viral disease has raised questions about the intersection of hygiene practices and respiratory disease, and, subsequently, ear ailments. Given these intersections, it , but also their overall health. This combined understanding of the impact of hygiene on ear health is complemented by the appropriate preventive measures necessary to counter ear diseases effectively (Figure 3.9).

3.4.3. Genetic Predispositions to Ear Conditions

Ear disease etiology illustrates the interaction between environmental factors and hereditary predisposition to be complicated, as well as the importance of considering hereditary influences. A few breeds are genetically predisposed to external ear disease, specifically otitis externa, a common disorder characterized by inflammation and infection of the external ear canal. The American Cocker Spaniel, for example, is markedly overrepresented among surgically treated breeds for such severe otitis externa. Studies have established that anatomical variations, such as ear conformation and canal structure, predisposing some breeds to chronic conditions and repeated infections, have a genetic origin. These genetic predispositions are crucial for breeders and veterinarians to know because they can assist in breeding practices to eradicate these debilitating conditions from vulnerable breeds like the American Cocker Spaniel (Kaimio et al., 2017). In addition, the German Shepherd Dog (GSD) is a breed in which genetics plays a significant role in ear health, particularly with respect to ear disorder frequencies. The clinical data from the VetCompass™ Programs indicate that GSD demographics and health disorder data can provide valuable insights into how genetic susceptibilities manifest clinically. A closer look at the genetic causes of ear infections in GSDs shows that some inherited characteristics can lead to structural defects in the ear, making it more susceptible to infection or other ear problems. This information can guide breeders in selecting against characteristics that contribute to ear issues, ultimately improving this popular working breed's health and illustrating the need for intensive genetic study (Agresti et al., 2017). Investigation of hereditary predispositions to ear complications not only guides breeding strategies but also enhances preventive veterinary care practices. By identifying breeds at higher risk of ear disease, veterinarians can implement earlier management in genetically targeted populations. For instance, breeds with identified prevalence rates for otitis externa can be provided with preventative ear care regimens, which exist with the aim of reducing infection incidence. Additionally, informing dog owners about the importance of routine ear cleaning and monitoring can mitigate genetic risk factors. In general, identifying the role of genetics in ear disease susceptibility emphasizes an integrated approach to understanding and managing external ear disease, combining breed-related information with holistic approaches to veterinary practice.

Test Your Knowledge

1. Explain the role of personal hygiene in maintaining ear health and preventing common ear diseases such as otitis externa and impacted cerumen.
2. Discuss the harmful effects of improper ear-cleaning practices and describe safe methods for maintaining ear hygiene.

3.5. Prevention Strategies

Learning Outcome

1. Proper Ear Care Practices
2. Importance of Regular Check-Ups
3. Education on Ear Health Awareness

An integrated prevention approach to external ear disease requires an understanding of the multifactorial determinants of such conditions. Even in Indigenous populations where chronic ear disease, like otitis media, is prevalent, prevention initiatives must be aimed at wider social determinants of health. Prevention of ear disease in such populations is also often complicated by poverty, limited access to medical care, and environmental factors that exacerbate health disparities. Education and community-based approaches are crucial for raising awareness about ear hygiene and health; these interventions can encourage people to take positive measures to prevent infection and further disease progression. In addition, collaboration with local health authorities will enhance the effectiveness of such programs in providing culturally specific health education in response to community needs (N/A). Additionally, intervention strategies ought to be evidence-based adaptive frameworks responding to the needs of the affected population. Previous programs intended to prevent ear diseases have been challenged, primarily due to poor planning or lack of scalability. The Northern Territory's Stronger Futures in the Northern Territory (SFNT) program is a positive step towards evidence-based practice, and it demonstrates that targeted health services can be highly effective in the prevention of rates of hearing loss and otitis media. Via a holistic system of health education, screening, and treatment, programs like these can create an environment conducive to prevention. Future directions , with the inclusion of feedback from community stakeholders, to ensure that they address the contextual realities of Indigenous communities (Astolfi et al., 2017). In addition to community-level efforts, collaboration between healthcare providers and public health authorities is essential for effective prevention of external ear diseases. This partnership can leverage resources and support innovative programs, such as telehealth services and mobile clinics, to expand access to ear health screenings and treatment. Utilization of technology may even further reduce outreach activities in far-flung areas, reducing wait time and increasing follow-through care adherence. Moreover, longitudinal studies would be needed to assess the long-term effectiveness of such measures, adjusting for demographic and health trends over time. With evidence-based strategies and the formation of ongoing partnerships, the healthcare community can make considerable progress in reducing the burden of ear disease among vulnerable populations (N/A).

3.5.1. Proper Ear Care Practices

Good ear care practices can help maintain ear health and prevent external ear infections. It is crucial to clean the auditory canal daily; however, cotton swabs are not recommended, as they push cerumen deeper into the canal and may cause clogging or injury. The outer ear should be cleaned with a washcloth during regular bathing to remove any debris or excess earwax. Besides, one should take precautions in areas where there is excessive exposure to water, that is, swimming pools or bathtubs, where water in the ear canal may make the ear vulnerable to becoming a breeding ground for infections like otitis externa. Earplugs or a swim cap can safeguard the ears from such activities. Taking these precautions reduces the risk of contracting common external ear infections and improves overall ear health. Ear care also involves monitoring for any change in hearing or signs of distress. Pain, itching, or unusual discharge may indicate an infection or other pathology requiring immediate medical consultation. Self-treatment and self-diagnosis must not be done, since improper use of over-the-counter drops or medications can make the situation worse. Additionally, understanding the benefits of regular visits to a healthcare provider can facilitate early identification of potential ear disease. Regular ENT checkups are critical, especially for individuals with a history of ear problems or who frequently engage in activities that increase the risk of outer ear infections. Such attention and knowledge can prevent little issues from becoming big medical concerns.

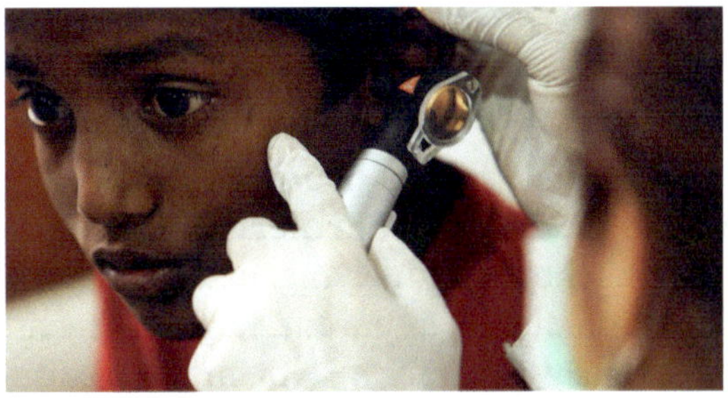

Figure 3.10. Proper ear care practices.

Source: https://external-content.duckduckgo.com/iu/?u=https%3A%2F%2Fcolinwilsonworld.co.uk%2Fwp-content%2Fuploads%2F2024%2F01%2Fboy-having-an-ear-checkup-1210x642.jpg&f=1&nofb=1&ipt=71088864d8426fb136d3a797dbb233aa5de1aa397266b0b08bd9119a2323fd7c.

Finally, proper education on ear-care procedures is also necessary, particularly for risk groups for ear disorders, such as children and the elderly. Public health interventions should focus on providing information on the necessity of ear protection in noisy environments and on proper ear-cleaning procedures. Also, teaching about the risk of harm from excessive earwax removal, which can lead to cerumen impaction and hearing loss, is essential. Lastly, studies highlighting the role of antimicrobial drugs, such as silver nanoparticles, in ear products can offer new avenues for preventing outer ear infections (A-Cşel et al., 2018). In general, comprehensive education on these practices will play an important role in preventing ear-related diseases in communities, fostering an ear-health-conscious culture (Figure 3.10).

3.5.2. Importance of Regular Check-Ups

Routine check-ups play a critical role in the prevention and early detection of external ear conditions. During these visits, healthcare providers have the opportunity to assess the ear's condition and identify issues such as ear infection, cerumen impaction, or external otitis, which can significantly affect hearing. By following a routine check-up program, patients benefit from early measures that prevent minor issues from developing into complete disorders. Furthermore, most ear conditions have underlying causes that may not be immediately apparent. Regular checkups provide early discovery, with more treatment options and possibly more favorable outcomes, and thus emphasize the value of preventive health care. Beyond encouraging individual health, regular visits also contribute to public health more broadly. Tracking the incidence and prevalence of external ear infections during such screening can yield valuable epidemiological data to inform resource allocation within the health system. The data informs public health interventions to increase awareness of ear health and can guide prevention activities. By analogy, recognizing trends in external ear infections can identify gaps in certain populations, informing the deployment of targeted education or vaccination programs. Ultimately, routine check-ups not only guard against specific ear illnesses at an individual level but also ensure public awareness and prevention of ear diseases. Secondly, the affordability and accessibility of regular check-ups significantly contribute to preventing individuals from neglecting their ears. Healthcare policy advancements, such as expanded insurance coverage for preventive services, have made such visits easier for patients to access without out-of-pocket costs. As Shindondola-Mote (2008) affirms, improved access to routine health checks is a cornerstone of effective health governance. The inclusion of ear checks in general health care plans leads individuals to prioritize their hearing health, particularly among populations at increased risk of ear disease. By integrating these check-ups as part of routine health care, we promote not only individual health but also a preventative culture of care that can lead to tremendous declines in external ear infections.

3.5.3. Education on Ear Health Awareness

Education plays a key role in fostering ear health awareness, particularly among populations disproportionately affected by conditions of the external ear. Information on risk factors for developing ear infections, such as otitis media, is of critical importance among groups with high prevalence. A significant proportion of Indigenous children, for instance, fight chronic ear disease owing to a combination of socio-economic deprivation and environmental characteristics. Successful educational interventions must address the urgency of awareness of ear health while also reconciling the specific cultural and socioeconomic realities of these populations. By prioritizing education on ear health, we not only alleviate the immediate burden of such diseases but also make strides toward long-term improvements in overall health status, thereby reducing associated conditions such as low educational attainment and unemployment, which are often concurrent effects of untreated ear infections (N/A). Moreover, targeted educational interventions can alleviate the occurrence of ear diseases and reduce their incidence. A majority of existing prevention interventions for ear disease are undermined by poor planning and by a lack of empirical evidence. As such, successful educational interventions must be evidence-informed to maximize health outcomes.

For instance, the Stronger Futures in the Northern Territory (SFNT) demonstrates how evidence-informed health services can achieve measurable declines in incidence and severity of outer ear diseases in high-risk populations. This highlights the necessity of community-level participation in learning interventions to enable individuals to take proactive steps to maintain ear health and respond to treatment as needed. Through concentration on joint responsibility between local populations and health authorities in the dispensation of ear health education, we can lay the ground for the successful alleviation of the burden of external ear disease (N/A). Finally, it is important to highlight that proper education about ear health awareness is not a matter of mere information transfer. The political and economic context also plays an important role in the success of these educational interventions. For example, communities with weak healthcare infrastructure can barely implement and sustain ear health education interventions, burden, thereby increasing the incidence of external ear infections. Thus, comprehension of the broader socio-political environment is vital for tailoring ear health education programs. Effective governance and resource allocation are essential to ensuring that program funds translate into tangible improvements in community health. As with the Cambodian avian influenza response, collaboration between health education policy and governance systems will determine the effectiveness of ear health programs. This overall strategy will promote a long-term commitment to ear health awareness and help reduce the incidence of diseases affecting the outer ear (Figure 3.11).

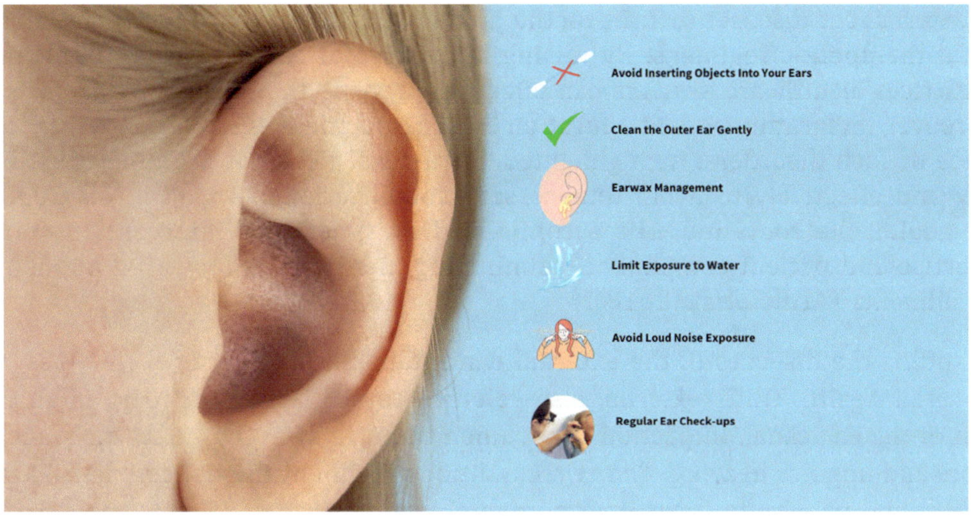

Figure 3.11. Education on ear health awareness.

Source: https://external-content.duckduckgo.com/iu/?u=https%3A%2F%2Fcrystalclearclinic.com.au%2Fwp-content%2Fuploads%2F2024%2F06%2FEssential-Ear-Care-Tips-blog-feature-image-1024x536.png&f=1&nofb=1&ipt=215867fda6d94802233dae02bf5bcc1e40d359877d9089a990e6145ee3c5da87.

Test Your Knowledge

1. What are proper ear care practices for maintaining healthy ears? Discuss safe cleaning methods, protection from noise, and prevention of ear infections.
2. Explain the do's and don'ts of ear care and their importance in preventing hearing loss and common ear disorders.

SUMMARY

The many diseases affecting the outer ear underscore the urgent need for immediate and appropriate medical attention. As observed in the course of studying diseases such as otitis externa, furuncles, and tick infestations, the external ear is not only a critical site for hearing but also an open area for infection and injury. The acute nature of the presentation of most of these conditions, particularly those like intra-aural tick infestation, dictates knowledge of immediate treatment to prevent complications and distress to the patient. In such cases, the role of specialist otolaryngologists is critical, as accurate diagnosis and intervention can significantly improve patient outcomes. The inference, therefore, from such information is that awareness, as well as prevention, the focal point of public health interventions. In consideration of certain conditions like Luc's abscess, it is clear that even infrequent complications of what at first glance would appear to be harmless diseases like otitis media can pose substantial health dangers. These scenarios demonstrate that, just as some external ear diseases are routinely treatable, others present hidden nuances that only careful clinical attention can prevent. The clinical care of such infections must be integrated, both to treat the short-term symptomatic condition and to ensure that potential complications are recognized and treated early. Awareness of such intricate interrelationships in ear pathology further underscores the importance of continuing education and training for health professionals, thereby empowering them to address the multifaceted presentations of ear disease more effectively. Lastly, the general overview of external ear diseases focuses on the pivotal interdependence between timely detection and successful therapeutic regimens. By raising awareness of ear health and implementing best treatment practices, healthcare systems can effectively reduce the incidence and severity of such diseases. Moreover, integrating patient education on ear care and hygiene is paramount for reducing the prevalence of such disorders. As highlighted, intra-aural ticks, for example, must be managed expeditiously and effectively to avoid unnecessary complications (Appaji et al., 2013). Thus, to improve ear health, the route must be accompanied by synergistic interventions that integrate medical expertise and patient compliance, culminating in a more empowered population against external ear ailments (Ardıç et al., 2018).

Understanding the diseases of the external ear entails a full study of their types, causes, and impact on overall health. Otitis externa, also referred to as "swimmers' ear," is an infection or inflammation of the ear canal. Impaction of cerumen because of overproduction of earwax is also uncomfortable and impairs hearing. The two conditions highlight the delicate balance required to favor ear health and bring into focus environmental factors such as water exposure and hygiene practices. Symptoms and case history are essential for identifying appropriate management strategies, underscoring the need for healthcare workers to remain vigilant in diagnosing and managing external ear infections. The association between external ear disease and overall health is also not exaggerated. As described, a strong history of childhood illness events has far-reaching adult health consequences. Chronic childhood of diseases, including otitis media, which are associated with an increased risk of ear problems in adulthood (Smith, 2025). Learning the developmental trajectory from childhood into adulthood can inform preventive interventions and strategies to mitigate the effects of early developmental events and to minimize the impact of later health outcomes. In that context, early diagnosis and therapy of external ear disease not only reduce existing pain but also potentially prevent more severe complications in later years. Finally, improvements in medical imaging techniques are transforming the assessment and management of external ear disease. Technologies such as high-spatiotemporal-resolution imaging enable accurate visualization of biological phenomena, thereby improving diagnostic accuracy and guiding treatment decisions. These technologies can reveal underlying structural changes or pathologic processes in the external ear, thereby enhancing clinicians' ability to tailor interventions appropriately (Cui et al., 2016). With technological development, it is imperative to again emphasize the necessity for ongoing research and adoption of better technologies in clinical practice, ultimately focusing on improving patient outcomes of patients with external ear disease.

KEY TERMS FROM THIS CHAPTER

Otitis Externa	Swimmer's Ear
Furunculosis	Impacted Cerumen
Cerumen Impaction	Otomycosis
Perichondritis	Cellulitis
Eczema	Dermatitis
Hematoma Auris	Cauliflower Ear
Traumatic Otitis Externa	Malignant Otitis Externa
Necrotizing Otitis Externa	Keratosis Obturans
External Auditory Canal Stenosis	Atresia

CRITICAL THINKING QUESTIONS

1. **Inflammation of the external auditory canal is called:**
   a) Otitis media
   b) Otitis externa
   c) Labyrinthitis
   d) Mastoiditis
2. **Swimmer's ear refers to:**
   a) Otitis media
   b) Otitis interna
   c) Otitis externa
   d) Mastoiditis
3. **A localized infection of the hair follicle in the ear canal is called:**
   a) Furunculosis
   b) Otomycosis
   c) Perichondritis
   d) Cellulitis
4. **Fungal infection of the external ear is known as:**
   a) Otitis externa
   b) Otomycosis
   c) Furunculosis
   d) Mastoiditis
5. **The most common cause of impacted cerumen is:**
   a) Overproduction of wax
   b) Narrow ear canal
   c) Improper ear cleaning
   d) All of the above

Short Answer Questions

1. What are the common diseases affecting the external ear, and how are they classified?
2. Define otitis externa and describe its causes, clinical features, and complications.
3. What is swimmer's ear? Explain its etiology and prevention.
4. Describe the signs, symptoms, and management of impacted cerumen (ear wax).
5. What are foreign bodies in the external auditory canal? Discuss their types and methods of removal.
6. Explain otomycosis (fungal infection of the external ear), including its causes, symptoms, and treatment.
7. What is perichondritis of the pinna? Discuss its causes, features, and complications.
8. Describe the congenital anomalies of the external ear and their clinical significance.

Answers to Critical Thinking Questions

1. (b) 2. (c) 3. (a) 4. (b) 5. (d)

REFERENCES

1. Abita, P., Alberti, G., Caminiti, F., Gargano, R., Gazia, F., Longo, P., & Loteta, S. (2019). *NICU Infants & SNHL: Experience of a Western Sicily Tertiary Care Center*. https://core.ac.uk/download/287858788.pdf (accessed on 7th August 2025).
2. O'Neill, D. G., Coulson, N. R., Church, D. B., & Brodbelt, D. C. (2017). Demography and disorders of German Shepherd Dogs under primary veterinary care in the UK. *Canine Genetics and Epidemiology*, *4*(1), 7. https://doi.org/10.1186/s40575-017-0046-4Akyol, M. U., Alden, T. D., Amartino, H., Ashworth, J., et al. (2019). *Recommendations for the Management of MPS IVA: Systematic Evidence- and Consensus-Based Guidance*. https://core.ac.uk/download/323075225.pdf (accessed on 7th August 2025).
3. Altissimi, G., Balla, M. P., Cianfrone, G., De Vincentiis, M., et al. (2017). *Work-related noise exposure in a cohort of patients with chronic tinnitus: Analysis of demographic and audiological characteristics*. https://core.ac.uk/download/98349325.pdf (accessed on 7th August 2025).
4. Anastasi, M. R., Rizzo, G., Nicita, F., Bramanti, A., Milardi, D., Macchi, V., Brunetto, D., et al. (2020). Microscopic reconstruction and immunohistochemical analysis of discomalleolar ligament. *Heliyon, 6*, e04651. https://doi.org/10.1016/j.heliyon.2020.e04651 (accessed on 7th August 2025).
5. Appaji, M., Devi, P. N., M. K., Goutham, Naik, S. V., et al. (2013). *Human otoacariasis: A common outbreak in rubber growing belt of Karnataka*. https://core.ac.uk/download/pdf/10806599.pdf (accessed on 7th August 2025).
6. Ardıç, F. N., Mengi, E., Sağtaş, E., Tümkaya, K., et al. (2018). *An Unusual Complication of Otitis Media: Luc's Abscess*. https://core.ac.uk/download/227066469.pdf (accessed on 7th August 2025).
7. Astolfi, L., Chicca, M., Danti, S., Franceschini, V., et al. (2017). *Nanoparticle Drug Delivery Systems for Inner Ear Therapy: An Overview*. https://core.ac.uk/download/80157791.pdf (accessed on 7th August 2025).
8. Australian Indigenous HealthInfoNet. (2025). *Overview of Australian Indigenous Health Status 2014*. https://core.ac.uk/download/pdf/30672220.pdf (accessed on 7th August 2025).
9. Aylin, P., Balinskaite, V., Bennett, P., Bottle, A., et al. (2016). *Estimating the risk of adverse birth outcomes in pregnant women undergoing non-obstetric surgery using routinely collected NHS data: An observational study*. https://core.ac.uk/download/77021205.pdf (accessed on 7th August 2025).
10. Badiu, D. C., Burcea-Dragomiroiu, G. T. A., Gherghiceanu, F., Hainarosie, R., et al. (2019). *Management Options in the Sudden Hearing Loss of a Diabetic Patient*. https://core.ac.uk/download/216811037.pdf (accessed on 7th August 2025).
11. Balasubramanian, T. (2025). *Revision Topics in Otology*. https://core.ac.uk/download/pdf/144787205.pdf (accessed on 7th August 2025).
12. Bánhidy, F., Czeizel, E., & Paput, L. (2014). *Association of drug treatments in pregnant women with the risk of external ear congenital abnormalities in their offspring: A population-based case-control study*. https://core.ac.uk/download/50566645.pdf (accessed on 7th August 2025).
13. Bell, N. J., Booth, R. E., Burge, M., Mahendran, M., et al. (2017). *Randomized positive control trial of NSAID and antimicrobial treatment for calf fever caused by pneumonia*. https://core.ac.uk/download/132194045.pdf (accessed on 7th August 2025).

14. Bian, F., Gale, D., Jiang, G. R., Lin, H., et al. (2016). *Delayed diagnosis of TownesBrocks syndrome with multicystic kidneys and renal failure caused by a novel SALL1 nonsense mutation: A case report.* https://core.ac.uk/download/81675732.pdf (accessed on 7th August 2025).

15. Boterberg, T., Cool, L., Debruyne, P. R., Lefebvre, J., et al. (2018). *Screening methods for age-related hearing loss in older patients with cancer: A review of the literature.* https://core.ac.uk/download/323056071.pdf (accessed on 7th August 2025).

16. Bowman, A. W., Katina, S., O'Tuathaigh, C. M. P., Waddington, J. L., et al. (2017). *Translational genetic modelling of 3D craniofacial dysmorphology: Elaborating the facial phenotype of neurodevelopmental disorders through the prism of schizophrenia.* https://core.ac.uk/download/132211200.pdf (accessed on 7th August 2025).

17. Brugada, J., Katritsis, D. G., Arbelo, E., Arribas, F., Bax, J. J., Blomström-Lundqvist, C., Calkins, H., et al. (2019). 2019 ESC guidelines for the management of patients with supraventricular tachycardia: The Task Force for the management of patients with supraventricular tachycardia of the European Society of Cardiology (ESC). *European Heart Journal, 41*, 655–720. https://doi.org/10.1093/eurheartj/ehz467 (accessed on 7th August 2025).

18. Burdușel, A. C., Gherasim, O., Grumezescu, A. M., Mogoantă, L., Ficai, A., & Andronescu, E. (2018). Biomedical applications of silver nanoparticles: An up-to-date overview. *Nanomaterials, 8*, 681. https://doi.org/10.3390/nano8090681 (accessed on 7th August 2025).

19. Busse, R., Martin, M., Schreyögg, J., Simon, M., et al. (2025). *Defining benefit catalogues and entitlements to health care in Germany: Decision makers, decision criteria, and taxonomy of catalogues.* https://core.ac.uk/download/pdf/6497859.pdf (accessed on 7th August 2025).

20. Chen, J. W., Vela, M. F., Peterson, K. A., & Carlson, D. A. (2023). AGA clinical practice update on the diagnosis and management of extraesophageal gastroesophageal reflux disease: Expert review. *Clinical Gastroenterology and Hepatology, 21*, 1414–1421.e3. https://doi.org/10.1016/j.cgh.2023.01.040 (accessed on 7th August 2025).

21. Cui, M., Germain, R., Kong, L., Lin, J., et al. (2016). *Continuous Volumetric Imaging Via an Optical Phase-Locked Ultrasound Lens.* https://core.ac.uk/download/144331254.pdf (accessed on 7th August 2025).

22. D'Aguanno, V., de Vincentiis, M., Greco, A., Ralli, M., et al. (2017). *Optimal Management of Cogan's Syndrome: A Multidisciplinary Approach.* https://core.ac.uk/download/144473159.pdf (accessed on 7th August 2025).

23. Ear, S. (2025). *Cambodia's Patient Zero: The Political Economy of Foreign Aid and Avian Influenza.* https://core.ac.uk/download/pdf/6935930.pdf (accessed on 7th August 2025).

24. Ezeanolue, B., Godwin, O., Ibiam, F. A., IJ, N., et al. (2013). *Acute otitis externa as seen at the University of Nigeria Teaching Hospital, Enugu.* https://core.ac.uk/download/pdf/10806603.pdf (accessed on 7th August 2025).

25. Ferrara, P., & Ferrara, S. (2012). *Patologie Rare Dell'orecchio.* https://core.ac.uk/download/53278734.pdf (accessed on 7th August 2025).

26. Fikenzer, S., Uhe, T., Lavall, D., Rudolph, U., Falz, R., Busse, M., Hepp, P., et al. (2020). Effects of surgical and FFP2/N95 face masks on cardiopulmonary exercise capacity. *Clinical Research in Cardiology, 109*, 1522–1530. https://doi.org/10.1007/s00392-020-01704-y.

27. Gall, L. S., & Riely, P. E. (2025). *Effect of diet and atmosphere on intestinal and skin flora.*

Volume II – Literature Survey. https://core.ac.uk/download/pdf/85249155.pdf (accessed on 7th August 2025).

28. Gragnolati, M., & Marini, A. (2025). *Health and Poverty in Guatemala*. https://core.ac.uk/download/pdf/6373323.pdf (accessed on 7th August 2025).
29. Groot, M., Hansma, H., Kleijer-Ligtenberg, G., van Asseldonk, M., et al. (2011). *Natural Dairy Cow Health*. https://core.ac.uk/download/10932083.pdf (accessed on 7th August 2025).
30. Houtsaeger, C., Pasmans, F., Claes, I., Vandenabeele, S., Haesebrouck, F., Lebeer, S., & Boyen, F. (2024). The role of the microbiome in allergic dermatitis-related otitis externa: A multi-species comparative review. *Frontiers in Veterinary Science, 11*. https://doi.org/10.3389/fvets.2024.1413684 (accessed on 7th August 2025).
31. Jamal, F. N., Dzulkarnain, A. A. A., Basri, N. A., Rahmat, S., Shahrudin, F. A., Azemin, M. Z. C., Sidek, S. N., et al. (2025). Influence of different types of contralateral suppression tones on otoacoustic emission in children with autism spectrum disorder. *Journal of Audiology & Otology, 29*, 49–56. https://doi.org/10.7874/jao.2024.00353 (accessed on 7th August 2025).
32. Johnson, D. E., Burtness, B., Leemans, C. R., Lui, V. W. Y., Bauman, J. E., & Grandis, J. R. (2020). Head and neck squamous cell carcinoma. *Nature Reviews Disease Primers, 6*. https://doi.org/10.1038/s41572-020-00224-3 (accessed on 7th August 2025).
33. Kaimio, M., Laitinen-Vapaavuori, O., & Saijonmaa-Koulumies, L. (2017). *Survey of Otitis Externa in American Cocker Spaniels in Finland*. https://core.ac.uk/download/84363697.pdf (accessed on 7th August 2025).
34. LeCouteur, R. A., & Vernau, K. M. (1999). *Feline vestibular disorders. Part II: Diagnostic Approach and Differential Diagnosis*. https://core.ac.uk/download/323068734.pdf (accessed on 7th August 2025).
35. Li, X., Wang, H., Wang, J., Duan, M., & Lyu, Y. (2025). Inner ear immunity and audio-vestibular dysfunction. *Sensory Neuroscience*. https://www.semanticscholar.org/paper/9bcb7f6386dba5b9c92c04bcc66fe15e2e9f66ba (accessed on 7th August 2025).
36. Majumder, S., Mondal, T., & Deen, M. J. (2017). Wearable sensors for remote health monitoring. *Sensors, 17*, 130. https://doi.org/10.3390/s17010130.
37. N/A. (2025). *Aerospace Medicine and Biology: A Continuing Bibliography with Indexes (Supplement 153)*. https://core.ac.uk/download/pdf/42883215.pdf (accessed on 7th August 2025).
38. N/A. (2025). *Ear Disease in Aboriginal and Torres Strait Islander children*. https://core.ac.uk/download/pdf/30673322.pdf (accessed on 7th August 2025).
39. Narayanan, A., & Sarvabhouma, G. V. S. S. N. (2023). *A review of Karnapaligata Rogas with possible contemporary correlation and pictorial representation*. https://core.ac.uk/download/617189583.pdf (accessed on 7th August 2025).
40. Nola, G., Ralli, G., Ralli, M., Sparvoli, M., et al. (2017). *Unilateral enlarged vestibular aqueduct syndrome and bilateral endolymphatic hydrops*. https://core.ac.uk/download/98349074.pdf (accessed on 7th August 2025).
41. Organization for Economic Co-operation and Development (OECD). (2018). *Stemming the Superbug Tide*. OECD Health Policy Studies. https://doi.org/10.1787/9789264307599-en (accessed on 7th August 2025).

42. Patra, J. K., Das, G., Fraceto, L. F., Campos, E. V. R., Rodriguez-Torres, M. P., Acosta-Torres, L. S., Díaz-Torres, L. A., et al. (2018). Nano-based drug delivery systems: Recent developments and future prospects. *Journal of Nanobiotechnology, 16.* https://doi.org/10.1186/s12951-018-0392-8 (accessed on 7th August 2025).

43. Popper, A. N., & Hawkins, A. D. (2019). An overview of fish bioacoustics and the impacts of anthropogenic sounds on fish. *Journal of Fish Biology, 94*, 692–713. https://doi.org/10.1111/jfb.13948 (accessed on 7th August 2025).

44. Ramadevi, C., Anasuya, K., & Priyanka, M. (2024). *Ayurvedic Approach Towards Karnagata Rogas.* https://core.ac.uk/download/617189912.pdf (accessed on 7th August 2025).

45. Sepehri, E., & von Unge, M. (2018). Congenital mastoidal cholesteatoma in an 87-year-old woman treated by watchful waiting. *OTO Open, 2.* https://doi.org/10.1177/2473974x18765700 (accessed on 7th August 2025).

46. Shindondola-Mote, H. (2008). *Uranium Mining in Namibia: The Mystery Behind 'Low Level Radiation.'* https://core.ac.uk/download/75779770.pdf (accessed on 7th August 2025).

47. Smith, J. P. (2025). *Re-Constructing Childhood Health Histories.* https://core.ac.uk/download/pdf/7152682.pdf (accessed on 7th August 2025).

48. Willems, A., Hetterich, J., Thöle, M., Pees, M., Fehr, M., & Reuschel, M. (2025). Evaluation of lateral ear canal ablation (LECA) as a surgical treatment option for external ear canal disease in lop-eared pet rabbits (*Oryctolagus cuniculus*). *Animals: An Open Access Journal from MDPI, 15.* https://www.semanticscholar.org/paper/877341b8d7a43640644d6b99adbcc3f2374f0c1d (accessed on 7th August 2025).

49. Zhou, N., Yang, J., Dong, L., Li, Y., An, X. J., Yang, J., Yang, J., et al. (2020). Prevention and treatment of skin damage caused by personal protective equipment: Experience of the first-line clinicians treating SARS-CoV-2 infection. *International Journal of Dermatology and Venereology, 3*, 70–75. https://doi.org/10.1097/jd9.0000000000000085.

MIDDLE EAR DISORDERS

4

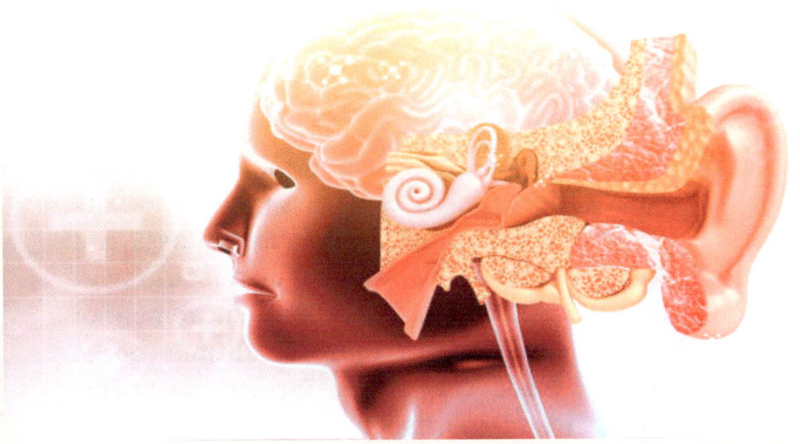

LEARNING OBJECTIVES

After studying this chapter, you will be able to:

1. Common middle ear disorders.
2. Causes of middle ear disorders.
3. Symptoms of middle ear disorders.
4. Diagnosis of middle ear disorders.
5. Treatment options for middle ear disorders.

Introduction

Middle ear diseases include a broad spectrum of conditions that significantly impact hearing and overall auditory health. Middle ear diseases can be precipitated by various causes, including infections, congenital anomalies, and autoimmune diseases, which makes their study complex but essential for proper management. The middle ear is an important component of the auditory system to facilitate the transmission of sound vibration from the surrounding environment to the inner ear. Hence, understanding the pathophysiology and clinical presentation of such diseases is crucial for the management of associated symptoms, including hearing loss, tinnitus, and balance impairment. Systematic research into middle ear disorders is needed, as it is the foundation for developing targeted treatments and optimizing patient outcomes. Middle ear disorders are associated with systemic illnesses, such as systemic lupus erythematosus (SLE), underscoring the intricate interplay between autoimmune disease and hearing symptoms. There is scientific evidence that SLE can cause extensive damage to the inner ear, leading to hearing and vestibular loss due to immune-mediated mechanisms and the deposition of immune complexes in ear structures (Stadio et al., 2017). The rationale for multidisciplinary diagnosis and treatment lies in the interaction between systemic disease and middle-ear pathology. Clinicians should take particular care to screen for hearing impairment in these patients, as early intervention can improve management and quality of life. Evaluation of the complications of systemic illnesses clarifies our knowledge of the complex issues of middle ear pathology. Beyond autoimmune conditions, congenital malformations, such as enlarged vestibular aqueduct (EVA) syndrome, are also a primary area of study in middle ear disorders. EVA syndrome is characterized by an enlarged vestibular aqueduct and is most commonly associated with all degrees of hearing loss and vestibular impairment. EVA patients may have mixed or sensorineural hearing loss; therefore, appropriate diagnostic tests, such as high-resolution imaging modalities (Nola et al., 2017), are essential. Treatment for EVA may also include new modalities, such as intratympanic corticosteroid injections, which have been shown to improve hearing outcomes. As research continues to explore the various aspects of middle ear disorders, it is evident that treatment plans must be individualized to optimize care and support enhanced auditory and vestibular function.

Definition of Middle Ear Disorders

Middle ear diseases encompass a range of conditions affecting the middle ear structures responsible for hearing. They most commonly result from infections, fluid accumulation, or congenital defects, thereby impeding sound conduction. One of the most prevalent middle ear illnesses is otitis media, which involves infection and swelling that can cause severe pain and, if left untreated, may result in hearing loss. The diseases should be differentiated, as they present not only challenges for auditory processes but also overlap with the complications of more severe health conditions such as tinnitus and other hearing problems. Therefore, understanding the etiology and definition of middle ear disorders is vital, as it enables the implementation of appropriate diagnostic and therapeutic strategies. In addition to otitis media, other causes such as cholesteatoma, eustachian tube dysfunction, and otosclerosis contribute to middle ear disorders.

Cholesteatoma, for instance, results in the pathological proliferation of skin cells in the middle ear, which may give rise to destructive pathology in the surrounding structures. Eustachian tube dysfunction impairs pressure equalization, which is necessary for optimal auditory function, and can cause fullness and pain. Otosclerosis involves irregular bone growth in the middle ear that resists the movement of the ossicles. Each of these conditions poses individualized challenges, for which further research and multispecialty management of diagnosis and treatment are needed, as reflected in the call for an informed knowledge base among healthcare providers (Pestel et al., 2017). Management of these disorders is of critical concern to clinical practice, particularly with regard to management approaches and their implications for affected individuals. The vulnerability to comorbidities, such as in the instance of auditory hallucinations in Musical Ear Syndrome, leads to the fact that middle ear diseases need to be treated with holistic therapy. In addition, identifying the psychological aspects associated with chronic ear ailments, such as distress associated with tinnitus, can lead to more integrated treatment approaches. Research has shown that psychiatric diseases often correlate with more severe forms of tinnitus, and therefore, the correlation between ear function and mental status is an important field of interest. On this basis, an accurate definition of middle ear disorders and their implications are essential not only for physicians and clinicians but also to enhance patient outcomes and quality of life (Altissimi et al., 2016) (Figure 4.1).

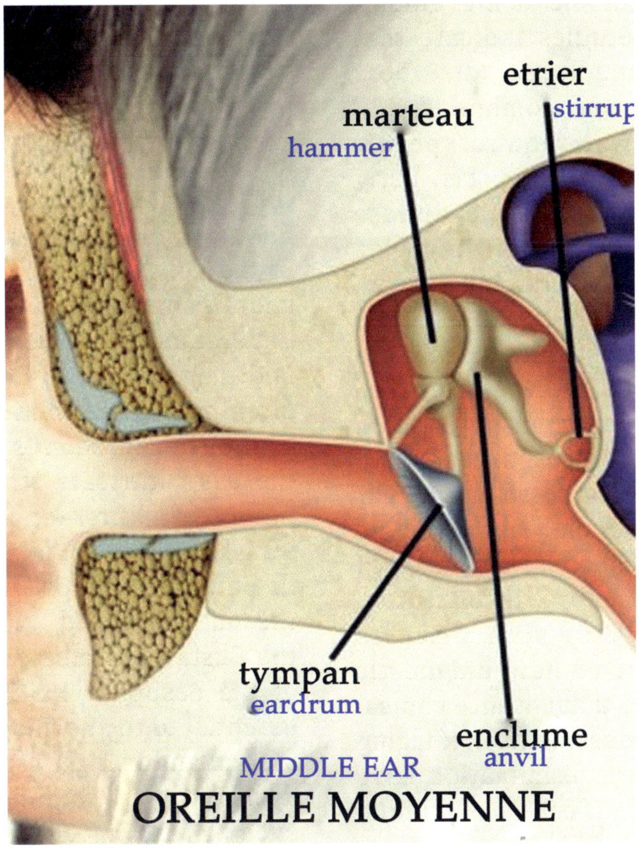

Figure 4.1. Anatomy of the middle ear.

Source: https://www.american-hospital.org/sites/default/files/styles/carousel_vertical_mobile/public/medias/images/2024/05/OREILLE-MOYENNE-FR-EN.jpg?h=4dbb47d6&itok=rlA11fX0.

Importance of Studying Middle Ear Disorders

Investigation of middle ear diseases is important not only for insights into hearing health but also for understanding the intricate relationship between the auditory system and systemic disease. Pathologies such as otitis media, characterized by inflammation and infection of the middle ear, can significantly impair hearing and result in long-term auditory dysfunction if left untreated. In addition, the involvement of the middle ear in systemic autoimmune disease is consistent with the nature of such disease. The findings suggest that immune-mediated inner ear disease may present as sensorineural hearing loss in patients with systemic disease; therefore, healthcare workers should be mindful of these associations. Identification of these patterns can enhance diagnostic accuracy and allow for early intervention, which should enhance patient outcomes and quality of life. This interdisciplinary foundation is critical to studying middle ear diseases and developing effective treatment protocols for a variety of patients. Furthermore, the impact of middle ear diseases extends beyond individual health and has implications for public health and the economy. Middle ear disease, if left untreated, typically leads to complications such as hearing loss, which significantly impacts child development, academic achievement, and social interactions. Studies indicate that children with chronic middle ear disorders may experience learning and communication issues, for which they will require specific educational interventions and supports. Early detection and treatment of middle ear disease not only prevent adverse outcomes but also reduce healthcare costs in the long term. Moreover, extensive research can inform the formulation of public health policies that ensure the prevention and control of these disorders, thereby contributing to a healthier population. Solving these issues, hence, reflects the extensive societal gains of careful research on middle ear disorders. Lastly, scientific analysis of middle ear disorders stimulates ongoing advances in medical science and technology. Investigation into the pathophysiology of such diseases informs the development of new diagnostic and therapeutic techniques that advance clinical practice. For example, advancements in imaging technology and audiometric examination have greatly improved the identification of middle ear pathology. Such continued advancement of knowledge enables a deeper understanding of the etiology and evolution of middle ear disease, thereby making the treatment protocol more personalized and effective. Furthermore, keeping up with new studies fosters a culture of continuous learning and adaptation among physicians, ultimately leading to improved patient outcomes. Therefore, studying middle ear disorders is not merely an academic exercise; it has far-reaching consequences for the development of medical science and for improving health outcomes for different populations.

Relationship Between the Middle Ear and Other Ear Parts

The middle ear is crucial to the auditory system and serves as a critical link between the inner and outer ears. Composed of three tiny bones known as the ossicles—the malleus, incus, and stapes—the role of which is to maximize sound waves received by the outer ear. These ossicles convert the tympanic membrane (eardrum) vibrations to mechanical energy to facilitate the conduction of sound into the inner ear, and more so, the cochlea. This connection reflects the interdependence of ear structures, as middle ear impairment can significantly affect sound conduction, leading to various types of auditory impairment. Hence, it is essential to understand this interaction for the treatment and diagnosis of middle ear disorders, which often present as conductive hearing loss when sound transmission is compromised, reflecting the ear's intricate structure. The middle and inner ears interact in ways beyond simple transmission of sound. The middle ear also helps in equilibrating pressure gradients between the outside world and the inner ear through the Eustachian tube connecting the middle ear to the nasopharynx. Pressure equilibration is essential to the normal function of the auditory system and is highly susceptible to infection or dysfunction, as commonly observed in diseases such as otitis media. These infections not only block the mechanical transmission of sound but may also complicate inner-ear processes and worsen hearing. Thus, it is essential to have a clear understanding of the functional interface between the middle and inner ear to effectively treat conditions that affect both areas, underscoring the importance of integrated ear health. Also, the role of the middle ear is closely related to that of the outer ear, particularly with respect to its form and function in sound collection. The outer ear, comprising the auricle and ear canal, directs the sound waves into the tympanic membrane, where they are converted into vibrations. The resonance characteristics of the outer ear resonate certain frequencies of sound, and these are then enhanced by the ossicular chain of the middle ear as they transmit vibrational energy to the inner ear. Any disruption of the highly sensitive process, whether due to structural abnormalities or pathologic mechanisms, can compromise auditory function. Therefore, the detection of abnormalities in any compartment of the ear is crucial for understanding middle ear disorders and their impact on overall hearing. The interconnectedness of such ear structures underscores the imperative of an integrative perspective both in diagnostics and treatment modalities in otology.

4.1. Common Middle Ear Disorders

Learning Outcome

1. Otitis Media
2. Eustachian Tube Dysfunction
3. Cholesteatoma

Middle ear illnesses are a broad group of disorders affecting the tympanic cavity and its associated structures, with a strong impact on hearing function. One of the most common issues encountered is otitis media, a middle ear inflammation caused by upper respiratory infections in most cases. It may lead to fluid accumulation behind the eardrum, resulting in conductive hearing loss and discomfort. Children are particularly susceptible duc to their anatomical predispositions and immature immune systems. The recurrent nature of otitis media may necessitate surgical interventions, such as tympanostomy tube insertion, to facilitate middle ear ventilation and prevent further complications. They emphasize the necessity of early diagnosis and treatment to prevent long-term auditory dysfunction and acute infection-related complications. A common feature of middle ear disorders is Eustachian tube dysfunction, in which the tube is unable to equalize the middle ear to external pressure. This can be caused by allergy, respiratory infection, or congenital defects and manifests as fullness, pain, and reduced hearing. Chronic Eustachian tube dysfunction also results in chronic otitis media, adding further complexity to the clinical picture. The concurrence of these disorders indicates that the dysfunction is not only symptomatic but also indicates a greater underlying issue that can include both environmental and physiological etiology. Providing patients experiencing such symptoms with comprehensive evaluation and treatment can help manage the condition and support long-term hearing health. Among the auditory phenomena of middle ear disease, Musical Ear Syndrome is a unique clinical enigma. Characterized by auditory hallucinations, the syndrome usually occurs when an individual suffers from sensory deprivation, frequently due to hearing loss. The affected individuals are likely to perceive music or other sounds that do not exist in reality, which creates puzzlement and discomfort.

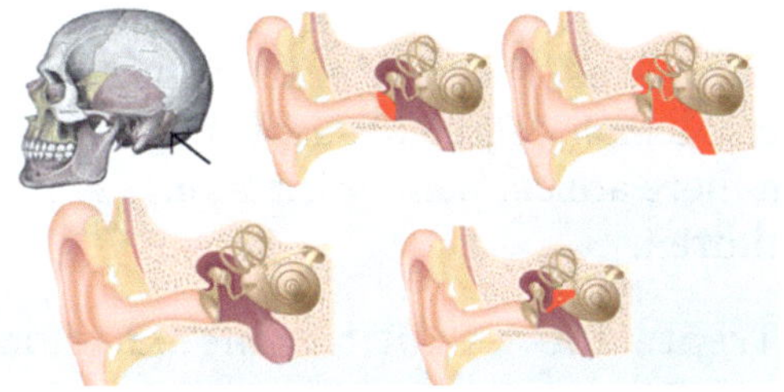

Figure 4.2. Common middle ear disorders

Source: https://study.com/cimages/videopreview/videopreview-full/middle-ear-disorder-terminology1_203673.jpg.

Although the condition is recognized, its pathophysiology remains incompletely elucidated, and it warrants further study of its etiology and treatment. This speaks to the broader context within which middle ear disease can cross-path with neurological and psychiatric illness, and for which interdisciplinary management is needed. Better understanding of Musical Ear Syndrome and its connection to hearing loss will allow health professionals to provide appropriate care for the victim, ensuring comprehensive treatment methods that address the physiological and psychological components (Pestel et al., 2017; Adelchi et al., 2018) (Figure 4.2).

4.1.1. Otitis Media

Otitis media, inflammation of the middle ear, is among the most prevalent middle ear disorders, particularly in children. The disorder can be classified into two categories: acute otitis media (AOM) and otitis media with effusion (OME). AOM is characterized by the sudden onset of symptoms, typically following an upper respiratory tract infection, while OME typically has a buildup of fluid in the middle ear without acute infection. It cannot be overstressed how important it is to understand the clinical presentations and potential complications of otitis media, because if left untreated, the condition can lead to long-term health issues, such as hearing loss and speech delay in children. Thus, medical practitioners need to exercise a high degree of suspicion, particularly when there are ear pain or irritability symptoms in children.

Treatment of otitis media remains controversial among physicians, particularly when antibiotics are involved. While antibiotics are commonly used for AOM due to pain and risk of complications from the disease, there is limited evidence that they are highly effective in pain relief. Systemic corticosteroids, for instance, have been studied as adjuvant treatments, hypothesized to reduce inflammation and produce symptomatic improvement, although supporting evidence is lacking. Based on current evidence, the evidence on whether corticosteroids reduce symptoms of AOM remains low quality and challenges their use in routine clinical practice (Beller et al., 2018). Hence, whether or not to initiate antibiotic therapy must be a cautious balancing of the assumed benefits and harms. While the management of otitis media is complex, several measures can be used to prevent and control it. Parents need to be educated on why vaccination is necessary because vaccination against certain pathogens, such as Streptococcus pneumoniae and Haemophilus influenzae type b, can reduce the incidence of otitis media. Additionally, preventing inadequate ventilation of the middle ear by eliminating secondhand smoke and ensuring breastfeeding are essential preventive measures. In recurrent cases, surgical intervention, such as the insertion of tympanostomy tubes, would be warranted to ensure drainage and aeration of the middle ear. By adopting a comprehensive approach that embraces an integrative strategy for preventive education with prudent therapeutic interventions, health care workers can significantly mitigate the impact of otitis media among affected individuals (LeCouteur et al., 1999) (Figure 4.3).

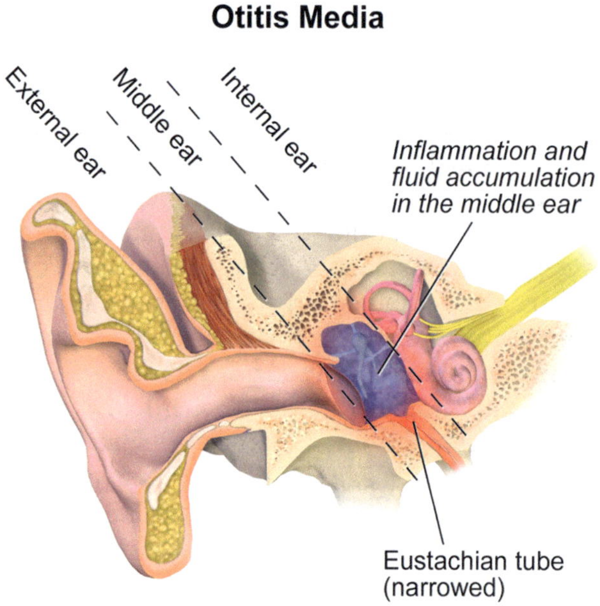

Figure 4.3. Otitis media.

Source: https://upload.wikimedia.org/wikipedia/commons/thumb/7/77/Otitis_Media.png/330px-Otitis_Media.png.

4.1.2. Eustachian Tube Dysfunction

Eustachian tube dysfunction (ETD) is one of the leading causes of middle ear abnormalities, often yielding a variety of complications, including hearing loss and chronic otitis media. The role of the Eustachian tube is to equilibrate barometric pressure and to adequately ventilate the middle ear. Dysfunction occurs when the tube fails to open and close as needed, which may be caused by a range of factors, including anatomical malformations, allergies, or infection. It is particularly true that those who have a history of upper respiratory infections or otitis media are most likely to develop ETD because the resulting inflammation may damage the normal functioning of the tubes. Evidence indicates that patients with a history of otological disease have a notable 21.4% expression of dysfunction of the Eustachian tube, compared to a control group in which no dysfunction existed, pointing to the relationship between infection history and ETD (Fukunaga et al., 2010). The clinical significance of Eustachian tube dysfunction is multifaceted. Patients may also experience ear fullness, changes in hearing, or ear pain, which can severely affect their quality of life. Chronic dysfunction may lead to more significant complications like fluid accumulation behind the eardrum, which can lead to permanent hearing loss. Also, disorders such as laryngopharyngeal reflux have been linked with ETD, and research has proven that acid reflux is linked with chronic Eustachian tube dysfunction symptoms. This connection accentuates that ETD treatment must be multidimensional and may involve dietary changes alongside traditional medical therapies. Such complexity of interactions calls for a well-tuned understanding of patient histories to identify potential causes of Eustachian tube dysfunction (Apisa et al., 2017). Management of Eustachian tube dysfunction varies widely depending on the underlying pathophysiology and symptom severity. In cases of minor conditions, conservative management with nasal decongestants, intranasal corticosteroids, or simple maneuvers such as the Valsalva maneuver can be beneficial by promoting tube opening. In cases of more chronic conditions in which conservative measures are ineffective, surgical interventions, such as tympanostomy tubes, can be used to restore normal middle ear function. The effectiveness of such interventions largely rests on the early diagnosis and tailored treatment plans suited to the patient's individual situation. As evidenced in clinical testing, preemptive testing of Eustachian tube function becomes paramount, particularly in those with a history of respiratory disease or ear infection, to offset the adverse effects associated with dysfunction (Fukunaga et al., 2010) (Figure 4.4).

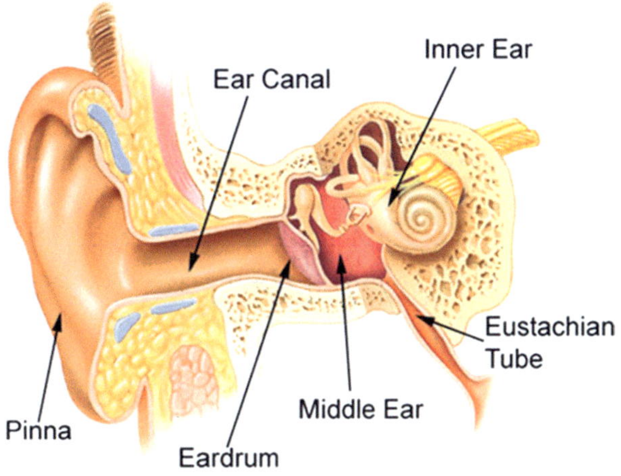

Figure 4.4. Eustachian tube dysfunction.

Source: https://www.chelwest.nhs.uk/your-visit/patient-leaflets/links/EUSTACHIANTUBEDYSFUNCTION.png/@@images/image-600-6b3f0c62550ba4430193cd26a9a14cca.png.

4.1.3. Cholesteatoma

Cholesteatoma is a serious yet often underestimated condition within the broader spectrum of middle ear diseases. It is characterized by the abnormal growth of skin cells in the middle ear and mastoid process and can lead to numerous complications without treatment. Typical symptoms in the patient include hearing loss, ear drainage, and pain that varies in intensity with the size of the cholesteatomas. The condition can present as a primary process or be secondary to chronic otitis media or other causes for disruption of the normal functioning of the tympanic membrane. Identifying the cause of ear canal blockage is crucial because it can lead to debris accumulation and create a conducive environment for cholesteatoma formation. The diagnosis of cholesteatoma requires a comprehensive evaluation, including a thorough medical history and physical examination, supplemented by advanced imaging techniques. As noted, the patient could have otalgia and hearing loss symptoms as the disease progresses, and hence it is challenging to diagnose at an early stage. A retrospective study enumerated a number of etiologies of external ear canal cholesteatoma as primary and secondary types, with an incidence rate relatively low at 0.30 cases per year per 100,000 residents. Typical manifestations of cholesteatoma, such as itching and ear fullness, underscore the need for careful assessment and appropriate interventions to prevent complications, including erosion of surrounding structures and middle ear disease, which can significantly impair a patient's quality of life (Sismanis et al., 2006). Treatment for cholesteatoma is largely surgical and involves the removal of the abnormal mass and anatomical repair of any damage caused by the disease. The operation not only seeks to remove the cholesteatoma but also to restore normal ear function and prevent recurrence. Appropriate postoperative care is essential because infection and further hearing loss may result if treatment is inadequate. Moreover, patients may require regular follow-up to identify signs of recurrence or other middle ear pathologies. The complexity of cholesteatoma reflects the need for a multidisciplinary team that includes otolaryngologists, audiologists, and primary care physicians to provide comprehensive care. Indeed, addressing the challenges posed by this disease requires an understanding of its etiology, symptomatology, and treatment modalities to avoid potential long-term consequences (Kaur, A., & Singh, A., 2013) (Figure 4.5).

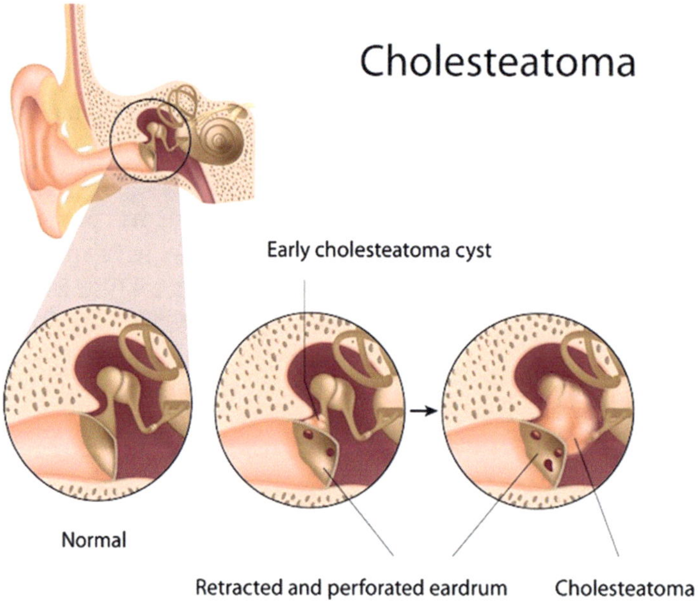

Figure 4.5. Development of cholesteatoma in the middle ear.

Source: https://entkidsadults.com/wp-content/uploads/2013/11/cholesteatoma1.jpg.

Test Your Knowledge

1. Describe the common middle ear disorders, including acute otitis media, chronic otitis media, and otitis media with effusion, highlighting their causes, clinical features, and complications.
2. Explain the diagnostic methods and basic management principles for common middle ear disorders in clinical practice.

4.2. Causes of Middle Ear Disorders

Learning Outcome

1. Infections and Inflammation
2. Allergies and Environmental Factors
3. Anatomical Abnormalities

Middle ear disease has numerous causes, including infection (otitis media). Middle ear infections can be acute or chronic and primarily result from bacterial or viral pathogens invading the middle ear following upper respiratory tract infections. The Eustachian tube, which connects the middle ear to the nasopharynx, is a key mechanism for ventilating the middle ear and equalizing pressure. Its dysfunction or blockage could lead to fluid retention, an optimal environment for infection. The condition is prevalent in children due to their anatomy, thus increasing their susceptibility to Eustachian tube dysfunction.

Having the knowledge of this process is significant, as repeated infections lead to not only hearing loss but also potential long-term complications if left untreated, thus timely medical attention is necessary in such cases. Another significant cause of middle ear conditions is the presence of anatomical defects or developmental abnormalities, which place the patients at risk of various complications. For instance, conditions such as cleft palate can lead to interference with the proper functioning of the Eustachian tube and the middle ear, as well as increased susceptibility to ear infections. Other structural issues may include a retracted eardrum or structural abnormalities of the auditory apparatus, which can lead to conductive hearing loss and increased susceptibility to infection. Along with congenital abnormalities, dysfunction can also be caused by acquired abnormalities from etiologic causes of trauma or inflammatory diseases. Addressing such intrinsic anatomical etiologies is important in good management, as these are often amenable to surgical intervention or targeted attention to reinstate normal hearing and prevent further complications. Finally, environmental factors should not be underestimated in middle ear diseases. Exposure to secondhand smoke, for example, is linked to an increased risk of otitis media in children because it can lead to irritation of the respiratory tract and make an individual susceptible to Eustachian tube dysfunction. Similarly, allergens and pollutants induce inflammation and exacerbate existing conditions, leading to chronic ear diseases. Socioeconomic status also plays a pivotal role, as access to healthcare has a profound impact on the management of ear diseases. In the majority of cases, patients with low socioeconomic status will have suboptimal access to preventive care, so middle ear disorders are more likely to remain untreated. By identifying these social and environmental determinants, healthcare providers can target interventions accordingly, ultimately reducing incidence and burden of middle ear disorders in at-risk populations (Figure 4.6).

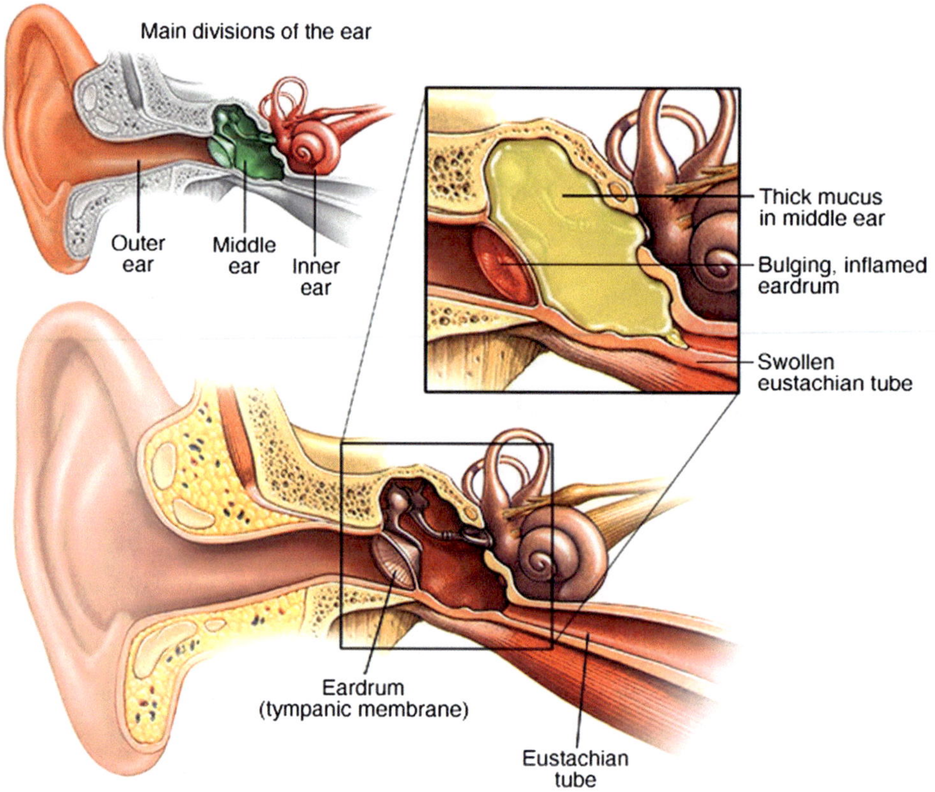

Figure 4.6. Causes of middle ear disorders.

Source: https://assets.mayoclinic.org/content/dam/media/en/images/2023/02/09/ear-infection.jpg.

4.2.1. Infections and Inflammation

Middle ear inflammation and infection (otitis media) is a serious health condition, particularly in children. It commonly occurs after an upper respiratory infection, when pathogens can ascend the Eustachian tube, triggering inflammatory processes that lead to fluid accumulation in the middle ear. This fluid not only creates a conducive environment for bacteria and viruses but also exacerbates inflammation, resulting in pain, fever, and other unpleasant symptoms. In children, because of the anatomical position of the Eustachian tube, which in them is shorter and horizontal rather than vertical as in adults, they become more susceptible to such infections. Effective management of middle ear disease requires an understanding of infectious and inflammatory processes, thereby guiding healthcare providers to formulate appropriate treatment regimens to relieve symptoms and reduce recurrence. The interplay of infection and inflammation in middle ear disease is also further entangled by the diversity of possible co-morbidities, like allergic rhinitis. Recent studies indicate that adenoid hypertrophy and sinusitis are significant contributing factors to the spread and recurrence of otitis media. In a study on allergic rhinitis, most patients reported secondary middle ear infections; therefore, an integrated treatment plan should address both the causative allergy and the resulting ear infections (Hardjojo et al., 2012). Systemic corticosteroids may be used to reduce secondary inflammation associated with allergic reactions, thereby potentially reducing the incidence of ear infections. Therefore, the detection and remediation of underlying causes are crucial to effective management of middle ear disorders. Regarding therapeutic action, antibiotics remain a common treatment for bacterial middle ear infections. However, the antibacterial efficacy of antibiotics may be undermined by the natural inflammatory process, as research has shown that inflammation prolongs symptoms regardless of antibiotic therapy (Beller et al., 2018). Interestingly, systemic corticosteroids have emerged as a potential adjunct therapy to antibiotics, aimed at curbing inflammation and promoting healing. Despite variable outcomes, recent research suggests that corticosteroids may enhance symptom resolution without necessarily reducing the course of the overall illness (Beller et al., 2018). Thus, although treatment of infection is vital, the inclusion of anti-inflammatory interventions may improve outcomes in individuals with recurrent middle ear disease (Figure 4.7).

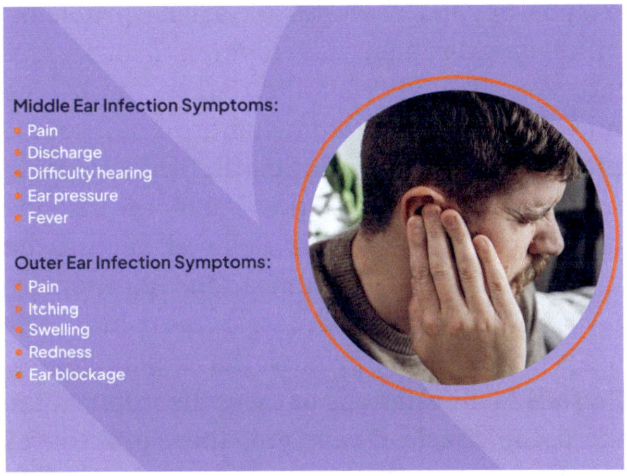

Figure 4.7. Common symptoms of middle and outer ear infections include pain, discharge, and swelling.

Source: https://www.health.com/thmb/4szIRyUfzBLv1AB-iomCV2riutg=/1500x0/filters:no_upscale():max_bytes(150000):strip_icc()/Health-ear-infection-symptoms-7497948_Hpriz-6a3c00ad254d4e088ccc6436daadbaee.jpg.

4.2.2. Allergies and Environmental Factors

Allergies significantly affect the incidence of middle ear diseases, particularly among children who are highly susceptible to allergic rhinitis. Allergic rhinitis is a common atopic condition characterized by an inflammatory condition of the nasal mucosa to specific allergens such as dust mites and pet dander. Allergic rhinitis has been identified across various populations, underscoring its epidemiological significance, as it accounted for 14.7% of patients presenting for otorhinolaryngology treatment, many of whom also had comorbidities such as adenoid hypertrophy and otitis media (Hardjojo et al., 2012). These conditions have serious morbidity potential because children with untreated allergic rhinitis have sleep-disturbed patterns and impaired quality of life, and timely intervention is necessary to avoid these outcomes. Environmental issues play an important role in exacerbating allergic reactions and the etiology of middle ear disease. The Eustachian tube, responsible for aeration and equilibration of middle ear pressure, can be compromised by inflammation caused by allergies and associated nasal illnesses. Research has identified patients with histories of respiratory illnesses, such as rhinitis, as having more dysfunctional Eustachian tubes than healthy controls, suggesting that such environmental factors precipitate or exacerbate middle ear infection (Fukunaga et al., 2010). This dysfunction may be particularly evident in populations with high allergen exposure, as continual inflammation may impair the protective role of the Eustachian tube and predispose them to infection and other ear health issues. Good allergy and environmental control is important in reducing the prevalence of middle ear disease. A multidisciplinary approach that includes allergen identification, environmental modification, and specific medical or surgical treatment can significantly alter the course in such patients. Public education about the necessity of treating allergies, particularly in children, can also help prevent delays in diagnosis and treatment, thereby precluding progression to more advanced middle ear pathology. For instance, a plan to limit exposure to known allergens, such as through the use of air purifiers and hypoallergenic bedding, has been found to alleviate symptoms of allergic rhinitis and, in turn, promote Eustachian tube function (Hardjojo et al., 2012). Overall approaches to the treatment of allergies not only seek to enhance patients' quality of life but also show promise in preventing chronic middle ear disease.

4.2.3. Anatomical Abnormalities

It is worth noting anatomical defects in the management of middle ear disease, particularly given that such abnormalities may affect multiple aspects of ear function. Anatomical defects, for instance, continuous osseous chain malformation or tympanic membrane malformation, can severely impair hearing function. Such malformations can be congenital in origin and are often accompanied by gene mutations or environmental influences during fetal development. Its importance is underscored by research suggesting a potential association between neurodevelopmental disorders and craniofacial dysmorphology.

For instance, research on genes associated with schizophrenia has found that abnormalities can lead to observable craniofacial dysmorphia, which may indicate more pervasive developmental deficiencies that may extend to the formation and function of the ears (Bowman et al., 2017). The correlation between such anomalies and the subsequent emergence of auditory disorders underscores the need for accurate anatomical assessments in these affected groups. Another notable clinical presentation of anatomical anomalies in middle ear disorders is the emergence of conditions such as enlarged vestibular aqueduct (EVA) syndrome. This congenital defect is coupled with abnormally dilated vestibular aqueducts, often leading to a variety of auditory dysfunction, ranging from mild hearing loss to profound deafness. EVA is clinically diagnosed with the assistance of advanced imaging techniques, including high-resolution CT scans and MRIs, which facilitate accurate measurement of the inner ear's anatomy. EVA-related symptoms may be mimicked by other vestibular conditions, and therefore, accurate diagnosis is imperative. Evidence indicates that patients with bilateral endolymphatic hydrops, which are also observed with EVA, may require targeted therapeutic strategies, such as intratympanic corticosteroid infusion, to improve auditory outcomes (NOLA et al., 2017).

This underscores the role of careful anatomical evaluation in appropriate management and treatment of middle ear disease. The impact of anatomical anomalies extends beyond short-term hearing problems, influencing broader developmental processes and overall quality of life. For example, the individuals suffering from malformations of the middle ear will have difficulties with learning and socialization on the basis of hearing loss, which leads to the delayed acquisition of language and communication. Additionally, new methods in geometric morphometric analysis hold great promise for explaining the physical manifestations of these disorders at the microscopic scale. By applying these procedures to animal models, researchers can elucidate the complex interactions between genetic and environmental factors in ear malformations (Bowman et al., 2017). Such information will not only improve understanding of the mechanisms underlying middle ear disorders but also inform the development of targeted interventions to mitigate the impact of these anatomical abnormalities on affected individuals.

Test Your Knowledge

1. Explain the common causes and predisposing factors of middle ear disorders, including Eustachian tube dysfunction, upper respiratory tract infections, allergies, and adenoid hypertrophy.
2. Discuss how anatomical, infectious, and environmental factors contribute to the development of acute and chronic middle ear diseases.

4.3. Symptoms of Middle Ear Disorders

Learning Outcome

1. Hearing Loss
2. Ear Pain and Discomfort
3. Fluid Drainage from the Ear

The symptoms of middle ear disorders can significantly impact patients' quality of life, including auditory and vestibular complaints. The patients complain of hearing impairments, which vary in degree from mild to profound, due primarily to Eustachian tube dysfunction or middle ear fluid. Hearing impairment can lead to speech difficulties, frustration, and social isolation. Furthermore, tinnitus, characterized by persistent ringing or buzzing in the ears, typically accompanies hearing loss and exacerbates distress and anxiety. The prevalence of these complaints underscores the need for early diagnosis and intervention, because untreated middle ear disease can result in permanent hearing loss and compromise general health, underscoring the relationship between otological health and well-being.

In addition to hearing loss and tinnitus, patients with middle ear disease may present with balance and spatial orientation symptoms. Because the vestibular apparatus is closely associated with the temporal bone, it is vulnerable to middle ear pathology, which can lead to dizziness or vertigo. These vestibular symptoms can cause significant disability in daily living activities, limiting the ability to perform simple activities and putting one at a higher risk for falls, particularly in older adults. Furthermore, the correlation of vestibular disturbance with psychiatric comorbidities like depression and anxiety is proven, which means these symptoms also affect not only the physical aspect but also the mental health of the patient. Effective management strategies, therefore, require a multidisciplinary approach to tackle both the psychological and the audiological components of middle ear disorders.

Contemporary studies have elucidated the pathophysiology underlying symptoms in middle ear disorders, including those in autoimmune diseases such as systemic lupus erythematosus (SLE). Immune-mediated processes can induce inflammation and injury to middle ear structures, thereby causing symptoms involving both auditory and vestibular dysfunction (Stadio et al., 2017). Tinnitus can be particularly burdensome, with severity ranging from mild to severe, prompting patients to seek medical care, especially in conjunction with the onset or progression of acute or chronic disease (Altissimi et al., 2016). Therefore, elucidating the etiology of such symptoms is imperative for the formulation of targeted therapeutic approaches. The confluence of diagnostic algorithms is capable of ensuring timely intervention and rehabilitation, and thus enhancing outcomes for those with middle ear disorders and emphasizing the need for global care in otolaryngology (Figure 4.8).

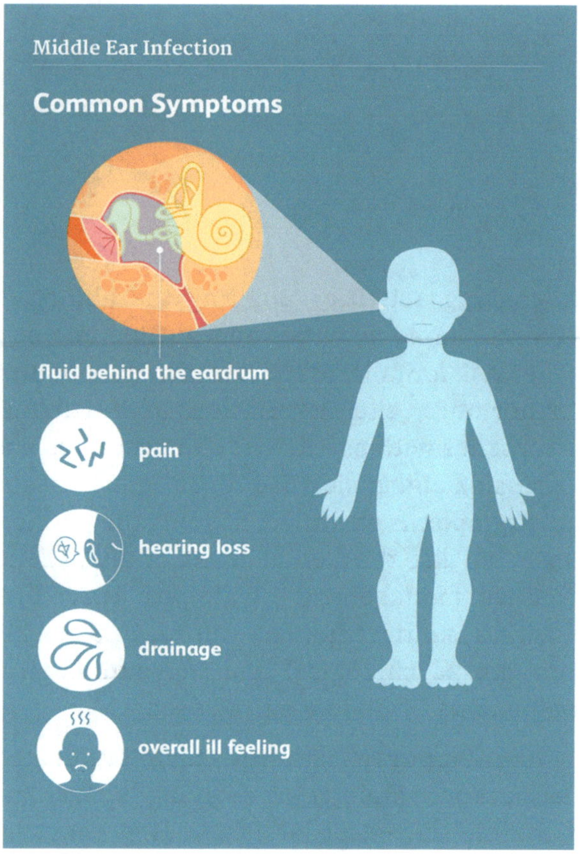

Figure 4.8. Symptoms of middle ear disorders.

Source: https://external-content.duckduckgo.com/iu/?u=https%3A%2F%2Fwww.verywellhealth.com%2Fthmb%2FzOT_vOQlsZ7Vk7RuTRiFC7FZV9c%3D%2F750x0%2Ffilters%3Ano_upscale()%3Amax_bytes(150000)%3Astrip_icc()%2Fear-infection-symptoms1-5b588c3746e0fb00250b9ef0.png&f=1&nofb=1&ipt=96d8ca263b7cf26f343db457c656c984534f18f16b21d918e0eaecac54c9b60e.

4.3.1. Hearing Loss

The problem of hearing impairment, particularly in cases of middle-ear conditions, has emerged as a global health concern. Quoted, an estimated 466 million individuals globally suffer from disabling hearing loss, most of which is preventable and is usually associated with middle ear infection. In developing nations, the burden is much higher due to insufficient access to ear and hearing care, fragile healthcare systems, and poor awareness of ear health. These conditions account for the high rates of untreated middle ear infections, which can lead to irreversible hearing loss. The World Health Organization is quick to call for public health campaigns to address this new problem, noting that a significant portion of hearing impairment is preventable through effective measures (Mulwafu et al., 2020). Middle ear disorders, such as otitis media and Eustachian tube dysfunction, are major causes of hearing impairment in children and adults. Otitis media, or infection or inflammation of the middle ear, is most frequently caused by nasal or throat infections and results in the accumulation of fluid and conduction impairment of sound. Otitis media is most prevalent in young children due to anatomical and physiological factors; therefore, early identification and treatment are essential to prevent permanent hearing impairment. Similarly, malfunction of the Eustachian tube disrupts the normal pressure balance, thereby increasing the risk of hearing difficulties. The interrelationship between ear health and overall health outcomes renders screening and prevention integral to primary health care, particularly in regions with high prevalence of ear disease, such as sub-Saharan Africa (Mulwafu et al., 2020). Furthermore, the socioeconomic impact of hearing impairment resulting from middle ear disease is significant. People with hearing impairments are generally challenged in communication, education, and social integration. Studies indicate that children with unaddressed hearing and ear conditions are least likely to attend school and have difficulties forming social relationships, ultimately affecting their overall quality of life. The World Health Organization's campaigns, such as World Hearing Day, revolve around raising awareness about the importance of hearing aids and embracing preventive strategies in the form of early detection and treatment of the middle ear. Legislative measures and training for community health workers are critical in enhancing the accessibility of ear care services, ultimately bridging the gap in healthcare delivery and the prevention of avoidable hearing impairment (Baycheva et al., 2022) (Figure 4.9).

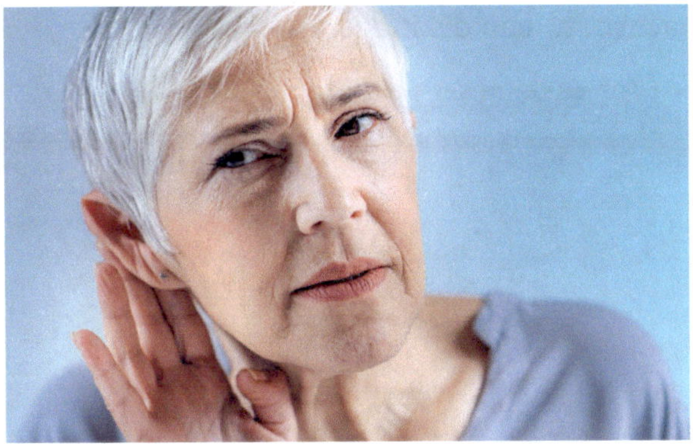

Figure 4.9. Hearing loss.

Source: https://external-content.duckduckgo.com/iu/?u=https%3A%2F%2Fveritascare.co.uk%2Fwp-content%2Fuploads%2F2023%2F03%2Fobraz-wyr%25C3%25B3zniajacy-1200x-628-px-7-1030x539.png&f=1&nofb=1&ipt=dd09c7a0c741ab40013c181bfc2f596db34a12c36d290300c83ab2e3124ab392.

4.3.2. Ear Pain and Discomfort

Pain and ear discomfort are common symptoms associated with middle ear conditions, significantly compromising quality of life. The middle ear, placed between the inner ear and eardrum, is in charge of transmitting sound during the assessment process thereof. For this reason, any dysfunction in the area can lead to symptoms such as sharp pains, pressure, or fullness. These feelings are often due to inflammation, infection, or fluid accumulation, which are known to change sound conduction and affect balance. The impact of such discomfort extends beyond hearing, encompassing activities of daily living, sleep disturbances, and mental states; therefore, in-depth evaluation and management are necessary to treat these painful symptoms. Secondly, otitis media, as a condition of sudden onset, demonstrates how middle ear disease can cause significant discomfort. This inflammation typically occurs after upper respiratory tract infections and is characterized by symptoms such as irritability, fever, and ear pain. Diagnosis typically involves a thorough examination by medical providers, who may also use diagnostic algorithms to determine the most appropriate interventions. Studies indicate that a substantial proportion of the population experiences these symptoms; thus, there is a need to identify acute attacks and perform early medical assessment.

Tinnitus, if it occurs alongside otitis media, further emphasizes the multifactorial nature of ear discomfort in that it may reflect a variety of conditions that may need to be dealt with on an urgent basis in order to avoid long-term morbidity and mortality risk, emphasizing the urgent requirement of effective and prompt management in such scenarios (Altissimi et al., 2016). In addition to infection, cerumen impaction is a common but often underrecognized cause of ear pain. As the ear normally secretes cerumen to protect against dirt and bacteria, excessive build-up will cause pain, hearing loss, and inflammation. Research indicates that approximately 4% of the population experience associated difficulties that must, in most cases, be treated. Primary care providers would typically assess this condition according to the SOAP (Subjective, Objective, Assessment, Plan) approach to maintain a methodical process that addresses the psychological and physical dimensions of discomfort. By understanding cerumen production and ear health, clinicians can develop appropriate management strategies to relieve symptoms and restore function, thereby playing a significant role in general ear care and the prevention of future complications from unresolved discomfort (Bickley et al., 2017) (Figure 4.10).

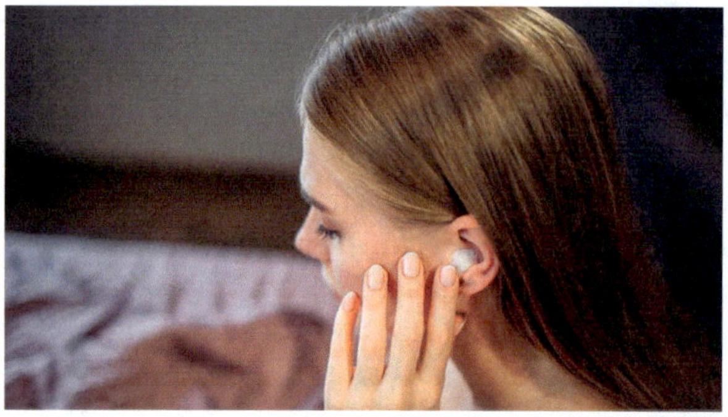

Figure 4.10. Ear pain and discomfort.

Source: https://external-content.duckduckgo.com/iu/?u=https%3A%2F%2Fwww.practostatic.com%2Ffit%2F32ff986e9e8f71ba00d681de0303a82de80456b3&f=1&nofb=1&ipt=a2416904b7656d91ace20045b4ac7ff3e61d82c3df282a9b16b9f98a5d29e689.

4.3.3. Fluid Drainage from the Ear

DRAINAGE OF THE EAR FLUID is a crucial topic in diagnosing and managing middle ear disease, particularly in otitis media. It refers to the accumulation of fluid in the middle ear, most often caused by infections, allergies, or upper respiratory tract infections. Fluid buildup may lead to changes in pressure and infection, causing pain and discomfort and, in some cases, hearing loss. Understanding the etiology of fluid drainage is crucial to treatment success. For instance, allergic rhinitis, as reported, is associated with a higher prevalence of ear disorders; therefore, assessing allergic conditions among patients with ear fluid accumulation is crucial (Hardjojo et al., 2012). The interaction between environmental factors, such as infections and allergens, can complicate the presentation of ear disorders and interfere with healing, necessitating detailed clinical evaluation. Diagnosis of drainage of fluid normally calls for a detailed history and assessment of presenting symptoms. Instruments like tympanometry and otoscopy are usually employed by medical professionals to assess whether fluid is behind the tympanic membrane or not. Where fluid is persistent, referral for further imaging studies, for example, A coronal CT scan, may be warranted to ascertain the gravity and nature of the problem (Kaur, A., & Singh, A., 2013). Careful examination of concomitant symptoms, including sinusitis, can provide insight into underlying conditions that exacerbate ear drainage.

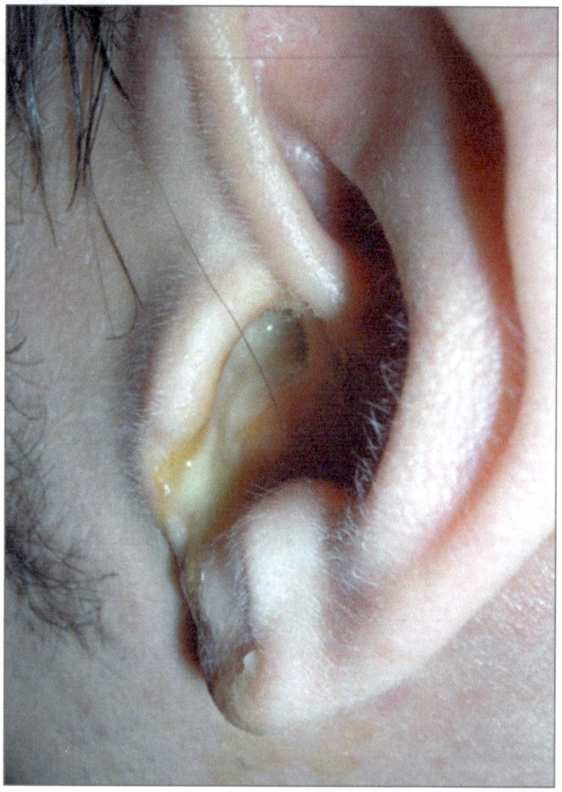

Figure 4.11. Fluid drainage from the ear.

Source: https://external-content.duckduckgo.com/iu/?u=https%3A%2F%2Fcdn.mdedge.com%2Ffiles%2Fs3fs-public%2FImage%2FSeptember-2017%2FRTEmagicC_PRF_101113.jpg.jpg&f=1&nofb=1&ipt=c9f0d47f93112511aa2e79babf167840322fac73cc292cbf3979ac0f0b6dbee4.

Moreover, the patients can also manifest with other rhizogenic symptoms such as nasal discharge and facial pain, which may overshadow the primary ear disorder. Therefore, multidisciplinary management using various diagnostic options is vital for appropriate diagnosis and effective management of ear fluid drainage. Therapeutic modalities for fluid drainage are primarily aimed at managing causes rather than treating symptoms. In otitis media acuta, antibiotic treatment may be necessary when a bacterial infection is suspected; however, in chronic conditions, the condition can be treated operatively by means such as implanting tympanostomy tubes to enable continuous drainage. Operative treatment may be most beneficial in children, who are particularly prone to recurrent middle ear infections due to their anatomical development (Hardjojo et al., 2012). Moreover, airway management by treating comorbidities—such as allergic rhinitis—has been shown to reduce the incidence of drainage complications and improve patients' overall health. Public education in prevention and the importance of early intervention can also play a significant role in reducing the incidence of such complications of fluid drainage from the ear (Figure 4.11).

Test Your Knowledge

1. What are the common symptoms of middle ear disorders? Describe ear pain, hearing loss, ear discharge, fever, and aural fullness, and explain their clinical significance.
2. Explain how symptoms differ between acute otitis media, otitis media with effusion, and chronic suppurative otitis media.

4.4. Diagnosis of Middle Ear Disorders

Learning Outcome

1. Physical Examination Techniques
2. Audiological Assessments
3. Imaging Studies

In otolaryngology, the diagnosis of middle ear disorders must be approached in a three-dimensional manner, using clinical evaluation, imaging, and audiometry. A complete patient history is initially required, as it highlights hearing loss, ear pain, and recurrent infection as key symptoms. This is particularly necessary for diagnoses such as otitis media, which remains prevalent among children. Comprehensive physical examinations, including otoscopic examinations, enable clinicians to visualize the tympanic membrane and identify abnormalities, such as fluid accumulation or perforations. Last but not least, early diagnosis not only allows for proper treatment but also minimizes the likelihood of associated complications, especially in high-risk populations such as children and individuals with developmental disorders, as seen in recent research highlighting the relationship between recurrent otitis media and language delay in children with Down Syndrome (Tenenbaum et al., 2025). High-technology imaging techniques, such as computed tomography (CT) scanning and magnetic resonance imaging (MRI), are valuable diagnostic tools in middle ear disease, particularly in complex cases where other methods may be insufficient. Cholesteatoma, a destructive bone lesion with potentially severe implications, generally requires meticulous imaging to assess disease extension into the middle ear and surrounding structures. Research has shown that early detection of complications of intracranial or extracranial cholesteatoma can significantly improve patient outcomes (Li et al., 2025). Audiometric tests are also important for determining the extent and nature of hearing loss, providing information that guides treatment (Li et al., 2025). These tests enable differentiation between conductive hearing loss, adopt specific management strategies depending on the cause of the condition. The prolonged diagnostic workup for middle ear disease often highlights the benefits of interprofessional collaboration among healthcare providers. Otorhinolaryngologists work alongside audiologists, speech therapists, and, when the case is complicated, neurosurgeons to develop a comprehensive treatment plan that addresses not only the patient's immediate medical needs but also the long-term developmental impacts.

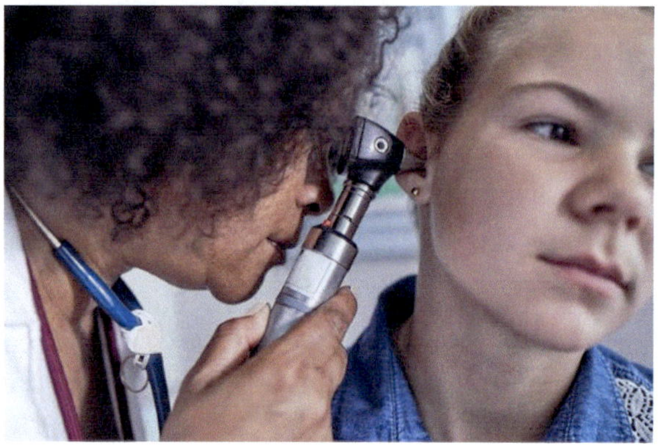

Figure 4.12. Diagnosis of middle ear disorders.

Source: https://external-content.duckduckgo.com/iu/?u=https%3A%2F%2Fedge.sitecorecloud.io%2Fmmanual-ssq1ci05%2Fmedia%2Fhome%2Fimages%2Ff%2F0%2F2%2Ff0253972-pediatrician-examining-ear-patient-spl-sized.jpg%3Fmw%3D2048%26thn%3D0%26sc_lang%3Den&f=1&nofb=1&ipt=a61c16442effd407553968e18fa00a235835c18e02f71f00818e4fbe24a9da86.

Particularly in children, where disorders of the middle ear significantly affect speech and language development, early intervention is essential. The integration of regular screening and examination into pediatrics has the potential to enable early identification of middle ear disease and prevention of associated complications such as conductive hearing loss and developmental delay, as identified in a study involving children with Down Syndrome (Tenenbaum et al., 2025). Through collaboration, healthcare professionals can enable patients to receive quality care that is best suited to improving their well-being and health (Figure 4.12).

4.4.1. Physical Examination Techniques

The physical examination technique used in the evaluation of middle ear disease focuses on establishing a diagnosis and developing treatment plans. One primary method of doing this is through otoscopic examination, which allows clinicians to view the outer ear canal and tympanic membrane (TM). Visual inspection can detect inflammation, perforation, or irregular fluid volumes characteristic of diseases such as otitis media. The technique of performing otoscopy is an essential skill, particularly in children, where middle ear disease is prevalent, as it guides the clinician in detecting abnormalities that may require treatment. As common as the middle ear disorders are in children with developmental issues, regular assessments by otorhinolaryngologists can guarantee early intervention and even avert future complications such as speech and language delay, thus demonstrating the value of detailed physical examination techniques in this group (Tenenbaum et al., 2025). In addition to otoscopy, audiometric testing is a crucial component of the physical examination for middle ear disorders. These tests typically involve pure-tone audiometry and tympanometry, which evaluate the functional integrity of the auditory apparatus. Pure-tone audiometry measures hearing sensitivity so that conductive hearing loss that is typically associated with middle ear effusion (MEE) or tympanic membrane perforation (TMP) can be detected. Tympanometry builds on this by measuring the compliance of the TM in response to changes in air pressure in the ear canal, a parameter that can indicate middle-ear fluid or stiffness. New technology, such as Wideband absorbance (WBA) tympanometry, provides a better prognosis with greater diagnostic precision by producing a consistent pattern to differentiate between varying middle ear disorders and is a valuable addition to the clinician's armory (Karuppannan et al., 2024). Lastly, the application of meticulous physical examination techniques on assessing middle ear disease and improve patient outcomes. Physicians' knowledge of the nuances of traditional and new examination methods is critical to accurate diagnosis of middle ear disorders. The ability to differentiate between middle ear disorders such as MEE and TMP using new parameters not only enables early and effective therapy but also reduces complications from undiagnosed hearing issues, including speech and language developmental delays. Focus on constant and systematic examinations, especially in risk groups such as children, illustrates the preventive capacity of proper physical examination techniques in preventing sequelae of long duration and therefore significance in otorhinolaryngologic practice (Karuppannan et al., 2024; Tenenbaum et al., 2025).

4.4.2. Audiological Assessments

The diagnosis of middle ear disease largely relies on audiological examination, which provides critical information about hearing function and auditory pathway pathology. The audiological test typically includes pure-tone audiometry, tympanometry, and auditory evoked potentials, each with a specific role in detecting middle ear pathologies. Pure-tone audiometry detects an individual's ability to perceive different frequencies and serves as the basis for conductive or sensorineural hearing loss. Tympanometry does, though, quantify middle ear pressure and tympanic membrane movement and allows audiologists to identify if fluid is building up or blockages are present. Both procedures, when combined, enhance diagnostic accuracy, thereby enabling individualized therapeutic interventions that specifically address dysfunctions within the middle ear. With advances in objective testing technologies, including the auditory steady-state response (ASSR), the discipline of audiological testing has undergone a significant transformation. ASSR is a method that provides more consistent information on auditory thresholds in uncooperative or otherwise problematic patient groups when tested using conventional methods. Research has demonstrated the feasibility of deriving clinically useful stopping rules for ASSR recording, enabling objective testing within a reasonable time without sacrificing accuracy. In a comparative study involving data for normal-hearing and hearing-impaired subjects, proposed stopping rules yielded comparable threshold estimates to standard multiple-ASSR studies, which implies that audiological testing with this procedure can successfully identify middle ear disease-associated hearing impairment. These developments underscore the need to use multiple assessment strategies to improve clinical outcomes. Furthermore, the implications of audiological assessment extend beyond transient diagnosis, encompassing long-term auditory status and adaptation interventions. Universal newborn hearing screening (UNHS) for the identification of permanent childhood hearing impairment (PCHI), for instance, underscores the need for early audiological evaluation in cases of middle ear dysfunction. Longitudinal analyses indicate that confirmation of PCHI at 9 months of age is associated with better reading comprehension in later childhood and adolescence. Such correlation underscores the need for early audiological testing to improve educational performance, further underscoring the necessity of early resolution of middle ear disorders. By incorporating these results into clinical interventions, health care professionals can promote improved auditory and general cognitive development in affected groups, underscoring the importance of audiological evaluations in the effective management of middle ear disorders.

4.4.3. Imaging Studies

Imaging studies have a critical function in the accurate diagnosis and management of middle ear conditions, especially in differentiating between conditions such as middle ear effusion (MEE) and tympanic membrane perforation (TMP). Routine tests, including immittance tests, are generally less than optimal in providing crisp differentiation of these conditions, and this can have implications for the treatment plan. Recent advances in imaging methods, particularly wideband absorbance (WBA) tympanometry, have demonstrated strong promise for ear condition classification based on individual WBA patterns. Research indicates that WBA can efficiently identify middle ear disorders through comprehensive analysis of absorbance patterns across frequencies, thereby enhancing diagnostic accuracy and enabling appropriate clinical treatment for affected individuals (Karuppannan et al., 2024). Additionally, imaging studies have revolutionized the treatment of middle ear cholesteatoma, a benign but debilitating disorder characterized by the accumulation of skin cells in the middle ear. CT is most commonly used as the first imaging modality for preoperative evaluation because it provides critical information on anatomical involvement and potential erosive complications of cholesteatoma. Visualization of bone structure and soft tissue may enable surgeons to plan precise surgical procedures, thereby minimizing risk and improving outcomes. Additionally, MRI plays an increasingly important role in postoperative imaging to search for residual disease in surgical candidates. This new imaging paradigm reduces the need for routine "second-look" procedures, thereby maximizing patient treatment and resource utilization (Touska et al., 2024). The availability of both CT and MRI in the diagnostic armamentarium enables physicians to circumvent most of the pitfalls of routine clinical evaluation of middle ear disease. As a case in point, the introduction of non-echoplanar DWI sequences, in particular, has markedly improved detection sensitivity for residual cholesteatoma, thereby informing patient follow-up protocols after surgery. These advancements underscore the relevance of modern imaging techniques for improving patient outcomes through earlier and more accurate diagnoses. Ongoing research on imaging not only enables the detection and treatment of middle ear disease but also advances understanding of the complex pathophysiological mechanisms involved, informing clinical practice and future research (Touska et al., 2024).

Test Your Knowledge

1. Describe the clinical methods used in diagnosing middle ear disorders, including history taking, otoscopic examination, tympanometry, and audiometric evaluation.
2. Explain the role of imaging techniques and laboratory investigations in confirming the diagnosis and assessing complications of middle ear diseases.

4.5. Treatment Options for Middle Ear Disorders

Learning Outcome

1. Medical Management
2. Surgical Interventions
3. Home Care and Preventive Measures

Treatment of middle ear disorders varies with the nature and severity of the disorder. Otitis media is among the most prevalent conditions and is managed by both medical and surgical interventions. Bacterial infection would be treated with antibiotics, while pain resulting from the condition can be alleviated with analgesics. Where drainage is continuous, myringotomy can be performed, inserting a tympanostomy tube to permit drainage and ventilation of the middle ear. Not merely symptomatic relief, it can also be preventative against chronic infection, significantly enhancing the patient's quality of life. Such rigorous management is especially crucial in children, whose recurrent otitis media may permanently affect hearing and speech, underscoring the necessity of effective, early treatment of middle ear disease. In addition to conventional therapeutic regimens, newer therapies have been investigated to control the complications of middle ear disease. Recent studies highlight the possible application of corticosteroids in the management of immune-mediated inner ear disease that may result in conductive hearing loss (Adelchi et al., 2018). In individuals presenting with symptoms indicative of autoimmune disease, the addition of immunotherapy to standard treatments can enhance overall prognosis. In addition, there is a greater awareness of psychological elements that go along with disorders such as Musical Ear Syndrome, where auditory hallucinations are added to the clinical presentation (Pestel et al., 2017). With the inclusion of multidisciplinary care practices involving audiologists, speech-language pathologists, and mental health professionals, providers can better meet the complex needs of individuals with these disorders. Long-term management plans for middle ear disorders must also address prevention and education. Follow-up consultations with medical specialists at regular intervals can monitor hearing status and identify any emerging complications early. Prevention of respiratory infections, such as influenza and pneumococcal infection, considerably reduces the frequency of otitis media. the signs and symptoms of ear infection can lead to early medical attention, thus avoiding any lasting effects. Nutritional supplements, particularly in populations with established deficiencies affecting immune function, are also important for preventing middle ear disease. A comprehensive, patient-centered approach that integrates medical management, education, and prevention is essential for effectively controlling middle ear disease.

4.5.1. Medical Management

Effective medical management of middle ear disease depends on an in-depth understanding of the multiple conditions that involve this anatomical site. Each disease, such as otitis media, eustachian tube dysfunction, and tinnitus, necessitates not just diagnostic expertise but also a treatment plan oriented towards the underlying pathology. For instance, otitis media, which is prevalent among children, may be treated with antibiotic therapy if bacterial infection is suspected, with close observation for complications. Decongestants or nasal corticosteroids can treat eustachian tube dysfunction, with the underlying cause addressed to restore middle ear function. Given the variety of possible disorders, tailored medical management is essential, as it can significantly influence patient outcomes by accelerating recovery and improving quality of life. The prominence of tinnitus as a symptom of middle ear disorders underscores the importance of integrated medical management strategies. Studies suggest that as many as

7% of individuals with tinnitus present for medical care, typically due to a change in their perception of hearing or an acute exacerbation of chronic conditions (Altissimi et al., 2016). Since severe tinnitus can be accompanied by frequent psychiatric comorbidities, physicians need to address not only the auditory but also the psychological needs. This combined approach can reduce the morbidity that accompanies tinnitus and contain associated risks like depression and anxiety, which can complicate the recovery process. The medical treatment of tinnitus and its attendant disorders thus necessitates the integration of audiological and psychological interventions, underscoring the need for a comprehensive treatment model. Furthermore, recognition of Auditory Processing Disorder (APD) underscores the importance of personalized medical management for middle ear dysfunction (Bamiou et al., 2017). APD imposes itself on individuals who might have average hearing acuity but processing deficits that have consequences for their communication abilities and overall psychosocial well-being. Effective medical management should thus involve rigorous diagnostic testing to distinguish APD from related auditory disorders. Treatment. At diagnosis, treatment may include auditory training, speech therapy, and environmental adaptations to improve functioning in natural communication environments. With ongoing research, establishing APD management protocols will become increasingly critical to bridge the gap between hearing perception and effective management. To this end, continuous investigation of the features of auditory processing can ultimately result in better therapeutic outcomes for patients with middle ear disorders.

4.5.2. Surgical Interventions

Surgical intervention is a crucial component of the management of middle ear disorders, particularly when non-surgical interventions do not provide relief or restore hearing. Perforation of the tympanic membrane and chronic otitis media, among other common disorders, will typically demand surgical intervention such as mastoidectomy or tympanoplasty. Surgical interventions aim to re-establish the tympanic membrane and remove infected tissue, thereby improving hearing and preventing recurrent infection. By employing advanced techniques, surgeons can enhance the quality of therapy for such disabled patients. Furthermore, the decision to perform surgical procedures must be guided by thorough clinical evaluations, with attention to each patient's needs and clinical history to optimize therapeutic outcomes. In addition to traditional interventions, emerging surgical techniques and technologies are enhancing treatment efficacy for middle ear pathology. Improved endoscopic surgery, for instance, allows less traumatic access to the middle ear with less trauma to the surrounding tissues, promoting quicker recovery. The use of 3D imaging and navigation devices also enhances the precision of such procedures, which is particularly beneficial in complex cases with anatomical variation. Additionally, the use of multidisciplinary teams as part of the surgical procedure, including audiologists and rehabilitation specialists, provides an all-encompassing approach to patient care. This coordination can assist not only in ensuring appropriate support for patients throughout the surgical procedure but also throughout their recovery and rehabilitation, ultimately improving overall health outcomes and well-being. Surgical procedures are also comparable to issues regarding systemic conditions that may affect persons with middle ear disorders. In congenital disorders, such as Apert syndrome, surgical intervention is a multidisciplinary process that targets functional and cosmetic problems (Caporlingua et al., 2015). In patients with mucopolysaccharidosis type IVA, surgical intervention must be based on the multidimensional nature of the condition (Akyol et al., 2019). Under these circumstances, there is a need for collaborative efforts among various healthcare professionals to design customized treatment regimens that minimize the risk of surgery, particularly anesthetic-related complications. Ultimately, by integrating advanced care methodologies and sophisticated surgical techniques, healthcare providers can enhance the efficacy of surgical interventions in patients with complex middle ear pathology.

4.5.3. Home Care and Preventive Measures

Management of middle ear conditions often extends beyond clinical care to include appropriate home care practices. Individuals with conditions such as otitis media should take extra precautions to ensure proper ear hygiene to avoid complications. Wiping the outer ear daily helps keep it free of wax and debris, which can cause infection. Application of warm compresses to the offending ear also ensures that pain is relieved and swelling is minimized. However, individuals should avoid inserting objects into the ear canal, as this can cause injury or complicate existing conditions. These measures form the foundation of home care, which prevents recurrent infections and facilitates accelerated recovery in patients with middle ear disorders. Identifying early symptoms associated with middle ear disorders is important for patient self-management. Ear pain, ear pulling, infection, and hearing loss should be addressed immediately to prevent further exacerbation of the condition. Home care practices involving the monitoring of such symptoms can have significant implications for the process of infection. Moreover, patients must be aware of the risk factors for ear disorders, such as exposure to smoke or allergens. Air purifiers and maintaining a smoke-free environment can serve as preventive measures to reduce the risk of middle ear disorders among susceptible patients, particularly children. This precaution can reduce the incidence and severity of middle ear disorders, thereby improving quality of life among affected individuals. In addition to the daily preventive regimen, parents and caregivers should ensure routine medical checkups to monitor ear health, particularly among children at risk of middle ear disorders. Continuous monitoring will more likely detect impending problems at their earliest stages before they become more complex to treat. Pairing vaccinations, such as the pneumococcal conjugate vaccine, with preventive actions also enhances protection against ear infections caused by bacterial pathogens. Education regarding these practices has been shown to significantly reduce the incidence of middle ear disorders in populations, highlighting the need for public health campaigns to raise awareness and disseminate knowledge. Thus, combining home care techniques with medical management constitutes an integrative system of prevention required for the efficient management of middle ear disorders (MacLean et al., 1957; Okoye et al., 2013).

Test Your Knowledge

1. Describe the medical and surgical treatment options for common middle ear disorders such as acute otitis media, otitis media with effusion, and chronic suppurative otitis media.
2. Explain the role of antibiotics, analgesics, ear drops, and surgical procedures (e.g., myringotomy, grommet insertion, and tympanoplasty) in the effective management of middle ear diseases.

SUMMARY

The study of middle ear disease raises the intricate relationship among anatomy, physiology, and the manifestation of auditory dysfunction. The middle ear is an important pathway for sound transmission, and any hindrance in this region can lead to crippling hearing disabilities and compromise general communication ability. Findings from certain studies provide evidence that early diagnosis and treatment are vital for managing diseases such as otitis media, eustachian tube dysfunction, and other conditions. As emphasized by recent studies, the auditory steady-state response (ASSR) technique, in addition to enhancing the accuracy of hearing threshold measurement, underscores the importance of formulating effective stopping criteria for precise evaluation. These developments in auditory diagnostics are vital to ensuring that individuals with hearing loss receive appropriate interventions tailored to their needs, thereby improving their quality of life. Also, therapeutic management for middle ear diseases has been greatly enhanced by a better understanding of their pathophysiology. Rehabilitation is typically provided in medical and surgical forms, which must be tailored to the individual patient profiles. Evidence currently available indicates that somatic tinnitus, particularly in patients with hyperacusis, requires differential management plans to improve symptoms appreciably. Studies have shown that hyperacusis-exhibiting patients with somatic tinnitus are more irritated and exhibit larger modulation rates for tinnitus, and therefore, a fine comprehension of their cases is required. Resolution of such complexities by personalized auditory therapy and education can be effective in optimizing treatment outcomes and mitigating middle ear disorder-related issues. Lastly, continued research is necessary for the ongoing improvement of best practices in the diagnosis and management of middle ear disorders. The marriage of novel technologies, namely the ASSR method, is paving the way toward more objective assessments that can be provided effectively across diverse populations, such as adults and children. Furthermore, awareness of the interrelationship between hyperacusis and somatic tinnitus underscores the need for interdisciplinary treatment modalities that account for psychological, acoustic, and physiological factors, as well as auditory well-being. Collectively, these results not only contribute to the theory of middle ear disorders but also endorse patient care in clinical practice. By promoting a thorough insight into these disorders, clinicians can ensure that the patients are provided with the most optimal and appropriate care following their individual needs.

Middle ear disease encompasses a cluster of disorders that significantly affect auditory function and global quality of life. The most prevalent condition is acute otitis media (AOM), particularly in children, which is chiefly characterized by heightened pain and discomfort. Even though antibiotics are the most commonly prescribed medications, studies document their limited capacity to alleviate pain in the first few days of treatment, thereby prompting the evaluation of other treatments such as systemic corticosteroids. The potential for such anti-inflammatory medicines, both in monotherapy and in combination with antibiotics, to act as therapeutics has been observed in recent research, although their effectiveness remains uncertain due to the poor quality of much of the current evidence (Beller et al., 2018). Hence, awareness of such implications and treatment shortcomings is highly significant for clinical practitioners treating middle ear conditions. Another integral part of middle ear disorders is the audiological assessment and its complexity. Audiologists often rely on behavioral tests to determine hearing thresholds, but more refined techniques, such as the auditory steady-state response (ASSR), have incorporated objective measures into clinical protocols. The application of ASSR is beneficial in limiting subjectivity in determining how to terminate recordings. Research has further identified stopping rules that optimize recording efficiency, yielding accurate threshold estimates within a reasonable time for healthy and hearing-impaired adults (D'Haenens et al., 2009). This innovation underscores the variability of auditory testing and the need for ongoing validation of testing methods to improve outcomes for patients with middle ear disorders. Lastly, the dynamic interaction between treatment approaches for middle ear disorders and advances in audio testing is a critical area of study. Despite advances in treatment, the multifactorial nature of AOM and other middle ear disorders necessitates an integrated approach that integrates medicine and sound diagnostic techniques. The need for further research into the long-term efficacy of systemic corticosteroids in the treatment of AOM provides a robust line of inquiry. These findings reveal that, although treatment is continually evolving, the core aim has not changed: improving patients' quality of life through effective symptom control and the best possible treatment (D'Haenens et al., 2009; Beller et al., 2018). Lastly, the deep insight into these disorders not only contributes to the practice in clinics but also to the ongoing debate about new solutions in the audiology practice.

KEY TERMS FROM THIS CHAPTER

Otitis Media
Chronic Otitis Media
Glue Ear
Eustachian Tube Dysfunction
Mastoiditis
Hemotympanum
Ossicular Discontinuity
Conductive Hearing Loss
Retraction Pocket
Acute Otitis Media
Otitis Media with Effusion
Tympanic Membrane Perforation
Cholesteatoma
Barotrauma
Tympanosclerosis
Otosclerosis
Aural Polyp
Adhesive Otitis Media

CRITICAL THINKING QUESTIONS

1. **The most common cause of acute otitis media is:**
   a) Viral infection
   b) Bacterial infection
   c) Fungal infection
   d) Allergic reaction
2. **The commonest organism causing acute otitis media is:**
   a) Staphylococcus aureus
   b) Streptococcus pneumoniae
   c) Pseudomonas aeruginosa
   d) Escherichia coli
3. **Glue ear is also known as:**
   a) Acute otitis media
   b) Chronic otitis media
   c) Otitis media with effusion
   d) Barotrauma
4. **The most common symptom of acute otitis media is:**
   a) Vertigo
   b) Ear discharge
   c) Ear pain
   d) Hearing loss
5. **Retraction of tympanic membrane occurs due to:**
   a) Increased middle ear pressure
   b) Decreased middle ear pressure
   c) Infection of inner ear
   d) Wax impaction

Short Answer Questions

1. What are the common disorders of the middle ear, and how are they classified?
2. Define acute otitis media (AOM) and describe its causes, clinical features, and complications.
3. Explain otitis media with effusion (OME) and its pathophysiology.
4. What is chronic suppurative otitis media (CSOM)? Differentiate between its tubotympanic and atticoantral types.
5. Describe the signs, symptoms, and complications of middle ear infections.
6. Explain the role of tympanometry and audiometry in diagnosing middle ear disorders.
7. Describe the pathogenesis, features, and complications of cholesteatoma.
8. Discuss the medical and surgical management options for middle ear disorders.

Answers to Critical Thinking Questions

1. (b) 2. (b) 3. (c) 4. (c) 5. (b)

REFERENCES

1. Woronowicz, K. C., & Schneider, R. A. (2019). Molecular and cellular mechanisms underlying the evolution of form and function in the amniote jaw. *EvoDevo, 10*(1), 17. https://doi.org/10.1186/s13227-019-0131-8Adelchi, C., Croce, A., D'Aguanno, V., De Vincentiis, M., De Virgilio, A., et al. (2018). *Audio-Vestibular Symptoms in Systemic Autoimmune Diseases.* https://core.ac.uk/download/188823057.pdf (accessed on 7th August 2025).
2. Akyol, M. U., Alden, T. D., Amartino, H., Ashworth, J., et al. (2019). *Recommendations for the management of MPS IVA: Systematic evidence- and consensus-based guidance.* https://core.ac.uk/download/323075225.pdf (accessed on 7th August 2025).
3. Altissimi, G., Attanasio, G., Cianfrone, G., De Vincentiis, M., et al. (2017). *Characteristics of somatic tinnitus patients with and without hyperacusis.* https://core.ac.uk/download/141695127.pdf (accessed on 7th August 2025).
4. Altissimi, G., Cianfrone, G., Ciofalo, A., Greco, A., et al. (2016). *When Alarm Bells Ring: Emergency Tinnitus.* https://core.ac.uk/download/54538689.pdf (accessed on 7th August 2025).
5. Apisa, P., Caruso, A. A., Cesari, U., Formisano, L., et al. (2017). *Role of Laryngopharyngeal Reflux in Eustachian tube Dysfunction in Adults.* https://core.ac.uk/download/80340755.pdf (accessed on 7th August 2025).
6. Bamiou, D. E., Barajas, J., Brechmann, A., Callimachou, A., et al. (2017). *A European perspective on auditory processing disorder—Current knowledge and future research focus.* https://core.ac.uk/download/144472883.pdf (accessed on 7th August 2025).
7. Baycheva, S., Konsulov, S., Milkov, M., Stoykov, S., et al. (2022). *History of the World Hearing Day.* https://core.ac.uk/download/539160243.pdf (accessed on 7th August 2025).
8. Beller, E. M., Del Mar, C. B., Pitoyo, Y., Ranakusuma, A., et al. (2018). *Systemic Corticosteroids for Acute Otitis Media in Children.* https://core.ac.uk/download/196606193.pdf (accessed on 7th August 2025).
9. Bickley, L. S., Douglas, G., Harkin, H., Nursing and Midwifery Council, Rodgers, R. W., et al. (2017). *Ear Care: An Update for Nurses (Part 1).* https://core.ac.uk/download/151172584.pdf (accessed on 7th August 2025).
10. Blythe, H. I., Kennedy, C. R., Kreppner, J., Mahon, M., et al. (2016). *The impact of universal newborn hearing screening on long-term literacy outcomes: A prospective cohort study.* https://core.ac.uk/download/228158961.pdf (accessed on 7th August 2025).
11. Bowman, A. W., Katina, S., O'Tuathaigh, C. M. P., Waddington, J. L., et al. (2017). *Translational genetic modelling of 3D craniofacial dysmorphology: Elaborating the facial phenotype of neurodevelopmental disorders through the prism of schizophrenia.* https://core.ac.uk/download/132211200.pdf (accessed on 7th August 2025).
12. Caporlingua, A., Di Giorgio, G., Fadda, M. T., Ierardo, G., et al. (2015). *Treatment Timing and Multidisciplinary Approach in Apert Syndrome.* https://core.ac.uk/download/54520953.pdf (accessed on 7th August 2025).
13. Deshpande, S., & Chhotala, D. (2023). Inner ear anomalies on HRCT and MR imaging of the temporal bone in children with sensorineural hearing loss. *International Journal of Science and Research (IJSR).* https://www.semanticscholar.org/paper/4cc52d2584859a66b4aea12d2b7699995a47ae6e (accessed on 7th August 2025).

14. D'Haenens, W., Dhooge, I., & Vinck, B. (2009). *Determination and evaluation of clinically efficient stopping criteria for the multiple auditory steady-state response technique.* https://core.ac.uk/download/55824629.pdf (accessed on 7th August 2025).

15. Di Stadio, A., & Ralli, M. (2017). *Systemic lupus erythematosus and hearing disorders: Literature review and meta-analysis of clinical and temporal bone findings.* https://core.ac.uk/download/98349075.pdf (accessed on 7th August 2025).

16. Fukunaga, J. Y., Gil, D., & Makibara, R. R. (2010). *Eustachian Tube Function in Adults with Intact Tympanic Membrane.* https://core.ac.uk/download/37709135.pdf (accessed on 7th August 2025).

17. Guo, M. H., Cai, J. X., Liu, Z. N., Mu, T. J., Martin, R. R., & Hu, S. M. (2021). PCT: Point cloud transformer. *Computational Visual Media, 7*, 187–199. https://doi.org/10.1007/s41095-021-0229-5.

18. Hardjojo, A., Shedden, A., Stuck, A., Cruz, A. A., Stevenson, A. N., Chauhan, B., Engel-Yeger, B., et al. (2012). *Allergic rhinitis and its associated co-morbidities at Bugando Medical Centre in northwestern Tanzania: A prospective review of 190 cases.* https://core.ac.uk/download/pdf/11307799.pdf (accessed on 7th August 2025).

19. Karuppannan, A., Barman, A., & Mamatha, N. (2024). Wideband absorbance pattern and its diagnostic value in adults with middle ear effusions and tympanic membrane perforation. *The Journal of International Advanced Otology, 20*, 158–163. https://www.semanticscholar.org/paper/802570b81c30b5706b0f67b4fcc9e6bafc2d816c (accessed on 7th August 2025).

20. Kaur, A., & Singh, A. (2013). *Headache—a Sinonasal Symptom and More... A Review Article.* https://core.ac.uk/download/201677922.pdf (accessed on 7th August 2025).

21. LeCouteur, R. A., & Vernau, K. M. (1999). *Feline Vestibular Disorders. Part II: Diagnostic Approach and Differential Diagnosis.* https://core.ac.uk/download/323068734.pdf (accessed on 7th August 2025).

22. Li, H., Zhu, X., Wang, L., Zhang, Y., Li, L., Wang, P., & Ye, F. (2025). Clinical data analysis of patients with middle ear cholesteatoma diagnosed with intracranial and extracranial complications as the first diagnosis. *Journal of Clinical Otorhinolaryngology Head and Neck Surgery, 39*(6), 548–552. https://www.semanticscholar.org/paper/30e171a2405e5ed92b95b1b7e583aec0b0e7699a (accessed on 7th August 2025).

23. MacLean, D. M., & Rice, V. R. (1957). *A Planned Program of Study and Guidance for Parents of Acoustically Handicapped Children.* https://open.bu.edu/bitstream/2144/24481/1/MacLean_Doris_et_al_1957_web.pdf (accessed on 7th August 2025).

24. Mulwafu, W. (2020). *Integration of ear and hearing care into primary health care in Malawi with special reference to task-sharing.* https://core.ac.uk/download/479079365.pdf (accessed on 7th August 2025).

25. Murray, C. J. L., Ikuta, K. S., Sharara, F., Swetschinski, L. R., Robles Aguilar, G., Gray, A. P., Han, C., et al. (2022). Global burden of bacterial antimicrobial resistance in 2019: A systematic analysis. *The Lancet, 399*, 629–655. https://doi.org/10.1016/s0140-6736(21)02724-0.

26. N/A. (2025). *Aerospace Medicine and Biology: A Continuing Bibliography with Indexes, Supplement 144.* https://core.ac.uk/download/pdf/42887122.pdf (accessed on 7th August 2025).

27. Nola, G., Ralli, G., Ralli, M., Sparvoli, L., et al. (2017). *Unilateral Enlarged Vestibular Aqueduct Syndrome and Bilateral Endolymphatic Hydrops.* https://core.ac.uk/download/98349074.pdf (accessed on 7th August 2025).

28. Okoye, B. C., Bugando Medical Centre (BMC), Trunkey, D., Kang, E. G., Orji, F. T., Matilda, I., et al. (2013). *Ear, nose, and throat injuries at Bugando Medical Centre in northwestern Tanzania: A five-year prospective review of 456 cases.* https://core.ac.uk/download/pdf/11307767.pdf (accessed on 7th August 2025).

29. Pereira, V., & Sell, D. (2023). How differences in anatomy and physiology, and other aetiologies affect the way we label and describe speech in individuals with cleft lip and palate. *International Journal of Language & Communication Disorders.* https://www.semanticscholar.org/paper/0798da623379abb9d028de7492da0d4e8bc57d96.

30. Pestel, C. D. (2017). *Musical Ear Syndrome: What Do We Know?* https://core.ac.uk/download/84120862.pdf (accessed on 7th August 2025).

31. Sismanis, A., Martin, D. W., Venkatraman, G., Brookes, G. B., Owen, H. H., Kemppainen, H. O., Farrior, J., et al. (2006). *Cholesteatoma of the external ear canal: Etiological factors, symptoms, and clinical findings in a series of 48 cases.* https://core.ac.uk/download/pdf/7517631.pdf (accessed on 7th August 2025).

32. Tenenbaum, A., Ben Yaakov, A., Peled, Y., Cohen-Cymberknoh, M., Averbuch, D., Brodie, R., & Gross, M. (2025). Middle ear disorders in children with Down syndrome: The detrimental effect on speech and language development. *Children, 12.* https://www.semanticscholar.org/paper/4bf8a6c4f11fb5d6ea9a5130481b279b72cefdb3 (accessed on 7th August 2025).

33. Touska, P., & Connor, S. (2024). ESR essentials: Imaging of middle ear cholesteatoma—Practice recommendations by the European Society of Head and Neck Radiology. *European Radiology, 35,* 2053–2064. https://www.semanticscholar.org/paper/b06880b885ca9f726a7ab5caba29286ea6b685c0 (accessed on 7th August 2025).

INNER EAR AND VESTIBULAR DISORDERS

5

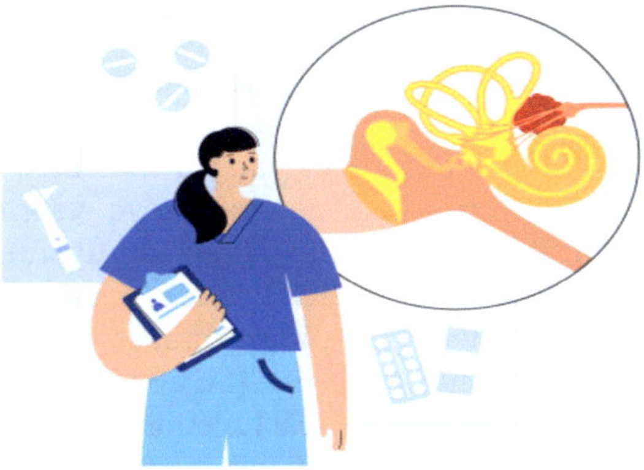

LEARNING OBJECTIVES

After studying this chapter, you will be able to:

1. Common inner ear disorders.
2. Symptoms of vestibular disorders.
3. Diagnosis of inner ear disorders.
4. Treatment options.
5. Impact on quality of life.

Introduction

The inner ear is involved in the function of maintaining balance and processing sound and is thus of utmost significance to the overall sense function. It comprises numerous structures, including the cochlea, which is involved in hearing, and the vestibular system, which contributes to balance. Inner ear and vestibular disorders have the potential to produce severely incapacitating symptoms such as vertigo, hearing loss, and tinnitus, severely impacting an individual's quality of life. Current studies have also highlighted the importance of examining these disorders in the context of broader health conditions, as they are often manifestations of underlying diseases. Vestibular disorders are a heterogenous collection of diseases, one of the most prevalent of which is vestibular migraine, which often presents as vertigo and dizziness as well as headaches. The disorder demonstrates the complex relationship between migraines and vestibular function, a relationship too frequently underestimated in clinical practice. Prevalence of vestibular migraine highlights increased sensitivity and appropriate diagnostic criteria due to the prevalence of misdiagnosis among affected populations (N/A, 2019). Vestibular migraine's ambiguous overlapping similarities with other diseases, such as Meniere's disease or transient ischemic attacks, pose challenges to the diagnostic and treatment landscape. Therefore, effective treatment of these conditions requires a multidisciplinary approach, supported by comprehensive patient history and examination, to enable early intervention. Understanding of the pathophysiology of inner ear and vestibular illnesses guides more precise research and clinical practice improvement. The intricate mechanisms underlying the development of vestibular migraine and the effect of systemic illness issues must be thoroughly explored. Recent meta-analyses have begun to illuminate the connection between singling out auditory and vestibular symptoms and broader health trends. For instance, studies reporting high rates of dizziness among COVID-19 patients underscore the need for further research to examine the potential long-term effects of these conditions on the vestibular system (Jafari et al., 2021). Not only does this search aid clinicians in helping more appropriately, but it also empowers patients by improving education regarding their illnesses, and consequently results in holistic treatment strategies.

Definition of the Inner Ear

The inner ear is a complex anatomical structure used in hearing and equilibrium. Comprising the cochlea, vestibule, and semicircular canals, the inner ear translates sound vibrations into nervous system signals as well as maintains the bodys equilibrium responses. The cochlea, which is spiral-shaped, is responsible for translating sound waves into electrical signals in the auditory system. Compared with that, the vestibular apparatus, that is, the vestibule and semicircular canals, senses head motion and position with respect to gravity, maintaining balance and spatial orientation. This dual functionality underscores the central role of the inner ear in sensory processing, making it the primary focus of research on most vestibular disorders. Additionally, pathologies of the inner ear have a significant impact on its normal functioning, leading to various vestibular disorders. Bilateral vestibulopathy (BVP), for example, has a defective vestibulo-ocular reflex (VOR) as its characteristic, required to sustain constant vision upon movement. Diagnosis of BVP involves careful assessment with patient history, laboratory testing, and bedside examination to determine the extent of vestibular dysfunction. Diagnostic standards must have reference values based on measures of VOR, so that a VOR gain of less than 0.6 at the higher frequency ranges indicates severe impairment. These diagnostic techniques identify how specific inner-ear dysfunctions can exert substantial effects on balance, thereby causing conditions that severely impact patients' quality of life (Strupp et al., 2017). Beyond its physiological functions, technological advancement has enhanced understanding of inner ear diseases. High-resolution computed tomography (HRCT) has been an invaluable tool for diagnosing acquired cochleo-vestibular conditions that are not readily detected by routine assessments. HRCT, with its enhanced focus, has highlighted labyrinthine dehiscences and other congenital structural abnormalities that can cause vestibular dysfunction. With advancing literature, the integration of HRCT findings into clinical practice is playing a substantial role for otologists in establishing accurate diagnoses. Knowledge of imaging in the diagnosis of inner ear disease not only enhances the quality of patient care but also advances research on the complexities of vestibular diseases (Pirodda et al., 2017).

Importance of the Vestibular System

The vestibular system, located in the inner ear, is in charge of balance and spatial location. It functions within a complex system of structures that detect head motion and gravity, enabling an individual to perceive their position in space. This intricate system not only maintains physical equilibrium but also helps keep the brain's functions in order. Vestibular system impairment can lead to significant disturbances that affect activities of daily living. In research conducted among 86 patients diagnosed with vestibular disorders, it was noted that 82.55% of subjects failed balance tests, indicating the widespread impact of these disorders on mobility and balance (Majeed et al., 2023). These revelations underscore the importance of considering the vestibular system's role in maintaining quality of life, as interference with it can severely debilitate individuals, particularly the elderly. Moreover, the vestibular system's contribution is much greater than mere balance; it is tightly coupled with cognitive processes, particularly spatial memory and navigation. The literature indicates that aging-related vestibular impairment is associated with deficits in spatial cognitive abilities, which are critical for daily navigation and situation awareness. Cognitive loss is particularly prevalent among older adults, who are often accompanied by concomitant vestibular impairment as well as cognitive loss, such as mild cognitive impairment and Alzheimer's disease (Agrawal et al., 2019). The common ground between vestibular health and cognitive status serves to highlight the importance of comprehensive testing that addresses both balance and neurological function. Vestibular disorder treatment not only aids physical stability but also helps to maintain cognitive health, thereby contributing to improved overall well-being in older adults. The impact of vestibular disorders is particularly undesirable from the viewpoint of their relationship to falls, one of the leading major health risks, especially in older adults. Falls can lead to serious injuries, loss of independence, and increased medical costs. The findings of the aforementioned research indicate that nearly one-fifth of participants in the study group reported a history of falls, and a substantial proportion reported varying degrees of vertigo (Majeed et al., 2023). This harmful trend requires early diagnosis and individualized interventions to regain vestibular functioning. Effective treatment strategies, including physical therapy exercises designed to promote vestibular recovery, can significantly reduce the risk of falls. The creation of a multidisciplinary management plan that addresses both physical and cognitive health can thus play a key role in enhancing the quality of life of individuals at risk of vestibular dysfunction and its sequelae (Figure 5.1).

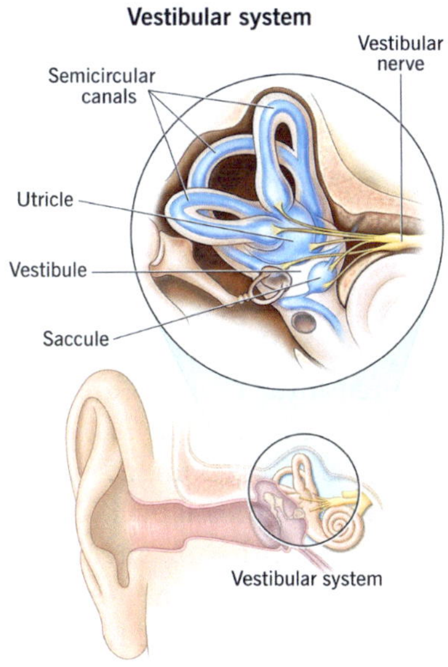

Figure 5.1. The vestibular system.

Source: https://my.clevelandclinic.org/-/scassets/images/org/health/articles/vestibular-system.

Overview of Vestibular Disorders

Vestibular disorders are a broad range of conditions that generally most frequently impact balance and orientation in space due to the disorder of the vestibular system located within the inner ear. Vestibular disorders can be demonstrated through signs and symptoms of vertigo, dizziness, imbalance, and sometimes hearing impairment. Understanding the anatomy and physiology of the vestibular system is crucial, as it involves complex structures, including the semicircular canals and the otolith organs, that respond to gravity and rotation. Because these structures are responsible for the body's balance and coordination, any derangement through inflammation, infection, or autoimmunity will result in serious symptoms. Among vestibular illnesses, Benign Paroxysmal Positional Vertigo (BPPV) is the most common, with brief episodes of dizziness triggered by head movements, underscoring the intimate connection between inner-ear function and vestibular health. Moreover, the pathogenesis of vestibular illnesses is multifactorial, as it is often driven by combined environmental, genetic, and pathological stimuli. For instance, autoimmune inner ear disease (AIED) is an uncommon yet significant disorder in which the immune system targets inner ear structures, resulting in progressive sensorineural hearing loss and concomitant vestibular symptoms such as vertigo and tinnitus. Based on recent reports, diagnosis of AIED might be particularly challenging due to the nonspecific nature of its symptomatology and the absence of distinctive biomarkers, necessitating meticulous clinical evaluation to exclude other causes of hearing loss. This multifaceted nature emphasizes the need for individually tailored diagnostic and treatment strategies, with immunosuppressive therapy used as a routine first-line intervention to reverse immune-mediated effects and restore auditory function in affected patients (Wang et al., 2025). Cross-talk between vestibular disorders and concomitant diseases, such as allergic diseases, suggests the need for a greater understanding of the inner-ear mechanisms at work. The data have shown the occurrence of some inner ear disorders, including Ménière's disease and sudden sensorineural hearing loss, with increased prevalence in patients with allergic disorders. This correlation raises important questions regarding immunological interactions between the vestibular system and allergic processes. For instance, increased serum IgE levels in such patients suggest an immunmediated mechanism contributing to their vestibular symptoms. Investigation of these connections may not only elucidate the pathophysiology of vestibular disorders but also suggest new therapeutic regimens, such as desensitization techniques, to address both allergy and vestibular manifestations simultaneously (Zeng et al., 2024).

5.1. Common Inner Ear Disorders

Learning Outcome

1. Meniere's Disease
2. Vestibular Neuritis
3. Benign Paroxysmal Positional Vertigo (BPPV)

Inner ear disease encompasses a broad range of conditions that can severely affect an individual's auditory and vestibular functions. Among these, immune-mediated inner ear disease is characterized by its complex relationship with systemic autoimmune illness. Sensorineural hearing loss is the most common auditory manifestation of these illnesses and can present in various patterns, including sudden, progressive, or fluctuating loss. Bilateral and asymmetric symptom presentation is frequent, making diagnosis and treatment challenging. Notably, corticosteroid treatment usually has positive effects, significantly restoring hearing in most patients. Tinnitus and aural fullness can also mimic primary inner-ear disorders, such as Meniere's disease, underscoring the importance of accurate diagnosis. Thus, understanding the association between systemic autoimmune diseases and inner-ear deficiencies is essential for effective patient management and care (Adelchi et al., 2018). Another common inner-ear condition is enlarged vestibular aqueduct

(EVA) syndrome, typically diagnosed by its characteristic anatomy and associated auditory impairment. This birth defect is characterized by a vestibular aqueduct greater than 1.5 mm in diameter, which causes sensorineural hearing loss ranging from mild to severe. Vestibular symptoms are also prevalent and present as ranging from mild imbalance to severe vertigo attacks. Higher-resolution imaging technologies, such as high-resolution CT and MRI, have recently been reported to be very important for the successful diagnosis of EVA. Additionally, other forms of treatment, such as intratympanic corticosteroid infusion, have shown promise in improving hearing outcomes, particularly in cases of endolymphatic hydrops.

However, EVA interactions with other vestibular disorders require careful diagnostic methods to implement appropriate management strategies (Nola et al., 2017). Lastly, Meniere's disease is a prevalent disorder of inner ear disorders that is known for its episodic and debilitating symptoms. Characterized by recurrent vertiginous attacks, tinnitus, and variable hearing loss, Meniere's disease is caused by aberrant fluid formation within the inner ear, interfering with the primary functions of hearing and balance. The disease typically affects individuals during the most productive period of their lives, resulting in significant psychosocial consequences. Even though the exact etiology remains elusive to scientists, potential offenders may be genetic predisposition, environmental factors, or immune responses. Treatment is generally broadened to lifestyle modifications, diet, and pharmacotherapy to minimize the severity of symptoms during an attack. Additionally, investigations for more therapeutic regimens remain a beacon of hope for individuals with Meniere's disease, highlighting the importance of acquainting oneself with this complex inner ear disorder (Adelchi et al., 2018).

5.1.1. Meniere's Disease

Meniere's disease, with its episodic vertigo, tinnitus, hearing loss, and ear fullness, remains a significant problem in the field of vestibular disorders. The pathogenesis of the disorder is due to an abnormal accumulation of endolymphatic fluid in the inner ear, developing excess pressure in the vestibular system and cochlea. This fluid imbalance affects not only hearing but also the vestibular responses critical to balance. Pathophysiology of Meniere's disease has been shown to be multifactorial, with possible involvement of genetic, environmental, and autoimmune factors, according to research. Also, certain evidence establishes the presence of a relationship between Meniere's disease and certain allergic disorders; that is, immune system malfunction might be accountable for an increase in symptoms of the disorder, as in the case of reports on the role of allergic disease in affecting inner ear health (Zeng et al., 2024). Diagnosis of Meniere's disease is traditionally a total clinical evaluation, including careful patient history and audiometric testing to measure patterns of hearing loss. The challenge in diagnosing the disease is the overlap of its symptomatology with that of other vestibular disorders, which complicates the clinical presentation. Differential diagnosis is thus essential to rule out conditions like vestibular migraine or vestibular paroxysmia. Also, the episodic nature of the presentation of Meniere's symptoms can lead to patients presenting late for medical care, and as a consequence, deteriorating their global auditory and vestibular function. It is exceedingly necessary that doctors can diagnose the classic patterns of Menieres disease early on so that the patients can be provided with appropriate management modalities to alleviate their symptoms and improve their quality of life. Meniere's disease is treated by using an array of treatment methods that range from lifestyle adjustments, through medication, to surgery, depending on the degree of the disease and attack frequency. Low-salt dietary management is often recommended to help reduce fluid retention, thereby alleviating symptoms. Pharmacotherapy may include the use of diuretics and medications for vertigo attack control. In refractory or more severe situations, more invasive treatments such as endolymphatic sac decompression or vestibular nerve section may be attempted. There is also new evidence of autoimmune causes of Meniere's disease, with some studies proposing a potential role for immunosuppressive therapy in inflammatory conditions (Wang et al., 2025). With the growing understanding of Meniere's disease comes an increasing need for personalized treatment protocols that account for each patient's unique clinical profile and the correlation between vestibular function and overall state.

5.1.2. Vestibular Neuritis

Vestibular neuritis is an inner ear disease with vertigo of sudden onset produced by vestibular nerve inflammation. It is typically caused by a viral infection, and most patients report an antecedent upper respiratory tract infection. Inflammation disrupts the vestibular system's signaling, creating an unbalanced response in the brain's neural circuitry and leading to misinterpretation of spatial position and movement.

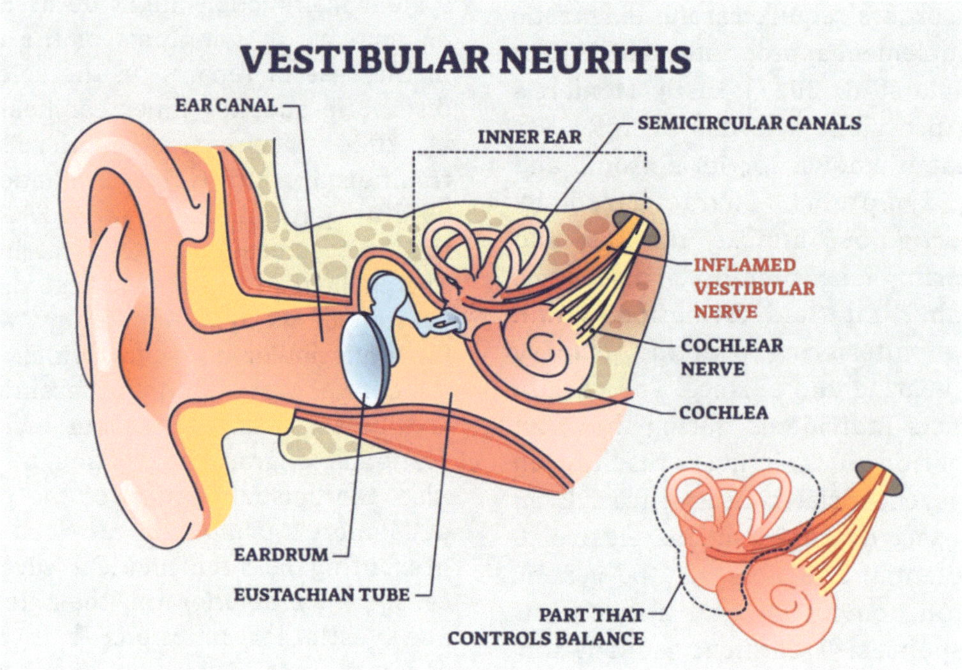

Figure 5.2. Vestibular neuritis is an inner ear disorder.

Source: https://www.thcp.co.uk/app/uploads/2025/01/vestibular-neuritis-diagram-ear.png.

Symptoms are also often characterized by severe spinning feelings, dizziness, and, in some cases, nausea, taking a serious toll on an individual's balance and coordination. Vestibular neuritis is not immediately life-threatening but significantly reduces quality of life, warranting in-depth study of its etiology and management protocols to optimize patient outcomes. Diagnosis of vestibular neuritis can be tricky in nature, as the condition tends to resemble other vestibular conditions.

Careful otologic examination, in conjunction with a complete patient history, is essential for successful diagnosis. A series of examinations, such as caloric testing or vestibular evoked myogenic potentials (VEMP), may be employed by clinicians to determine the integrity of the vestibular system. Early detection is essential for effective treatment, as early intervention may reduce symptom duration and severity. It may, in exceptional cases, present in concert with autoimmune inner ear disorders, making diagnosis and treatment more problematic. Definition of the specific etiology and pathogenic mechanisms of vestibular neuritis enables more targeted therapy, thereby maximizing the potential for recovery in affected patients. Treatment of vestibular neuritis is typically symptomatic and rehabilitative, with primary objectives including restoring balance and reducing vertigo. Corticosteroids are frequently employed to decrease inflammation in the vestibular nerve to improve the recovery periods. Vestibular rehabilitation therapy (VRT) is also a part of the management plan, and these exercises are particularly directed at helping compensate for vestibular loss. These treatments are intended to retrain the brain's capacity for deciphering sensory information related to balance and movement. Emerging studies are left to identify underscoring the evolving nature of this discipline. The use of multiple-faceted treatment modalities holds a great deal of promise to optimize patient recovery and minimize long-term disability with this disabling illness (Figure 5.2).

5.1.3. Benign Paroxysmal Positional Vertigo (BPPV)

Benign paroxysmal positional vertigo (BPPV) is a frequent vestibular disorder characterized by attacks of vertigo triggered by changes in head position. It results from the displacement of otoconia, minute calcium carbonate crystals, out of the utricle into the semicircular canals within the inner ear. The resulting disturbance with regular fluid movement within such canals could produce spurious signals to the brain regarding the position and motion of the body, inducing dizziness. BPPV occurs most commonly in elderly patients, but can occur after head trauma or otologic surgeries. Its clinical management requires knowledge of its pathogenesis, along with effective diagnostic techniques to distinguish it from other vestibular disorders, and underscores its implications for clinical practice and surgery (Kamal et al., 2025).

BPPV diagnosis is usually achieved by clinical testing that assesses for the presence of nystagmus—a swift eye motion reaction against a change in head position. The diagnosis and definition of nystagmus can be particularly challenging due to its variable presentation, including horizontal, vertical, and torsional components. Accurate identification of these movements is required for accurate diagnosis and subsequent management. Recent studies have shown that more sophisticated methods, like template matching methods, could potentially refine the examination of torsional nystagmus, which has been observed to be more intricate than other types of nystagmus in BPPV. As insights into these diagnostic hurdles advance, it becomes increasingly clear that early treatment and accurate diagnosis play a leading role in positive patient outcomes and recovery experiences (Dogru et al., 2024). Treatment of BPPV usually includes the use of specialized therapeutic maneuvers, like the *Epley maneuver*, which is intended for repositioning displaced crystals in the vestibular apparatus. Further, there is evidence to indicate that some oral and maxillofacial surgical procedures can incidentally cause BPPV, and thus, proper caution should be exercised on the part of health care professionals. Studies have identified a correlation between procedures such as ridge augmentation and TMJ surgery and subsequent BPPV diagnosis, suggesting underlying mechanisms involving mechanical stress or vibration on the vestibular apparatus. As clinicians gain greater awareness of how various dental and surgical procedures relate to vestibular disorders, interdisciplinary care integration is required to ensure optimal patient safety and minimize BPPV-related complications (Kamal et al., 2025).

Test Your Knowledge

1. Describe the anatomy of the nasal cavity, including its boundaries, blood supply, and nerve supply.
2. Explain the anatomical relations of the thyroid gland and recurrent laryngeal nerve.

5.2. Symptoms of Vestibular Disorders

Learning Outcome

1. Dizziness and Vertigo
2. Balance Issues
3. Nausea and Vomiting

The symptoms of vestibular disorders vary and can significantly impact a person's quality of life. Common presentations include vertigo, an illusory sense of movement or spinning, typically increased with head movement or a change in position. The feeling of disorientation may be accompanied by imbalance, which leads to difficulty with walking or standing. Many patients also report dizziness, a symptom that encompasses a wide range of sensations, from lightheadedness to unsteadiness. Tinnitus, or ear ringing, can further complicate these disturbances, providing additional distress and often occurring together with hearing loss. Identification of these symptoms is critical, as they may be associated with a number of underlying conditions, like autoimmune inner ear disorders that may lead to progressive sensorineural hearing loss and vertigo, as reported in literature (Wang et al., 2025). Moreover, the diagnostic pathway for vestibular disorders is particularly challenging given their nonspecific signs. The affected patients frequently mention episodes of vertigo or severe dizziness, at times for minutes but more frequently for hours, accompanied by resultant anxiety or panic attacks. The nature of the symptoms sometimes makes accurate diagnosis difficult, as many tests are conducted on numerous patients to identify the exact cause. Conditions such as Ménière's disease, acute low-tone hearing loss, and sudden sensorineural hearing loss have been associated with elevated immunological markers, including IgE, suggesting an immune-mediated component contributing to heightened vestibular symptoms. Thus, information on the interaction between immune responses and vestibular function is relevant to diagnosis and management (Zeng et al., 2024). Furthermore, the effects of vestibular disorders extend beyond somatic symptoms to influence psychological well-being and everyday functioning. Avoidance of movement or phobic responses to situations precipitating symptoms can have consequences for lifestyle that may cause social isolation and depression. The chronic status of vestibular neuritis or acoustic neuroma may lead to persistent trouble maintaining employment and social relationships. Early intervention methods, including vestibular rehabilitation therapy and cognitive-behavioral intervention, are essential to treating both physical and psychological implications of the disorders. By developing a comprehensive understanding of symptoms and broader contexts, medical professionals are best positioned to help individuals with vestibular disorders and to develop individualized treatment approaches (Figure 5.3).

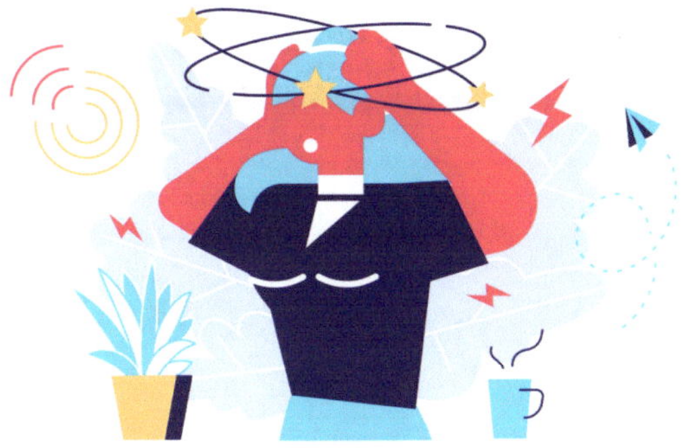

Figure 5.3. The symptoms of vestibular disorders.

Source: https://www.avcphysio.com.au/wp-content/uploads/2023/09/dizzy-scaled.jpeg.

5.2.1. Dizziness and Vertigo

Vertigo and dizziness are common symptoms in individuals with vestibular and inner-ear conditions, typically causing significant distress and functional impairment. Appreciation of the complexity of these conditions should involve discussion of their underlying mechanism. The vestibular system, consisting of major structures in the inner ear, is critical for balance and space orientation. When this system is disturbed—either by peripheral disorders, such as benign paroxysmal positional vertigo (BPPV), or by central disorders, such as vestibular migraines—patients typically present with spinning, lightheadedness, and unsteadiness. Extensive evaluation by otolaryngologists and neurologists is required because these symptoms may reflect multiple underlying pathologies. The multifactorial nature of dizziness calls for an integrated approach to diagnosis and management, underscoring the need for ongoing research to elucidate the therapeutic implications of these disorders (N/A, 2025). Recent studies have identified a wide range of etiologies for dizziness and vertigo, underscoring the need for accurate diagnostic criteria. A clinical cohort study determined benign paroxysmal positional vertigo to be the most common etiology, present in a high percentage of the patients in different age groups and genders. This is particularly notable because BPPV demonstrates how much even minor disturbances in the vestibular apparatus can create dominating symptoms. Vestibular migraine, another of the top causes of vertigo, was also highly gendered, with higher rates of prevalence among females. These other etiologies, such as primary unilateral peripheral vestibular dysfunction and psychogenic dizziness, add to the diagnostic pathway complexity. This diversity of etiological bases leads to multiple management pathways, depending on patient-specific factors, underscoring that a single pathway is insufficient for the treatment of dizziness and vertigo (Xing et al., 2024). Practitioners must place the utmost importance on an all-encompassing treatment approach that combines symptomatic relief with long-term management strategies for patients with dizziness and vertigo. Management may include vestibular rehabilitation exercises to improve balance and reduce motion sensitivity. Pharmacologic treatment, including the use of vestibular sedatives or migraine prophylactics, can also be an important part of symptom management. As the specialty of neurotology has advanced, greater emphasis is placed on the importance of an interdisciplinary model among specialists in providing comprehensive treatment to patients. It is also necessary to conduct patient education and counseling since patients feel anxious and frustrated as their symptoms are unreliable. Having a multidisciplinary team will enable healthcare practitioners to better meet the multifaceted needs of patients with vestibular disorders, thereby improving health outcomes and overall quality of life (N/A, 2025).

5.2.2. Balance Issues

Inner ear and vestibular disorders are one of the primary reasons for balance disorders, which tend to disrupt individuals quality of life and capacity to live normally. The vestibular mechanism, located in the inner ear, is used for balancing and spatial orientation. Dysfunction of the vestibular apparatus may be a cause of dizziness, vertigo, and unsteadiness, which occur commonly among individuals of all ages, including older adults and those with hearing impairment. Recent studies indicate that these symptoms are not merely single conditions but are also associated with sound processing and overall motor function. For example, children with hearing impairment often come with concomitant vestibular dysfunction, which may hinder their motor development and balance function.

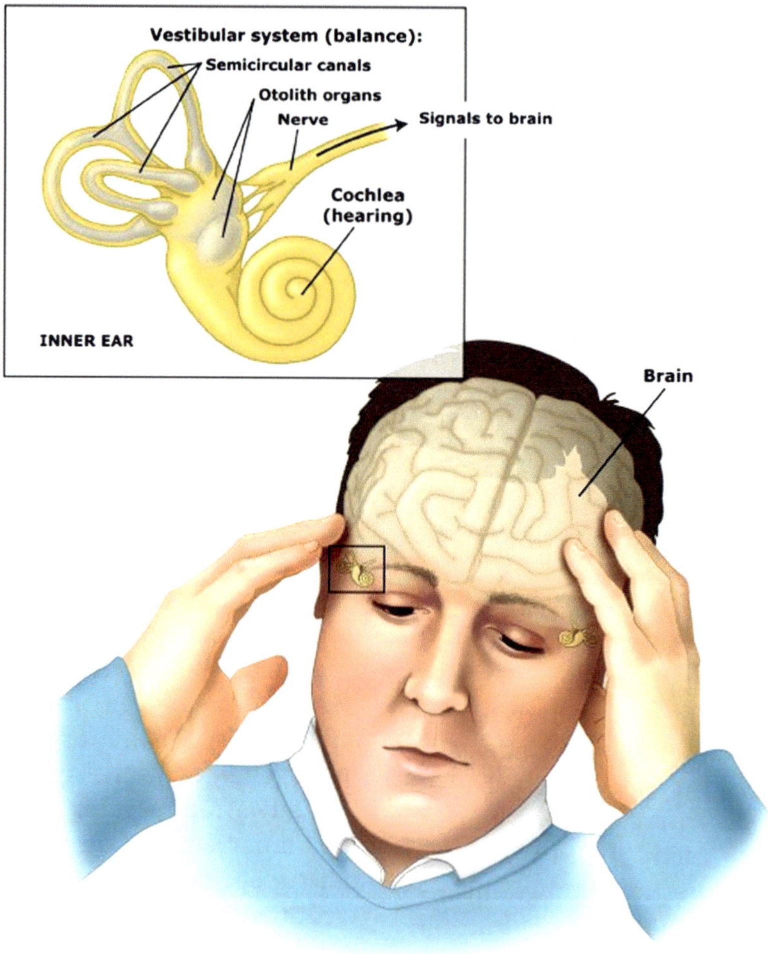

Figure 5.4. Balance issues are a significant consequence of inner ear and vestibular disorders.

Source: https://physiotherapyvictoria.ca/wp-content/uploads/2012/08/vestibular_system_pi.jpg.

This connection underscores the need for comprehensive evaluation of both auditory and vestibular functions to enable early intervention and coordinated care (Muzammil et al., 2025).

The prevalence of vestibular disorder-induced balance disturbances is particularly suggestive in specific groups, that is, deaf children. As per recent research, a high proportion of deaf children show vestibular dysfunction, and screening tests revealed 61.0% showed disturbance of balance in norm-referenced tests. The prevalence of disturbances highlights a critical gap in healthcare practice, given that balance assessment is seldom conducted in deaf children despite its significant developmental implications. Accurate detection of vestibular involvement can lead to rehabilitation methods tailored to enhance motor function and prevent secondary complications resulting from balance impairment. It also emphasizes the need for clinical practice recommendations that incorporate regular vestibular evaluation within pediatric populations predisposed to balance disorders to ensure that interventions are effective and timely (Muzammil et al., 2025). The relationship between hearing loss and balance disorders remains a complex area of investigation, with significant implications for treatment and diagnosis. Research indicates that distinct audiometric phenotypes correspond to distinct vestibular dysfunctions, suggesting that patients with balance disorders can be categorized according to their auditory profiles. This categorization offers a way toward tailored management protocols that address hearing loss and vestibular issues. For instance, studies have indicated that central pathologies are more likely to be linked with older patients with hearing loss, while others may have vestibular migraine or other balance conditions, irrespective of hearing impairment. Knowing these correlations enables a more differentiated treatment plan in which specific therapies can address auditory and balance challenges concurrently, thereby enhancing overall patient outcomes and quality of life (Figure 5.4).

5.2.3. Nausea and Vomiting

The nausea and vomiting experience is typically associated with several internal as well as external stimuli, particularly with inner ear and vestibular disorders. The inner ear is implicated in balance and space orientation, and malfunction of the system can cause significant sensory conflicts. Mechanisms such as vertigo exemplify this conflict in that patients may experience moving without actually moving, and subsequently, feel ill. Nausea is a visceral response to any vestibular system imbalance because the brain attempts to make sense of sensory input from visual, vestibular, and proprioceptive sources. This inconsistency has the potential to result in vomiting as a reflexed reaction, creating a cycle of distress that has the potential to seriously impact the quality of life of such patients. Accounting for the impact of vestibular disorders on the incidence of nausea and vomiting yields very important information regarding patient management strategies. Ménière's disease, vestibular neuritis, and bilateral vestibular loss have been found to trigger vestibular symptoms like severe dizziness and unsteadiness spells. These symptoms can escalate to severe nausea and vomiting, which can further worsen the patient's condition. The physiological rationale for this is overstimulation of vestibular pathways that input to the vomiting center in the brainstem. Treatment approaches typically involve pharmacologic reduction of underlying vestibular dysfunction, such as antiemetics that alleviate nausea and vomiting but do not address the underlying cause of vestibular disturbances. Research into autoimmune inner ear disease (AIED) has also clarified the association between vestibular impairment and nausea. Patients with AIED typically present with a syndrome of sensorineural hearing loss and other vestibular dysfunction, including vertigo and imbalance. The condition will provoke violent nausea due to the incongruity of input. In AIED, where complex immunological processes contribute to inner-ear damage, relief may be achieved through a successful treatment plan aimed at reducing immune function. Glucocorticoids and immunosuppressive therapy are generally employed to abate vestibular symptoms and to reduce inflammation. Thus, appropriate evaluation of vestibular disorder and the associated nausea and vomiting is important, pointing to an all-encompassing modus operandi of care that both engages the vestibular system and patient care, as tended to by Pérez-Fernández et al. (2023) and Wang et al. (2025).

Test Your Knowledge

1. What are the common symptoms of vestibular disorders? Explain how vertigo, dizziness, imbalance, and nausea affect a patient's daily activities.
2. Differentiate between peripheral and central vestibular disorder symptoms, giving examples of clinical features that help in diagnosis.

5.3. Diagnosis of Inner Ear Disorders

Learning Outcome

1. Clinical History and Physical Examination
2. Audiometric Testing
3. Imaging Studies (e.g., MRI, CT Scans)

Diagnosis of inner ear disease is a complex, multifaceted process that typically involves a synergy between clinical evaluation and advanced diagnostic technologies. Dizziness, a hallmark symptom of these diseases, often leads patients to consult multiple specialists before receiving an accurate diagnosis. Not only does this hinder timely access to proper treatment, but it also places enormous pressure on healthcare resources. To better distinguish conditions such as Ménière's disease, vestibular migraine, and benign paroxysmal positional vertigo, continuous ambulatory vestibular assessment (CAVA) trials have been developed. The trials aim to utilize wearable technology for collecting data on eye movements when people are dizzy, thus enhancing diagnostic accuracy and enabling intervention in a timely fashion. Early detection of certain conditions can significantly improve patient outcomes and reduce the burden on healthcare services, underscoring the need for novel diagnostic methods (Phillips et al., 2024). In recent years, research has more and more emphasized the multifaceted relationship between vestibular disorders and cognitive impairment. Patients with inner ear disease also tend to report not only bodily symptoms such as unsteadiness and vertigo but also cognitive impairments, particularly in attention, spatial memory, and executive function. From the clinician's point of view, in diagnosing these disorders, a detailed understanding of cognitive impact becomes extremely important. There does, however, seem to be a noteworthy deficiency in addressing the cognitive realms of vestibular disorders in clinical care. Through the inclusion of cognitive assessment in diagnosis, clinicians can apply a more comprehensive strategy that identifies the multidimensional characteristics of vestibular disorders. This comprehensive strategy is essential for developing effective treatment plans that integrate physical rehabilitation and cognitive therapy (Smith et al., 2024). Furthermore, interdisciplinary collaboration among audiologists, neurologists, psychologists, and other physicians is crucial for the diagnosis and treatment of inner ear disease. Available methods have evolved towards preferring this interdisciplinary environment to enable a more comprehensive approach to the knowledge of vestibular disease in relation to cognitive function. As practice guidelines evolve, clinicians are urged to keep abreast of new studies endeavoring to delineate the mechanistic substrates underlying vestibular-related cognitive dysfunctions. Such emphasis on collaboration not only promotes refinement of diagnostic criteria but also enables the development of individualized rehabilitation interventions targeted at both the vestibular and cognitive components of the disorders. These advancements will enhance patients' quality of care overall, providing an integrated view that improves their lives (Phillips et al., 2024; Smith et al., 2024) (Figure 5.5).

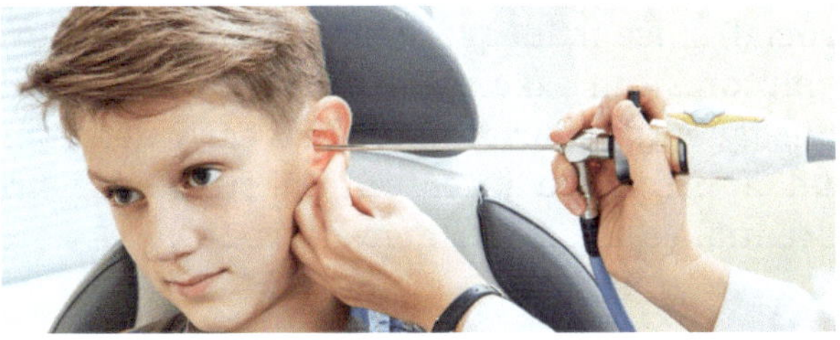

Figure 5.5 The diagnosis of inner ear disorders.

Source: https://www.harleystreetent.com/sites/default/files/field/image/What%20are%20the%20Symptoms%20of%20Inner%20Ear%20Problems.jpg.

5.3.1. Clinical History and Physical Examination

Detailed physical examination and a thorough clinical history are essential for the diagnosis of inner-ear and vestibular diseases. Not only does the clinical history assist in interpreting the patient's symptoms, but it also assists in differentiating various vestibular pathologies. Vertigo, dizziness, imbalance, and hearing disturbance typically require careful evaluation. For instance, an in-depth interview of the patient might clarify the nature of vertiginous attacks, their frequency and duration, and associated symptoms such as tinnitus or hearing loss. Additionally, examination of the patient's medical history can uncover previous conditions or trauma to the inner ear, which would be likely to exert a significant influence on presentation. Understanding these factors clarifies differential diagnoses and guides further investigation, resulting in a more effective management plan for the patient, particularly in complex situations involving auditory and vestibular loss (Zamora, E., & Zamora, C., 2025). In addition to clinical history, physical examination is a useful tool for evaluating vestibular function. Examination may reveal important signs that guide clinicians in diagnosing certain disorders. Core components of this evaluation include standardized tests such as the Romberg test, the Dix-Hallpike maneuver, and gait testing, which assist in distinguishing between central and peripheral vestibular disorders. Neurological testing may also determine concomitant disorders such as central nervous system lesions. Abnormal findings on the physical examination are often reproduced on imaging studies, enabling clinicians to make a more comprehensive diagnosis. This combination of clinical history, physical examination, and corresponding imaging ensures that the assessment of chronic conditions, acute syndromes, and etiologies is sequential and well informed (Xing et al., 2024). Synthesis of clinical history and physical examination findings is crucial for differentiating among various vestibular and inner-ear disorders. Illnesses like Benign Paroxysmal Positional Vertigo (BPPV) may have specific presentations involving precipitating circumstances and elicited symptoms on provocative maneuvers, whereas central vestibular diseases are usually less dramatic presentations in the form of atypical dizziness or neurological phenomena. Thus, clinicians can more effectively allocate resources by making selective diagnoses based on historical patterns and physical findings. Moreover, recognition of stable patterns facilitates pedagogic advancement in practitioners and enhances patient communication related to their illness and expected clinical courses. Finally, a better understanding of clinical history and physical examination leads to more accurate diagnoses and targeted therapeutic approaches in individuals afflicted with inner ear and vestibular disease (Xing et al., 2024; Zamora, E., & Zamora, C., 2025).

5.3.2. Audiometric Testing

Audiometry is a significant tool for assessing hearing impairment, particularly when used in the context of inner-ear and vestibular diseases. Audiometry is a form of testing that assesses various parameters of auditory function by measuring the individual's reaction to a sound stimulus at different frequencies and intensities. In patients with balance and hearing complaints, for example, those with AIED, audiometric measures can provide extremely valuable information regarding the functional status of the auditory and vestibular systems. The two systems are interdependent; once pathology occurs in one, it will usually affect the other. Notably, AIED is characterized by rapidly evolving bilateral neurosensorial hearing loss, complicating diagnosis since the symptoms may vary and therefore necessitate accurate audiometric tests to inform treatment and monitor disease progression (Bustos-Merlo et al., 2024). Audiometric testing is not only pertinent for diagnosis but also for clinical management and outcomes. Audiologic examination can show significant changes in hearing thresholds, providing the physician with the patient's full auditory picture. This is particularly significant in vestibular disorders, as compromised hearing can exacerbate dizziness and balance dysfunction. Some patterns of hearing loss on audiometry are recognizable and may be helpful in establishing causation and planning for therapeutic intervention towards enhancing the quality of life of the affected. Additionally, data from such tests may be vital for further studies on the correlation between vestibular dysfunction and audiometric findings, which are important for advancing knowledge in the area (Majeed et al., 2023). In particular, the addition of audiometric testing to the diagnostic workup of vestibular disorders can improve the diagnosis of autoimmune disorders of auditory function. For instance, the detection of antiphospholipid antibodies in patients with AIED not only underscores the autoimmune nature of the condition but also highlights the importance of specialized audiometric examination to assess prognosis and guide treatment. By employing a multidisciplinary approach that includes audiometric testing, clinicians can better understand how inner-ear diseases affect the vestibular apparatus and therefore treat both hearing and balance symptoms in affected patients. This is especially crucial, since inadequate management of these symptoms can exacerbate the risk of falls and, consequently, injuries; therefore, early detection and appropriate intervention strategies are essential (Bustos-Merlo et al., 2024).

5.3.3. Imaging Studies (e.g., MRI, CT Scans)

Imaging studies, particularly CT scans and MRIs, are of immense value in diagnosing and managing inner ear and vestibular disease. With these advanced imaging techniques, clinicians can visualize the inner ear's complex structures with high precision, enabling identification of congenital malformations, tumors, and other pathological conditions. For instance, conditions such as enlarged vestibular aqueduct (EVA) can be diagnosed using high-resolution CT, which defines the pathologic dilatation of the vestibular aqueduct. This is important because EVA is often associated with severe hearing loss and vestibular dysfunction, necessitating early and accurate diagnosis to implement effective therapeutic measures (Nola et al., 2017). Additionally, MRI enables assessment of soft-tissue structures and can detect diseases such as endolymphatic hydrops, providing a general overview of both the membranous and integumentary labyrinths. In clinical practice, the addition of imaging studies significantly contributes to the understanding of the anatomical and functional specifics of the inner ear, especially among patients with sensorineural hearing loss. MRI and CT scans not only assist in the diagnosis of these conditions but also inform treatment planning for procedures such as cochlear implantation.

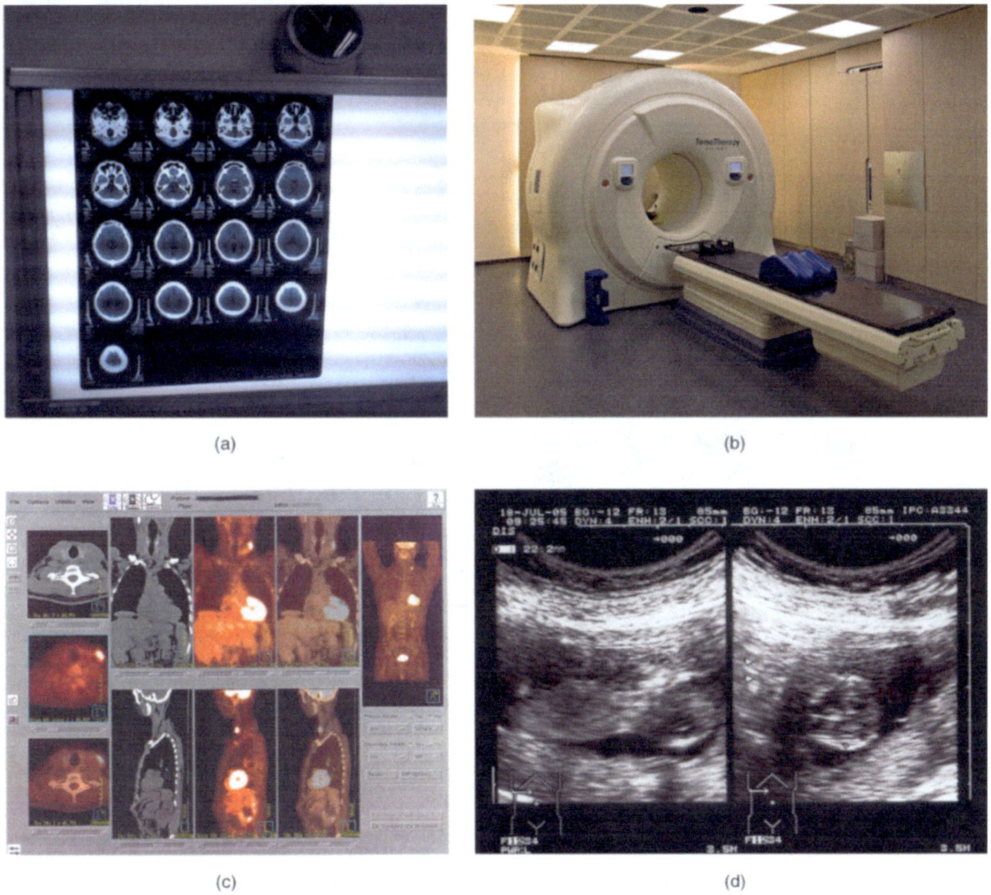

Figure 5.6. Imaging studies, particularly MRI and CT scans.

Source: https://s3-us-west-2.amazonaws.com/courses-images-archive-read-only/wp-content/uploads/sites/198/2014/10/20082407/113abcd_Medical_Imaging_Techniques.jpg.

Research indicates that imaging of anatomical abnormalities of the inner ear influences the performance of cochlear implants. In cases of ear deformity or brain abnormalities, visualization of these abnormalities with high-resolution imaging plays a major role in predicting surgical outcome and postoperative language function (Aimoni et al., 2015). Imaging studies are thus an essential component of the decision-making process for audiologists and otolaryngologists to obtain adequate knowledge of the individual patient's unique auditory system. Additionally, advances in imaging technology have improved diagnostic accuracy for inner-ear pathology. CT scans and MRI provide complementary information; while CT is capable of detecting bony pathology, MRI excels when detecting changes in soft tissues. With this method, physicians prevent the omission of important findings that could affect treatment outcomes. For example, the diagnosis of vestibular disorders such as endolymphatic hydrops by MRI can directly affect the choice of interventions, either medical therapy or rehabilitation. With the reality that the majority of vestibular disorder patients experience disabling symptoms with significantly impaired quality of life, urgent and accurate imaging is crucial in guiding effective management strategies and improving long-term outcomes. The convergence of these imaging modalities increasingly strengthens the association between diagnostic accuracy and therapeutic efficacy in the diagnosis and management of inner ear and vestibular diseases (Figure 5.6).

Test Your Knowledge

1. What are the main clinical methods used in the diagnosis of inner ear disorders? Describe the role of history taking, physical examination, audiological tests, and vestibular function tests.
2. Explain the importance of audiometry, tympanometry, and imaging techniques (CT and MRI) in diagnosing common inner ear disorders such as Ménière's disease, labyrinthitis, and acoustic neuroma.

5.4. Treatment Options

Learning Outcome

1. Medications for Symptom Relief
2. Vestibular Rehabilitation Therapy
3. Surgical Interventions

Vestibular and inner-ear disorders present a complex, multidimensional nature, given that their etiologies require specific, individualized therapeutic interventions. Immunosuppressive therapy is among the most promising treatments, particularly for conditions such as autoimmune inner ear disease (AIED). The disorder is characterized by immune-mediated injury that leads to sensorineural hearing loss, accompanied by vestibular manifestations such as vertigo and tinnitus. Treatment usually begins with glucocorticoids and is successful in around 70% of cases. When patients are resistant or partially responsive, physicians may use alternative medications, such as methotrexate or biologics that target inflammatory mediators, to improve outcomes. These personalized approaches are vital, as they emphasize the need to value the patient's own immunologic status, thus demanding tailored treatment regimens to permit optimal recovery and improved quality of life in such patients (Wang et al., 2025). Leaving the pharmacologic arena aside, recent advances have emphasized the role of vascular health in the management of inner ear disorders. Pericytes, which are integral to preserving microvascular integrity, have also faced scrutiny over their potential contribution to the pathophysiology of various inner ear diseases, including Meniere's disease and vestibular neuritis. Understanding pericytes' function can pave the way to new therapeutic strategies for enhancing blood supply and neuronal care in the microenvironment of the inner ears. Early research indicates that treatments targeting pericytes may trigger angiogenesis and provide trophic support that could reverse hearing loss and balance disorders. Therefore, developing pericyte-targeted therapies may represent a major breakthrough, transforming treatment paradigms and improving patient outcomes in a market traditionally characterized by limited options (Maniaci et al., 2024). Finally, the landscape of management of inner ear and vestibular disorders is evolving rapidly. It is a combination of standard immunosuppressive therapies, novel biologic therapies, and targeted therapies to promote vascular health. With an increase in treatment modalities, clinicians can manage the heterogeneity of these disorders better and maximize their treatment regimens and outcomes in those patients. Future studies will need to further elucidate the pathophysiology of these conditions, particularly the role of vascular components such as pericytes. Such an understanding will not only enhance current therapies but also drive the development of new treatments that can ultimately improve the quality of life of individuals with severe inner-ear and vestibular pathology (Maniaci et al., 2024; Wang et al., 2025).

5.4.1. Medications for Symptom Relief

The management of inner ear and vestibular disease usually involves drugs to improve symptoms of vertigo, nausea, and imbalance disturbances. These disturbances in balance, while they may significantly affect patients' quality of life, can be controlled with a variety of pharmacologic approaches. Antihistamines such as meclizine and dimenhydrinate are commonly used to suppress vertiginous sensations by blocking histamine receptors in the vestibular apparatus. In addition, drugs like prochlorperazine, which are antiemetics, are also employed to treat nausea and vomiting due to vestibular disorder. The drug generally relies on the specific disorder diagnosed, since different conditions may respond differently to different forms of treatment, further emphasizing the need to fully understand the underlying pathology when planning therapy. Where vestibular symptoms are linked to more complex interactions, such as those involving allergies and inner-ear disorders, symptom relief may require a multifaceted treatment approach. Examples include a systematic review that reported a correlation between allergic illness and conditions such as Ménière's disease and idiopathic sudden sensorineural hearing loss, in which overlapping symptoms in patients were observed. This cross-reactivity indicates that medications that target allergy symptoms, such as corticosteroids and antihistamines, may also alleviate inner-ear disturbance, particularly when accompanied by high serum IgE levels (Zeng et al., 2024). Treatment regimens should therefore be modified not only for the vestibular symptom but also for any superimposed allergic condition present among patients to maximize overall efficacy.

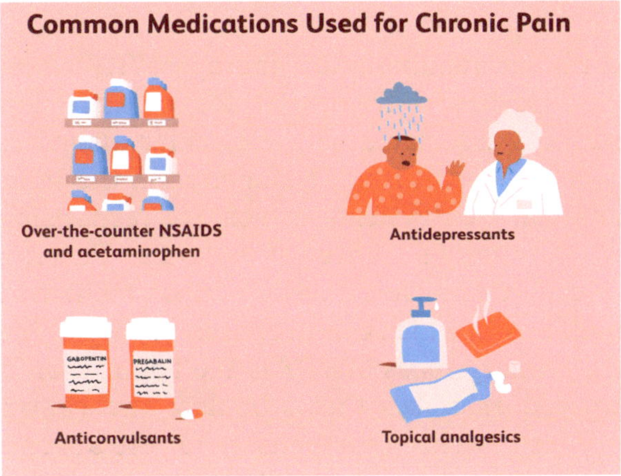

Figure 5.7. Medications for symptom relief.

Source: **https://www.verywellhealth.com/thmb/mLohaOeW2XPdSW0JeQpgMK3-TAw=/1500x0/filters:no_upscale():max_bytes(150000):strip_icc()/commonly-used-pain-medication-2564482_FINAL_V2-5c5dad1cc9e77c0001d92b06.png.**

In addition, ongoing research on the pathophysiology of disorders such as SSCD has the potential to uncover novel pharmacologic modalities to reduce symptoms. SSCD is characterized by excessive vestibular signs and symptoms, and studies indicate an appreciable incidence among patients with vestibular disorders (Tran et al., 2024). Whereas surgical treatment may be indicated for severe cases, medication can manage mild to moderate conditions by reducing acute dizziness and balance impairment. These measures could also complement vestibular rehabilitation therapy, which emphasizes a comprehensive treatment plan. With more knowledge, the union of targeted drugs with surgical or rehabilitative treatment may yield improved outcomes for patients suffering from the disabling effects of inner ear and vestibular disease (Figure 5.7).

5.4.2. Vestibular Rehabilitation Therapy

Vestibular rehabilitation therapy (VRT) is an evidence-based treatment for balance and dizziness associated with vestibular disorders. Disorders result from dysfunction in the inner ear's complex systems, which are responsible for the body's sense of balance. Patients typically demonstrate severe impairment with equilibrium, which compromises quality of life. The primary focus of VRT is the application of targeted exercises that stimulate the central nervous system to compensate for the absence of vestibular function. Through vestibular compensation mediated by adaptive mechanisms, patients can recover from symptoms such as vertigo and disequilibrium. Numerous studies support the use of individualized exercise programs, emphasizing the role of rehabilitation in promoting functional stability and improving patient outcomes. Drawing on recent advances in neuroplasticity, modern VRT methods emphasize multisensory integration as central to optimizing outcomes. The previous inclination towards habituation and adaptation procedures has given way to recognition that a broader set of methods can lead to improved recovery. More recent modalities, such as sensorimotor substitution, optokinetic stimulation, and cognitive-motor dual-tasking, have become essential components of contemporary rehabilitation programs. These techniques are not only for restoring balance but also for optimizing dynamic gaze stability, which is crucial for daily living. With increased advances in VRT, current research highlights that individually designed treatment protocols that meet the unique requirements of each patient are crucial to maximize functional outcomes and overall well-being. The clinical benefit of vestibular rehabilitation exceeds that of mere relief of symptoms, as evidenced by more recent studies linking vestibular dysfunction with broader health issues. For instance, vestibular disorders have been shown to be associated with increased risk of falls, social isolation, and psychological impacts such as depression and anxiety. By making a comprehensive VRT available beyond conventional methods, clinicians can provide more holistic patient care. Recent advances in gene therapy, including research on the ATP6V1B2 gene and its role in hearing and vestibular function, further suggest that genetic knowledge could enhance standard rehabilitation protocols (Wei et al., 2025). Hence, the future of vestibular rehabilitation will be based on a combination of established intervention strategies and innovative research, leading to more effective interventions and improved quality of life for patients with inner-ear and vestibular diseases (Tramontano et al., 2025).

5.4.3. Surgical Interventions

Surgical interventions for inner-ear disorders are critical components of the care and treatment of numerous vestibular disorders. A case in point is the way individuals manage patients with an enlarged vestibular aqueduct (EVA), a congenital defect that causes sensorineural hearing loss and vestibular dysfunction. Early diagnosis, commonly by multispiral computed tomography (MSCT), is important for preventing unnecessary surgery, which can cause additional complications, such as gusher syndrome. Surgery is typically reserved for severe hearing loss or when quality of life is significantly compromised due to severe vestibular impairment. Thus, the identification of the anatomical and functional effects of EVA not only guides effective surgical treatment but also underscores the importance of personalized treatment to avoid the risks associated with surgical intervention in the inner ear's thin structures (Astashchenko et al., 2024). SSCD is another common surgical procedure used to correct, which drastically alters vestibular function due to an additional movable window in the optic capsule. This condition is characterized by symptoms such as sound-induced dizziness, autophony, and balance dysfunction. The surgical procedures are aimed at sealing the defect and restoring normal pressure dynamics within the inner ear. Animal model studies have demonstrated that surgical fenestration effectively models the condition and contributes to understanding of vestibular function after surgery and recovery of balance. These studies recognize a reversible postoperative period of impairment, necessitating rigorous observation and rehabilitation. These connections between surgical procedures and outcomes underscore the need for greater familiarity with the complexity of the vestibular system when developing treatment plans (Hong et al., 2024). For inner-ear and vestibular system disorders, surgery must be performed with a high risk-to-benefit ratio. Some improve a great deal and have an improved quality of life after surgery, but others will experience complications or partial function recovery. Among the most crucial elements of surgical planning is thorough preoperative assessment through extensive testing to ensure that the underlying cause of the disorder has been accurately identified. The evolution of techniques to minimize invasiveness and maximize recovery supports the trend towards more comprehensive and individualized treatment modalities. Ultimately, ongoing study of the efficacy of these procedures is needed to streamline protocols and improve patient outcomes, such that the subtlety of inner ear disease is addressed with targeted, optimized interventions (Astashchenko et al., 2024; Hong et al., 2024) (Figure 5.8).

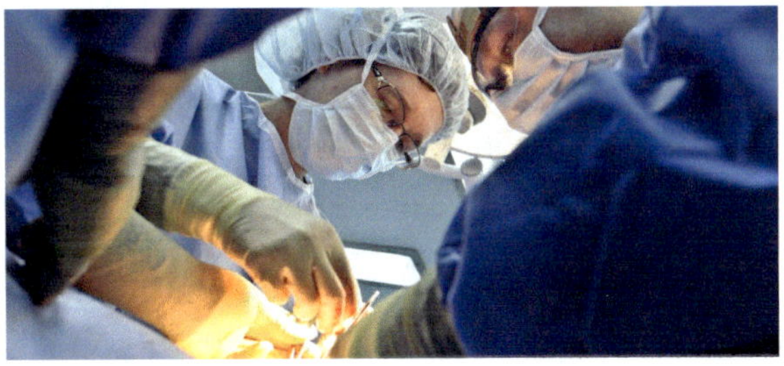

Figure 5.8. Surgical interventions for inner ear disorders.

Source: https://www.policyforum.net/wp-content/uploads/2015/06/v2.jpg.

Test Your Knowledge

1. What are the main treatment options for managing inner ear and vestibular disorders? Discuss the roles of medications, vestibular rehabilitation therapy, and lifestyle modifications.
2. Describe the commonly used medications for symptom relief in vestibular and inner ear disorders, including antiemetics, antihistamines, vestibular suppressants, and corticosteroids.

5.5. Impact on Quality of Life

Learning Outcome

1. Psychological Effects of Vestibular Disorders
2. Social Implications and Isolation
3. Coping Strategies for Patients

The impact of vestibular and inner ear disease on the quality of life in an individual is extreme and reaching. These conditions, such as Meniere's disease and vestibular neuritis, most often lead to debilitating symptoms like dizziness, imbalance, and hearing loss. These patients are thus left with issues that extend beyond the disease's physical impact. Emotional well-being is usually lost since the patient is more anxious and depressed due to the symptoms. The incapacitation that results in difficulties with daily living, social relations, and even the workplace feeds back into a significant loss of quality of life. As newer innovations in otoneurology improve diagnostic results, the need for early detection becomes crucial. Efficient and timely diagnoses will enable appropriate interventions, thereby mitigating the negative effects of these disorders on people's lives and restoring their ability to engage in daily activities. Understanding the basic pathophysiology of inner ear disorders is essential for devising effective treatments aimed at enhancing patients' quality of life. New studies reveal that pericytes, or vascular mural cells, are key to ensuring the integrity of the microvasculature of the inner ear. Not only does their presence have significant implications for diseases that cause hearing impairment and balance disturbances, but it may also exacerbate symptoms, as compromised vascular function can worsen these conditions. By elucidating the pathophysiology underlying these disorders, we can pave the way for novel therapies that target their underlying causes. The study of pericyte-targeting approaches not only offers hope for augmenting existing therapies but also opens up avenues for novel therapeutic interventions. These findings indicate that patients can experience significant symptom relief, which is associated with improved quality of life, allowing them to re-establish their positions in society and reduce feelings of isolation. Furthermore, the evolving landscape of treatment and diagnostic options underscores the importance of interdepartmental collaboration to enhance patient care. With advances in technology, such as imaging examinations and genetic testing, practitioners are better equipped to understand complex cases of inner ear diseases.

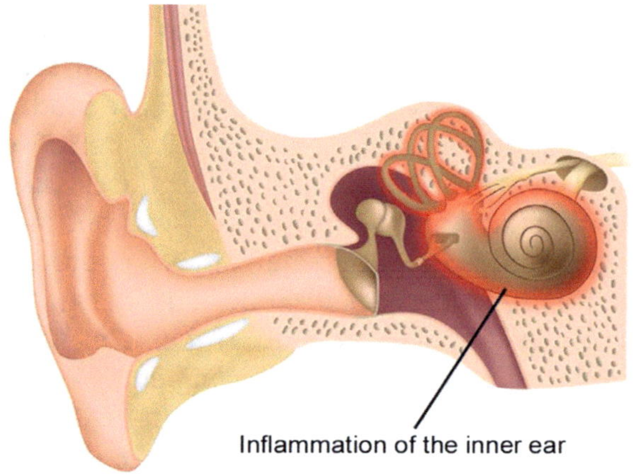

Figure 5.9. The impact of inner ear and vestibular disorders on an individual's quality of life.

Source: https://media.healthdirect.org.au/images/inline/original/labyrinthitis-illustration-80290b.jpg.

This enhanced understanding is translated into treatment regimens tailored to each patient's needs. These tailored interventions aim not only to reduce physical pain but also to address the psychosocial aspects of a patient's life. More support structures, including rehabilitation and counseling, are critical in addressing the patients' integral needs. As science learns more about the complexities of inner ear illness, a commitment to the integration of scientific inquiry with compassionate care will be paramount in promoting an enhanced quality of being for those afflicted with these crippling conditions, so that advances in treatment may have a meaningful and lasting impact on their daily lives (Figure 5.9).

5.5.1. Psychological Effects of Vestibular Disorders

Vestibular disorders exert a tremendous impact not only on patients' bodily functions but also on their psychological state. Patients report a wide range of psychological symptoms, including anxiety, depression, and social isolation. These states are a consequence of the inherent vagueness and variability of balance dysfunction, which can limit activities of daily living and reduce quality of life. Vestibular patients tend to complain of elevated levels of anxiety before attacks, which might set in motion a vicious cycle. By staying away from situations in which the symptoms tend to arise— for example, in public places or during social gatherings—their alienation and hopelessness can be exacerbated, further feeding their psychopathology. Thus, it is of primary importance to address psychological outcomes to support integrative patient care and underscores the necessity of integrative treatment that engages physical and psychological care. The connection between vestibular disorders and mental health has also been discussed in studies, which list the impact of chronic vestibular disorders like benign paroxysmal positional vertigo (BPPV) on emotional status. Research has indicated that individuals who have BPPV are more likely to report greater use of diuretics compared to individuals with no such conditions, which suggests an intrinsic relationship between vestibular symptom control and its broader implications (Li et al., 2025). The psychological impact of vestibular disorders can lead to a loss of mastery and self-esteem since patients have a hard time coping with symptoms that are unpredictable and disrupt their regular day-to-day activities. Thus, the lifestyle of suffering from such conditions demands not only medical treatment but also psychological support and coping. Interventions to improve patients' sense of control can contribute to better adjustment to illnesses and lower psychological distress. Moreover, vestibular disorders' interaction with psychological status is also expressed in conditions such as Restless Legs Syndrome (RLS), where patients report a substantial impairment in their quality of life induced by both physical and associated psychological discomfort. The Pearlin Mastery Scale provides a model for explaining mastery and control as potential mediators of the psychological effect of chronic illness, such as RLS, and thus demonstrates its relevance to vestibular disorders as well (Hellström et al., 2024). Improving patients' adaptive capacities may be an incredibly effective means of infusing resilience against the psychological effects of these disorders. Getting individuals engaged in emotional and cognitive skill-based therapeutic treatments may not only be helpful in symptom control but also in general mental health, and thus lead to a complete treatment strategy for vestibular disorders and their psychological effects.

5.5.2. Social Implications and Isolation

The symptoms of inner-ear and vestibular disorders have a profound impact on one's social life and participation in society. Conditions like Benign Paroxysmal Positional Vertigo (BPPV) and hearing impairment can make one feel insecure and vulnerable, thus withdrawing into one's shell and avoiding social interactions. Such withdrawal is usually due to the fear of an episode of dizziness or getting lost in public, which can be embarrassing as well as socially isolating. Since social interaction forms the foundation of human well-being, reduced participation can lead to isolation and psychological distress. Furthermore, this isolation may exacerbate the disorder itself, thereby creating a self-fulfilling prophecy in which the individual's condition may deteriorate due to a lack of social support and interaction. The social impact of vestibular disorders is made all the more difficult by the variability of the symptoms and their unpredictability. Patients with such conditions often find themselves not only grappling with physical limitations but also with misconceptions from their friends and family members. Such misconceptions could result from a lack of awareness about the intricacies involved with balance disorders, translating to less sympathy and support. In the vast majority of cases, patients who suffer from such disorders will find it impossible to verbalize their symptoms and only remain frustrated and lonely.

The impact of such disorders does not restrict itself to bodily symptomatology but seeps into emotional and psychological areas where patients are stigmatized and misunderstood. Raising awareness about vestibular disorders can contribute to building an accommodating environment and hence decreasing the social impacts of such diseases. Management and treatment of inner ear diseases, as per research, yield hopeful results in the enhancement of quality of life. Successful treatments not only alleviate the physical condition but also significantly enhance social interaction and mental status. The literature available currently indicates that intensive management programs can lead to spectacular improvement in the overall quality of life in hearing loss and BPPV patients. With the right interventions, patients also experience reduced anxiety concerning social interactions, and they are able to feel confident again. In this sense, the implementation of treatment practices highlighted in research is critical in addressing not only the physical states of the disorders but also their accompanying social consequences of loneliness. Whereas these aspects are given prominence by clinicians and support systems, a totalistic perception of treatment sets in and opens doors to constructive social change as well as better interpersonal relationships (Miller, 2011) (N/A) (Figure 5.10).

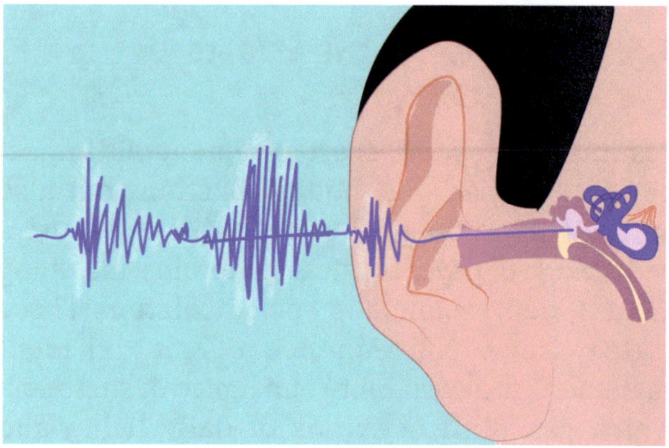

Figure 5.10. The experience of inner ear and vestibular disorders significantly affects an individual's social interactions and community engagement.

Source: https://creakyjoints.org//wp-content/uploads/0619_Hearing-Loss-and-Arthritis.jpg.

5.5.3. Coping Strategies for Patients

Symptoms of inner ear and vestibular pathology often produce severe psychological distress and therefore warrant addressing with coping skills to enhance the quality of life of patients. Cognitive-behavioral therapy (CBT) has been an effective therapy for reducing anxiety and depression, which are common comorbid conditions associated with tinnitus and dizziness, among others. CBT is helpful by altering maladaptive thought patterns and facilitating adaptive coping skills so that patients can take control of their symptoms. Furthermore, psychoeducation is highly significant; it provides patients with information about their illness and the range of coping mechanisms available to promote resilience. Familiarity with the psychological impact of these disorders is able to help the patient cope with their condition better and remove feelings of loneliness. Not only does this intervention promote psychological health, but it also enhances compliance with medical therapy, resulting in improved physiological outcomes. In addition to therapy interventions, self-management skills are components of patients' coping processes for inner-ear and vestibular disorders. Mindfulness skills such as yoga and meditation have also gained popularity as effective tools for stress management and symptom alleviation. These skills place an individual in a relaxed state, which relaxes the nervous system, something that is overactive in inner ear disorder patients. Typical engagement in such practices has also been linked to reductions in perceived loudness of tinnitus and improvement in general emotional functioning. Furthermore, the presence of a healthy social support network can also augment coping, in addition to offering emotional support and a sense of belonging. Open discussion with friends and family, besides facilitating the patient's ability to relay their experiences, enhances understanding and therefore reduces the burden of these often disabling conditions. Lastly, the addition of pragmatic lifestyle modification can add much to coping strategies for vestibular disorder patients. Proper nutrition and routine physical exercise enhance general well-being, which may ease some of the symptoms associated with inner ear issues. For example, vestibular rehabilitation therapy (VRT) is able to offer some individualized exercises that improve balance and reduce dizziness so that patients can engage more actively in everyday activities. Additionally, avoiding known precipitants, such as foods or activities, will reduce symptom worsening. Paying attention to environmental precipitants, such as noise for tinnitus patients, reinforces patients' ability to change the environment to enhance their ability to manage conditions. As the patients begin to take a more active role in their health by adjusting their lifestyle, they voice a greater sense of control and satisfaction over their coping mechanisms for their inner ear disorders, which ultimately translates to improved overall quality of life.

Test Your Knowledge

1. What are the common psychological effects experienced by patients with vestibular disorders? Discuss anxiety, depression, fear of falling, and social withdrawal in relation to chronic dizziness and imbalance.
2. Explain how long-term vestibular disorders can impact a patient's mental health, quality of life, and daily functioning.

SUMMARY

In characterizing the multifarious presentation of inner ear and vestibular disorders, it is apparent that diagnosis is essential in guaranteeing effective management and good patient outcomes. The totalizing symptoms of dizziness, vertigo, and balance impairment, caused primarily by various vestibular dysfunctions, need a rigorous approach in diagnosis. Existing literature indicates that there is no consensus on which tests are effective. As a result, patients receive delayed diagnosis or have poor health care, much to the need for an organized vestibular patient care pathway. The integration of rigorous anamnesis and thorough vestibular testing, as outlined in current studies, can be a way forward in improving the recognition of vestibular lesions, eventually leading to personalized treatment methods that enhance quality of life for those affected (Lennox-Bowley, A., & Dasgupta, S., 2024). Research on conditions such as bilateral Ménières disease (BMD) provides substantial evidence of the complexity of vestibular disorders. Research indicates that BMD is associated with distinct clinical features relative to unilateral cases, particularly with respect to disease duration and degeneration of inner-ear function. A high percentage of BMD patients have existing vestibular disorders and demographic factors complicating the clinical profile. For instance, statistics indicate that patients with BMD may have a longer course of disease and higher frequencies of family history of vertigo, which emphasizes the heterogeneity of the condition. These observations emphasize the necessity of personalized diagnostic methods taking into account disease heterogeneity, which remains important for the management of vestibular disorders (Shi et al., 2022). Overall, the prevalence of inner ear and vestibular disorders among the general population necessitates a push from all directions towards enhanced diagnosis and treatment strategies. As explicated, the inclusion of sophisticated neuro-vestibular diagnostic tests has the potential to enhance patient care pathways, enabling clinicians to more effectively diagnose the vestibular dysfunctions underlying patients' symptoms. This solution is key to addressing the pressing issues of misdiagnosis and poor outcomes of treatment. Furthermore, identification of the unique offerings provided by each disorder, such as BMD, helps to emphasize the ongoing need for research and education in the field. By focusing on accurate diagnosis and individualized treatment, clinicians can promote management strategies that not only alleviate symptoms but also maximize overall quality of life for individuals with inner-ear and vestibular disorders (Shi et al., 2022; Lennox-Bowley, A., & Dasgupta, S., 2024).

The inner ear maintains balance and sound, but the malfunction of this complex system may lead to different vestibular disorders. The most significant vestibular disorder feature is vertigo and dizziness, which contribute significantly to patients' quality of life reduction. The disease can be caused by multiple etiologies, including inner ear infections, structural abnormalities, or neurological conditions. Considering the frequent presentation of dizziness in the emergency department, approximately 4.4 million visits annually in the United States, definite enhanced diagnostic processes are required. Enhanced diagnostic accuracy is being achieved by healthcare providers, who recognize the need to develop effective tools to identify the causes of vertigo and dizziness, enabling more accurate management (Jentsch, T. J., & Pusch, M., 2018). Apart from this, the anatomical intricacy of the inner ears also emphasizes the interactive nature of vestibular and auditory function. These conditions are particularly brought to the fore by the localization of CLC anion transporters, which not only regulate ion homeostasis but also contribute to the functionality of various cellular processes within the inner ear. The transports facilitate the transmembrane movement of anions, a mechanism that plays a significant role in the maintenance of electrochemical gradients that account for sensory cell excitability. The diverse biological activities that are undertaken by CLCs are supplemented by the spectrum of disorders that result from genetic mutations in their genes, resulting in disruptions in ion transport processes to hearing and balance disorders (Jentsch, T. J., & Pusch, M., 2018). An understanding of these associations is central to articulating an integrated approach to the diagnosis and management of inner-ear and vestibular disorders. In addition, vestibular disorder pathophysiology often reveals far-reaching implications for health and welfare. Vestibular system disorders do not include isolated symptoms; they can be representative of more general conditions, such as neurodegenerative disease or vascular disease. The immediate association between vertigo and significant underlying pathology, like strokes, warrants urgent assessment and intervention. The economic burden of dizziness-related emergency department visits exceeds $10 billion annually, and excessive neuroimaging utilization underscores the need for more efficient diagnostic pathways (Tehrani et al., 2018). A better understanding of the interaction between inner-ear structures and their physiological responses will be required to advance therapeutic interventions and patient outcomes in vestibular disorders through ongoing research.

KEY TERMS FROM THIS CHAPTER

- Sensorineural Hearing Loss
- Tinnitus
- Ménière's Disease
- Vestibular Neuritis
- Acoustic Neuroma
- Endolymphatic Hydrops
- Noise-Induced Hearing Loss
- Perilymph Fistula
- Motion Sickness
- Presbycusis
- Vertigo
- Benign Paroxysmal Positional Vertigo
- Labyrinthitis
- Vestibular Schwannoma
- Ototoxicity
- Sudden Sensorineural Hearing Loss
- Autoimmune Inner Ear Disease
- Vestibular Migraine

CRITICAL THINKING QUESTIONS

1. **ENT stands for:**
   a) Ear, Nose, Throat
   b) Eye, Nose, Throat
   c) Ear, Neck, Tongue
   d) Eye, Neck, Throat
2. **The medical specialty dealing with ENT is called:**
   a) Neurology
   b) Otorhinolaryngology
   c) Cardiology
   d) Ophthalmology
3. **Which part is NOT included in ENT?**
   a) Ear
   b) Nose
   c) Throat
   d) Heart
4. **The study of ear diseases is known as:**
   a) Rhinology
   b) Laryngology
   c) Otology
   d) Audiology
5. **The study of nasal diseases is called:**
   a) Otology
   b) Rhinology
   c) Laryngology
   d) Pharyngology

Short Answer Questions

1. What is meant by ENT and Head & Neck Surgery, and what are the main areas it covers?
2. Describe the anatomical divisions of the ear and state the functions of each part.
3. Explain the basic anatomy of the nose and paranasal sinuses.
4. What are the common diagnostic tools used in ENT practice?
5. Discuss the common symptoms that indicate ENT disorders.
6. What is the role of endoscopy in ENT and head & neck surgery?
7. Explain the importance of asepsis and sterilization in ENT surgical procedures.
8. Describe the basic principles of patient evaluation and examination in ENT and head & neck surgery.

Answers to Critical Thinking Questions

1. (a) 2. (b) 3. (d) 4. (c) 5. (b)

REFERENCES

1. Agrawal, Y., Smith, P. F., & Rosenberg, P. B. (2019). Vestibular impairment, cognitive decline and Alzheimer's disease: balancing the evidence. *Aging & Mental Health*, *24*(5), 705–708. https://doi.org/10.1080/13607863.2019.1566813Aimoni, C., Busi, M., Calzolari, F., Castiglione, A., et al. (2015). *Cochlear implant outcomes and genetic mutations in children with ear and brain anomalies*. https://core.ac.uk/download/53523126.pdf (accessed on 7th August 2025).
2. Altissimi, G., Cianfrone, G., Ciofalo, A., Greco, A., et al. (2016). *When Alarm Bells Ring: Emergency Tinnitus*. https://core.ac.uk/download/54538689.pdf (accessed on 7th August 2025).
3. Alves, S., & Morais Martin, M. G. (2024). Anatomy and embryology of the middle ear, labyrinth, and intracranial vestibular pathways. *Seminars in Ultrasound, CT, and MR*. https://www.semanticscholar.org/paper/7e25f9abd01581cb70454c8d63b8f9d073fd2017 (accessed on 7th August 2025).
4. Astashchenko, S., Goncharov, O. I., Kalyapin, D. D., Shcherbakova, Y. L., & Valkova, A. A. (2024). Case report of a patient with an enlarged vestibular aqueduct. *Russian Otorhinolaryngology*. https://www.semanticscholar.org/paper/e53ec2fe8f2a5750e3367db4b0e13f62c2527079 (accessed on 7th August 2025).
5. Axon, P., Coulson, C., Donnelly, N., Forge, A., et al. (2015). *Characterizing human vestibular sensory epithelia for experimental studies: New hair bundles on old tissue and implications for therapeutic interventions in ageing*. https://core.ac.uk/download/29410918.pdf (accessed on 7th August 2025).
6. Azevedo, A., Binetti, A. C., Coelho, C., de Ridder, D., et al. (2012). *Trauma-Associated Tinnitus: Audiological, Demographic, and Clinical Characteristics*. https://core.ac.uk/download/224999466.pdf (accessed on 7th August 2025).
7. Bustos-Merlo, A., Ortíz-Parra, A., Rosales-Castillo, A., Espinosa-Sánchez, J. M., & Navarrete-Navarrete, N. (2024). Autoimmune inner ear disease associated with antiphospholipid antibodies. *Clinical and Experimental Rheumatology*. https://www.semanticscholar.org/paper/8030b171d793f9d2430be2ef5040e1d75db04d03 (accessed on 7th August 2025).
8. Croce, A., D'Aguanno, V., De Vincentiis, M., De Virgilio, A., et al. (2018). *Audio-Vestibular Symptoms in Systemic Autoimmune Diseases*. https://core.ac.uk/download/188823057.pdf (accessed on 7th August 2025).
9. D'Aguanno, V., De Vincentiis, M., Greco, A., Ralli, M., et al. (2017). *Optimal Management of Cogan's Syndrome: A Multidisciplinary Approach*. https://core.ac.uk/download/144473159.pdf (accessed on 7th August 2025).
10. Dogru, H. B., Kaplan, A., Zengin, A. T., & Ozkul, T. (2024). Image-based nystagmus analysis in BPPV disorders: Polar coordinate system and template matching. In *2024 IEEE 3rd International Conference on Computing and Machine Intelligence (ICMI)*. https://www.semanticscholar.org/paper/fed3dc28879986c371c907b1dbc12edce76f7627 (accessed on 7th August 2025).
11. Hellström, A., Pakpour, A., Odzakovic, E., Björk, M., Ulander, M., Knutsson, S., Sandlund, C., et al. (2024). The psychometric properties of the Pearlin Mastery Scale in persons living with restless legs syndrome. *PLOS ONE*, 19. https://www.semanticscholar.org/paper/7d33e324996e35d04cfde0842256e82e9a42f757 (accessed on 7th August 2025).

12. Hong, S. S., Wackym, P. A., Murphy, D. J., Peci, E., Kiel, M. Y., Tucker, A., Carayannopoulos, N. L., et al. (2024). Model of superior semicircular canal dehiscence: Asymmetrical vestibular dysfunction induces reversible balance impairment. *Frontiers in Neurology, 15.* https://www.semanticscholar.org/paper/56457fac88fee7bc786cc03c6572832632d48d90 (accessed on 7th August 2025).
13. Ishiyama, A., Ishiyama, G., Ishiyama, P., & Lopez, I., et al. (2017). *The blood labyrinthine barrier in the human normal and Meniere's disease macula utricle.* https://core.ac.uk/download/323076450.pdf (accessed on 7th August 2025).
14. Jafari, Z., Kolb, B., & Mohajerani, M. H. (2021). Hearing loss, tinnitus, and dizziness in COVID-19: A systematic review and meta-analysis. *Canadian Journal of Neurological Sciences / Journal Canadien des Sciences Neurologiques, 49*, 184–195. https://doi.org/10.1017/cjn.2021.63 (accessed on 7th August 2025).
15. Jentsch, T. J., & Pusch, M. (2018). CLC chloride channels and transporters: Structure, function, physiology, and disease. *Physiological Reviews, 98*, 1493–1590. https://doi.org/10.1152/physrev.00047.2017 (accessed on 7th August 2025).
16. Kamal, N., Verma, R. K., Singhal, G. L., Mohod, P., Joya, V. A., & Kasliwal, R. (2025). Benign paroxysmal positional vertigo (BPPV) following maxillofacial procedures and trauma: A rare but real complication – Review and case report. *International Journal of Advanced Research.* https://www.semanticscholar.org/paper/18c51f5420f5d8b6c0524d6d3729e9954733022f (accessed on 7th August 2025).
17. Koch, E. D., Vilela, L. F. C., Destefani, A. C., & Destefani, V. C. (2024). Revolutionizing otoneurology: A comprehensive review of advanced diagnostic techniques and their long-term impact on patient care. *Revista Ibero-Americana de Humanidades, Ciências e Educação.* https://www.semanticscholar.org/paper/147d46ff257015d4d16baa0314adc2be32950812 (accessed on 7th August 2025).
18. Lahlou, H., Zhu, H., Zhou, W., & Edge, A. (2024). Pharmacological regeneration of sensory hair cells restores afferent innervation and vestibular function. *The Journal of Clinical Investigation, 134.* https://www.semanticscholar.org/paper/5d024b6d60210ba8197555177e858ca01bd8b0d1 (accessed on 7th August 2025).
19. Lennox-Bowley, A., & Dasgupta, S. (2024). Modernizing vestibular assessment. *The Journal of Laryngology & Otology, 138*(Suppl. 1), S3–S7. https://www.semanticscholar.org/paper/7a108b7f666c058c05070007db511474022451bb (accessed on 7th August 2025).
20. Li, M., Chiffer, R. C., & Li, H. (2025). Risk of benign paroxysmal positional vertigo modified by diuretics—A population-level case-control study. *Otolaryngology--Head and Neck Surgery: Official Journal of the American Academy of Otolaryngology-Head and Neck Surgery.* https://www.semanticscholar.org/paper/37d467c022bb8ff67a60ffcb32c610473f8a26ed (accessed on 7th August 2025).
21. Liu, J., Wang, C., & Liu, S. (2025). *Recent advances in the diagnosis of autoimmune inner ear disease: A scoping review.* https://www.semanticscholar.org/paper/3652d13226ac2c58d2231961dbe453e6b373dddf (accessed on 7th August 2025).
22. Majeed, S., Farooqi, S., & Jamshed, A. (2023). Vestibular disorders and their impact on balance and mobility. *Pakistan Journal of Medical and Health Sciences, 17*, 686–688. https://doi.org/10.53350/pjmhs2023173686 (accessed on 7th August 2025).

23. Majeed, S., Farooqi, S., & Jamshed, A. (2023). Vestibular disorders and their impact on balance and mobility. *Pakistan Journal of Medical and Health Sciences*. https://www.semanticscholar.org/paper/35de113b71a9db20e59f23b9461dd5c2a201e042 (accessed on 7th August 2025).

24. Maniaci, M., Briglia, F., Allia, F., Montalbano, G., Romano, G. L., Zaoualí, M., H'Mida, D., et al. (2024). The role of pericytes in inner ear disorders: A comprehensive review. *Biology, 13*. https://www.semanticscholar.org/paper/d6b888e34de5472787aaa7b94de726df7061c0c0 (accessed on 7th August 2025).

25. Mencia, A., Subramanian, A., Postigo, A. A., Biedlingmaier, A., Griffith, A. J., Morrisson, A., Lewis, B. P., et al. (2011). *Cell type–specific transcriptome analysis reveals a major role for Zeb1 and miR-200b in mouse inner ear morphogenesis*. https://core.ac.uk/download/pdf/8622458.pdf (accessed on 7th August 2025).

26. Miller, E. (2011). *Quality of life and the benefits of remediation in patients with hearing loss or peripheral vestibular disorders*. https://core.ac.uk/download/159573912.pdf (accessed on 7th August 2025).

27. Muzammil, M., Rasool, A., & Zaheer, R. (2025). Prevalence of vestibular disorder among deaf children. *Insights—Journal of Health and Rehabilitation*. https://www.semanticscholar.org/paper/b781ba218a5effb14f77582ca6433c4a1bb8ad44 (accessed on 7th August 2025).

28. N/A. (2025). *Aerospace Medicine and Biology: A Continuing Bibliography with Indexes, Supplement 130, July 1974*. https://core.ac.uk/download/pdf/42893215.pdf (accessed on 7th August 2025).

29. Nicolas-Puel, J., Bourien, J., Nouvian, R., Puel, J., & Ceccato, J. (2025). Audiometry as a predictive proxy for balance dysfunction. *Scientific Reports, 15*. https://www.semanticscholar.org/paper/a425188b369b054f92fed0dfeecfb727a8c5db62 (accessed on 7th August 2025).

30. Nola, G., Ralli, G., Ralli, M., Sparvoli, L., et al. (2017). *Unilateral Enlarged Vestibular Aqueduct Syndrome and Bilateral Endolymphatic Hydrops*. https://core.ac.uk/download/98349074.pdf (accessed on 7th August 2025).

31. Pérez-Fernández, N., & Ramos-Macías, Á. (2023). Recent advances in the diagnosis and treatment of vestibular disorders. *Journal of Clinical Medicine, 12*. https://www.semanticscholar.org/paper/62f11383e3b6ab8434b1b994ac35e66dcda94937 (accessed on 7th August 2025).

32. Phillips, J., Cox, S. J., Howard, G., High, J., Murdin, L., Nunney, I., Rea, P., et al. (2024). Development of the continuous ambulatory vestibular assessment (CAVA) system to provide an automatic diagnosis for vestibular conditions: Protocol for a multicenter, single-arm, non-randomized clinical trial. *BMJ Open, 14*. https://www.semanticscholar.org/paper/d4794291b9e3532b4dbf4b75a253ce742e647fe0 (accessed on 7th August 2025).

33. Pirodda, A., Savastio, G., Stagni, S., Ferri, G. G., Brandolini, C., & Zompatori, M. (2017). The role of high-resolution computed tomography in the diagnostic protocol of cochleo-vestibular disorders. *Hearing Balance and Communication, 15*, 48–53. https://doi.org/10.1080/21695717.2017.1286085.

34. Saber Tehrani, A. S., Kattah, J. C., Kerber, K. A., Gold, D. R., Zee, D. S., Urrutia, V., & Newman-Toker, D. E. (2018). Diagnosing stroke in acute dizziness and vertigo. *Stroke, 49*, 788–795. https://doi.org/10.1161/strokeaha.117.016979.

35. Shi, S., Li, W., Wang, D., Ren, T., & Wang, W. (2022). Characteristics of clinical details and endolymphatic hydrops in unilateral and bilateral Ménière's disease in a single Asian group. *Frontiers in Neurology, 13*. https://www.semanticscholar.org/paper/ba2a396b8d2efad566e049eca34109a09b8f4fc4 (accessed on 7th August 2025).

36. Smith, L. J., Wilkinson, D., Bodani, M., Surenthiran, S., VanRullen, R., & Smith, P. (2024). Cognition in vestibular disorders: State of the field, challenges, and priorities for the future. *Frontiers in Neurology, 15*. https://www.semanticscholar.org/paper/71cd35f7a8673eb0976b10c2a6ea3669f957784c (accessed on 7th August 2025).

37. Strupp, M., Kim, J.-S., Murofushi, T., Straumann, D., Jen, J. C., Rosengren, S. M., Della Santina, C. C., et al. (2017). Bilateral vestibulopathy: Diagnostic criteria consensus document of the classification committee of the Bárány Society. *Journal of Vestibular Research, 27*, 177–189. https://doi.org/10.3233/ves-170619 (accessed on 7th August 2025).

38. Tramontano, M., Haijoub, S., Lacour, M., & Manzari, L. (2025). Updated views on vestibular physical therapy for patients with vestibular disorders. *Healthcare, 13*. https://www.semanticscholar.org/paper/cf9f2788f9e8f7647267ce6fd7d2aeeb9685b457 (accessed on 7th August 2025).

39. Tran, C. T., Le, T., Hang, T. T. T., Ma, N., Phuong, H. H., & Thuy, T. P. (2024). Correlation between vestibular disorders and superior semicircular dehiscence on high-resolution computed tomography at Tam Anh Ho Chi Minh General Hospital. *Medeniyet Medical Journal, 39*, 117–121. https://www.semanticscholar.org/paper/7d3adc15b0bc436560b7d5d5ddd85079840ba363 (accessed on 7th August 2025).

40. Virk, S. M., Trujillo-Provencio, C., & Serrano, E. (2024). *Transcriptomic analysis identifies candidate genes for differential expression during Xenopus laevis inner ear development*. bioRxiv. https://www.semanticscholar.org/paper/a34a5afb67f3ee5626b30b32d87bd7e7065b0017 (accessed on 7th August 2025).

41. Wang, M., Zhang, P., Li, Q., & Kong, C. (2025). Investigating the process of autoimmune inner ear disease: Unveiling the intricacies of pathogenesis and therapeutic strategies. *International Journal of Medical Sciences, 22*, 179–187. https://www.semanticscholar.org/paper/625a813dc804c8c339402997e1f3b01f81473e18 (accessed on 7th August 2025).

42. Wei, G., Qiu, S., Gao, X., Zheng, L., Chen, Y., Ma, Y., Feng, H., et al. (2025). Single administration of AAV-mAtp6v1b2 gene therapy rescues hearing and vestibular disorders caused by Atp6v1b2-induced lysosomal dysfunction in hair cells. *Advanced Science*. https://www.semanticscholar.org/paper/2b206087e948ea6f86039f701ec2c73c12d0da25 (accessed on 7th August 2025).

43. Xing, Y., Si, L., Zhang, W., Wang, Y., Li, K., & Yang, X. (2024). Etiologic distribution of dizziness/vertigo in a neurological outpatient clinic according to the criteria of the International Classification of Vestibular Disorders: A single-center study. *Journal of Neurology, 271*, 2446–2457. https://www.semanticscholar.org/paper/29a0bc2ecad98f07b20fd2742fb3c93b9836968f (accessed on 7th August 2025).

44. Zamora, E., & Zamora, C. (2025). The inner ear: A primer for radiologists: Part 2, congenital anomalies, inflammatory disease, trauma, and neoplasms. *Neurographics*. https://www.semanticscholar.org/paper/f40ab9a78cd7850afeeeff246660f9549fcc5575 (accessed on 7th August 2025).

HEARING ASSESSMENT AND REHABILITATION

6

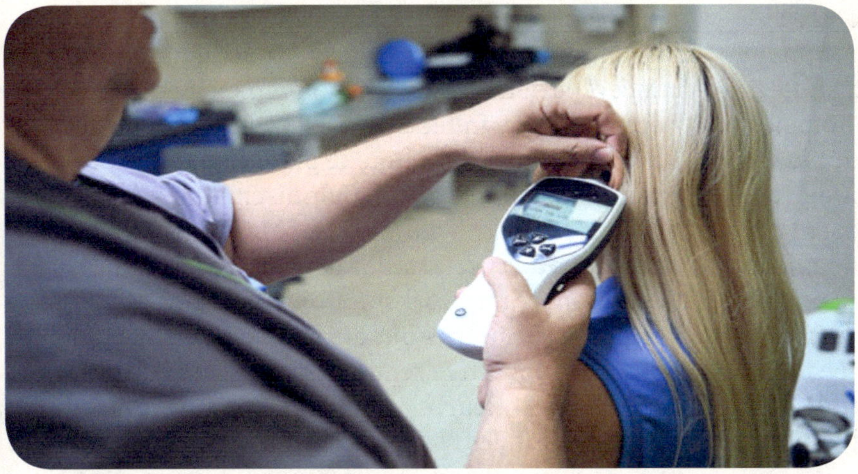

LEARNING OBJECTIVES

After studying this chapter, you will be able to:

1. Anatomy relevant to ENT and head and neck surgery.
2. Common conditions treated in ENT.
3. Surgical techniques in head and neck surgery.
4. Diagnostic tools in ENT and head and neck surgery.
5. Patient management and care.
6. Advances and innovations in ENT and head and neck surgery.

Introduction

The otolaryngology specialty, which encompasses ear, Nose, and Throat surgery, plays a vital role in comprehensive hearing evaluation and management of rehabilitation. Aside from managing and diagnosing hearing disorders, the specialty also covers general head and neck diseases with a direct influence on patients' quality of life. Surgeons in this field are trained to address everything from chronic ear infections to complex surgical interventions for tumors of the head and neck region. As advanced technologies and techniques are employed by practitioners, they enhance their ability to restore hearing and improve overall patient outcomes. A realization of the interdisciplinary nature of ENT surgery means coordination that must be accomplished among specialists, including audiologists and speech therapists, to offer integrated care to individuals with hearing impairments. In the rehabilitation of hearing, ENT specialists are the most prominent actors in assessing auditory function and developing effective treatments. As part of multidisciplinary management, these specialists use a range of diagnostic tools and tests to evaluate hearing impairment and accordingly plan treatments. With the increased recognition of the impact of hearing loss on cognitive development and emotional stability, treatment protocols among ENT specialists play a significant role in enhancing the quality of life for affected individuals. The collaborative strategy observed among physicians, as affirmed in the guidelines issued for the management of MPS VI, insists on the importance of combined care for patients with hearing impairment (Akyol et al., 2019). In addition, advances in ENT surgical treatment modalities shed light on emerging trends in hearing rehabilitation. Emerging technologies, such as cochlear implants, tympanoplasty, and other surgical procedures, demonstrate the remarkable capacity to restore hearing in patients with congenital or acquired deafness. These surgical treatments are supported by non-surgical interventions, such as auditory training and hearing aid use, which help patients maximize auditory potential. The need for ongoing clinical trials and studies is necessary to develop new treatments and improve existing practices. As evidenced by current evidence-based practice guidelines, the role of a multidisciplinary team in managing conditions such as X-linked hypophosphatemia, which indirectly affects hearing through skeletal deformities, underscores the interconnectedness of various health issues. These advances affirm the commitment of the ENT specialty towards fostering innovation while maintaining patient-centered care (Haffner et al., 2019).

Importance of Head and Neck Surgery in Medical Practice

Head and neck surgery is part of the medical practice context, particularly the management of conditions that have a quantifiable effect on hearing and rehabilitation. Surgeons within this department treat a variety of disorders, including those involving tumors, congenital abnormalities, and traumatic injury, which have an effect on the processes of hearing within the head and neck regions. Complication-free surgery often calls for a multi-disciplinary assault since liaison with otolaryngologists, audiologists, and speech-language pathologists is required. Only by this liaison can patients be assured of being offered overall management, addressing not only the immediate surgical needs but also follow-up auditory rehabilitation necessary for restored function and quality of life. Additionally, innovations in head and neck surgery have dramatically improved the patient outcome, particularly for head and neck cancer patients and other complex head and neck patients. Indeed, as observed under head and neck cancer treatment planning, decision-making is facilitated by a multidisciplinary group of professionals who assess definite sites and stages of a disease to tailor therapies accordingly. Such team frameworks not only ensure precise surgical procedures but also maximize support with post-operative rehabilitation, which is vital for optimal hearing restoration. Therefore, coordination of surgical expertise in head and neck medicine is paramount, highlighting the intricate relationship between surgical procedures and rehabilitation regimens that effectively address the hearing effects of these conditions (Pfister et al., 2020). Furthermore, head and neck surgery implications extend beyond simple anatomical corrections; they also embrace substantial psychosocial dimensions. Patients undergoing these operations are often faced with speech, swallowing, and quality-of-life issues. Rehabilitation efforts post-operatively must then overcome such factors through appropriately coordinated audiological assessment and intervention. For example, CP patients may have concomitant auditory processing disorders, and this would necessitate targeted rehabilitation programs that merge auditory and occupational therapies. This explains why there is a need for a more holistic approach to management, because rehabilitation of the patients hinges on breaking physical as well as communicative barriers.

The integration of neck and head surgery with hearing rehabilitation is thus essential, exemplifying how surgical advances can improve hearing outcomes and enhance patients' overall health (Patel et al., 2020).

Historical Development of ENT and Head and Neck Surgery

The history of Ear, Nose, and Throat (ENT) and head and neck surgery has evolved from ancient times, when simple procedures were being performed in a state of ignorance of anatomy. Early practitioners used primarily observational methods in which they would diagnose and manage the diseases of the head and neck. The craft evolved significantly with the Renaissance, an age of sophisticated surgical techniques and additions to knowledge of human physiology. Pioneers like Ambroise Paré and Giovanni di Lorenzo formed the basis of developing surgical practices that resulted in modern-day ENT. These advancements have deepened understanding of ear and throat diseases, serving as an entry point for future research. This evolution points towards having to continually refine hearing assessment and treatment, as historical perspective affects clinical practice today and dictates current practice in the management of ear disorders. The beginning of specialized training in ENT and head and neck surgery began in the 19th century, when there were outstanding developments in medical education. It was at this period that institutions began to introduce specialized programs through which physicians could receive comprehensive training in such specialized fields. This specialization was required because it appreciated the complexity of disease conditions taking place in the ear, nose, and throat that required more specialized treatment approaches. The 20th-century surgical boom further revolutionized the specialties as surgical and anesthesia technologies advanced, enabling more invasive interventions with lower patient morbidity. Increased research and clinical trial focus also became common during this time, more profoundly informing preventive care and treatment practices. As such, present hearing testing techniques and rehabilitation methods have immensely benefited from the developments in the past, repeatedly reshaping the patient's course from diagnosis to therapy. Furthermore, current developments in ENT and head and neck surgery are largely the result of past cooperation and data sharing among physicians worldwide. Better globalization facilitated faster knowledge transfer, enabling developing nations to harness the benefits of advanced training programs that have been created as a reaction to health disparities. Training programs that promote fellowship training overseas, as outlined in comparable studies, have led to skilled practitioners coming back home to improve local healthcare systems. According to recent studies, ongoing continuing education among healthcare professionals in developing regions correlates positively with improved subspecialty outcomes of care in such conditions as hearing impairment and rehabilitation (Hickey, 2023). This historical orientation places the imperative for continued education and training at the forefront in developing future ENT practices and highlights the value of integrating historical progress into contemporary healthcare policy for hearing health (Figure 6.1).

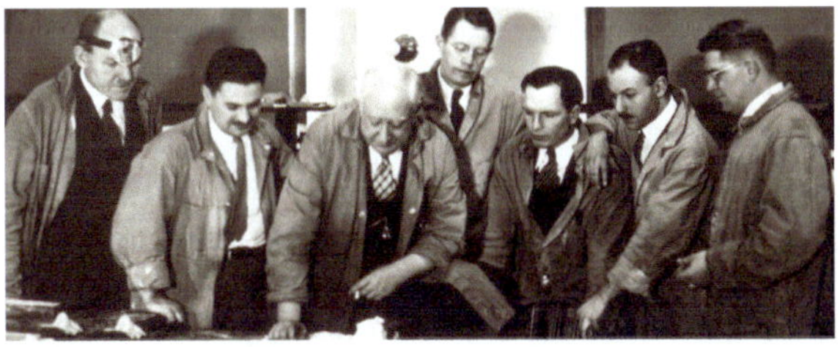

Figure 6.1. The historical development of Ear, Nose, and Throat (ENT) and head and neck surgery has roots that trace back to ancient civilizations.

Source: https://oto.hms.harvard.edu/sites/g/files/omnuum8391/files/oto/files/history2.png.

6.1. Anatomy Relevant to ENT and Head and Neck Surgery

Learning Outcome

1. Anatomy of the Nasal Cavity and Paranasal Sinuses
2. Overview of the Throat and Laryngeal Structures

Understanding the anatomy of ear, nose, and throat (ENT) and head and neck surgery is crucial for accurate hearing assessment and rehabilitation. The ear itself can be divided into three components: the outer ear, the middle ear, and the inner ear, with each having specific functions in the process of hearing. The outer ear, made up of the pinna and the external auditory canal, collects sound waves and funnels them towards the tympanic membrane (eardrum). Sound passes through the middle ear, which has the ossicles—malleus, incus, and stapes—that increase the vibrations of sound. Aside from this mechanical function, the intricate structure of the inner ear, or the cochlea, plays a vital role in converting these vibrations into neural impulses understandable by the brain, which illustrates the co-interdependence of anatomical structures in hearing. The interplay between the hearing apparatus and the neighboring anatomical elements is also necessary to understand the complexity of hearing disorders. Maladies such as tinnitus often necessitate knowledge of both the anatomy and physiology of the auditory system. The organization of the cochlea, its basilar membrane and hair cells, reinforces the physiological basis of sound perception and diversity, which may lead to hearing impairment. Moreover, the anatomy extends to neuroanatomy, where cranial nerves, specifically the vestibulocochlear nerve (CN VIII), convey auditory input to the brain. Ensuring complete knowledge of the relationship facilitates improved diagnostic and therapeutic management, particularly in handling disorders like tinnitus, which may require quick medical intervention owing to its psychological as well as physiological impact on patients (Altissimi et al., 2016). Additionally, applications of surgery in ENT practice ensure the significance of precise anatomical data for an intended result. Surgical procedures such as tympanoplasty, cochlear implantation, and others depend on a thorough understanding of the ear and adjacent structures. For instance, a proper understanding of the temporal bones' anatomy is essential in cochlear implantation cases to avoid complications and ensure correct electrode placement in the cochlea. In addition, the involvement of the head and neck anatomies, such as the pharynx and larynx, depicts the cross-sectional nature of these systems since both are central to the functionality of the auditory and overall patient rehabilitation. By combining approaches from all facial plastic and reconstructive surgery specialties within ENT, medical professionals can develop comprehensive plans that enhance patient care through customized treatment protocols (Akyol et al., 2019).

6.1.1. Anatomy of the Nasal Cavity and Paranasal Sinuses

The anatomy of the nasal cavity and paranasal sinuses is a key determinant for various physiological processes, such as hearing-related ones. The nasal cavity is divided into the right and left chambers and is lined with a mucous membrane that is involved with olfactory senses as well as the filtration of airborne particles. Besides, it possesses structures such as the turbinates that enhance air flow and offer increased surface area for heating and humidifying air one inhales. The paranasal sinuses, which are air chambers in the head bones, possess many functions such as reducing the weight of the skull, resonating sound, and perhaps influencing one's sense of hearing. Furthermore, they are also connected to the nasal cavity, providing an airway for pressure balance, which is crucial for enhanced hearing functionality. Such anatomical structures thus directly link the respiratory and auditory systems, demonstrating an interdependence in their specific function (Niedzielski et al., 2023). Adenoid tissues, often considered part of the lymphatic system, have a dominant role in the anatomy of the nasal cavity. Located on the posterior surface of the nasal cavity, the adenoids play a critical immunological role in children, responding to pathogens that enter via the nasopharynx. Adenoid status influences respiratory health, and adenoid hypertrophy, in which the tissues enlarge, is widespread. It may lead to obstructive symptoms, which in turn give rise to altered dynamics of airflow and affect the functionality of the Eustachian tubes, causing middle ear effusion or otitis media. Such a connection between adenoids and auditory health makes it important to understand nasal cavity anatomy, particularly in children, as it may have a ripple effect on hearing and all respiratory processes (Niedzielski et al., 2023). The paranasal sinuses, including the maxillary, frontal, ethmoid, and sphenoid sinuses, also illustrate the dependency between nasal anatomy and hearing health. The arrangement of these sinuses around the nasal cavity allows for effective drainage and exchange of air, which is crucial to preventing respiratory infections that can affect sound pathways. In the context of hearing assessment and treatment, effective sinus function is critical; blockages or infections can cause complications that impede normal auditory processing. Current studies on oropharyngeal dysphagia in head and neck cancer patients illustrate the clinical relevance of becoming familiar with such anatomical correlations because variability in management tends to arise from nuances of individual anatomy. Hence, a comprehensive approach to hearing tests should consider the implications of nasal and sinus health to enable more effective rehabilitation in patients with auditory disorders.

6.1.2. Overview of the Throat and Laryngeal Structures

The laryngeal elements and the throat play important roles in both sound production and respiratory tract processes. The throat is further categorized into three main divisions: the oropharynx, the nasopharynx, and the laryngopharynx, which together enable air, food, and sound to travel through. The larynx, which is located at the intersection point of the pharynx and trachea, serves as a vital component in controlling airflow and voice production through the movement of vocal cords. These bodily structures not only permit basic biological functions but also enable the nuances of communication, making them significant in the context of hearing assessment and rehabilitation. Anatomy and physiology of the larynx and throat are essential for professionals dealing with individuals who have voice disorders or dysphagia because both are serious impairments of both communication and swallowing function. For hearing evaluation and rehabilitation, the interrelationships among structures of the throat and larynx are particularly crucial, particularly in populations affected by oropharyngeal dysphagia. This status, prevalent in head and neck cancer patients, may complicate rehabilitation, as it impacts safe swallowing of food and fluid, aspiration pneumonia risk, and eventually auditory and sensory loss. Thus, interdisciplinary methods are now increasingly regarded as crucial where the medical professionals integrate speech-language pathology and audiology to address the various challenges in such patients. Given there are significant variations in management of the conditions across Europe, as highlighted by recent attempts to establish common guidelines, formulation of a harmonious treatment approach can significantly enhance patient quality of life and outcomes and ensure that all concerned aspects of care, for example, hearing, are integrated into the rehabilitation process (Baijens et al., 2020). Furthermore, symptoms of neurodegenerative disorders, such as those included under Sanfilippo syndrome, underscore the intricacy of managing patients with complicated impairments, such as those of the throat and larynx. Patients diagnosed with such conditions may experience a progressive loss of cognitive and physical functions, best addressed by an integrative plan of care that addresses the neurological and physiological functions. The importance of an interdisciplinary approach in such scenarios is of top priority since professionals from various branches of expertise work together to address the extensive demands of the patient. Through setting evidence-based practices that serve to mark the boundaries of best practices in clinical management, medical practitioners are able to make timely diagnoses and interventions feasible, resulting ultimately in improved patient outcomes for hearing and communication disorders (Muschol et al., 2022).

Test Your Knowledge

1. Disuss the Anatomy of the Paranasal Sinuses
2. Explain Cranial Nerves and Neck Surgery

6.2. Common Conditions Treated in ENT

Learning Outcome

1. Otitis Media and Its Implications
2. Sinusitis and Its Treatment Options
3. Disorders of the Larynx, Including Vocal Cord Nodules

Among the many conditions encountered in otolaryngology, hearing loss is among the most prevalent in patients across all age groups. Hearing loss may be observed in several forms, including conductive, sensorineural, and mixed hearing loss, each with its own unique challenges in diagnosis and treatment. Conductive hearing loss, most often resulting from physical obstructions like earwax or fluid within the middle ear, can frequently be corrected by straightforward medical or surgical procedures. Unlike sensorineural hearing loss, which most often results from trauma to cochlear hair cells or the auditory nerve, frequently more advanced rehabilitation tactics are needed, such as the placement of hearing aids or cochlear implants. Given the basic significance of effective communication to quality of life, treatment of such hearing impairments is a component of general healthcare policy. Tinnitus, ringing and buzzing in the ears, is also a common complaint managed by ENT specialists. Easily associated with hearing loss, profound ear injury, or exposure to noise, tinnitus can be debilitating in character, significantly impairing the capacity of an individual to concentrate and engage in social activities. Understanding the multifaceted character of tinnitus is the most important factor in effective management. Treatment today ranges from counseling and sound therapy to the prescription of hearing aids that mask noise perception. Because of the complexities involved, combined audiological and psychological interventions have been successful in alleviating the distress of this symptom. Successful tinnitus management, then, is not only therapeutic to hearing symptoms but also enhances functioning and well-being. Sinusitis is another common condition managed in otolaryngology and is typically associated with other ENT disorders, such as allergies and respiratory infections. This inflammatory response within the sinus cavities can be very uncomfortable, involving facial pain, nasal congestion, and alteration of the sense of smell. Acute sinusitis is usually treated with medicine, such as antibiotics or intranasal corticosteroids, whereas chronic sinusitis might require more forceful intervention, such as endoscopic sinus surgery, to re-establish drainage and normal function. The simultaneous occurrence of sinusitis with other ENT issues highlights the importance of proper coordination of care among medical professionals in order to offer holistic treatment plans. Even when hearing loss co-occurs with sinus issues, treating the sinuses is essential to ensuring optimal performance of hearing tests and subsequent therapy, thereby highlighting the holistic nature of ENT care (Figure 6.2).

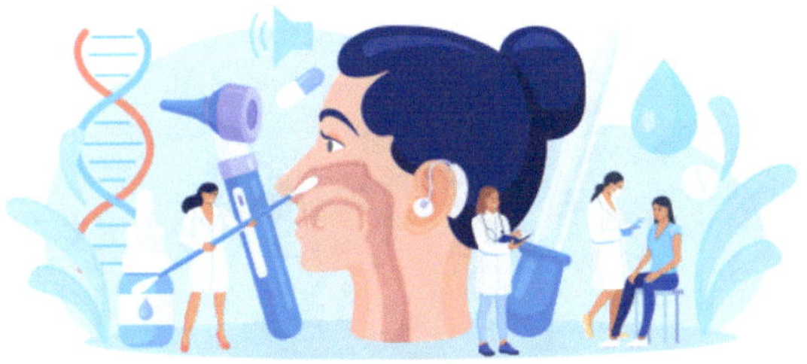

Figure 6.2. Common conditions treated in ENT.

Source: https://www.manipalhospitals.com/uploads/blog/top-5-ENT-conditions-symptoms-and-treatment.png.

6.2.1. Otitis Media and Its Implications

Otitis media, or inflammation of the middle ear, is a frequent condition that presents a significant issue with hearing, particularly in children. The condition can progress to acute and chronic infection, leading to fluid accumulation in the ear and interfering with normal hearing processes. This interference can present as temporary or permanent hearing loss, which, if left untreated, has profound impacts on speech and language development. Evidence shows that early management and treatment are essential in avoiding the adverse consequences of otitis media since early treatment can reinstate the hearing function and avert delayed long-term development. Also, an understanding of the epidemiological trends of otitis media is important in the formulation of proper hearing assessment protocols and rehabilitative measures, particularly in high-risk populations such as Aboriginal and Torres Strait Islander children who are disproportionately affected by the condition (Leach et al., 2021). In addressing the effects of otitis media on sound perception, it is necessary to consider its role in everyday communication and social interaction. Those with frequent episodes of otitis media will not only have difficulty in school but also in their social lives, as their delayed speech will hinder peer relationships and self-esteem. Appropriate hearing-assessment tools must then be used to appropriately diagnose the disparate levels of hearing loss associated with otitis media. Sophisticated methods, including the digits-in-noise test (DIN), can be useful in optimizing sensitivity to conductive as well as sensorineural hearing losses, emphasizing the need for proper audiological evaluation in patients with otitis media (Sousa et al., 2019). These tests drive targeted rehabilitation so that treatment is individualized and useful in remedying specific auditory impairments. The implications of otitis media do not simply stop at thc prcvailing hearing problems; the condition is a public health concern that necessitates continued research and intervention. Effective management practices must provide for preventive controls in order to reduce incidence rates, particularly in more vulnerable populations. Education on the importance of early detection and treatment of otitis media must be continued on both the caregiver and healthcare provider sides. Improvements in screening tests, such as the antiphase digit presentation screening tests discussed above, are a promising trend in hearing assessment methods. Using these new methods, clinicians can achieve early detection of hearing impairment due to otitis media and implement rehabilitation interventions that enhance the auditory well-being and quality of life of affected individuals, resulting in positive developmental outcomes (Sousa et al., 2019; Leach et al., 2021).

6.2.2. Sinusitis and Its Treatment Options

Sinusitis, or an infection of the sinus cavities, is a common and often incapacitating disorder that detracts from the overall well-being of individuals. The symptoms are generally nasal congestion, facial pain, and headache, which restrict daily activity and quality of life. Chronic sinusitis, lasting more than 12 weeks, is particularly vexing and can be associated with other diseases, including respiratory infections and allergies. Since the sinuses lie close to the ears anatomically, sinusitis has effects that extend beyond sinus discomfort and can affect the acuteness of hearing. The interconnectedness of the sinus and auditory systems indicates that a clearer understanding of how sinusitis may be involved in hearing loss or other audiological difficulties requires an interdisciplinary treatment and rehabilitation model, particularly for patients with both hearing and sinus difficulties (Greenhalgh et al., 2022). Various types of management are available for the management of sinusitis, depending on the severity and chronicity of the condition. For acute illness, symptomatic cure may be addressed by saline nasal irrigation and intranasal corticosteroids, which reduce inflammation and clean out the nasal passages. For chronic illnesses, long-term therapy with antibiotics, if bacterial infection is considered a risk factor, could be indicated. Furthermore, hyperbaric oxygen therapy (HBOT) has become an adjunctive treatment for sinusitis. HBOT promotes greater oxygenation of tissues and may potentially facilitate healing and reduce inflammation in sinus cavities. This therapy is promising in its antimicrobial and immunomodulatory action, highlighting the importance of new therapy in the management of sinusitis, especially when treatment with conventional means fails (Ortega et al., 2021). Moreover, preventive measures and lifestyle modifications can play a vital role in managing recurrent sinusitis. Patients might be advised to abstain from known allergens and irritants, ingest sufficient fluid, and practice good nasal hygiene to reduce sinusitis attacks.

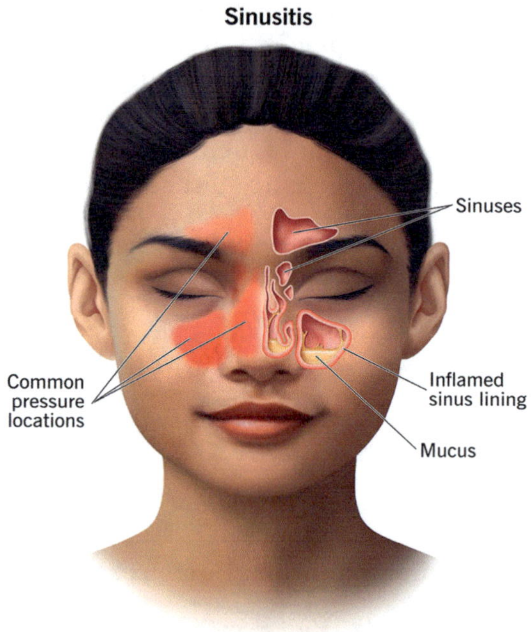

Figure 6.3. Sinusitis and its treatment options.

Source: https://my.clevelandclinic.org/-/scassets/images/org/health/articles/17701-sinusitis.

Together with a patient-focused model of care, these interventions not only decrease the incidence of sinusitis attacks but also potentially have positive impacts on auditory wellbeing. Treatment of both ears and sinus together can allow practitioners to develop a more comprehensive approach, ultimately enhancing the overall quality of life in patients with comorbid conditions. Future research that further investigates the overlap between sinusitis and hearing loss will be crucial to refine these strategies and optimize patient benefit in both fields (Greenhalgh et al., 2022) (Figure 6.3).

6.2.3. Disorders of the Larynx, Including Vocal Cord Nodules

Laryngeal diseases, particularly vocal cord nodules, are significant problems for voice as well as overall communication and can interfere with hearing assessment and rehabilitation. Vocal cord nodules are benign growths on the vocal cords and typically occur due to habitual abuse or misuse of the voice. The lesions manifest as hoarseness, breathy voice, and voice strain. Since individuals can strive to maintain their voice capabilities, they may withdraw from social interactions or work tasks that require effective communication. The withdrawal may therefore exacerbate the sense of isolation and anger, necessitating an interdisciplinary intervention in the evaluation and treatment of hearing that is not only tailored to the physical aspects of voice but also the psychosocial components of these disorders. The effects of vocal cord nodules extend beyond the complaint of voice quality alteration. The relationship between the larynx and hearing may be intricate; abnormal vocalization may disrupt clear auditory communication, priceless in most situations. Patients with vocal cord disorders may employ compensatory communication strategies that, conversely, complicate their hearing experiences. For instance, because individuals with laryngeal disorders may unconsciously alter their speech, doctors need to recognize the way these alterations can influence hearing tests without realizing it. Understanding the relationship between vocal health and one's ability to hear is significant, particularly when designing multidimensional rehabilitation programs aimed at restoring the best forms of communication. Management of laryngeal disorders, such as vocal cord nodules, requires an interprofessional effort from the healthcare community, including otolaryngologists, speech-language pathologists, and audiologists. Early management can quite effectively result in a favorable outcome, further underlining the importance of education regarding vocal hygiene and prevention measures. In high-risk populations, such as teachers and public speakers, awareness of effective vocal practice is of particular importance to avert the development of such disorders. Moreover, rehabilitative treatment to specific areas can enable patients to regain their voice function with retained auditory clarity. By integrating techniques that enhance both vocal health and auditory processing, practitioners can implement an approach to full cure that overcomes the disruption to quality of life associated with laryngeal illnesses.

Test Your Knowledge

1. Describe the anatomy of the nasal cavity, paranasal sinuses, pharynx, and larynx, and explain their clinical importance in ENT and head & neck surgical procedures.
2. Explain the anatomical relations of the carotid sheath, thyroid gland, and major cranial nerves in the neck, highlighting their significance in head and neck surgeries and prevention of complications.

6.3. Surgical Techniques in Head and Neck Surgery

Learning Outcome

1. Endoscopic Procedures and Their Applications
2. Open Surgical Techniques for Tumor Removal
3. Reconstructive Surgery in Head and Neck Cases

In head and neck surgery, the surgical environment has evolved significantly, particularly with respect to disease processes affecting hearing. Operations such as microsurgical excision and reconstruction are central in the treatment of tumors originating from the auditory apparatus or overlying tissues. The accuracy of these operations is imperative not only for tumor extirpation but also for preserving fundamental functions such as hearing. Additionally, intraoperative monitoring of neurologic status is standard to minimize complications associated with operations on or around the auditory pathways. Such improvements enable surgeons to intervene more effectively, with patients undergoing surgery for hearing disease optimally prepared for postoperative management and rehabilitation of their auditory function. Cochlear implantation (CI) is an extensive operation for those with severe hearing impairments, especially when conventional hearing aids are ineffective. According to the description in recent studies, CI surgery success largely relies on preoperative tests and tailored surgical interventions, particularly in syndromic hearing loss, which is often burdened with anatomical variations and functional impairments. Care for the exact choice of electrode types and technique that honors individual anatomy is essential to optimizing auditory outcomes. Moreover, incorporation of lengthy perioperative management strategies—such as careful monitoring of facial nerve integrity and fluid status—underscores the delicate balance between surgical expertise and patient protection in achieving successful rehabilitation outcomes for the hearing-impaired population (Yuan et al., 2025). Rehabilitation following surgery in the head and neck region is quite significant to ensure maximum quality of life, particularly among patients who develop dysphagia or other speech issues. Operations such as resection or reconstruction near the oropharynx can cause difficulties in swallowing and speech production. In such cases, treatment using a multidisciplinary team that includes speech therapy and swallowing rehabilitation is the first priority. For instance, head and neck surgical patients with synchronous squamous cell carcinomas usually present with anastomotic strictures that need complex therapeutic management to preserve swallowing functions. Clinical rehabilitation programs provide evidence that swallowing dysfunction should be treated early to ensure safe oral intake and improve the quality of life of head and neck surgical patients (Xue et al., 2024).

6.3.1. Endoscopic Procedures and Their Applications

Endoscopic methods have considerably advanced the art of auditory assessment and therapy, transforming clinicians' ability to visualize and manage ear disease. With flexible endoscopes, clinicians can visually examine the middle ear anatomy, tympanic membrane, as well as the nasopharynx with unprecedented clarity. This direct visualization not only aids in the accurate diagnosis of diseases such as otitis media but also facilitates minimally invasive surgery, enhancing patient comfort and reducing recovery time. In particular, endoscopic ear surgery allows for more focused intervention, which can be vital when operating on complex pathologies, thereby optimizing the efficacy of hearing rehabilitation treatment. It is partially driven by advances in technologies behind sensors, creating the foundation for structural health monitoring and non-destructive testing, as contextualized by the systematic review of sensor sensing technologies (Hassani, S., & Dackermann, U., 2023). In addition, endoscopic procedures are more than simple diagnostics. Incorporating endoscopy with advanced technology has opened doors to new treatments personalized according to the specific patient needs. For instance, in conjunction with 3D printing, clinicians can design custom prostheses and implants using anatomical data obtained from imaging techniques such as CT and MRI. The custom approach is particularly advantageous in cases of complicated auditory reconstruction, such as ossicular chain reconstruction, where size and fit are absolutely essential in order to restore hearing functionality. Furthermore, endoscopic interventions are being explored for possible use of augmented reality, with the potential to enhance preoperative planning and intraoperative guidance, ultimately with even better hearing rehabilitation outcomes (Cornejo et al., 2022).

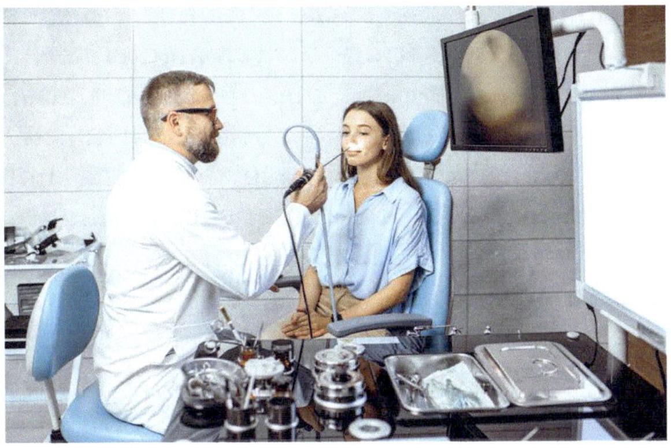

Figure 6.4. Endoscopic procedures have significantly advanced the field of auditory assessment and treatment.

Source: https://www.otorrinoicic.com/sites/default/files/styles/gesdi_row_image/public/2020-12/endoscopia-nasal-servicio-de-exploraciones-instituto-de-cabeza-y-cuello-icic.jpg?h=8ab0b107&itok=KPiDEhrp

The use of endoscopic interventions in hearing diagnosis and treatment is ongoing, showcasing a critical convergence of technology and clinical practice. The greater reliance on multifunctional endoscopes emphasizes the importance of precise anatomical visualization for successful patient care. As endoscopic techniques become more prevalent in clinics and operating rooms, their effects on hearing health cannot be overstated. The capability to conduct comprehensive assessments and implement personalized interventions creates new avenues for improved patient experience and outcomes in hearing rehabilitation. Ultimately, future progress in the field will likely be prompted by ongoing advancements in endoscopic applications, providing a foundation for improved treatment of hearing loss and related disorders and ultimately enhancing quality of life for millions of individuals (Figure 6.4).

6.3.2. Open Surgical Techniques for Tumor Removal

The application of open surgical techniques in tumor resection, particularly in cases involving hearing impairments, constitutes a pivotal boundary crossing between oncologic surgery and sound rehabilitation. Open surgery is advantageous in that it offers direct access to tumors that could be affecting life-critical structures like auditory pathways and facial nerves. These procedures typically employ advanced microsurgical techniques to maximize the potential for tumor resection while minimizing damage to adjacent neural tissues. In case of giant vestibular schwannomas, for instance, intraoperative neuromonitoring has proven to be unavoidable; it allows for facial nerve and cochlear function preservation that is vital for postoperative hearing and global quality of life. Meticulous surgical planning, including thorough evaluation of tumor grading, is critical, as recent research underscores the importance of systematic grading in patients' perioperative management of such tumors. Postoperative outcomes would often be about the primary surgical procedure performed, making the choice of open surgery a critical consideration for both surgeons and audiologists. Rehabilitation strategies after tumor removal may involve auditory training and hearing aids or cochlear implantation, depending on the degree of loss of hearing incurred during surgery.

The success of such rehabilitation methods is typically attributed to the degree of surgical resection and maintenance of auditory function. Indeed, as evidenced by current literature, multidisciplinary treatment protocols embracing surgical and rehabilitative intervention bear witness to high-quality patient outcomes and quality of life measures. By closely monitoring postoperative hearing thresholds and facial nerve function, healthcare providers can tailor rehabilitation protocols to individual patient needs, facilitating a more unified recovery process (Baijens et al., 2020). Furthermore, open surgical approaches require collaboration among otolaryngologists, audiologists, and rehabilitation therapists to provide comprehensive care following tumor excision. For instance, oropharyngeal dysphagia, more commonly a result of head and neck cancers, points to the heterogeneity of postoperative recovery and rehabilitation procedures (Baijens et al., 2020). This interdisciplinary cooperation allows for an insidious adjustment to individual challenges presented by patients after tumor surgery, for example, the assessment and enhancement of auditory function. While progress in surgery does much to accomplish oncologic control, the incorporation of hearing assessment into the protocol for rehabilitation is key to restoring overall patient function. The collaborative model demonstrates greater recognition of quality-of-life issues in surgical oncology, reaffirming the need for ongoing assessment and refinement of rehabilitation planning to meet evolving patient needs.

6.3.3. Reconstructive Surgery in Head and Neck Cases

In the context of hearing assessment and management, head and neck reconstructive surgery is a critical part in restoring both functional and aesthetic integrity. Such patients presenting with significant deformity or functional compromise due to congenital malformation, trauma, or oncologic resections will typically require advanced reconstruction. These procedures not only reestablish anatomical complexes but also serve as mechanisms of hearing, that is, the tympanic membrane and ossicular chain. Since psychological impacts of facial and neck deformities can also significantly contribute to quality of life impairment, as evidence shows, reconstructive surgery is a key element of overall rehabilitation treatment. Furthermore, the best outcomes of surgery can lead to improved auditory function and enable patients to communicate more effectively in communicative and social situations. Besides that, the integration of telemedicine has transformed pre- and postoperative patient care following head and neck reconstructive surgery. Telehealth technology was vital amid the pandemic to continue care without a significant risk of COVID-19 spread. However, telemedicine challenges such as technical issues and difficulties in the doctor-patient relationship cannot be overlooked (Ftouni et al., 2022). The inability to perform good physical examinations remotely, for instance, can interfere with accurate assessment of surgical candidacy or postoperative complications. Therefore, while telemedicine is a useful addition, it should not entirely supplant in-person evaluation, particularly in complicated cases that require thoroughly elaborated and highly nuanced plans of care with direct bearing on the rehabilitation of the ears. Moreover, cutting-edge treatments such as HBOT hold the potential to enhance outcomes in head and neck reconstructive surgery patients. HBOT may improve oxygen delivery to hypoxic tissues, promote angiogenesis, and likely minimize the risk of necrosis in surgical flaps, thereby promoting better healing and possibly supporting auditory recovery (Ortega et al., 2021). As research into the therapeutic potential of HBOT continues, it becomes progressively more important to assess its integration within holistic, comprehensive surgical and rehabilitation programs. With the use of new surgical techniques combined with adjunctive treatments like HBOT, health professionals can optimize the rehab process for patients to finally achieve improved hearing results and general wellbeing (Figure 6.5).

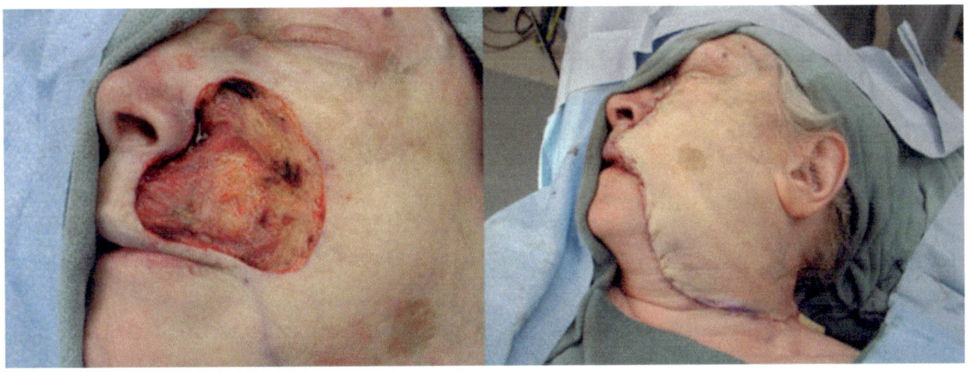

Figure 6.5. Reconstructive surgery for head and neck cases plays a pivotal role in restoring both functional and aesthetic integrity.

Source: https://www.google.com/url?sa=i&url=https%3A%2F%2Fwww.bradgarber.com%2Fplastic-reconstructive-surgery%2Freconstructive%2Fhead-neck-cancer-treatment.asp&psig=AOvVaw3itIlD2b8ClCTBSm7CL479&ust=1757981106017000&source=images&cd=vfe&opi=89978449&ved=0CBUQjRxqFwoTCKDnso282Y8DFQAAAAAdAAAAABAR

Test Your Knowledge

1. Describe the common surgical techniques used in head and neck surgery, including incision planning, dissection methods, hemostasis, and wound closure.
2. Discuss the principles and steps involved in major head and neck surgical procedures such as thyroidectomy, neck dissection, and laryngectomy, highlighting potential complications and their prevention.

6.4. Diagnostic Tools in ENT and Head and Neck Surgery

Learning Outcome

1. Role of Imaging Techniques (CT, MRI)
2. Importance of Endoscopy in Diagnosis
3. Audiological Assessments and Their Relevance

The process of hearing test and rehabilitation is greatly assisted by advanced diagnostic tools utilized in ENT and head and neck surgery. The key among these diagnostic methods is audiometry, specifically pure-tone and speech audiometry, which measure a person's hearing sensitivity across various frequencies. This diagnostic test can be a major criterion in identifying the occurrence and severity of hearing loss and guiding clinicians towards appropriate measures of rehabilitation. Early detection is important in the instance of presbycusis, with guidelines emphasizing the treatment of hearing loss symptoms in the early stages. Particularly, the use of questionnaires in conjunction with audiometry enhances patient disability measurement and enables more personalized forms of rehabilitation, such as hearing aids or cochlear implants, which have the potential to aid in cognitive preservation and enhance quality of life (Thai-Van et al., 2023). Moreover, imaging modalities such as CT and MRI complement the diagnostic roles of ENT practitioners. These modalities are a godsend when investigating pathologies that can lead to hearing loss, such as cholesteatoma or vestibulopathies. In dizziness and vertigo, for instance, the utility of imaging is achieved, especially in distinguishing between peripheral and central vestibulopathies. HINTS is a must-see bedside examination employed to differentiate these conditions without an emergent indication for imaging. Combining clinical tests with high-technology imaging allows for a complete understanding of the underlying pathology, which in turn ensures prompt, effective treatment choices that support hearing rehabilitation measures (Thong, G., & Casserly, P., 2019).

Moreover, newer technologies such as telehealth and mobile applications have transformed the era of hearing assessment. Remote monitoring systems enable audiologists to test patients' hearing and rehabilitation level remotely outside clinics, promoting follow-up care. These digital platforms can also include interactive hearing-testing tools for patient assessment, enabling active participation in their own treatment. By providing accessible resources that promote auditory rehabilitation and training exercises, these tools facilitate a more holistic approach to addressing hearing loss. Thus, the evolution of ENT and head and neck surgery diagnostic equipment not only enhances routine evaluation procedures but also supports cutting-edge practice that improves patient outcomes and advances hearing restoration (Thong, G., & Casserly, P., 2019; Thai-Van et al., 2023).

6.4.1. Role of Imaging Techniques (CT, MRI)

Imaging techniques such as computed tomography (CT) and magnetic resonance imaging (MRI) play crucial roles in diagnosing and treating hearing loss. These newer technologies can provide high-resolution images of the temporal bone and adjacent anatomical structures, which are critical for diagnosing most ear disorders. For instance, CT scans are superior for identifying bony abnormalities, such as cholesteatomas or otosclerosis, that cause hearing loss. Furthermore, MRI is important in the diagnosis of soft tissue lesions like acoustic neuromas or other tumors of the auditory nerve. With the use of these imaging technologies, clinicians can formulate targeted treatment strategies responding to the specific etiology of the patient's hearing disorder, leading to more effective rehabilitative procedures. In hearing assessment, integrating CT and MRI data is invaluable in planning surgical interventions as well as therapeutic interventions. For example, in head and neck cancer patients, imaging supports the multidisciplinary team in completing treatment plans based on individual needs. In accordance with supportive care guidelines, accurate imaging facilitates optimal treatment decisions in complex cases involving auditory structures. Also, advancements in imaging technologies have further enhanced the precision of these diagnostic devices to enable clinicians to see minute changes in anatomy, which can compromise hearing. Hence, these modalities are not just crucial for initial evaluation but also for monitoring disease and treatment during the course of rehabilitation (Pfister et al., 2020). The use of imaging techniques in hearing rehabilitation is also increasing, particularly as studies highlight their role in treating systemic disorders that affect hearing. For instance, conditions like X-linked hypophosphatemia (XLH) present severe effects on bone health and consequently hearing as a result of related complications such as osteocalcin. Imaging plays a vital role in the diagnosis of such pathologies, with the detection of pathology leading to hearing loss or other types of auditory dysfunction. With guidelines set for multisystemic diseases, concurrent evaluation of hearing and systemic status using advanced imaging may lead to improved outcomes. By facilitating the completion of a comprehensive patient assessment, imaging technologies ensure that the processes of rehabilitation are appropriately informed and targeted, eventually optimizing the qualitative aspects of life in patients (Haffner et al., 2019) (Figure 6.6).

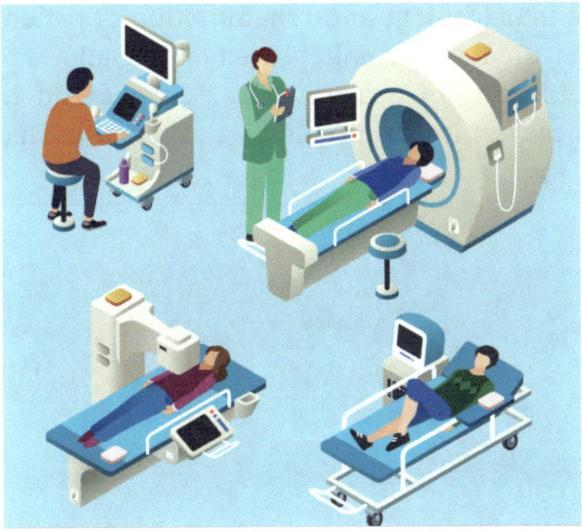

Figure 6.6. Role of imaging techniques (CT, MRI).

Source: https://i0.wp.com/averagejoemed.com/wp-content/uploads/2020/01/Medical-Imaging.png?resize=916%2C800&ssl=1.

6.4.2. Importance of Endoscopy in Diagnosis

The contribution of endoscopy to the process of hearing testing and rehabilitation cannot be overstated, particularly in diagnosis and therapy for auditory disorders. Endoscopic procedures allow ear experts to view the ear components with unparalleled precision, so that a complete examination of the outer ear canal, eardrum, and middle ear is possible. This visualization is also essential for the identification of obstructions, tumors, or abnormalities that could influence hearing. Moreover, endoscopy has been helpful in diagnosing diseases such as cholesteatoma or otitis media with effusion that could require immediate intervention to prevent further hearing loss. Direct visualization of these inner structures enhances the strength of diagnosis and makes way for more personalized treatment plans, ultimately improving patient outcomes in the audiology field. In addition, advances in endoscopy technology have added to its utility as a diagnostic aid. Modalities such as transnasal endoscopy are being used more commonly to explore the interaction between upper respiratory tract disease and hearing impairment. Not only does this technique enhance visualization, but it also allows for the biopsies to be taken, providing histological data that is essential in making an accurate diagnosis. Aside from its use in diagnosis, endoscopy can also be applied in guiding therapeutic intervention, for example, middle ear effusion drainage or removal of obstructive lesions that might be compromising auditory function. The inclusion of such new procedures indicates the evolving dynamics of auditory diagnostics, wherein endoscopy comes to serve as an essential instrument for both otolaryngologists and audiologists in maintaining patients' optimal rehabilitation plans. Lastly, endoscopy, coupled with advanced imaging modalities such as three-dimensional printing and augmented reality, holds significant promise for future hearing diagnosis and rehabilitation. Collaboration among researchers from various medical imaging and surgical fields has resulted in the development of models that assist with preoperative planning and patient-specific treatment. By taking advantage of the exact anatomical information obtained from CT and MRI scans, doctors are able to employ endoscopic techniques more precisely, delivering treatments specific to the individual anatomical quirks of each patient. As explained in recent studies, such advancement not only increases the success of surgery but also is a significant development towards more personalized care in the field, with focus on the very crucial role of endoscopy in enhancing the overall efficiency of hearing assessment and rehabilitation techniques (Lin et al., 2019; Cornejo et al., 2022).

6.4.3. Audiological Assessments and Their Relevance

Audiological assessments are basic elements in the diagnosis and treatment of hearing health. Audiological assessments determine the nature and extent of a person's hearing loss, thereby informing diagnosis and subsequent rehabilitation. For instance, hearing loss due to aging, known as presbycusis, entails gradual alterations in auditory function, which can extensively impact an individual's lifestyle. Among the complexities of aging and hearing processing, most elderly individuals experience a concurrent reduction in cognitive processes along with peripheral hearing impairment. Audiological assessments thus play an important role in identifying the nuances of auditory processing disorders, particularly among the elderly. Through accurate diagnosis of such issues, healthcare practitioners can adjust intervention strategies that not only address the physiological condition of hearing loss but also mitigate subsequent cognitive impairment, thereby enhancing overall well-being and communicative ability (Sardone et al., 2019).

In addition to diagnosing hearing loss, audiological testing plays a crucial role in the assessment of specific disorders, such as Meniere's disease, that create complexities in diagnosis and treatment. The insidious onset of Meniere's disease necessitates extensive audiometric evaluation to distinguish between its different stages and its influence upon auditory function. Enhanced diagnostic techniques and equipment have facilitated the identification of this disease more precisely. Present-day research, particularly that of the European Academy of Otology and Neurotology, emphasizes an organized diagnostic approach that links clinical findings to appropriate treatment modalities. The integration of these diagnostic results with audiological assessments drives the clinician's ability to develop treatment plans that address the various severities and presentations of Meniere's disease, with the ultimate aim of maximizing patient outcomes (Magnan et al., 2018). The use of audiological assessments goes beyond diagnosis and treatment planning and is also essential in the management and rehabilitation of patients over the long term. Repeated testing allows for monitoring of hearing status change and the efficacy of interventions as a function of time.

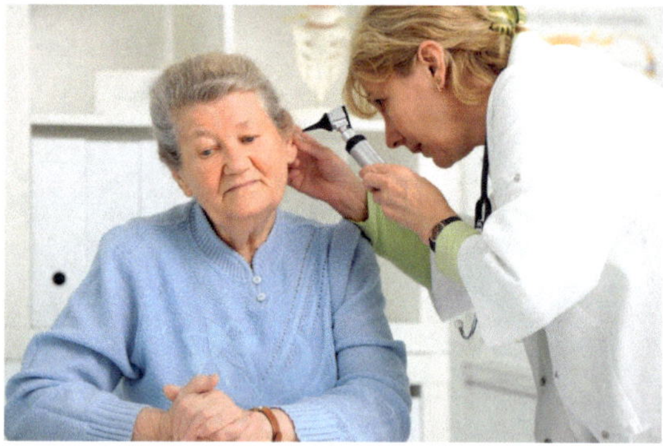

Figure 6.7. Audiological assessments are critical to understanding and managing hearing health.

Source: https://s3.amazonaws.com/media.audiologydesign.com/wp-content/uploads/sites/312/2024/02/01142616/audiologist-using-hearing-instrument-to-examine-inner-ear-canal-of-her-patient.jpg.

Regular assessment is especially needed in progressive disorders, as it allows for timely adjustments in therapeutic interventions. Audiologic testing is also used in health education to empower patients and their families to appreciate the impact of hearing impairment, as well as the benefit of early detection and treatment. By creating an awareness and proactive response to one's hearing, these tests facilitate both physical rehabilitation and a more active approach to overall health, enabling patients to maintain social interactions and quality of life despite auditory challenges (Figure 6.7).

Test Your Knowledge

1. What are the common diagnostic tools used in ENT and head & neck surgery, and what is the clinical importance of each?
2. Explain the role of endoscopy and imaging techniques (CT, MRI, and ultrasound) in the diagnosis of ENT and head & neck disorders.

6.5. Patient Management and Care

Learning Outcome

1. Preoperative Assessment and Preparation
2. Postoperative Care and Recovery
3. Multidisciplinary Approach to Patient Management

Effective patient management and care are central in the context of hearing assessment and rehabilitation. A patient management approach tailored to the individual ensures that each person receives targeted support that directly addresses their auditory issue. This is particularly important for people who have conditions like tinnitus, which is an affliction of millions worldwide. Sound therapy remains a central element in the majority of tinnitus treatment programs, employing a variety of techniques to minimize the salience of the condition in patients. Advances in cell phone technology have also expanded access to sound therapy software, enabling patients to incorporate self-help techniques into their daily lives. However, it has been observed in research that many individuals are yet to learn about such resources, further reiterating the need for health professionals to actively make patients aware of aids that support management strategies (Sereda et al., 2019). Management of congenital aural atresia is also one of the subspecialties of auditory rehabilitation that comes with early diagnosis and individualized interventions. Bilateral atresia patients benefit most from early amplification interventions, and bone conduction hearing aids play a central role in facilitating speech development. Rehabilitation is a difficult process; for only specific candidates, there are surgical options available, but much controversy still exists over the optimal age of intervention and for choosing ideal candidates for successful outcomes. For less-than-ideal surgical candidates, alternatives such as bone-anchored hearing aids are valuable alternatives that do not take away from future options. The strategy is to judiciously select surgical candidates and employ evidence-based techniques that incorporate patient-specific requirements to avoid unnecessary surgery while maximizing potential auditory gain (Declau et al., 1999). Patient care beyond hearing rehabilitation starts and moves into the stage of ongoing care and adjustment. Ongoing follow-up with rehabilitation therapists and audiologists helps clinicians monitor progress and modify treatment protocols as necessary. The incorporation of psychological counseling can enhance patient results even more, especially in cases where tinnitus treatment presents significant emotional or psychological factors. By fostering an interactive relationship with patients and an integrative care model, practitioners can address both auditory and psychosocial factors that contribute to overall well-being. Not only is this the key to aiding patients' existing hearing needs, but it also leads to patients taking more of an active role in their rehabilitation, leading to improved quality of life and hearing (Sereda et al., 2019).

6.5.1. Preoperative Assessment and Preparation

Preoperative assessment and preparation for cochlear implantation are critical elements in the prediction of the likelihood of successful auditory rehabilitation results. Thorough evaluation begins with a thorough medical history and audiological assessment, which aid in the identification of specific factors that influence both candidacy for the implant as well as potential recovery patterns. In situations involving children with conditions such as prelingually sensorineural deafness (PLSND), the extent of cerebral white matter lesions (CWMLs) has a significant impact on auditory, speech, and non-verbal cognitive outcomes following surgery. Studies have established that about 15% of PLSND children have CWMLs, with the severely affected ones having reduced auditory function prior to and following cochlear implantation. Thus, the refinement of preoperative assessments to take such aspects into account enhances the process of surgical candidate selection and facilitates individualized rehabilitation strategies in the future (Li et al., 2025). In addition to the medical aspect, the psychosocial aspect is part and parcel of preoperative assessments, particularly in children who are to undergo cochlear implantation. Evaluation of family dynamics, social support, and attitudes of caregivers can influence both the process of decision-making and the anticipated success of the rehabilitation process. Parents are likely to provide critical information about a child's communication demands and daily problems that might not be evident by clinical evaluation alone. Moreover, information about the home life of the child before surgery can inform planning to optimize postoperative rehabilitation optimally. Evidence shows that intensive counseling prior to implantation facilitates families to develop realistic expectations regarding outcomes and support mechanisms and to enhance commitment to continuing auditory and speech therapy and surgical intervention (Friis et al., 2024). Interdisciplinary collaboration is critical during the preoperative stage, and care must be taken to ensure that a child's unique needs are met in a holistic manner. Audiologists, otolaryngologists, speech therapists, and psychologists should collaborate on an integrated strategy to treat both medical and rehabilitative problems effectively.

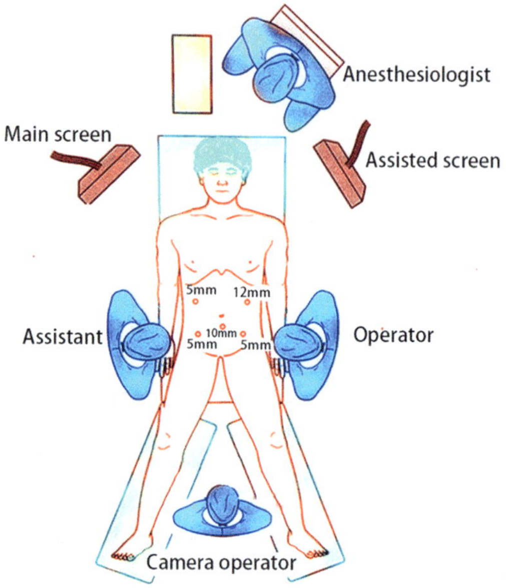

Figure 6.8. The preoperative assessment and preparation for cochlear implantation play a crucial role in determining the likelihood of successful auditory rehabilitation outcomes.

Source: https://www.researchgate.net/publication/336569594/figure/fig1/AS:814495635079180@1571202300213/Preoperative-preparation-the-position-of-patient-surgeon-screen-and-trocar.png.

This multidisciplinary process enables teams to identify such factors as age during implantation and potential etiologic factors for hearing loss that influence success in the long term. For instance, children with congenitally sensorineural hearing loss are likely to benefit from earlier implantation than those with acquired sensorineural hearing loss. By employing a thorough preoperative evaluation that combines these various perspectives, health professionals can develop an integrated rehabilitation plan that not just treats the surgery but also readies the child for the complex challenges and support required in the child's hearing process following implantation (Friis et al., 2024; Li et al., 2025) (Figure 6.8).

6.5.2. Postoperative Care and Recovery

Postoperative care is also crucial to overall recovery in patients undergoing hearing-related surgeries. The surgeries could be tympanoplasty, cochlear implant, or tympanostomy tube insertion, with the aim of improving auditory function. Effective postoperative care is not just essential in minimizing complications but in maximizing auditory outcomes. This involves close monitoring of the patient's vital signs and the wound site for evidence of infection or reaction. Proper pain control is also essential, as pain can slow the rehabilitation process. Follow-up schedules on a regular basis are necessary to check on the progress of healing and compliance with rehabilitation exercises. By controlling these critical factors, medical personnel can provide a more uneventful recovery course, ultimately guaranteeing that patients maximally utilize their post-surgical auditory capabilities. In the area of hearing rehabilitation, both post-operative therapy and continued audiological management cannot be overstated. Postoperatively, patients often require audiological evaluation to assess hearing status and guide rehabilitation. This can involve the selection of hearing aids or cochlear device programming to optimize auditory function. Audiologists are at the core of this stage, as they work to take their patients through the complex process of auditory training and adaptation to novel hearing sensations. In addition, patient and family member education and counseling are essential in informing them about the rehabilitation process and the importance of ongoing follow-up treatment. Postoperative rehabilitation ultimately leads to effective rehabilitation outcomes since adherence to prescribed practice can have a direct impact on the effectiveness of auditory treatments and quality of life for individuals with hearing disabilities. Psychological and emotional support must also be included in postoperative care and recovery in hearing assessment and rehabilitation. Patients often experience anxiety and uncertainty following surgical interventions, making counseling and support services essential. This psychological aspect is particularly critical as emotional well-being can directly influence a patient's motivation to engage in rehabilitation practices. The collaborative efforts among audiologists, speech therapists, and mental health professionals can address these concerns holistically. Furthermore, support groups and community resources can provide additional encouragement and connection, which are invaluable during recovery. By identifying and treating the emotional component of postoperative recovery, healthcare professionals can produce strong patients with good outcomes and successful rehabilitation (ElSayed et al., 2022; Óskarsdóttir et al., 2023).

6.5.3. Multidisciplinary Approach to Patient Management

Patient care, particularly in hearing testing and rehabilitation settings, is increasingly guided by a multidisciplinary approach. This type of system integrates a number of specialists, including audiologists, speech-language pathologists, and occupational therapists, who collaborate to meet the multifaceted challenges of hearing-impaired patients. Not only does this cooperative process enhance diagnosis, but it also allows for integrated treatment plans customized to every patient case. For example, the speech-language pathologist may focus on cognition-communication functions impaired by hearing loss, as outlined in guidelines for cognitive rehabilitation in adult acquired brain injury (Panel et al., 2022). Engaging multiple professionals simultaneously may enhance the overall perception of a patient's issue, thereby positively influencing rehabilitation outcomes and quality of life in patients with hearing impairment. The blending of various perspectives from different fields significantly strengthens the rehabilitation process and responds to the intricate nature of hearing loss. Clinicians can offer observations that inform better patient care strategies, particularly considering the relationship between hearing loss and associated conditions such as cognitive impairment or risk of falling. Research has also shown that older patients with hearing loss are at higher risk of falls and functional decline, underscoring the need for an organized interdisciplinary strategy (M-Odasso et al., 2022). With good communication among practitioners, patients are likely to undergo early interventions that minimize the risks and maximize their ability to participate socially and occupationally. This holistic model of care not only addresses urgent issues related to hearing loss but also supports overall well-being and health. Building a highly coordinated multidisciplinary team highly benefits patients by ensuring care continuity throughout their recuperation process. Well-coordinated communication among the team members gives them the opportunity to continually adjust treatment plans based on patients' evolving needs and desires. Interdisciplinary regular sessions enable such collaboration to take place, and they are able to address any emerging issues in a creative manner. Thus, patients struggling with the complexities of hearing loss can receive better assistance as they undergo rehabilitation. Further, a multidisciplinary model promotes patient empowerment through involvement in decision-making, hence putting their concerns and preferences first. Hence, the adoption of this model is advantageous not only for clinical practice but also promotes a patient-centered approach to hearing assessment and treatment, ultimately improving the quality of life for those affected (Figure 6.9).

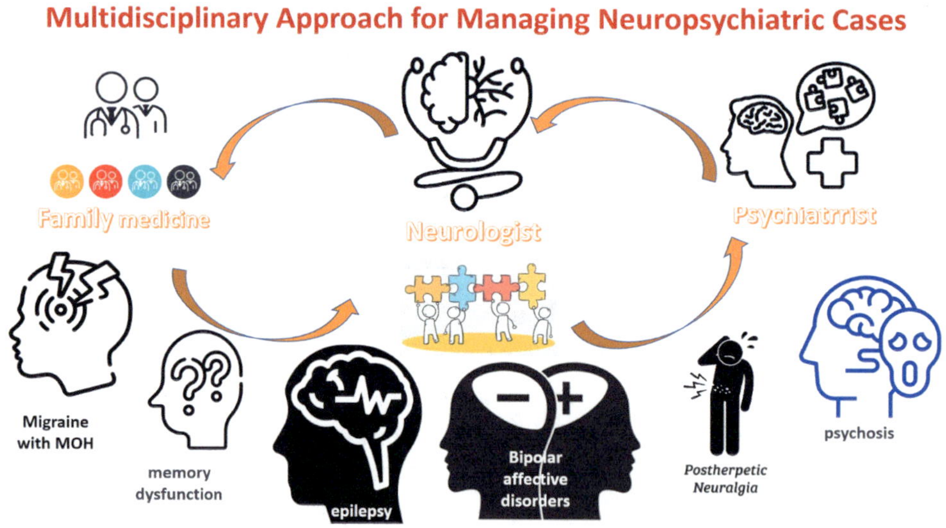

Figure 6.9. Multidisciplinary approach to patient management.

Source: https://www.mdpi.com/jcm/jcm-12-05754/article_deploy/html/images/jcm-12-05754-g001.png.

Test Your Knowledge

1. What are the essential steps in evaluating and managing a patient with ENT or head and neck disorders?
2. Explain the principles of preoperative and postoperative care, including patient counseling and follow-up in ENT surgery.

6.6. Advances and Innovations in ENT and Head and Neck Surgery

Learning Outcome

1. Technological Advancements in Surgical Tools
2. Emerging Treatments and Therapies
3. Research Trends and Future Directions in the Field

The field of otolaryngology, and hearing assessment and rehabilitation in particular, has experienced remarkable advances that enhance patient care. Diagnostic technology advances, such as sophisticated audiometric assessment and genetic testing, have become key drivers for the prompt diagnosis of presbycusis, a condition of hearing deterioration associated with aging. These developments are indicative of an integrated reaction advocated by multi-disciplinary teams of hearing professionals, which illustrates the importance of early identification and effective rehabilitation techniques. Notably, the application of free-field speech audiometry makes it easier to test hearing under a more naturalistic listening environment, thus optimizing intelligibility testing in patients with hearing loss. Incorporation of questionnaires with audiometry permits an overall understanding of patients' hearing ability and disabilities and thus guides interventions as per individual requirements (Thai-Van et al., 2023). Improvements in equipment, as well as medication in the ENT scenario, also play an important role in managing hearing impairments. The FDA's approval of over-the-counter hearing aids is a giant leap, providing auditory rehabilitation to the masses at an affordable price. The democratization of hearing technology provides individuals with options tailored to their individual and financial needs and facilitates rehabilitation adherence. Besides, advances in cochlear implant technology have enhanced the outcome for persons with severe to profound sensorineural hearing loss. These technologies not only improve the sound quality but also support cognitive preservation in patients, disrupting the relationship between untreated hearing loss and cognitive decline (Choi et al., 2022). As a result, ongoing technological improvements continually redefine the way healthcare providers engage with hearing testing and rehabilitation. As the dynamics of ENT and head and neck surgery evolve, the integration of digital technology in hearing rehabilitation becomes increasingly relevant. Apps accessible on tablets and smartphones enable independent practice and sustained engagement in auditory and cognitive training and can supplement traditional therapy sessions. The potential for remote management and telehealth consultation is a paradigm shift toward more patient-centered and flexible care. With the use of these new applications, clinicians are better able to treat each patient's special needs while overcoming barriers to in-office visits. As testified by ongoing and emerging research, the future of auditory rehabilitation is ensured through technology, which not only optimizes the efficacy of interventions but also that of patient satisfaction and adherence. Taken together, these advances herald a new era for the practice, one committed to developing integrative, patient-centered plans for hearing loss (Thai-Van et al., 2023) (Figure 6.10).

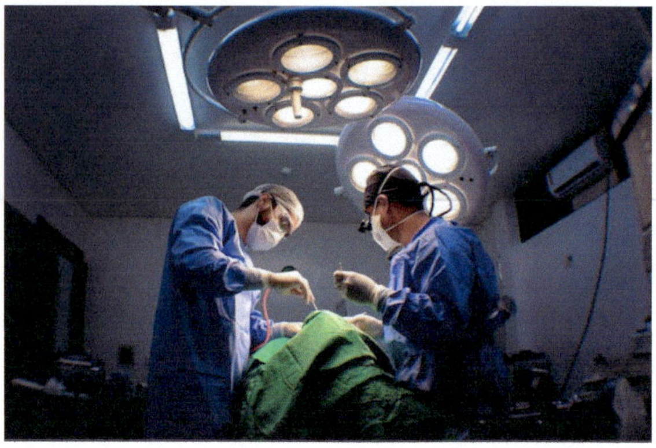

Figure 6.10. Advances and innovations in ENT and head and neck surgery.

Source: https://www.bestentdoctor.nyc/wp-content/uploads/2024/05/pexels-weverton-oliveira-927931218-20217787.jpg.

6.6.1. Technological Advancements in Surgical Tools

The field of hearing testing and rehabilitation has seen significant advances in surgical instrumentation, driven by technological developments. The instrumentation has developed a lot to enhance surgical precision and patient outcomes, particularly for otolaryngology surgeries aimed at correcting hearing disabilities. For instance, sophisticated imaging technology like high-resolution computed tomography and magnetic resonance imaging allows detailed visualization of the ear anatomy. This aids surgeons in more accurately diagnosing and planning interventions, minimizing risks, and improving procedure success rates, such as tympanoplasty or cochlear implantation. As the anatomy is better comprehended, the surgeon can use these advanced tools to achieve improved esthetic and functional results, aligning interventions with better-suited individual patients' needs. These advances underscore the necessity of integrating technology into surgery to optimize hearing restoration techniques and improve patient quality of life. Parallel to advances in imaging, surgical instruments engineered with precision technologies, such as robotic-assisted instruments, have transformed surgical techniques in hearing rehabilitation. These instruments offer improved dexterity and control and allow surgeons to perform intricate procedures with unprecedented accuracy. For instance, robotic systems can minimize trauma to surrounding tissues during soft ear surgeries, shortening recovery and postoperative complication time. Augmented reality overlays can also assist in providing real-time information in the operating room, enhancing situational awareness and enabling the surgeon to make more informed decisions. Such tools not only facilitate the surgical process but also improve the safety profile of such procedures. The use of these technologies is part of a broader trend toward minimally invasive surgery, leading to greater patient comfort and faster recovery, and attests to the significant change in hearing restoration surgery. Moreover, the integration of artificial intelligence (AI) into diagnosing and monitoring hearing diseases is a revolutionary innovation within the development of surgical devices. Computer-savvy algorithms search vast databases to identify patterns in the operation of hearing, allowing for more precise assessments and individualized therapy alternatives. Machine learning, for example, is revolutionizing the interpretation of audiometric testing, enabling clinicians to provide tailored treatment plans based on individual hearing profiles. These advancements extend to rehabilitation, where sensor systems and mobile accelerometers, as reported in research, enable improved monitoring of rehabilitation exercises and postoperative recovery. Through the application of next-generation sensor technologies and AI, providers of treatment outcomes can enhance overall treatment outcome effectiveness, providing patients with the most appropriate interventions. Together, these developments suggest an increasingly cohesive approach to hearing analysis and treatment, integrating surgical precision with advanced monitoring practices (Procházka et al., 2024; Shetty, S., & Kasrija, R., 2025).

6.6.2. Emerging Treatments and Therapies

The field of hearing assessment and therapy is evolving rapidly, and new therapies and treatments are being developed to address various auditory issues. One area of advancement is the use of auditory brainstem implants (ABIs) for individuals with hearing loss resulting from cochlear nerve damage. Unlike traditional cochlear implants, ABIs bypass the cochlea altogether and stimulate the auditory pathway in the brainstem directly. This discovery brings new hope to patients who previously had little recourse, especially those with extreme sensorineural hearing loss. As research continues, the potential for using ABIs as an addition to rehabilitation treatments may enhance auditory perception and improve the quality of life for those affected. These advancements represent a giant leap toward tailoring more effective intervention methods that address individual patient needs. In addition, the use of pharmacological therapy is increasingly relevant in the rehabilitation of hearing. New drugs, in particular, which target chosen molecular mechanisms involved in auditory function, are under investigation for their therapeutic potential. Therapeutic drugs that target the neurotrophin levels are, for example, potentially useful in promoting hair cell regeneration and neural recovery following acoustic trauma. These drug therapies not only aim to restore auditory function but also to preserve residual hearing, thereby enhancing the overall efficacy of auditory rehabilitation programs. With the accumulation of more data on the efficacy of these new therapies, it becomes imperative to incorporate these treatments into existing rehabilitation frameworks so that patient outcomes can be optimized. The integration of pharmacology and auditory therapy can revolutionize the treatment of hearing loss in clinical settings. Additionally, innovative technologies such as virtual reality (VR) are beginning to transform clinical practice in hearing rehabilitation. Virtual reality applications generate advanced environments designed to facilitate auditory training, allowing one to practice sound localization and improve speech perception in the presence of background noise. Because they simulate normal listening environments, these treatments facilitate active engagement in therapy and can be tailored to address varied levels of auditory processing. With increased use of VR in rehabilitation. It is important to assess the effectiveness of these interventions and their contribution to overall hearing rehabilitation outcomes. Enabling this, interdisciplinary research exploring the neurophysiological effects of such technology may provide insight into their long-term benefits, providing avenues to comprehensive auditory rehabilitation programs that incorporate the most current technological advancements (Figure 6.11).

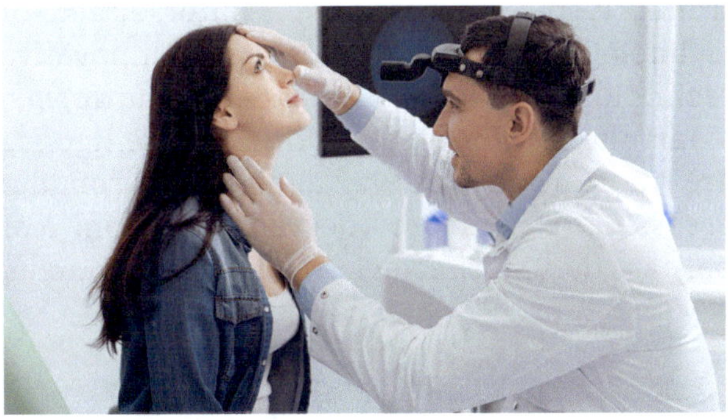

Figure 6.11. The field of hearing assessment and rehabilitation is evolving rapidly, with emerging treatments and therapies being developed to address a range of auditory impairments.

Source: https://www.entandallergyspecialists.com/wp-content/uploads/2017/09/checking-nose.jpg.

6.6.3. Research Trends and Future Directions in the Field

The field of hearing disability assessment and rehabilitation is undergoing a revolutionary change as researchers have become increasingly interested in the pivotal application of the International Classification of Functioning, Disability and Health (ICF). This framework attempts to establish a general plan for comprehending how hearing impairment affects individuals' everyday living. Existing literature identifies that the ICF suggests a multi-dimensional approach to allow further nuanced classification of hearing loss and its resulting challenges. In audiology, researchers aim to enhance clinical practice and rehabilitation outcomes through its use. However, its application has remained limited in practice with the recent World Health Organization approval of the ICF. As this model becomes integrated into practice and research, the expectation is that future studies will increasingly refer to it in order to address varying patient populations and enhance the holistic approach toward hearing rehabilitation (Bruyere et al., 2005). Furthermore, one of the predominant research trends is the interest in the intersection of technology and hearing assessments. Innovative technologies such as telehealth platforms, smartphone apps, and artificial intelligence are transforming the way audiologists conduct assessments and provide rehabilitation. Not only are these technologies making assessments more accessible, but they also offer real-time data collection to create customized treatment plans. Initial research indicates that the use of technology can increase patient engagement and outcomes. With the growing popularity of telehealth, future studies should focus on developing standardized protocols to integrate these technologies into conventional practice. Continued research of these technologies can help close service delivery gaps and impact populations traditionally underserved for hearing health (Neill et al., 2004). Finally, the psychosocial impacts of hearing loss are an increasingly significant area of research in hearing rehabilitation. Research is increasingly focusing on hearing impairment co-morbidities, such as social isolation and depression, and on the need for holistic models of care. Through research into these associations, researchers are advocating holistic intervention, including mental health care as well as traditional auditory rehabilitation. Interdisciplinary collaboration among audiologists, psychologists, and social workers is advocated to address the broader consequences of hearing loss. Future research can also be focused on developing intervention techniques not only for improving auditory function but also for improving the overall quality of life for hearing-impaired people. Such an integrated approach may also lead to more effective rehabilitation outcomes and thereby promote inclusion for victims of hearing loss (Bruyere et al., 2005).

Test Your Knowledge

1. What are some recent technological advances in ENT and head & neck surgery, and how have they improved patient outcomes?
2. Explain the role of minimally invasive techniques, robotic surgery, and laser applications in modern ENT practice.

SUMMARY

The implication of this chapter is the essential importance of early hearing assessment and timely rehabilitation in establishing the optimal developmental results in children. Evidence cited here indicates that congenital hearing loss affects a significant proportion of infants, with one such prevalence of approximately 5% from a recent report clearly illustrating the significance of early identification by methods like Automated Auditory Brainstem Response (AABR) screening (Huang et al., 2025). Intervention at an early stage can counteract the potential impairment of language acquisition, socialization, and intellectual development. By prioritizing systematic newborn hearing screening, healthcare systems can ensure follow-up for those at risk and maximize lifelong outcomes for affected individuals. Beyond the clinical aspects of hearing assessment, the integration of cutting-edge strategies, such as tele-practice, offers a thrilling platform for expanding access to rehabilitation services. Recent research has enlightened the possibility of tele-practice to address the shifting needs of families and ensure that children with hearing loss are provided with proper diagnostic and therapeutic interventions. Parents have shown strong interest in this approach and have requested a hybrid model combining face-to-face encounters and off-site consultations (Jesudass et al., 2025). Through adopting tele-practice, particularly among rural or underserved populations, speech-language pathologists and audiologists have the ability to maximize service delivery, ultimately allowing greater numbers of families access to necessary rehabilitation services and enhancing children's developmental trajectories. Finally, the problems that were noted within the literature, that is, greater awareness among the community and training on hearing loss and rehabilitation services, cannot be omitted. Parent and stakeholder education must be part of intervention strategies, including information about resources, the benefits of early intervention, and the benefits of new models of service delivery. To be effective, community engagement is essential to the implementation of these interventions, particularly given the multifactorial nature of risk for hearing impairment and the social and emotional impact on families (Huang et al., 2025). Therefore, collective efforts toward public awareness and access to hearing evaluation and rehabilitation are critical to developing a supportive infrastructure that promotes healthy development in children with hearing impairment.

In the field of hearing rehabilitation and evaluation, the critical evaluation of treatments has been under tremendous criticism. The roles of various modalities, such as repetitive transcranial magnetic stimulation (rTMS), have been brought into the limelight in recent studies, emphasizing their potential therapeutic applications in a range of neurological diseases, which would have spin-off benefits for auditory rehabilitation as well. High-frequency rTMS of the primary motor cortex proved to be unequivocally effective in the treatment of neuropathic pain, whereas low-frequency rTMS proved to be effective in facilitating motor recovery after strokes, a condition usually associated with difficulties in the performance of auditory processes. The evidence that rTMS can lead to beneficial effects in disorders like depression and motor disability further lends itself to its use in hearing rehabilitation, especially for those patients who may have dual issues of auditory loss and emotional distress (Jean-Lefaucheur et al., 2020). In addition, successful stroke rehabilitation measures have been at the center of the European Stroke Action Plan with a multidisciplinary care focus, including management, rehabilitation, and ongoing evaluation of stroke outcome. The plan also brings into focus specific priorities that not only can be used for the patient with stroke but can also be applied to the patient with auditory difficulties since both of them can benefit from an evidence-based, structured rehabilitation strategy. The focus on coordinated care and early intervention underscores the need for hearing experts to collaborate with other healthcare practitioners to deliver comprehensive care to patients. In addition, the appeal for national action and quality measurement further emphasizes the necessity of not only making auditory rehabilitation services available but also effective, in order to enhance overall outcomes for patients in this integrated healthcare field (Norrving et al., 2018). Finally, integration of new discoveries in research into the practice of hearing evaluation and rehabilitation is important to advancing the practice of hearing evaluation and treatment. Continued review of the latest techniques, such as the applications of rTMS in audiology, informs best practice and encourages creative solutions for particular requirements. Not only does this enhance therapeutic results, but it also opens up inquiry into inter- and cross-disciplinary approaches that can more effectively enhance auditory outcomes. By cooperation and openness to new evidence, healthcare professionals are better able to address the complexities of hearing loss, especially in the context of comorbidities like stroke or depression. Such a wide-ranging strategy is essential to creating a comprehensive platform for hearing rehabilitation, ultimately attaining a better quality of life for patients with auditory impairments (Norrving et al., 2018; Jean-Lefaucheur et al., 2020).

KEY TERMS FROM THIS CHAPTER

- Pure Tone Audiometry
- Tympanometry
- Audiogram
- Air Conduction Testing
- Otoacoustic Emissions (OAE)
- Impedance Audiometry
- Diagnostic Audiometry
- Masking
- Auditory Training
- Speech Audiometry
- Acoustic Reflex Testing
- Bone Conduction Testing
- Free Field Testing
- Auditory Brainstem Response (ABR)
- Screening Audiometry
- Hearing Threshold
- Recruitment
- Hearing Aid

CRITICAL THINKING QUESTIONS

1. **Pure tone audiometry is used to assess:**
   a) Middle ear pressure
   b) Hearing threshold
   c) Speech understanding
   d) Balance
2. **The graphical representation of hearing sensitivity is called:**
   a) Audiometer
   b) Audiogram
   c) Tympanogram
   d) Sonogram
3. **Tympanometry mainly evaluates:**
   a) Inner ear function
   b) Middle ear function
   c) Auditory nerve function
   d) Cochlear function
4. **The normal hearing threshold range is:**
   a) 0–10 dB
   b) 0–20 dB
   c) 20–40 dB
   d) 40–60 dB
5. **Which test assesses cochlear outer hair cell function?**
   a) ABR
   b) OAE
   c) PTA
   d) Tympanometry

Short Answer Questions

1. What is meant by hearing assessment, and why is it important in clinical practice?
2. Describe the basic methods of hearing evaluation, including subjective and objective tests.
3. Explain the principles of pure tone audiometry and its clinical significance.
4. What is speech audiometry? Discuss its role in hearing assessment.
5. Describe the impedance audiometry (tympanometry) and its applications.

Answers to Critical Thinking Questions

1. (b) 2. (b) 3. (b) 4. (b) 5. (b)

REFERENCES

1. Akyol, M. U., Co-Chairs, M. C. P., Alden, T. D., Amartino, H., Ashworth, J., Belani, K., Berger, K. I., Borgo, A., Braunlin, E., Eto, Y., Gold, J. I., Jester, A., Jones, S. A., Karsli, C., Mackenzie, W., Marinho, D. R., McFadyen, A., McGill, J., Mitchell, J. J., . . . Scarpa, M. (2019). Recommendations for the management of MPS VI: systematic evidence- and consensus-based guidance. *Orphanet Journal of Rare Diseases, 14*(1), 118. https://doi.org/10.1186/s13023-019-1080-yAkyol, M. U., Alden, T. D., Amartino, H., Ashworth, J., et al. (2019). *Recommendations for the management of MPS IVA: Systematic evidence- and consensus-based guidance.* https://core.ac.uk/download/323075225.pdf (accessed on 7th August 2025).

2. Altissimi, G., Cianfrone, G., Ciofalo, A., Greco, A., et al. (2016). *When Alarm Bells Ring: Emergency Tinnitus.* https://core.ac.uk/download/54538689.pdf (accessed on 7th August 2025).

3. Baijens, L. W. J., Walshe, M., Aaltonen, L. M., Arens, C., Cordier, R., Cras, P., Crevier-Buchman, L., et al. (2020). European white paper: Oropharyngeal dysphagia in head and neck cancer. *European Archives of Oto-Rhino-Laryngology, 278*, 577–616. https://doi.org/10.1007/s00405-020-06507-5 (accessed on 7th August 2025).

4. Bruyere, S. M., Peterson, D., & VanLooy, S. (2005). *The International Classification of Functioning, Disability and Health: Contemporary Literature Overview.* https://core.ac.uk/download/5124461.pdf (accessed on 7th August 2025).

5. Choi, A. M., Brenner, M., Gorelik, D., Erbele, I. D., Crowson, M. G., Kadkade, P. P., Takashima, M., et al. (2022). New medical device and therapeutic approvals in otolaryngology: State of the art review of 2021. *OTO Open, 6.* https://www.semanticscholar.org/paper/9b78bfff11f6163ba7dc8fe66074d489b4e33744 (accessed on 7th August 2025).

6. Christensen, P., Baeten, C. I. M., Espín, E., Martellucci, J., Nugent, K., Zerbib, F., Pellino, G., et al. (2021). Management guidelines for low anterior resection syndrome – The MANUEL project. *Colorectal Disease, 23*, 461–475. https://doi.org/10.1111/codi.15517 (accessed on 7th August 2025).

7. Cornejo, J., Cornejo, J., Vargas, M., Helguero, C. G., Andrade, R. M., Torres, S., Asensio-Salazar, J., et al. (2022). Anatomical engineering and 3D printing for surgery and medical devices: International review and future exponential innovations. *BioMed Research International, 2022*, 1–28. https://doi.org/10.1155/2022/6797745 (accessed on 7th August 2025).

8. De Sousa, K. C., Swanepoel, D. W., Moore, D. R., Myburgh, H. C., & Smits, C. (2019). Improving sensitivity of the digits-in-noise test using anti-phasic stimuli. *Ear and Hearing, 41*, 442–450. https://doi.org/10.1097/aud.0000000000000775 (accessed on 7th August 2025).

9. Declau, F., Cremers, C., & Heyning, P. (1999). Diagnosis and management strategies in congenital atresia of the external auditory canal. *British Journal of Audiology, 33*, 313–327. https://www.semanticscholar.org/paper/0ab6fae9a43290d1e36d783838b72e9a7a741933 (accessed on 7th August 2025).

10. Ebrahimi-Madiseh, A., Nickbakht, M., Eikelboom, R. H., Bennett, R. J., Friedland, P., Atlas, M. D., & Jessup, R. (2023). Models of service delivery in adult cochlear implantation and evaluation of outcomes: A scoping review of delivery arrangements. *PLoS ONE, 18*, e0285443. https://doi.org/10.1371/journal.pone.0285443 (accessed on 7th August 2025).

11. ElSayed, N. A., Aleppo, G., Aroda, V. R., Bannuru, R. R., Brown, F. M., Bruemmer, D., Collins, B. S., et al. (2022). 4. Comprehensive medical evaluation and assessment of comorbidities: *Standards of care in diabetes—2023. Diabetes Care, 46*, S49–S67.2. https://doi.org/10.2337/dc23-s004 (accessed on 7th August 2025).

12. Friis, I. J., Aaberg, K., Edholm, B., Jørgensen, K. F., Britze, A., Thrane, J. F., & Devantier, L. (2024). Cochlear implantation in children with single-sided deafness: Preoperative assessment and device use. *Annals of Otolaryngology and Rhinology.* https://www.semanticscholar.org/paper/32e6f59b1bcecd73894cd6958b5c3b48c37b5776 (accessed on 7th August 2025).

13. Ftouni, R., AlJardali, B., Hamdanieh, M., Ftouni, L., & Salem, N. (2022). Challenges of telemedicine during the COVID-19 pandemic: A systematic review. *BMC Medical Informatics and Decision Making, 22.* https://doi.org/10.1186/s12911-022-01952-0 (accessed on 7th August 2025).

14. Greenhalgh, T., Sivan, M., Delaney, B., Evans, R. A., & Milne, R. (2022). Long COVID—An update for primary care. *BMJ.* https://doi.org/10.1136/bmj-2022-072117 (accessed on 7th August 2025).

15. Guideline Development Panel, Brown, J., Kaelin, D. L., Mattingly, E., Mello, C., Miller, E. S., Mitchell, G., et al. (2022). American Speech-Language-Hearing Association Clinical Practice Guideline: Cognitive rehabilitation for the management of cognitive dysfunction associated with acquired brain injury. *American Journal of Speech-Language Pathology, 31*, 2455–2526. https://doi.org/10.1044/2022_ajslp-21-00361 (accessed on 7th August 2025).

16. Haffner, D., Emma, F., Eastwood, D. M., Biosse, D. M., Bacchetta, J., Schnabel, D., Wicart, P., et al. (2019). Clinical practice recommendations for the diagnosis and management of X-linked hypophosphatemia. *Nature Reviews Nephrology, 15*, 435–455. https://doi.org/10.1038/s41581-019-0152-5 (accessed on 7th August 2025).

17. Hassani, S., & Dackermann, U. (2023). A systematic review of advanced sensor technologies for non-destructive testing and structural health monitoring. *Sensors, 23*, 2204. https://doi.org/10.3390/s23042204 (accessed on 7th August 2025).

18. Hickey, H. (2023). International Congress on Academic Medicine: 2023 medical education abstracts. *Canadian Medical Education Journal.* https://doi.org/10.36834/cmej.77628 (accessed on 7th August 2025).

19. Huang, M., Jing, Y., Peng, X., Xie, J., Zhao, Q., Yin, J. L., Xiao, W. D., et al. (2025). Neonatal hearing loss risk factors and miRNA biomarkers identified through AABR screening. *Journal of Multidisciplinary Healthcare, 18*, 2541–2550. https://www.semanticscholar.org/paper/2375e7132ead785290ac34dd9559def946670043 (accessed on 7th August 2025).

20. Jesudass, N., Ramkumar, V., Kumar, S., & Venkatesh, L. (2025). Parents' perceptions regarding needs and readiness for tele-practice implementation within a public health system for the identification and rehabilitation of children with hearing and speech–language disorders in South India. *International Journal of Environmental Research and Public Health, 22.* https://www.semanticscholar.org/paper/60523394803eceb36b23fc95edbe6d5d84323a3e (accessed on 7th August 2025).

21. Kawecki, D., & Majewska, A. (2021). Pneumonia in the COVID-19 era – Emergency room physician's perspective. Part II – Diagnosis and therapy. *Emergency Medical Service, 8*, 179–189. https://doi.org/10.36740/emems202103109 (accessed on 7th August 2025).

22. Leach, A., Morris, P. S., Coates, H., Nelson, S., O'Leary, S., Richmond, P., Gunasekera, H., et al. (2021). Otitis media guidelines for Australian Aboriginal and Torres Strait Islander children: Summary of recommendations. *The Medical Journal of Australia, 214*, 228–233. https://doi.org/10.5694/mja2.50953 (accessed on 7th August 2025).
23. Lee, J., Ishihara, S., Ishihara, K., & Ito, K. (2024). Proximal auditory AR rehabilitation: System integration and wellness applications—from hearing support up toward vestibular rehabilitation. *Frontiers in Rehabilitation Sciences, 5.* https://www.semanticscholar.org/paper/ed788188723af881caf5684a5d3fd25645852d45 (accessed on 7th August 2025).
24. Lefaucheur, J. P., Alemán, A., Baeken, C., Benninger, D., Brunelin, J., Di Lazzaro, V., Filipović, S. R., et al. (2020). Evidence-based guidelines on the therapeutic use of repetitive transcranial magnetic stimulation (rTMS): An update (2014–2018). *Clinical Neurophysiology, 131*, 474–528. https://doi.org/10.1016/j.clinph.2019.11.002 (accessed on 7th August 2025).
25. Li, H., Tang, W., Li, T., Wang, S., Li, H., Yun, M., Xu, J., et al. (2025). Outcomes and prognostic factors in prelingually sensorineural deaf children with cerebral white matter lesions following cochlear implantation: A multicenter, retrospective study. *Scientific Reports, 15.* https://www.semanticscholar.org/paper/5464e31a0937a3ba73b0bf934da9fab0fb72cf64 (accessed on 7th August 2025).
26. Lin, A. E., Prakash, S. K., Andersen, N. H., Viuff, M., Levitsky, L. L., Rivera-Dávila, M., Crenshaw, M., et al. (2019). Recognition and management of adults with Turner syndrome: From the transition of adolescence through the senior years. *American Journal of Medical Genetics Part A, 179*, 1987–2033. https://doi.org/10.1002/ajmg.a.61310 (accessed on 7th August 2025).
27. Magnan, J., Özgïrgïn, O. N., Trabalzini, F., Lacour, M., Lopez Escamez, A., Magnusson, M., Güneri, E. A., et al. (2018). European position statement on diagnosis, and treatment of Meniere's disease. *The Journal of International Advanced Otology, 14*, 317–321. https://doi.org/10.5152/iao.2018.140818 (accessed on 7th August 2025).
28. Montero-Odasso, M., van der Velde, N., Martin, F. C., Petrović, M., Tan, M. P., Ryg, J., Aguilar-Navarro, S. G., et al. (2022). World guidelines for falls prevention and management for older adults: A global initiative. *Age and Ageing, 51.* https://doi.org/10.1093/ageing/afac205 (accessed on 7th August 2025).
29. Muschol, N., Giugliani, R., Jones, S., Muenzer, J., Smith, N., Whitley, C. B., Donnell, M., et al. (2022). Sanfilippo syndrome: Consensus guidelines for clinical care. *Orphanet Journal of Rare Diseases, 17.* https://doi.org/10.1186/s13023-022-02484-6 (accessed on 7th August 2025).
30. Niedzielski, A., Chmielik, L. P., Mielnik–Niedzielska, G., Kasprzyk, A., & Bogusławska, J. (2023). Adenoid hypertrophy in children: A narrative review of pathogenesis and clinical relevance. *BMJ Pediatrics Open, 7*, e001710. https://doi.org/10.1136/bmjpo-2022-001710 (accessed on 7th August 2025).
31. Norrving, B., Barrick, J., Dávalos, A., Dichgans, M., Cordonnier, C., Guekht, A., Kutluk, K., et al. (2018). Action plan for stroke in Europe 2018–2030. *European Stroke Journal, 3*, 309–336. https://doi.org/10.1177/2396987318808719 (accessed on 7th August 2025).
32. O'Neill, G., & Sutherland, M. (2004). *Training and Employment of People with Disabilities: Australia 2003.* https://core.ac.uk/download/5120538.pdf (accessed on 7th August 2025).
33. Ortega, M. Á., Fraile-Martínez, O., García-Montero, C., Callejón-Peláez, E., Sáez, M. A., Alvarez-Mon, M. Á., García-Honduvilla, N., et al. (2021). A general overview on the hyperbaric oxygen

therapy: Applications, mechanisms and translational opportunities. *Medicina, 57*, 864. https://doi.org/10.3390/medicina57090864 (accessed on 7th August 2025).

34. Óskarsdóttir, S., Boot, E., Crowley, T. B., Loo, J. C. Y., Arganbright, J. M., Armando, M., Baylis, A. L., et al. (2023). Updated clinical practice recommendations for managing children with 22q11.2 deletion syndrome. *Genetics in Medicine, 25*, 100338–100338. https://doi.org/10.1016/j.gim.2022.11.006 (accessed on 7th August 2025).

35. Patel, D. R., Neelakantan, M., Pandher, K., & Merrick, J. (2020). Cerebral palsy in children: A clinical overview. *Translational Pediatrics, 9*, S125–S135. https://doi.org/10.21037/tp.2020.01.01 (accessed on 7th August 2025).

36. Pfister, D. G., Spencer, S., Adelstein, D. J., Adkins, D. R., Anzai, Y., Brizel, D. M., Bruce, J. Y., et al. (2020). Head and neck cancers, version 2.2020, NCCN Clinical practice guidelines in oncology. *Journal of the National Comprehensive Cancer Network, 18*, 873–898. https://doi.org/10.6004/jnccn.2020.0031 (accessed on 7th August 2025).

37. Procházka, D., Martynek, M., Vitujová, M., Janáková, D., Charvátová, H., & Vyšata, O. (2024). Mobile accelerometer applications in core muscle rehabilitation and pre-operative assessment. *Sensors (Basel, Switzerland), 24.* https://www.semanticscholar.org/paper/0638244e31cf41c2c8a752537fb2b1ede828b4f0 (accessed on 7th August 2025).

38. Sardone, R., Battista, P., Panza, F., Lozupone, M., Griseta, C., Castellana, F., Capozzo, R., et al. (2019). The age-related central auditory processing disorder: Silent impairment of the cognitive ear. *Frontiers in Neuroscience, 13.* https://doi.org/10.3389/fnins.2019.00619 (accessed on 7th August 2025).

39. Sereda, M., Smith, S. N., Newton, K., & Stockdale, D. (2019). Mobile apps for management of tinnitus: Users' survey, quality assessment, and content analysis. *JMIR mHealth and uHealth, 7.* https://www.semanticscholar.org/paper/83cbecc5a0a6c451d8389c59d5c857e586144b7e (accessed on 7th August 2025).

40. Seylanova, N., Chernyavskaya, A. S., Degtyareva, N., Mursalova, A., Ajam, A., Xiao, L., Aktulaeva, K., et al. (2024). Core outcome measurement set for research and clinical practice in post-COVID-19 condition (long COVID) in children and young people: An international Delphi consensus study "PC-COS Children." *European Respiratory Journal, 63*, 2301761. https://doi.org/10.1183/13993003.01761-2023 (accessed on 7th August 2025).

41. Shetty, S., & Kasrija, R. (2025). Analog to digital diagnosis and planning in orthognathic surgery: A narrative review. *Cureus, 17.* https://www.semanticscholar.org/paper/5d01fd9cb63d6db96d4de54e728ddb2b9520d267 (accessed on 7th August 2025).

42. Siggaard, L. D., Jacobsen, H., Hougaard, D. D., Khaled, M. S., & Høgsbro, M. (2023). Cross-cultural translation and adaptation of the Consumer Ear Disease Risk Assessment (CEDRA) Questionnaire in Danish. *Audiology Research, 13*, 859–870. https://doi.org/10.3390/audiolres13060075 (accessed on 7th August 2025).

43. Stachurski, J., Kaczyńska, A., & Czaplińska-Paszek, Z. (2021). Implementing the regulation of the Minister of Health by Polish emergency departments in 2020. *Emergency Medical Service, 8*, 144–149. https://doi.org/10.36740/emems202103104 (accessed on 7th August 2025).

44. Starnoni, D., Giammattei, L., Cossu, G., Link, M. J., Roche, P. H., Chacko, A. G., Ohata, K., et al. (2020). Surgical management for large vestibular schwannomas: A systematic review, meta-analysis, and consensus statement on behalf of the EANS Skull Base Section. *Acta*

Neurochirurgica, 162, 2595–2617. https://doi.org/10.1007/s00701-020-04491-7 (accessed on 7th August 2025).

45. Thai-Van, H., Mosnier, I., Dejean, F., Ambert-Dahan, E., Bakhos, D., Belmin, J., Bonnard, D., et al. (2023). Early management of presbycusis: Recommendations from the French Society of Otorhinolaryngology and Head and Neck Surgery, the French Society of Audiology, and the French Society of Geriatrics and Gerontology. *Gériatrie et Psychologie Neuropsychiatrie du Vieillissement.* https://www.semanticscholar.org/paper/7abc1e471dc68a0af55cd2c66e0c70c0c82c2566 (accessed on 7th August 2025).
46. Thong, G., & Casserly, P. (2019). A case of acute peripheral vertigo: Using the HINTS exam to guide diagnostic workup. *Archives of Case Reports.* https://www.semanticscholar.org/paper/84c38abd0e94c7fa4b5e2e0972536b658750eb16 (accessed on 7th August 2025).
47. Xue, X., Azman, A., Zhang, C., Chen, Y., Ni, J., & Wang, Z. Y. (2024). Rehabilitation for complicated dysphagia after synchronous head-and-neck and esophageal cancer surgery: A case report. *Medicine, 103.* https://www.semanticscholar.org/paper/3923035a74fcc785b5620dc5645e0f1f27ecd861 (accessed on 7th August 2025).
48. Yuan, Y. Y., Li, X. G., Gao, B., Bi, Q., Yang, S. M., Han, D., & Dai, P. (2025). [Perioperative management of cochlear implantation and analysis on the influencing factors of efficacy in patients diagnosed as hereditary syndromic hearing loss]. *Zhonghua er bi yan hou tou jing wai ke za zhi = Chinese Journal of Otorhinolaryngology Head and Neck Surgery, 60*(2), 153–165. https://www.semanticscholar.org/paper/01824d451d646930e76a8ab5296f9dd11e9d0c4a (accessed on 7th August 2025).
49. Zheng, Q., Wu, Y., Zhu, J., Cao, L., Bai, Y., & Ni, G. (2024). Cochlear implant artifacts removal in EEG-based objective auditory rehabilitation assessment. *IEEE Transactions on Neural Systems and Rehabilitation Engineering, 32*, 2854–2863. https://www.semanticscholar.org/paper/4c9e262abf953742d5d89c40a442ddc5b7649ff2 (accessed on 7th August 2025).

ANATOMY AND PHYSIOLOGY OF THE NOSE AND PARANASAL SINUSES

7

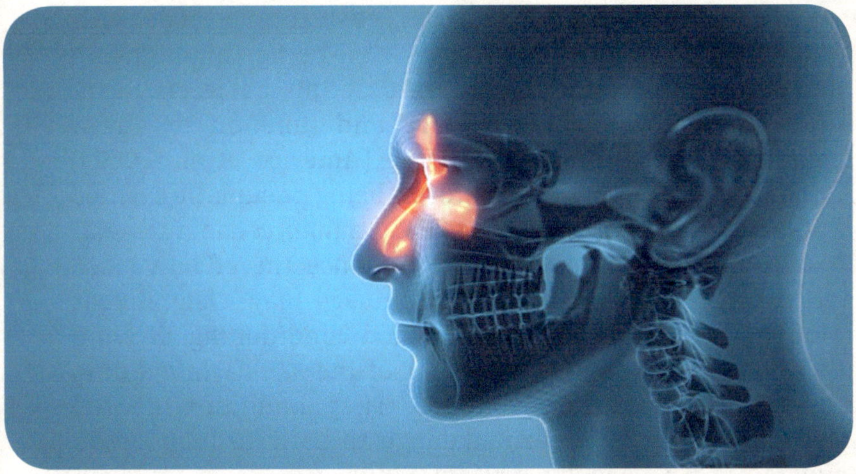

LEARNING OBJECTIVES

After studying this chapter, you will be able to:

1. Anatomy of the nose.
2. Physiology of the nose.
3. Anatomy of the paranasal sinuses.
4. Physiology of the paranasal sinuses.
5. Common disorders of the nose and sinuses.
6. Diagnostic techniques.

Introduction

The paranasal sinuses and the nose play a significant role in the human respiratory system, not only as passageways for air flow but also as primary contributors to numerous physiological functions. The nose has complex structure with numerous structures including the nostrils, nasal cavity, and turbinates. These structural elements facilitate the filtering of particulates, the regulation of air temperature, and assist in the maintenance of humidity. Moreover, the paranasal sinuses, which are air cavities within the skull, allow resonance during speech and serve as the most important factor in reducing the overall weight of the skull. Understanding this intricate anatomy is essential for the diagnosis and treatment of a range of disorders that can take place in the upper respiratory tract, such that it renders an intensive study of the anatomical as well as functional elements of these systems essential (Américo et al., 2007). At the level of physiology, the nose and paranasal sinuses are part of the body's immune defense mechanism. The nasal mucosa, which is rich in goblet cells and cilia, serves to trap pathogens and particulates and sweep them away through mucociliary clearance. This defense mechanism is essential, as it contributes to infection prevention and respiratory well-being. The sinuses are also involved in the process of olfaction, where the olfactory receptors held within the upper nasal cavity sense odorants, thus allowing for the sense of smell. These physiological functions emphasize the nose and sinuses' functions as more than mere airflow regulation, directing toward participation in the quality of life and general well-being. Furthermore, current advances in medical therapies and surgical interventions targeted at these areas exhibit a shifting understanding of their complexities (Azimonti et al., 2018). With the ongoing expansion of the field in otorhinolaryngology, it is apt to reflect on how developments in the past have shaped current practice in terms of understanding the anatomy and physiology of the nose and paranasal sinuses. Acquainting oneself with past achievements helps one better appreciate how treatments for various conditions in these regions have evolved, from nasal obstruction to chronic sinusitis. Techniques such as endoscopic surgery and balloon catheter dilations have revolutionized how experts handle chronic rhinosinusitis, proving the evolution from uncouth means to sophisticated ones that yield beneficial clinical results. The application of modern technology in the diagnosis, treatment, and investigation of nasal and sinus diseases not only enhances care but also reflects the dynamic nature of medical science in dealing with emerging challenges and discoveries (Américo et al., 2007; Azimonti et al., 2018).

Importance of the Nose and Paranasal Sinuses in the Respiratory System

The nose is the first site of air entry into the respiratory tract and plays a crucial role in the filtration, humidification, and warming of inhaled air. When air passes through the nasal cavity, it encounters a complicated mucous membrane and microscopic hairs known as cilia. These structures capture particles, pathogens, and irritants such that they are not carried to the lower part of the respiratory tract and thereby protect lung health. Furthermore, the nose also enables olfaction, or the ability to smell, an integral component of taste and of significance to appetite and nutrition. This multifunctional character of the nose supports not only its pivotal function in respiratory processes but also in overall well-being, highlighting the multifaceted interaction between nasal anatomy's structure and function to attain respiratory well-being (Américo et al., 2007). The paranasal sinuses, being pneumatic cavities within the bones of the cranium, collaborate with the nasal cavity to enhance the effectiveness of respiration. The sinuses play a significant role in air filtration and conditioning, striving to reduce the weight of the skull while aiding in voice resonance. They humidify inhaled air to prevent damage to delicate lung tissue caused by dry air. Sinuses are also involved in drainage and mucociliary clearing, which ensures that rubbish and mucus do not block airflow. This anatomical confluence of the nose and paranasal sinuses is typical of the upper respiratory system's complexity and reflective of the vital role these structures play in allowing normal respiratory function as well as overall well-being (Djupesland, 2012). Furthermore, the effects of nasal and sinus pathology are not only local but also systemic and extend into disease susceptibility. These conditions will compromise the effective filtering and humidifying of air, with an ensuing downstream cascade of effects on lung health and increased exposure to respiratory pathogens. Chronic diseases, such as allergic rhinitis, describe the intricate relationship between the nasal cavity and overall respiratory health. Therapeutic agents are routinely administered via nasal delivery systems, as the nose's architecture facilitates rapid drug uptake and distribution.

Note, however, that the nasal airway's primary role is as protection of the lungs, and therapeutic action should be mindful of these physiological processes in treating problems with such nasal drug therapy (Américo et al., 2007; Djupesland, 2012) (Figure 7.1).

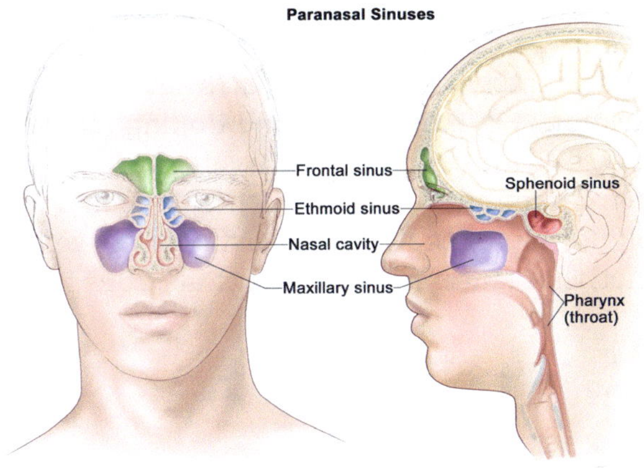

Figure 7.1. The nose and paranasal sinuses in the respiratory system.

Source: https://nci-media.cancer.gov/pdq/media/images/713969.jpg.

Overview of the Anatomy and Physiology

The physiology and anatomy of the nose and the paranasal sinuses are significant to understanding their function and clinical relevance. The nose is a highly specialized organ designed to perform an array of functions, including air filtration, humidification, and warming, and thus protect the lower respiratory airways. Its complicated structure includes the nasal cavity, divided into two nostrils, and is linked to the nasal conchae—bony structures that extend into the nasal cavities. Not only does this structure promote surface area for better airflow conditioning, but it also plays a critical role in the olfactory process, allowing airborne chemicals to be sensed. Thus, the nose is a vital first line of defense against extrinsic pathogens and pollutants, underscoring its role in respiratory physiology and overall health and informing the suitability of nasal drug delivery systems (Djupesland, 2012). Paranasal sinuses, such as the maxillary, frontal, ethmoid, and sphenoid sinuses, also support nasal functions. These air-filled cavities decrease the weight of the skull, enrich the resonance of the voice, and contribute to the mucosal immune system. Anatomically, the sinuses are lined with a mucus membrane that continually produces mucus, which secretes particles and pathogens. The mucus is transported to the nasal cavity by cilia action, a function significant in maintaining a healthy respiratory system. Nonetheless, there are certain anatomical variations in certain individuals that result in issues such as chronic sinusitis, which is usually related to blockages and inflammation caused by infections or allergies (N/A, 2022).

Understanding such variations and their influence provides insights into varied treatment procedures and surgical interventions for sinus diseases. The union of sophisticated imaging and diagnostic technologies has greatly enhanced our understanding of nasal and sinus system anatomy and physiology. Technologies such as computed tomography (CT) scans have provided a three-dimensional visualization of the nasal cavity and paranasal sinuses and enabled clinicians to assess anatomical abnormalities and plan appropriate interventions. Recent work highlights the potential of nasal drug delivery devices that leverage the region's unique physiologic properties to provide more effective treatment of sinusitis, as indicated by new bidirectional delivery technologies (Djupesland, 2012). Such advancements not only improve therapeutic efficacy but also augment the possibility of use in vaccination and systemic drug delivery through the nasal path. By incorporating the subtleties of sinus and nasal physiology, the discipline can more effectively accommodate preventative as well as therapeutic modalities, which are bound to increase patient outcomes.

7.1. Anatomy of the Nose

Learning Outcome

1. External Structures of the Nose
2. Internal Nasal Cavity and Its Components
3. Nasal Septum and Its Significance

The anatomy of the nose is functional and complex, made up of several structures that are necessary for respiration, smelling, and overall protection of the airway. The cartilage-supported bony framework constitutes the outside of the nose, giving it its external shape and making it lovely. The nasal cavity is shared internally by two chambers as a result of the cartilaginous and bony nasal septum. This division not only contributes to the overall structure but also enables proper regulation of airflow and humidification of inspired air. Within the cavity, the intricate nasal conchae, or turbinates, anatomy helps to maximize air filtration, warming, and conditioning, thereby protecting the sensitive lung tissue from harmful environmental stimuli, which represents the double role of the nose in aesthetic as well as functional features (Américo et al., 2007).

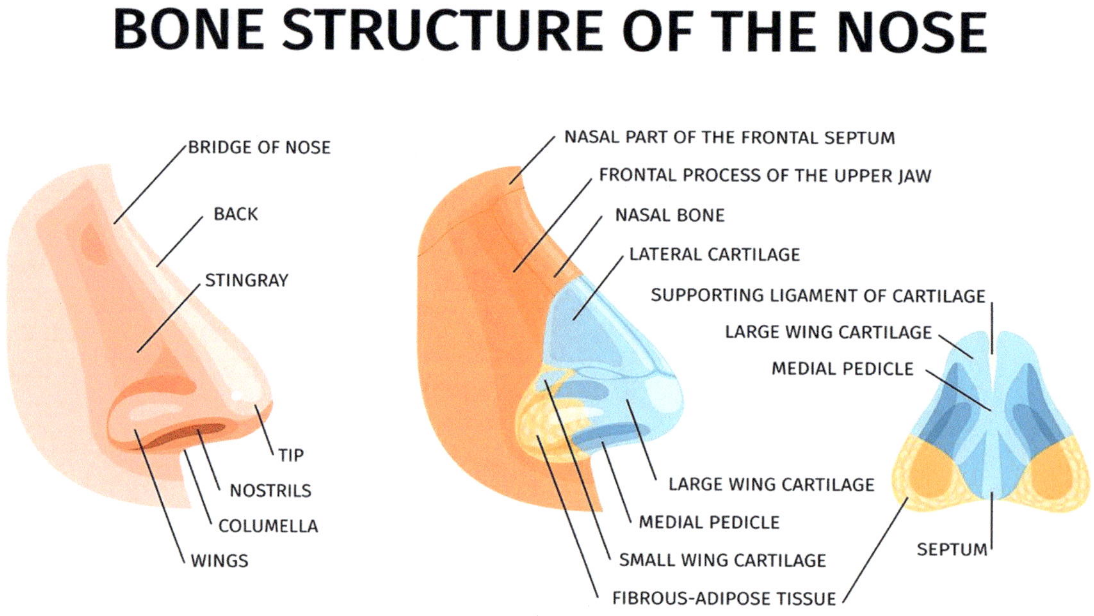

Figure 7.2. The anatomy of the nose is both complex and functional.

Source: https://nosecontour.com/wp-content/uploads/2024/05/Anatomy-of-the-Nose-Structure-1024x538.jpg.

Moreover, the nasal passages are lined by a specialized epithelium that contains olfactory receptors, which play a critical role in the sense of smell. Olfactory epithelium is situated at the uppermost part of the nasal cavity and is also remarkable due to its regenerative ability. The relevance of olfaction extends far beyond sensory input; it is critical to taste, memory, and emotional response. In addition, the dynamic functioning of the nasal cavity, including its rapid air pressure and temperature alterations, facilitates effective gas exchange. Understanding the anatomical complexity of the nose enhances the significance of its location within the respiratory system and its role in an individual's overall health and well-being, depicting the nose as a multi-purpose organ (Djupesland, 2012). The anatomy of the nose is also closely related to a series of paranasal sinuses, air-filled spaces within the bones of the face. The sinuses have several functions, including reducing the weight of the skull, enhancing voice resonance, and contributing to humidification and filtration of the inspired air. The frontal, maxillary, ethmoid, and sphenoid sinuses all drain through the nasal cavity, which gives an open channel that is vital for the health of the nasal passages and sinuses. Obstruction or inflammation of these routes of drainage can create conditions such as sinusitis, hence the importance of understanding nasal and sinus anatomy. As advances in medical technology move forward, there is a need to comprehend the nose and sinuses in developing effective interventions and treatment, thus the need for this anatomical study in clinical practice (Américo et al., 2007) (Figure 7.2).

7.1.1. External Structures of the Nose

The external nasal units are vital anatomical components that have crucial functions both in function and in aesthetics. The nose can be grossly separated into different parts: the tip, the bridge, the root, and the nostrils, which are surrounded by facial integument. The bridge of the nose, consisting primarily of bone and cartilage, is what provides rigidity to the structure and supports the nasal passages below. Besides, nostrils, or nares, are the primary entry points for air while carrying complex elastic and muscular structures that enable them to regulate airflow. This active function equips the nose to perform its primary function in respiration as well as its involvement in olfactory functions. Understanding these structures is essential, as they are not only cosmetic structures but structural components that allow for critical physiological functions of the respiratory system (Américo et al., 2007). In studying the external nose structures, one should consider how important they are in regard to overall health and treatment strategies. For instance, the nasal valve shape—the narrowest part of the nasal airway—will directly influence airflow dynamics and can have significant physiological consequences. This area is also significant for efficient air conditioning and filtration that protects the lungs from environmental danger. Any nasal structural abnormalities on the outside can lead to greater susceptibility to infections like sinusitis or rhinitis. Besides this, when treatment modalities are being discussed, it is clear that these external features are considered during medical treatments, both surgical and non-surgical treatments (Djupesland, 2012).

Through this, a thorough insight into the external nasal anatomy equips healthcare practitioners with the needed knowledge to enable effective diagnosis as well as treatment. Additionally, the interface between the external parts of the nose, as well as their functional capabilities, extends even to therapeutic delivery systems. The nasal region, due to its unique anatomical characteristics, has emerged as a promising route of drug delivery, particularly in local diseases such as allergic rhinitis. The nasal delivery systems benefit from the rich blood supply of the nose and permeable mucous membranes to enhance bioavailability, which results in rapid absorption into systemic circulation. Yet, this path is drawn back by the central protection of the nose to the lungs, which can impede efficient drug delivery. The pragmatic aspect of this contrast exposes both the benefits and limitations that clinicians must contend with when using these external bodies for therapeutic purposes (Djupesland, 2012). Therefore, careful study of external nasal anatomy not only enriches anatomical knowledge but also improves clinical practice by informing optimal treatment.

7.1.2. Internal Nasal Cavity and Its Components

The internal nasal cavity is a fundamental anatomical characteristic of the respiratory system that serves primarily as a passageway for air and as the site for the preliminary processes of smell. It is divided by the nasal septum into the right and left nostrils, each of which leads into its own airway passage. The lining of the cavity is primarily made up of mucous membranes that play an important role in humidifying as well as heating the air inhaled. Secondly, the epithelial cells that are part of the lining are responsible for trapping particulates and microbes and thus forming a protective covering over inner structures. As described in the literature, familiarity with the morphological aspects of the nasal cavity and the paranasal sinuses is essential to improve clinical outcomes and surgical interventions for associated conditions (N/A, 2022). In the internal nasal cavity, there are certain important structures that contribute to its function and anatomical integrity. Of particular note are the turbinate, or nasal conchae, striking bony structures that maximize the surface area available for humidifying, warming, and filtering air inhaled. The turbinate combined with the meatus, creates complex airflow dynamics that promote efficient nasal respiration and efficient pathogen clearance.

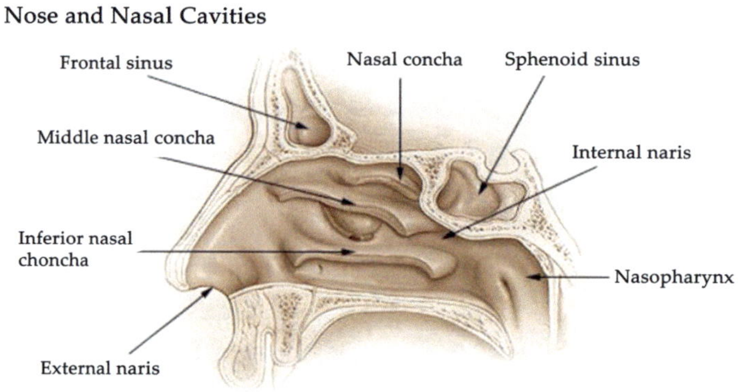

Figure 7.3. The nasal cavity is a fundamental anatomical structure of the respiratory system.

Source: https://training.seer.cancer.gov/images/anatomy/respiratory/nose_nasal_cavities.jpg.

Moreover, the olfactory bulbs, found at the superior aspect of the nasal cavity, are intimately related to the sense of smell. Their location near the nasal cavity underscores the intimacy of respiratory and sensory functions in this anatomy (Alsaied, 2017). Understanding the intricacy of their design and functions is crucial for the diagnosis and management of nasal pathologies. The role of the internal nasal cavity extends beyond managing airflow; it is critical to phonation and olfaction. The nasal cavities' architecture influences resonance in speech, also contributing to the quality and clarity of vocal sounds. Also, olfactory receptors located in the roof of the nasal cavity play a crucial role in detecting odors, influencing taste and perception of environmental stimuli further. The complex interplay between the nasal cavity and the paranasal sinuses surrounding it cannot be overstated, as these structures have anatomical and physiological correlations that affect conditions such as sinusitis (N/A, 2022). Elaborate appreciation of the interaction underscores the significance of precise anatomical knowledge, particularly in surgery, where variations and landmarks should be meticulously navigated so as to minimize complications (Alsaied, 2017) (Figure 7.3).

7.1.3. Nasal Septum and Its Significance

The nasal septum is a key anatomical characteristic of the human nasal passage that divides the left and right nostrils. It consists primarily of bone and cartilage and is significant in the general functioning of the nasal apparatus because it facilitates smooth airflow and optimizes the conditioning of incoming air. A properly shaped nasal septum provides significant physiological functions, such as humidification, filtration, and temperature regulation, all of which are essential for lung defense against environmental risks. A deviated septum or crooked septum may result in a variety of problems, ranging from compromised airflow to frequent infections and chronic sinusitis. A deviated nasal septum has been documented as among the most common anatomical variations in the paranasal sinus region and most commonly accompanies other variations that are a cause for concern for surgical operations (Kardam, N. K., & Tiwari, T. N., 2019). The nasal septum not only contributes to the structural function but also influences the effectiveness of therapeutic medication, particularly with regard to drug administration through the nose. With its intricate anatomy, the nose is increasingly being discovered to be a valuable method of drug delivery, especially for diseases involving nasal and sinus function, that is, rhinitis or sinusitis. The intricate nasal architecture, with septum, prevents ease of drug absorption but also has protective functions to consider in therapy planning. For instance, nasal airflow dynamic behavior and anatomical variations can influence how effectively drugs reach their sites of action in the nasal cavity and paranasal sinuses (Djupesland, 2012). Understanding these points to a necessity to understand and respect the anatomical nuances of the nasal septum when designing and optimizing nasal treatment delivery systems. Moreover, the implication of anatomical variations, including septal ones, and the risk of intraoperative complications cannot be exaggerated. Research offers evidence that while variations do not predispose persons to sinus pathology, variations will clearly alter the risk profile significantly during surgeries (Kardam, N. K., & Tiwari, T. N., 2019). Anatomical variations must be recognized by surgeons using preoperative imaging and tests to minimize the risk of complications. Precise appreciation of anatomy, including understanding the septum's role within the overall nasal cavity design, is important for the development of personalized surgical planning. Thus, the nasal septum's significance is multifaceted, impacting both clinical effectiveness as a function of pathophysiology and enabling new treatment paradigms for otolaryngology.

Test Your Knowledge

1. Describe the structural divisions of the nose, including the external nose, nasal cavity, and nasal septum, and their functions.
2. What are the paranasal sinuses, and how do they relate anatomically and functionally to the nasal cavity?

7.2. Physiology of the Nose

Learning Outcome

1. Functions of the Nose in Respiration
2. Role of the Nose in Olfaction
3. Mechanisms of Filtration and Humidification of Air

The nasal physiology is at the core of its primary function in the respiratory system: humidification, warming, and filtration of inhaled air. The nasal cavity is lined with respiratory mucosa, which has specialized cells involved in mucociliary clearance. This role is significant in trapping inhaled particulate matter, pathogens, and allergens, thereby protecting the lower respiratory tract. Furthermore, the mucosa also secretes mucus, a sticky secretion that catches these unwanted guests, while cilia, tiny hair-like structures, move and push the mucus down the throat for elimination. This coupling of mucus production and ciliary action is not only used to maintain the nasal passages in a clean state but also to be part of the overall defense mechanism of the respiratory tract, an illustration of the great physiological forces that come into play in this modest but significant organ (Beule, 2011). The complex physiology of the nose also applies to the system of smell, which perceives odors. The olfactory epithelium lining the roof of the nasal cavity is made up of sensory neurons that are chemically sensitive. When molecules enter the nasal cavity, they bind to receptors on these neurons, triggering nerve impulses that get relayed to the brain for interpretation. This olfactory pathway is significant to the sense of smell and also plays a significant part in taste, and adds to the overall sensory experience of eating. Through olfaction, the nose enables perception of the world by detecting possibly harmful chemicals and thereby serving as a crucial evolutionary adaptation (Américo et al., 2007). Awareness of such physiological processes demonstrates the fact that the nose is not only an air tube but a complex organ engaged in sensory reception and protective processes. Second, the nose regulates airflow and pressure during inspiration to facilitate effective lung function.

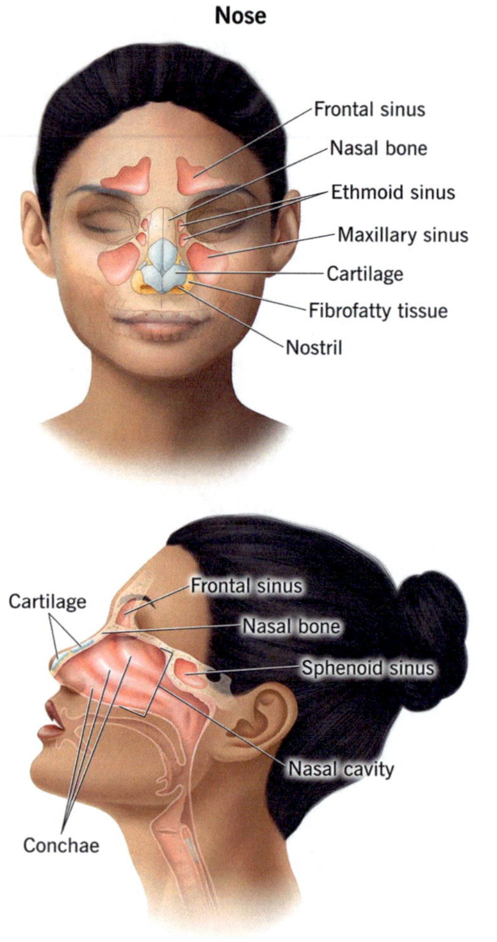

Figure 7.4. The physiology of the nose.

Source: https://my.clevelandclinic.org/-/scassets/images/org/health/articles/21778-nose.

The nasal turbinates, which are nasal bones, create turbulence as air moves through them to ensure more contact of the inhaled air with the mucosal surface. More contact results in effective warming and humidification of the air prior to entering the lower respiratory system. The function of the nose is facilitated by the existence of blood vessels within the nasal mucosa, which contribute to this process because they are able to dilate in order to increase blood flow, thus increasing the passage of heat and moisture to inspired air. This physiological adaptation accentuates the role of the nose in respiratory mechanics, pointing out its role in ensuring effective gas exchange and optimizing the quality of air supplied to the lungs (Beule, 2011) (Figure 7.4).

7.2.1. Functions of the Nose in Respiration

The nose is a central part of the respiratory system and the main point of entry for air into the lungs. This anatomical feature supports many key functions that are important for successful respiration. The first function of the nose is to filter the incoming air via its complex network of hairs, or cilia, and mucus membranes. These systems catch harmful particles, allergens, and pathogens, so they are not able to penetrate the lower respiratory tract. Consequently, the nose is the respiratory system's first line of defense against respiratory illness and infection, and highlights the importance of its filtering function in the maintenance of respiratory health. Additionally, nasal structures assist in warming and humidifying the air before it reaches the lungs and prep it for optimal conditions for gas exchange. In addition to its filtering capacity, the nose is also crucial in the olfactory apparatus, a component of sensation and response to much in the environment. The upper nasal cavity contains olfactory receptors that detect airborne molecules, enabling olfactory perception, which is important for flavor perception and for triggering protective reflexes. For example, exposure to stinky odors might cause immediate responses to ward off poisonous substances and thereby indirectly safeguard the respiratory system. The interface between the olfactory tracts and the respiration reflexes further evinces the multi-purpose function of the nose in keeping alive and healthy, and demonstrates that the functions of the nose extend beyond air control to incorporate the intricate sensory interactions determining response behavior and overall well-being. Aside from that, the paranasal sinuses' anatomical and physiological connection to the nose and the rest of the breathing apparatus cannot be omitted. The paranasal sinuses are also involved in voice resonance and skull weight loss. The paranasal sinuses' anatomical disposition enhances the breathing efficiency through intensified airflow dynamics in the nasal cavity. As pointed out in recent research, ailments like sinusitis have been found to have a serious bearing on respiratory well-being, testifying to the interrelatedness of the nasal structures and the overall respiratory system. Specifically, the co-existence of sinus disease and respiratory disorders like asthma testifies to the urgent need for integrative therapies targeting both. Appropriate treatment of sinusitis can lead to improved respiratory function, which highlights the basic need to know about the anatomical and physiological function of the nose for breathing and overall health (Balaji, 2017; N/A, 2022).

7.2.2. Role of the Nose in Olfaction

The nose is a significant anatomical structure in the olfactory process and the primary site of entry for airborne chemical molecules. The odorant molecules are directed through the nasal passages when inhaled and contact the olfactory epithelium, which is a specialized tissue within the upper nasal passage. The epithelium houses olfactory receptor neurons that are highly sensitive to detecting particular chemical molecules. When odorants are attached by receptors on these neurons, the process initiates a train reaction of neural impulses that ultimately reach the olfactory bulb within the brain. This complex process not only presents the nose as a physical organ of airflow but also as a highly evolved sensory organ, crucial for detecting odors indispensable for survival, perceiving flavor, and regulating social conduct. Moreover, the nasal cavity's structural characteristics are significant for its olfactory function. The complex geometry of nasal passages enables efficient trapping and processing of odorant molecules, making the sensitivity of olfactory receptor detection higher. The provision of turbinates, bony extensions in the nasal cavity, increases the surface area where olfactory epithelium can attach, making the chances of odor detection more likely.

Additionally, the mucous layer of the olfactory epithelium facilitates odorant binding and protects against pathogens to ensure the integrity of the olfactory system. All these anatomical components together optimize olfactory sensitivity and acuity and enable the detection of minute concentrations of volatile chemicals in the air, an imperative function that has implications for food habits as well as environmental perception. The interplay between olfaction and the other physiological functions of the body is particularly noteworthy. Evidence in recent times has highlighted the connection between nasal function and respiratory disease, such as sinusitis and asthma. For instance, inflammation of the nose is likely to jeopardize olfactory function and lead to diminished ability for odor detection. In patients with asthma, sinusitis can exacerbate respiratory symptoms and form a vicious cycle for both overall health and quality of life. Appropriate medical or surgical therapy for nasal health may then restore olfactory function and improve respiratory status, underscoring the nose's dual role in sensory perception and respiratory physiology. This intricate relationship profoundly establishes the crucial importance of maintaining nasal integrity not only for smell but also for general physiological health, as claimed by Balaji (2017) (Figure 7.5).

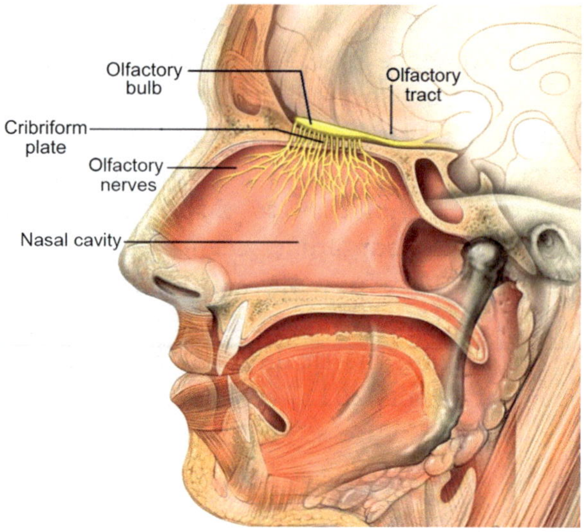

Figure 7.5. Role of the nose in olfaction.

Source: https://upload.wikimedia.org/wikipedia/commons/3/34/Head_Olfactory_Nerve_Labeled.png.

7.2.3. Mechanisms of Filtration and Humidification of Air

The nose plays important functions in the human respiratory system, foremost among these being the humidification and filtering of air to the lungs. The intricate anatomy of the nasal passages involving the turbinate bones and mucosal surfaces is vital to the functions. Air coming through the nostrils is confronted by a dense collection of mucous membranes that remove particulate material, pathogens, and other types of contaminants. The cilia covering these membranes help transport this caught detritus to the pharynx, from where it is able to be swallowed or expelled. This filtration is important not only to maintain respiratory health but also to prep the air for optimal gas exchange in the lungs. The need for effective filtration is further urgent in diverse environmental conditions, particularly highlighting the nose as a primary defense organ against inhaled irritants and pathogens (Keck, T., & Lindemann, J., 2011). In addition to filtration, the nose is also important in humidifying the inspired air. When air is inhaled and traverses the nasal passages, it becomes exposed to moist mucosal surfaces, which facilitate absorption of water vapor. This humidification is significant since it maintains the respiratory tracts as thin tissues, which otherwise can lead to irritation or infection. The nasal anatomy's intricacies, including the extensive surface area provided by the turbinates and the rich vascular supply, enable effective heating and humidification of the air. Optimal nasal air conditioning is essential for maximal gas exchange within the lungs, emphasizing the nose's structural and functional interdependence. In the absence of adequate humidification, desiccation of alveolar tissue and resulting pathology have a significantly increased probability, illustrating the nose's vital role beyond reductive air passage (Cooper, 2024). Moreover, the significance of the nose in humidification and filtration translates to the impact on global respiratory health and functioning. Well-oxygenated air is required not only to be effective in gas exchange but also to prevent chronic sinusitis and rhinitis, which are enhanced by the malfunctioning of nasal functions. Malfunction in such processes leads to a series of pulmonary complications that affect overall health. This is compounded by the need for effective medical techniques, such as intranasal anesthetics used in various procedures, and by potential effects on nasal anatomy and physiology. It serves as the foundation for mechanisms of filtration and humidification that inform clinical practices and merits the maintenance of nasal health in order to obtain proper respiratory function (Keck, T., & Lindemann, J., 2011; Cooper, 2024).

Test Your Knowledge

1. Explain the functions of the nose, including olfaction, respiration, filtration, humidification, and temperature regulation of inspired air.
2. Describe the physiology of nasal airflow and mucociliary clearance, and their role in protecting the respiratory tract.

7.3. Anatomy of the Paranasal Sinuses

Learning Outcome

1. Types of Paranasal Sinuses and Their Locations
2. Structure and Lining of the Sinuses
3. Relationship Between Sinuses and Nasal Cavity

The paranasal sinuses form a complex system of air spaces within the skull bones, the frontal, maxillary, ethmoid, and sphenoid sinuses. They lie in close relation to the nasal cavity and form a significant component of the overall upper respiratory tract anatomy and physiology. Sinuses have mucous membranes that produce mucus, which is essential in trapping pathogens and particulate matter and thus contributes to the respiratory defense mechanism. In addition, the paranasal sinuses enable voice resonance as well as help in reducing skull weight after birth. Their structure also plays a role in normal respiration and may significantly influence the presentation of certain nasal diseases in the event of obstruction and resultant cascades of clinical manifestations, such as sinusitis or chronic rhinitis (Américo et al., 2007). Each of the sinuses is unique in terms of its location and form, which leads to its roles and clinical significance. The frontal sinuses, which are located above the eyes, drain initially into the nasal cavity via the frontonasal duct. The maxillary sinuses are the most conspicuous of the sinuses and are located in the cheeks and open into the nasal cavity in a manner that can easily clog and cause infection. The ethmoid sinuses, composed of a number of small air cells between the nose and the eyes, and the sphenoid sinuses, located deep within the skull, serve similarly in drainage and airflow. The intricacy of their drainage pathways highlights the necessity for sinus health, for anything that obstructs them can have negative physiological effects, which reaffirms the necessity for clear comprehension in otorhinolaryngology, a progressively dynamic specialty with advances in medical technology and surgery (Américo et al., 2007). Upon learning about the anatomy of the paranasal sinuses, one needs to consider their clinical relevance, particularly in pathophysiology. Diseases such as non-allergic rhinitis and chronic sinusitis underscore the importance of identifying anatomical as well as physiological factors. Effective mucociliary clearance, a critical protective mechanism of the respiratory mucosa, plays a central role in avoiding sinus infection. Failure of the system may lead to the overproduction of mucus, promoting bacterial proliferation.

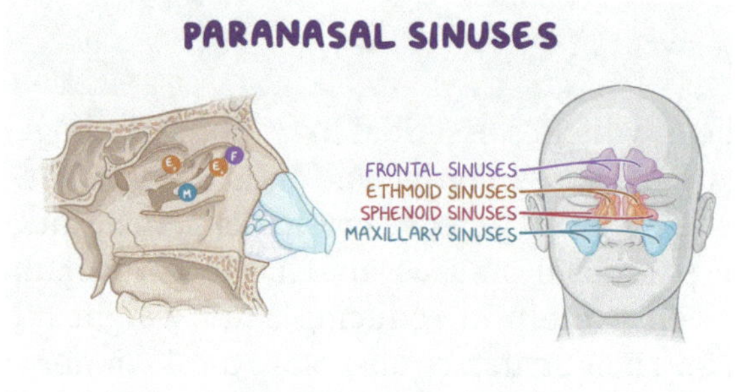

Figure 7.6. Anatomy of the paranasal sinuses

Source: https://d16qt3wv6xm098.cloudfront.net/oWXLhA3eQcOzSAwJX_HwCn5rSI_q1qnX/_.jpg.

Further, interaction of several anatomical structures, such as the ostiomeatal complex, becomes relevant in diagnostic evaluation as well as treatment modalities, such as endonasal procedures to restore normal sinus function (Beule, 2011). Identification of these nuances is key to treatment modalities and improved patient outcomes in respiratory illness (Figure 7.6).

7.3.1. Types of Paranasal Sinuses and Their Locations

The paranasal sinuses, a system of air spaces, are strategically positioned within the skull bones and play a critical role in the physiology of the upper airways. The paranasal sinuses have four main groups: maxillary, frontal, ethmoid, and sphenoid. They vary in location and function. Maxillary sinuses, the largest among them, are positioned below the eyes, in the maxillary bones. These sinuses contribute to the resonance of the voice, as well as assist with the drainage of mucus into the nasal cavity. Familiarity with the specific anatomical locations of these sinuses is significant to sinus-related sickness diagnosis and treatment since their close association with key structures dictates both medical and surgical intervention within the region, supporting the case that the correct understanding of sinus anatomy is required for proper clinical practice (Alsaied, 2017). The frontal sinuses in the forehead area above eye level are two paired cavities that can be significantly different in size between individuals. The sinuses are located in the frontal bone and empty into the nasal cavity by means of the frontonasal duct, which can sometimes become clogged and cause frontal sinusitis. Their anatomical position makes them susceptible to trauma and infection, highlighting the need for healthcare professionals to have a clear grasp of their anatomical variation and conditions associated with them. As highlighted in contemporary publications, advances in imaging modalities have improved visualization of these sinuses, thereby enhancing diagnostic accuracy and treatment planning. This information is not only critical to alleviate sinusitis but also to research their role in dental and overall respiratory function (N/A, 2022). Ethmoid sinuses between the eyes are an aggregation of complex patterns of small airspaces referred to as the ethmoid labyrinth. The function of these sinuses is crucial for mucus drainage and to overall morphology of the sinus cavity. Their single anatomical position, close to the orbit and nasal cavity, makes them a common site of inflammation and infection. The sphenoid sinuses, being deeper in the skull and hidden, are located posterior to the nasal cavity and are most poorly understood due to their intricate anatomy. This limited understanding during surgical procedures is problematic, even more so with the emphasis on advanced anatomical knowledge in sinus surgery. Accurate management of conditions that involve the paranasal sinuses necessitates detailed information regarding their locations and types, which in turn highlights the significant contribution these structures have towards the nose anatomy and physiology, as well as surrounding structures (Alsaied, 2017).

7.3.2. Structure and Lining of the Sinuses

The paranasal sinuses, which include the frontal, maxillary, ethmoid, and sphenoid sinuses, are component structures of the upper respiratory tract intended only for reducing the skull's weight and enhancing voice resonance. The cavities, which are air-filled, are positioned strategically within and near the nasal cavity, and their development is a complex arrangement of bone walls that define their shape and location. The unique configuration of these sinuses not only allows air to flow through but also assists in filtering, humidifying, and warming the incoming air. The locations of these sinuses in relation to one another also allow protective barriers against infection and facilitate drainage of mucus, which is an important factor in maintaining overall nasal health and functioning. Sinus anatomy and its association with adjacent structures are of clinical significance for the diagnosis and treatment of sinus-related problems, which highlights the relevance of sinus anatomy in practice. Sinus linings are primarily made up of pseudostratified ciliated columnar epithelium, a layer of cells that plays an essential role in sinus respiratory function. This ciliated epithelium is equipped with cilia, which are useful in moving mucus towards the drainage system, leading to the expulsion of particulate matter and pathogens. Underneath this layer of epithelium is a vascular network as well as mucous glands that are tasked with the secretion of mucus as well as protecting the lining from dehydration and irritation. Also, goblet cells that are distributed all over the epithelium secrete mucus that traps dust and microorganisms, making the sinus cavity a vital protection against respiratory infection. Therefore, the form and lining of the sinuses are not only crucial for air conditioning but also for protection against infection, underscoring their significance in respiratory physiology.

The consequences of sinus structure and lining reach into other health states, notably sinusitis, which has a substantial impact on quality of life. Inflammation of the sinus linings, frequently caused by infection or allergy, interferes with normal drainage and may result in mucus accumulation, providing a fertile ground for bacteria. This phenomenon forms a vicious circle as chronic sinusitis can then be linked to other diseases, such as chronic otitis media, whose middle ear infection is due to sinus issues. Functional endoscopic sinus surgery (FESS) has been found by studies to have an important part to play in alleviating such conditions by improving drainage pathways and removing inflammation in the sinuses (Kumar, 2012). For that reason, it is imperative to have knowledge of the architecture and histological structure of the sinuses when creating effective therapy and diagnosis approaches in treating these more common disorders in the population (Américo et al., 2007) (Figure 7.7).

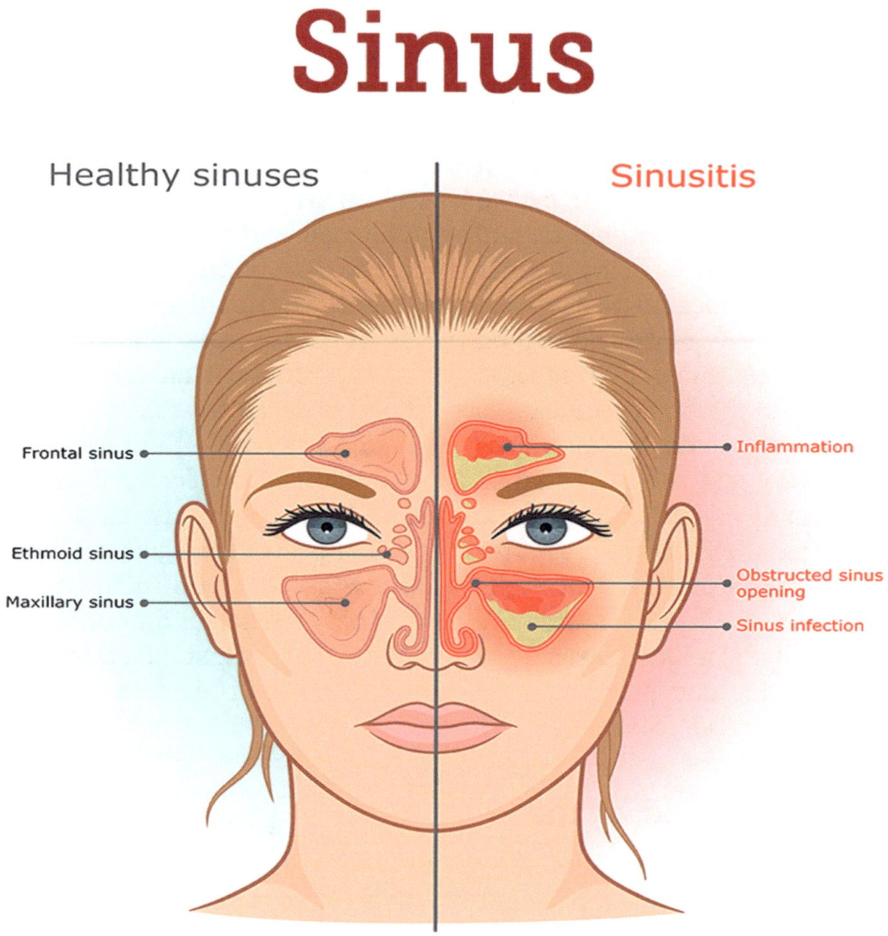

Figure 7.7. Structure and lining of the sinuses.

Source: https://assets.lybrate.com/imgs/tic/enadp/image-of-the-sinus.jpg.

7.3.3. Relationship Between Sinuses and Nasal Cavity

The intricate relationship between the sinuses and the nasal cavity is central to optimal respiratory function. The paranasal sinuses, made up of the maxillary, frontal, ethmoid, and sphenoid sinuses, are air-filled cavities that surround the nasal cavity. The sinuses empty into the nasal cavity through small openings known as ostia, which offer an avenue for air and mucus exchange. This connection serves several physiological functions, for example, humidifying and cleaning the air entering the lungs, and is vital for respiratory health. Moreover, the presence of sinuses helps reduce the load on the skull, another structural benefit. Thus, an understanding of the anatomy of these spaces is important not only for comprehending how they function but also for diagnosing potential pathologies due to their interconnected nature. Such an association of sinuses and the nasal cavity is further emphasized under inflammation and infection. Acute and chronic sinusitis are typically the consequence of inappropriateness of mucus drainage due to blockage of the channels between the paranasal sinuses and the nasal cavity. When such channels are obstructed, bacteria or viruses proliferate, causing inflammation and infection, which manifest as nasal congestion, facial pain, and difficulty in breathing. With the exploration of the anatomical details of these linkages, researchers have been able to demarcate specific risk factors that may result in sinus-based issues, such as anatomical variation or intrinsic medical conditions. Morphological features of the maxillary sinus and anatomical variations occupy central positions in elucidating these conditions in accordance with the literature (N/A, 2022). Besides, advancements in medical technology have enhanced our capability to diagnose and cure sinus and nasal cavity illnesses. Techniques such as endoscopy allow direct vision exploration of the nasal passages and sinuses, making the identification of obstructions or abnormalities easy. All these are because of the great historical development of otorhinolaryngology, the branch of medicine dealing with the exploration of the ear, nose, and throat (Américo et al., 2007). By integrating anatomical knowledge with cutting-edge clinical techniques, clinicians can craft targeted treatment plans for conditions caused by the complex interdependence between the sinuses and the nasal cavity. This new information calls for further research in this evolving field, offering a window of opportunity to improve patient outcomes.

Test Your Knowledge

1. Name the paranasal sinuses and describe their location, structure, and relationship to the nasal cavity.
2. Explain the anatomical variations of the paranasal sinuses and their clinical significance in sinus disease and surgery.

7.4. Physiology of the Paranasal Sinuses

Learning Outcome

1. Functions of the Paranasal Sinuses in the Respiratory System
2. Role in Voice Resonance and Sound Production
3. Contribution to the Immune Defense System

Paranasal sinus physiology is of critical significance in the general operation of the nasal system, an expression of the close interdependence between structure and function. Air-filled sinuses, that is, maxillary, frontal, ethmoid, and sphenoid sinuses, are covered with mucous membranes that are of crucial significance for respiratory health. Mucous membranes secrete mucus that captures airborne particles and pathogens to be cleared from the airways by mechanisms of mucociliary clearance. This physiological action is supplemented by the action of the sinuses in conditioning the air for temperature and humidity, thus maximizing the conditions for the more distal airways. Being aware of the physiological functions of the paranasal sinuses marks their importance in keeping the respiratory potency intact and preventing infection and, by extension, the intricacy of their functional and anatomical relationships (Américo et al., 2007). Moreover, the paranasal sinuses serve multiple purposes in defense mechanisms in the nasal cavity. The unique anatomy of each sinus facilitates specialized function, such as resonation of sound and pressure regulation, that can optimize vocalization and even impact olfactory senses. In normal functioning sinuses, they facilitate the body's defense against pathogens and contribute to the immune system by producing antimicrobial products. The physiological role of the paranasal sinuses also includes intricate neural reflexes, which are responsible for the reflex reactions caused by nasal mucosal irritation. Such reflexes may bring about sneezing, a protective reflex which is vital to clear irritants from the nasal airway (Américo et al., 2007). Therefore, a thorough understanding of sinus physiology is necessary to explore useful treatments for upper respiratory tract conditions. In clinical settings, paranasal sinus dysfunction can present in several forms, a point that serves to emphasize the clinical significance of their normal physiology. Sinusitis, or mucosal inflammation of the sinus, is one such example of abnormal sinus physiology that has significant implications for health. Dysfunction of this function can give rise to defective mucociliary clearance and favor infection-prone conditions and chronic congestion. Therapeutic interventions focus on normalizing sinus function through medical therapy, such as topical therapy, which emphasizes physiological recuperative processes and aims to stop the inflammatory processes. Understanding the physiological underpinning of the paranasal sinuses thus not only adds to our knowledge of their intrinsic role in respiratory health but also is an essential foundation for creating clinical solutions to the management of sinus disease (Beule, 2011) (Figure 7.8).

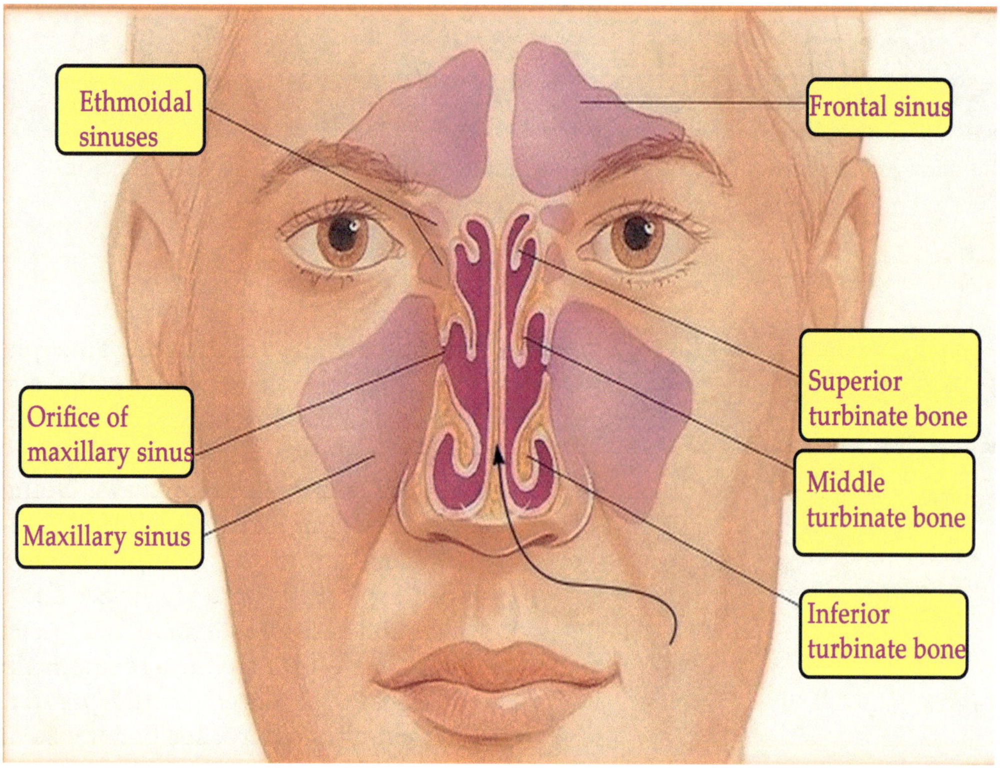

Figure 7.8. The physiology of the paranasal sinuses.

Source: https://slideplayer.com/12315300/73/images/slide_1.jpg.

7.4.1. Functions of the Paranasal Sinuses in the Respiratory System

Paranasal sinuses play a number of important roles in the respiratory system that result in normal nasal physiology. The first is that these air spaces, which are housed in the frontal, maxillary, ethmoid, and sphenoid bones, assist in humidifying and warming the entering air. This serves the purpose of protecting the delicate tissue of the lower respiratory tract, as appropriately conditioned air enhances mucosal condition and assists in maintaining respiratory efficiency. Second, the sinuses are also responsible for minimizing the skull's weight as a whole, providing structural support with minimal loss of strength. This anatomical feature enhances head and neck mobility, which is advantageous for activities such as communication and feeding. These functions serve to prove that the paranasal sinuses are not vestigial but functional components of the respiratory system's anatomy and physiology. Secondly, the paranasal sinuses also function to keep nasal airflow and pressure. They achieve this by their connection to the nasal cavity, into which the sinuses drain through the nasal meatuses. The connection facilitates the flow of air across the entire nasal passage as well as draining away excess mucous from the sinuses themselves. Acting in concert, the paranasal sinuses contribute to ideal airflow dynamics that enhance olfaction by routing air appropriately onto the olfactory epithelium located in the superior nasal cavity. This collaboration between the sense of smell and airflow is what makes the importance of the sinuses to the respiratory system so notable. In case of an occluded sinus drainage, however, it could lead to sinusitis, disrupting these processes and leading to other respiratory problems. The role of the paranasal sinuses is more than mechanical; they also play a role in immune protection. The mucous covering of the sinuses contains immune cells and produces mucus, which catches pathogens and particulate matter from the air. It is the first line of defense against respiratory infections, notably acute and chronic sinusitis, which are prevalent conditions associated with sinus dysfunction. Besides, with growing understanding of morphology and anatomical sinus variations of the paranasal sinuses, their clinical significance has been better realized. As discussed in recent studies, knowledge of these variations can inform treatment approaches in otorhinolaryngology to assist in the management of diseases of the sinonasals (N/A, 2022). The paranasal sinuses are thus pivotal in respiratory function, alongside immunity, further cementing their position in the overall health of the respiratory system.

7.4.2. Role in Voice Resonance and Sound Production

The sinuses and paranasal sinuses are also very important elements in sound resonance and voice production, and these are integral parts of the vocal tract. When a person talks, air generated by the lungs passes through the vocal cords in the larynx and gets modulated to create a sound. Nasal cavity and sinuses, due to their anatomical structure, add timbre and quality to this sound as resonating cavities. By vibrating microphones at certain frequencies but inhibiting others, these environments amplify the depth and richness of the vocal sound, which is crucial to effective word communication. For instance, the size and shape of an individual's nasal cavities significantly alter their unique vocal characteristics, resulting in identifying factors like resonance and pitch. Thus, a better knowledge of the sinuses and nasal anatomy is necessary to be able to value their impact on voice projection and clarity. Aside from being resonating cavities, nasal cavities and paranasal sinuses also contribute to sound production by modulation of airflow and the humidification functions they serve. The nasal cavities are channels that regulate the flow of air into the larynx and thus influence vocal output. Resonating is a dynamic process, based on airflow alterations, which can be controlled by vocal habits, that is, nasal sound or pitch modulation. The paranasal sinuses also play a part in warming and humidifying inhaled air for smoother airflow compatible with optimal voice production. This relationship between air flow and anatomy underlines a more profound correspondence between nasal passage shape and sound quality created, illustrating the significance of these anatomical features in singing. Furthermore, the correlation among the nasal cavity, paranasal sinuses, and voice resonance extends to many illnesses that can significantly affect vocal quality. For example, sinusitis or nasal obstructions can prevent the proper functioning of these anatomical structures, resulting in the decreased vocal resonance characterized by a nasal quality. These changes can affect not only the appearance of the voice but also clarity and communicative efficiency. This connection underscores the significance of why ear, nose, and throat (ENT) doctors focus on maintaining healthy and functioning nasal passages and sinuses to help provide the best possible vocal performance. As such, it is crucial to become familiar with the anatomy and physiology of the nose and paranasal sinuses, not only for singers and actors but also for anyone whose daily communication rides on effective sound production (Figure 7.9).

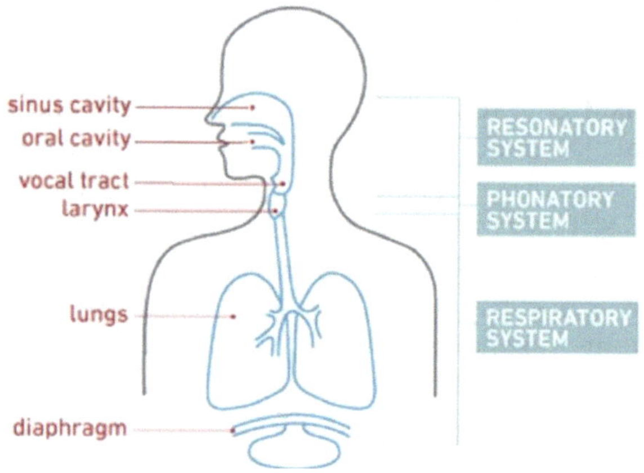

Figure 7.9. Role in voice resonance and sound production.

Source: https://www.templehealth.org/sites/default/files/styles/without_crop/public/TH-180180-THNI-VoiceDiagram-cropped%20%281%29.jpg?itok=tsyVIhT2.

7.4.3. Contribution to the Immune Defense System

Nose and paranasal sinuses are critical components of the immune defense system, as they clean and condition air taken into the respiratory tract. The intricate anatomy of the nasal cavity, for example, the nasal mucosa, plays a role in trapping pathogens and particulate matter. This is done by ciliated epithelial cells and mucus-secreting glands, which work together to remove foreign elements. Through warming and humidification of inhaled air, the nasal tissues provide protection for the lungs against environmental irritants, reducing the risk of respiratory infections such as sinusitis and bronchitis.

The secondary advantage lies in the location of immune cells in the nasal mucosa, which provides an additional line of defense by enabling localized immune responses to hazards (Djupesland, 2012). Another key aspect of the immunoprotection offered by the nose relates to its role in mucociliary clearance, a process that is responsible for the removal of pathogens and debris. The respiratory mucosa of the nose and paranasal sinuses harbors a highly regulated system that relies upon the coordinated activity of the cilia in propelling mucus towards the pharynx, where it may be swallowed or expelled. This system, aside from clearing out noxious particles, also ensures the optimal amount of moisture within the respiratory tract in order to facilitate peak immune function. The efficiency of mucociliary clearance is particularly clear when one considers the anatomical constraints of the nasal cavity, such as its complex geometry, which increases airflow turbulence and increases contact time with the mucosal surface (Beule, 2011). Such dynamics underscore the importance of the nasal passages in maintaining an effective immune defense mechanism.

Furthermore, the nose also presents itself as a viable route for the administration of immunomodulatory therapies to induce systemic immunity. Being easily accessible, the nasal cavity is a viable route for vaccines and drugs that are designed to induce immune responses without the use of painful traditional needle-injected vaccinations. There have been some recent studies into new nasal delivery technology that can avoid gastrointestinal breakdown and avoid first-pass metabolism, and this shows the potential for the use of the nose in preventive medicine. However, it must be pointed out that while there are many advantages to drug delivery by the nose, the anatomical configuration is usually one of protective function (Djupesland, 2012). This duality underscores the nose's importance within the continuum of immune defense, and it is implied that any therapeutic approach must account for these inherent biological functions (Beule, 2011).

Test Your Knowledge

1. Explain the functions of the paranasal sinuses, including their roles in humidifying air, voice resonance, reducing skull weight, and protecting facial structures.
2. Describe the mechanism of sinus drainage and mucociliary clearance and its importance in preventing sinus infections.

7.5. Common Disorders of the Nose and Sinuses

Learning Outcome

1. Rhinitis and Its Types
2. Sinusitis: Causes and Symptoms
3. Nasal Polyps and Their Implications

The nose and paranasal sinuses are susceptible to a number of conditions that have extensive impacts on respiratory well-being and lifestyle. These conditions include nasal polyps, allergic rhinitis, and sinusitis. The most prevalent condition is allergic rhinitis, which is typically caused by environmental allergens such as pollen, dust mites, and pet dander. Allergic rhinitis is characterized by sneezing, nasal congestion, and watery eyes. This condition results from a hyperactive immune response by IgE antibodies, leading to inflammation of the nasal mucosa. Sinusitis secondary to an upper respiratory viral infection can be either acute or chronic and presents symptoms with overlap of similar symptoms presented by allergic rhinitis, but also including facial pain, purulent nasal discharge, and fever. This interaction of conditions highlights the need for a comprehensive understanding of nasal anatomy and physiology to best treat and manage these common conditions. Progressing further into sinusitis, care must be taken to distinguish between its acute and chronic presentations so as to offer appropriate therapeutic interventions. Acute sinusitis is typically a self-limiting illness of fewer than four weeks' duration, which is often self-limiting and resolves without the need for antibiotics in viral infections. Chronic sinusitis, however, lasts more than 12 weeks and may involve recurrent attacks. Chronic rhinosinusitis also has a tendency to complicate the medical history of the patient, particularly among those who are suffering from asthma or other respiratory diseases. Further, fungal rhinosinusitis, particularly among immunocompromised individuals, is of significant risk, varying from non-invasive to invasive forms that need emergency medical care (Cojocari et al., 2018). Identification of these differences offers directed management alternatives, which may include nasal corticosteroids, saline irrigations, or surgery, depending on etiology and severity. Nasal polyps are another prevalent issue that results from chronic mucosal inflammation of the nasal and sinus mucosa and are often associated with diseases such as asthma, cystic fibrosis, and allergic rhinitis. Such benign growths can obstruct nasal flow and cause a range of symptoms, from difficulty breathing to loss of olfaction and recurrent sinusitis. The occurrence of nasal polyps suggests an underlying inflammatory dysregulation, which implies the need for medical management aimed at eradicating chronic inflammation and preventing recurrence. Polypectomy or other surgical procedures may be indicated in cases with serious obstruction. Understanding the anatomical and physiological basis of these conditions enables healthcare providers to implement preventive measures and therapeutic interventions more effectively, leading to improved patient outcomes (Américo et al., 2007). The complexity of these common conditions requires ongoing research and study into treatment modalities to help treat individuals afflicted by them better (Figure 7.10).

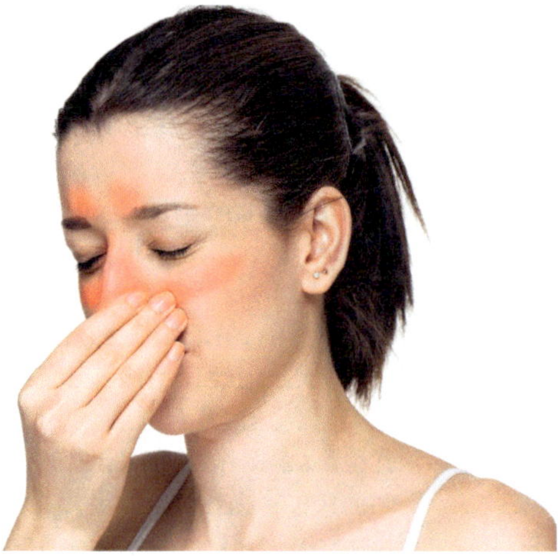

Figure 7.10. Common disorders of the nose and sinuses.

Source: https://www.entlubbock.com/wp-content/uploads/2022/06/sinus-issues.jpg.

7.5.1. Rhinitis and Its Types

Rhinitis, an inflammation of the nasal mucosa, is a frequent condition and produces a significant effect on the paranasal sinuses and the anatomy and physiology of the nose. It could be classified into different types including allergic rhinitis, non-allergic rhinitis, and infectious rhinitis, with unique pathophysiological characteristics. Allergic rhinitis is most often caused by environmental allergens such as pollen, dust mites, and pet dander, resulting in IgE-mediated immune responses that manifest as sneezing, nasal congestion, and itching. The complex interaction between allergens and the immune system reveals the complexity of nasal physiology, illustrating the significance of nasal tissues in mediating responses to environmental contacts, and illustrating the nose's function in protecting the respiratory tract and conditioning inspired air. Non-allergic rhinitis, however, is caused by non-allergic factors such as irritants, pungent odors, or hormonal changes. This form shares the same symptoms as allergic rhinitis but does not involve the characteristic immunological response. The distinction between these two forms of rhinitis is important if they are to be effectively treated and managed. For instance, knowledge of the cytokine response that occurs with allergic rhinitis can make targeted therapy possible, targeting the resulting inflammation. Studies on human nasal epithelial cells have shown that baseline levels of cytokines like IL-6 and IL-8 are noticeably dissimilar in allergic rhinitis compared to chronic rhinosinusitis, emphasizing the need for targeted approaches depending on the nature of rhinitis (Kuchai, 2009). It is central to this data for the creation of effective treatment plans with consideration of the intricacies of nasal and paranasal sinus function. Moreover, infectious rhinitis, more often caused by viruses, is typically associated with symptoms proportional to mucosal changes and immune responses against the invading pathogens. As compared to allergic rhinitis, infectious rhinitis might have more pronounced systemic symptoms such as fever and malaise. Lastly, awareness of the pathophysiology of infectious rhinitis serves to heighten the nuances of the nasal airway as the initial defense mechanism against pathogens. The nose's geometric anatomy, which entails complex geometry, not only allows for air filtration but also plays a crucial role in enhancing the efficacy of potential therapeutic interventions for conditions such as rhinitis. This observation underscores the potential to explore new mechanisms for nasal drug delivery, as outlined in the context of emerging nasal delivery technologies that can optimize therapeutic impact while circumventing the physiological barriers inherent to the nasal pathway (Djupesland, 2012).

7.5.2. Sinusitis: Causes and Symptoms

Sinusitis, a paranasal sinus infection and inflammation, results from multiple infectious agents and, to a lesser extent, noninfectious irritants. Acute sinusitis is most commonly initiated by respiratory infections such as the common cold, which are capable of causing swelling and occlusion of the sinus tract. This blockage may lead to the development of mucus accumulation, hence providing ground for bacterial growth. Conversely, chronic sinusitis may result from persistent infection, allergy, or anatomical sinus capes of decreased drainage.

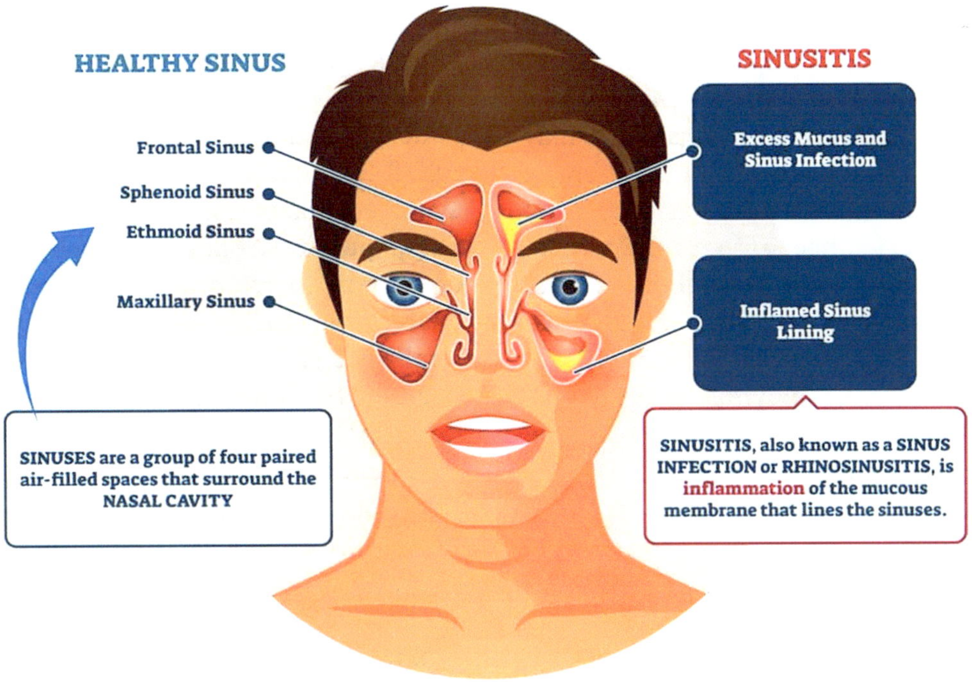

Figure 7.11. Sinusitis: causes and symptoms.

Source: https://allergyasthmanetwork.org/wp-content/uploads/2024/10/Infographic-of-sinuses.jpg.

Paranasal sinus anatomical variations, like morphologies, play a major role in comprehending these conditions, and thus thorough study becomes essential in understanding sinusitis and its etiology (N/A, 2022). Sinusitis symptoms are diverse and may disrupt one's quality of life. Nasal obstruction, facial pain or pressure, thick yellow or green nasal secretions, and loss of the sense of smell are common presentations. Patients often report facial fullness, predominantly over the cheeks and forehead, that worsens with forward bending. In chronic cases, symptoms last for weeks to months and lead to fatigue and irritability. Furthermore, sinusitis commonly co-exists with other respiratory illnesses, such as asthma, and is thus complicated to diagnose and treat. A critical analysis of the relationship between these illnesses reveals shared pathological pathways, as indicated by eosinophil and mast cell recruitment (Balaji, 2017). This overlap underscores the need to understand sinusitis symptoms in the context of general respiratory illness. Effective management of sinusitis relies on the determination of its causes and symptomatology to direct treatment modalities from medical to surgical. Treatment may start with the eradication of causative infectious agents by antibiotics, while nasal corticosteroids ease inflammation and improve drainage of the sinuses. In cases of sinusitis with allergy or asthma, total management strategies may involve allergen avoidance and immunotherapy. The link between sinusitis and asthma is of particular interest since optimal control of sinusitis can greatly improve asthma control and lung function. This cross-link emphasizes the importance of screening for sinusitis in asthmatic patients, employing medical and surgical treatments when indicated, to optimize patient outcomes and quality of life (Balaji, 2017) (Figure 7.11).

7.5.3. Nasal Polyps and Their Implications

Nasal polyps are benign neoplasms that often arise from the mucosal lining of the nasal airway and sinuses. Nasal polyps are secondary to chronic inflammation and could be secondary to underlying diseases such as asthma, allergic rhinitis, and cystic fibrosis. Nasal polyps can significantly alter the normal anatomy and physiology of the nasal cavity and paranasal sinuses, and various complications can follow. When nasal polyps obstruct sinus drainage tracts, they are the cause of chronic sinusitis, which is an ongoing infection and inflammation of the sinuses. The anatomical effects of polyps should be recognized, as their formation can lead to facial pain, loss of smell, and nasal obstruction, which can significantly affect quality of life (N/A, 2022). The management of nasal polyps is similarly multi-modal, so it is essential to address the anatomical and physiological sides of the condition. Treatment usually involves the use of corticosteroids, which decrease polyp size and inflammation, but in whom these do not work, surgery can be considered. FESS is presently a mainstay of treatment in patients with chronic rhinosinusitis with or without polyposis.

A recent prospective study measured the efficacy of FESS, and it reported considerable improvement in the patient's quality of life after undergoing the procedure, as expressed in the SNOT 22 questionnaire. The study provided average gains of approximately 20.8 points for polyp patients, emphasizing the importance of surgery in restoring nasal functioning and overall well-being (Sunny, 2013). Long-term implications of nasal polyps are significant, necessitating ongoing monitoring and therapy. Nasal polyp patients are at higher risk for recurrence, thereby validating that treatment protocols should encourage both surgical and medical management to minimize relapse rates. Nasal polyp occurrence is also often related to other systemic diseases, again adding complexity to patient management. Gaining the ability to deal with these complexities relies on understanding the interconnectedness of nasal anatomy and general well-being. Treatment should focus not only on the short-term benefits of surgery but also on preventive care to reduce the risk of complications and improve long-term outcomes, thereby synthesizing medical and surgical understanding in the diagnosis of nasal polyps and their implications (N/A, 2022).

Test Your Knowledge

1. What are the most common disorders affecting the nose and paranasal sinuses, and what are their typical causes and clinical features?
2. Explain the diagnosis and management of conditions such as rhinitis, sinusitis, nasal polyps, and deviated nasal septum.

7.6. Diagnostic Techniques

Learning Outcome

1. Physical Examination of the Nose and Sinuses
2. Imaging Techniques: CT and MRI
3. Endoscopic Evaluation of Nasal Passages

In otorhinolaryngology, diagnosing conditions of the nose and paranasal sinuses calls for a multidisciplinary approach that involves both established and novel means. Advances made in the past have led to the development of current diagnostic strategies, such as endoscopy and imaging technology. Endoscopy, specifically, enables clinicians to view the nasal cavities and sinus ostia in direct sight, making the diagnosis of diseases like chronic rhinosinusitis and mucosal abnormalities possible. In addition, imaging techniques such as computed tomography (CT) and magnetic resonance imaging (MRI) provide accurate anatomical information that supports the evaluation process.

These tools play an important role not only in the diagnosis of the structural and functional issues in the nasal and sinus anatomy but also in the planning of upcoming therapeutic treatment, showing significant evolutions in diagnostic techniques over the years (Américo et al., 2007). The application of imaging in the diagnosis of diseases affecting the paranasal sinuses cannot be overstated. CT scans are especially invaluable in assessing the severity of sinus disease, revealing acute and chronic inflammation, mucosal thickening, and anatomical variations to influence treatment. Moreover, advances in imaging technology have increased scan resolution, thereby improving diagnostic accuracy. For instance, high-resolution CT can adequately differentiate between types of sinusitis, including allergic fungal rhinosinusitis and acute invasive fungal rhinosinusitis, which is primarily seen in immunocompromised individuals (Cojocari et al., 2018). Therefore, careful evaluation by imaging not only leads to diagnosis but also supports the selection of appropriate care plans, showing the interconnectedness between the diagnostic process and adherence to therapeutic decisions. Also, the examination of nasal secretions and testing for allergens are crucial diagnostic tools in sinus-related disorder research. Rhinologic assessment would normally begin with a comprehensive history and physical exam that leads to secondary investigations on the basis of the presenting symptoms. Analysis of nasal secretions may reveal allergens or pathogens, and the findings can help establish a diagnosis of allergic rhinitis or bacterial or fungal infection. In addition to that, immunologic evaluation is crucial in the case of recurrent sinusitis, particularly in the history of atopy or compromised immune status. By identifying specific triggers or pathogens through these tests, doctors are able to prescribe customized treatment protocols that address both symptoms and root causes (CITE50). Thus, an integrated diagnostic approach emphasizes developing a comprehensive understanding of nasal and paranasal sinus anatomy and physiology to optimize patient outcomes (Figure 7.12).

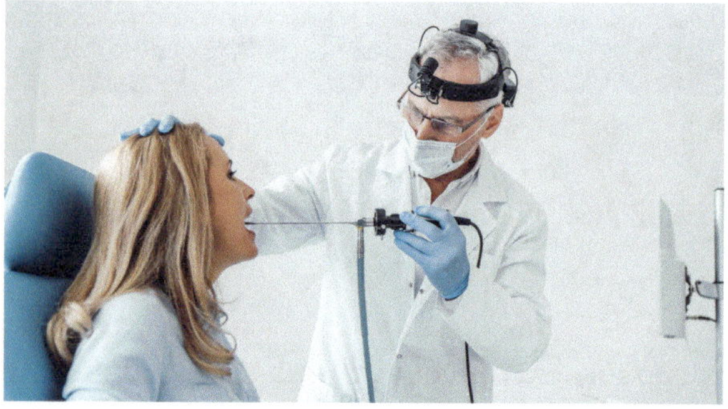

Figure 7.12. The otorhinolaryngology.

Source: https://grandgenesishealth.com/wp-content/uploads/2022/10/Otorhinolaryngology.jpg.

7.6.1. Physical Examination of the Nose and Sinuses

Physical inspection of the nose and sinuses is an essential component of clinical examination whose aim is to identify underlying pathology that can affect respiratory well-being. The first inspection is often in the shape of the external appearance of the nose, and asymmetry, swelling, or deformity here may indicate trauma or chronicity. Nasal bridge and sinus palpation together may detect the tender areas, which may be suggestive of sinusitis or other inflammatory conditions. The nasal obstruction and discharge are also normally assessed in the patient for color, texture, and amount of secretions. This multi-dimensional assessment provides valuable information about the condition of both the nasal cavity and adjacent paranasal sinuses, which is important to achieve the best respiratory performance as well as overall health. An extensive assessment of the nose often exceeds plain observation and comprises various techniques such as otoscopy, rhinometry, or nasal endoscopy. Nasal endoscopy, in particular, offers direct visualization of sinuses and nasal passages and enables clinicians to examine for potential obstruction, abnormalities, or polyps. Nasal endoscopy is paramount to examine the anatomy and physiology of the nasal mucosa, which is indeed primarily accountable for the response to allergens and pathogen filtration. A mucosal health checkup may also inform treatment through the identification of swelling or inflammation that compromises mucociliary clearance. Accurate recording of these findings enhances understanding of the role that anatomical differences or pathological changes may have in chronic issues like sinusitis or associated disorders like asthma, and the interconnectedness of nasal and sinus health. Of most relevance to the physical assessment of the nose and sinuses is understanding specific conditions that may arise, including fungal rhinosinusitis. Immunocompromised individuals are at higher risk of developing such a condition, and it may manifest as invasive or non-invasive disease. On physical examination, there may be obvious manifestations of allergic fungal rhinosinusitis, including mucosal thinning and typical secretions. Moreover, understanding the complicated associations of sinus infection with respiratory disorders, that is, asthma, necessitates practitioners to evaluate such associations on physical examination. Screening asthmatic patients for sinus involvement has significant implications for the outcome of treatment, in that successful treatment of sinusitis appears to enhance the control of asthmatic symptoms, and hence the importance of a comprehensive examination strategy in diagnosing and treating these interrelated conditions (Balaji, 2017; Cojocari et al., 2018).

7.6.2. Imaging Techniques: CT and MRI

Imaging techniques, that is, Computed Tomography (CT) and Magnetic Resonance Imaging (MRI), are of critical significance in the understanding of the nasal and paranasal sinus anatomy and physiology. CT is used to obtain high-resolution cross-sectional images of these complexes with X-rays and yields high-definition data on bony anatomy and sinus opacification. This is particularly useful for the diagnosis of sinusitis or anatomical deformities that may impede airflow or drainage. MRI, in contrast, employs powerful magnets to generate images according to tissues' water content and is especially useful for imaging soft tissue such as mucosal linings and any associated lesions without the use of ionizing radiation. By the combination of both modalities, clinicians can achieve complete evaluation of nasal and sinus pathologies, opening the gates to improved treatment outcomes. The new imaging technology has significantly enhanced our ability to do virtual simulation and three-dimensional paranasal sinus reconstructions. Computer-aided design models have recently been brought to the forefront of literature as having the ability to better visualize these complex anatomical regions. For instance, the union of Surf driver software and Cinema 4D has led to photorealistic 3D models that provide unprecedented virtual endoscopy capabilities. These developments not only support medical professionals during preoperative planning but also serve as educational tools for students and researchers. This imaging modality, particularly when used in combination with the traditional approach, offers a detailed insight into anatomy and pathology and hence improves surgical precision and patient management of conditions affecting the nose and sinuses, as emphasized by recent research findings (Kapakin, 2016). Furthermore, an understanding of the implications of fungal infections of the paranasal sinuses highlights the importance of accurate imaging in making decisions for treatment and diagnosis. Fungal rhinosinusitis poses particular challenges, particularly in immunocompromised patients, where early diagnosis can prevent severe complications, including orbital and intracranial extension. CT and MRI are invaluable for the detection of these pathologic changes by showing sinus anatomy and assessing mucosal thickening and consequent fungal ball formation. These imaging findings directly influence treatment, as they determine the need for medical versus surgical care. As we further understand the complex interrelationship between pathology and anatomy of the nose and paranasal sinuses, comprehensive imaging remains an essential part in developing therapeutic strategies, particularly in complex cases of chronic rhinosinusitis (Cojocari et al., 2018) (Figure 7.13).

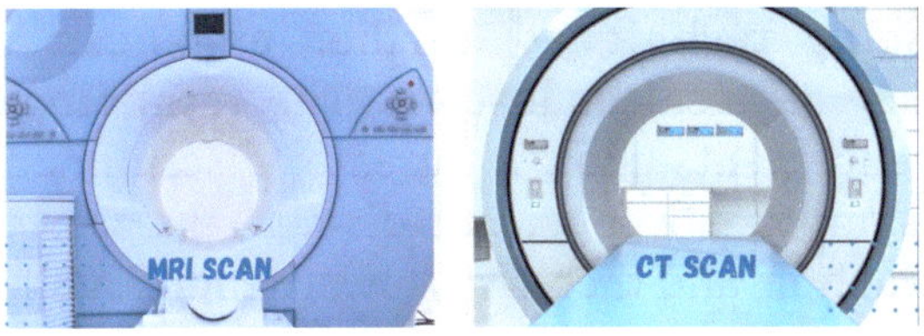

Figure 7.13. The application of imaging techniques, particularly Computed Tomography (CT) and Magnetic Resonance Imaging (MRI).

Source: https://www.usmanpuraimaging.com/images/resource/mri-scan-and-ct-scan.jpg.

7.6.3. Endoscopic Evaluation of Nasal Passages

Endoscopic examination of the nasal passages has revolutionized otorhinolaryngology, enabling direct visualization of nasal anatomy and disease. This fiber-optic camera-based minimally invasive method makes it possible to explore the intricate nasal cavities and paranasal sinuses. Earlier, physicians relied on external visual inspections or crude instruments, which compromised diagnostic precision. However, with the advent of nasal endoscopy, the understanding of illnesses such as chronic rhinosinusitis, nasal polyps, and other inflammatory diseases has been enhanced, and clinicians have obtained valuable information about the condition of their patients. Moreover, direct visualization of anatomical variations within the osteomata complex affects the treatment modalities, which in most cases determine the indications for surgery or management (Américo et al., 2007). Aside from its application to diagnosis, endoscopic examination is therapeutic as well, and various procedures such as biopsy, polypectomy, and even drainage of abscesses related to sinusitis are possible. With direct access to areas of interest within the nasal cavities, otorhinolaryngologists are able to operate where open surgery had hitherto excluded them from, with low patient morbidity and hospital stay. The addition of technology, such as high-definition video and improved imaging techniques, further enhanced the utility of nasal endoscopy. The technological advancements allow for greater discrimination in symptomatology and disease progression evaluation, and therefore, toward individualized treatment protocols. Therefore, endoscopic treatment has been the signature of modern-day therapy for the majority of conditions affecting the sinonasal tract, standing as a significant leap in surgical technique alongside patient outcome (Kandukuri, R., & Phatak, S., 2017). In addition, endoscopic evaluation of the nasal passages has been complemented by imaging technology advancements, namely computed tomography (CT). CT scans are also an important part of pre-operative assessment, providing excellent anatomical detail that complements the detail observed with endoscopy. This synergy of imaging and direct vision enables physicians to diagnose and treat difficult sinonasal pathologies with greater accuracy. Current research highlights the utility of such diagnostic tests, with high sensitivity and specificity rates of CT in chronic sinusitis and other inflammatory diseases (Kandukuri, R., & Phatak, S., 2017). The addition of these diagnostic devices not only enhances the clinician's ability to make an educated decision but also facilitates improved surgical planning and postoperative management, ultimately leading to improved patient care for the specialty of rhinology and sinonasal health (Américo et al., 2007).

Test Your Knowledge

1. What are the common diagnostic techniques used in ENT practice, including clinical examination, endoscopy, and imaging, and how do they aid in diagnosis?
2. Explain the role of audiological tests, nasal endoscopy, CT, MRI, and laboratory investigations in diagnosing ENT and head & neck conditions.

SUMMARY

The involved physiology and anatomy of the nose and paranasal sinuses are crucial to respiratory well-being and the facilitation of various physiological processes. The nasal cavity houses diverse structures, including the nasal septum and turbinates, which are designed to optimize air flow, humidify the air we breathe in, and remove dust and other particulates. Understanding such complexities simplifies how it is possible to appreciate how afflictions such as chronic rhinosinusitis (CRS) progress and impact overall well-being. Current studies indicate that interventions such as balloon catheter dilation (BCD) and traditional endoscopic sinus surgery (ESS) are effective in alleviating symptoms of frontal sinusitis, as noted by a statistically significant difference in symptom control among individuals with moderate to severe CRS (Azimonti et al., 2018). Furthermore, the nasal physiological therapeutic importance is more than simple filtration and humidification. The nose is also an important route of delivery for drugs, particularly in the management of local diseases of the upper respiratory tract, for instance, sinusitis and rhinitis. Nasal delivery exploits the unique anatomy of the nasal cavity, which allows for immediate absorption and action and the potential to avoid first-pass metabolism, thereby improving drug efficacy (Djupesland, 2012). However, with this capability comes a cost; defensive nasal passageway functions can be an obstacle to effective drug delivery, necessitating the continuing discovery of delivery systems attuned to these physiologic constraints. By overviewing the anatomy and physiology of the nose and paranasal sinuses, it is apparent that their functions are complex and of significance to respiratory health as well as successful medical treatment. The subtle interplay of structure and function must be savored in full to proceed with clinical outcomes in treatment options related to the sinuses. The future research must continue to explore the interconnection between anatomical parameters and therapy approaches, specifically since developing technologies introduce opportunities for enhanced solutions for paranasal and nasal pathology patients. This combined understanding emphasizes not only the significance of anatomical data but also the impact of physiological ideas on clinical practice in this field.

Anatomy and physiology of the nose and paranasal sinuses play a significant role in understanding the respiratory system's health and concomitant disorders. The nose is the primary doorway for air to enter the respiratory system, with certain specialized structures called turbinates to warm, humidify, and filter air to render the respiratory system more effective. The paranasal sinuses, like the maxillary, frontal, ethmoid, and sphenoid sinuses, are air cavities that minimize skull weight and facilitate speech resonance. Their highly designed passageways enable mucous drainage and olfactory purposes. Irritation or infection in these cavities can lead to illnesses like chronic rhinosinusitis, and this illustrates the nasal passage and sinus interdependence, which calls for medical procedures that require a comprehensive understanding of this anatomy. Functional endoscopic sinus surgery (FESS) is now a standard of treatment for both chronic sinusitis with and without nasal polyposis, by addressing structural impediments to optimal sinus function. Studies indicate significant improvement in patient quality of life measures, particularly those measured using the SNOT 22 questionnaire. A notable consequence of such interventions is an important elevation in endoscopic score, stressing that not only do operative corrections help alleviate symptoms, but also enhance measurable anatomical status. Such implications serve to underscore the principal role of precise anatomical knowledge and technique, demonstrating how creative developments in surgical procedure can enhance chronic conditions limiting nasal and sinus function. Thus, the relationship between theory and actual usage in the therapeutic setting becomes pivotal. The delivery of anesthetics intranasally has become pivotal in improving patient comfort during nasal endoscopy procedures, a step toward patient-centered care in otolaryngology. Analysis of different studies indicates divergent outcomes as regards pain relief during endoscopy, but it points toward the enhancement in procedural ease for practitioners in employing anesthetics. The methods of anesthetic administration then emerged as the most significant consideration to shape outcomes, as contrasted with the choice of specific anesthetic agents. Moreover, findings suggest that the development of effective masking agents could improve patient experience. Overall, the use of intranasal anesthetics, guided by meticulous procedural protocols, improves not only the efficiency of nasal examinations but also patient satisfaction, underscoring the need for continued research in this field to enhance care in nasal and sinus procedures.

KEY TERMS FROM THIS CHAPTER

- External Nose
- Nasal Septum
- Turbinates
- Middle Turbinate
- Meatus
- Olfactory Epithelium
- Cribriform Plate
- Hard Palate
- Maxillary Sinus
- Nasal Cavity
- Vestibule
- Inferior Turbinate
- Superior Turbinate
- Nasal Valve
- Respiratory Epithelium
- Olfactory Bulb
- Soft Palate
- Frontal Sinus

CRITICAL THINKING QUESTIONS

1 **The nasal septum is made of:**
   a) Bone only
   b) Cartilage only
   c) Bone and cartilage
   d) Muscle

2. **The main function of nasal turbinates is:**
   a) Smell detection
   b) Warming, humidifying, and filtering air
   c) Producing mucus
   d) Voice resonance

3. **Which sinus is located above the eyes?**
   a) Maxillary sinus
   b) Frontal sinus
   c) Ethmoid sinus
   d) Sphenoid sinus

4. **The largest paranasal sinus is:**
   a) Frontal sinus
   b) Ethmoid sinus
   c) Maxillary sinus
   d) Sphenoid sinus

5. **The olfactory epithelium is located in the:**
   a) Nasal vestibule
   b) Superior part of nasal cavity
   c) Middle meatus
   d) Inferior turbinate

Short Answer Questions

1. Describe the anatomical divisions of the nose, including the external nose, nasal cavity, and nasal septum, and their primary functions.
2. What are the paranasal sinuses, and how are they connected to the nasal cavity?
3. Explain the functions of the nose in respiration, olfaction, filtration, humidification, and temperature regulation of inspired air.
4. Describe the physiology of sinus drainage and mucociliary clearance, and its role in preventing sinus infections.
5. Discuss the anatomical variations of the paranasal sinuses and their clinical significance in sinus disease and surgical procedures.

Answers to Critical Thinking Questions

1. (c) 2. (b) 3. (b) 4. (c) 5. (b)

REFERENCES

1. Abdalla, M. A. (2022). Human maxillary sinus development, pneumatization, anatomy, blood supply, innervation and Functional Theories: An update review. *Siriraj Medical Journal/San Sirirat, 74*(7), 472–479. https://doi.org/10.33192/smj.2022.56Alsaied, A. S. (2017). *Paranasal Sinus Anatomy: What the Surgeon Needs to Know.* https://core.ac.uk/download/322431348.pdf (accessed on 7th August 2025).
2. Américo, R. dos R., Barauna Filho, I. S., Hermann, D. R., Nogueira Júnior, E., et al. (2007). *A Brief History of Otorhinolaryngology: Otology, Laryngology, and Rhinology.* https://core.ac.uk/download/37707315.pdf (accessed on 7th August 2025).
3. Azimonti, D., Cavaliere, C., Dragonetti, A., Franzetti, A., et al. (2018). *Use of balloon catheter dilation vs. traditional endoscopic sinus surgery in management of light and severe chronic rhinosinusitis of the frontal sinus: A multicenter prospective randomized study.* https://core.ac.uk/download/153367692.pdf (accessed on 7th August 2025).
4. Balaji, C. (2017). *The Impact of Sinusitis Management in Asthmatic Patients.* https://core.ac.uk/download/288215760.pdf (accessed on 7th August 2025).
5. Beule, A. G. (2011). *Physiology and pathophysiology of the respiratory mucosa of the nose and the paranasal sinuses.* https://core.ac.uk/download/pdf/8632753.pdf (accessed on 7th August 2025).
6. Cooper, C. (2024). *Examining the benefits and risks of using an intranasal local anesthetic for nasal endoscopy: A review of the literature.* https://open.bu.edu/bitstream/2144/47967/6/Cooper_bu_0017N_18416.pdf (accessed on 7th August 2025).
7. Djupesland, P. G. (2012). *Nasal Drug Delivery Devices: Characteristics and Performance in a Clinical Perspective—A Review.* https://core.ac.uk/download/pdf/81263903.pdf (accessed on 7th August 2025).
8. Kandukuri, R., & Phatak, S. (2017). *Computed Tomographic Evaluation of Inflammatory Sinonasal Diseases.* https://core.ac.uk/download/544390498.pdf (accessed on 7th August 2025).
9. Kapakin, S. (2016). *The paranasal sinuses: Three-dimensional reconstruction, photo-realistic imaging, and virtual endoscopy.* https://core.ac.uk/download/268451302.pdf (accessed on 7th August 2025).
10. Kardam, N. K., & Tiwari, T. N. (2019). *CT evaluation of anatomical variations of the paranasal sinus region and their clinical importance.* https://core.ac.uk/download/539910737.pdf (accessed on 7th August 2025).
11. Keck, T., & Lindemann, J. (2011). *Numerical Simulation and Nasal Air-Conditioning.* https://core.ac.uk/download/pdf/8632756.pdf (accessed on 7th August 2025).
12. Kuchai, R. (2009). *The effect of macrolides on allergic rhinitis versus chronic rhinosinusitis—An in-vitro study.* https://core.ac.uk/download/30695215.pdf (accessed on 7th August 2025).
13. Kumar, S. (2012). *A study on chronic otitis media active mucosal type with sinusitis as focal sepsis.* https://core.ac.uk/download/235654452.pdf (accessed on 7th August 2025).
14. N/A. (2022). *Paranasal Sinuses Anatomy and Conditions.* https://core.ac.uk/download/534899812.pdf (accessed on 7th August 2025).

NASAL AND SINUS DISORDERS

8

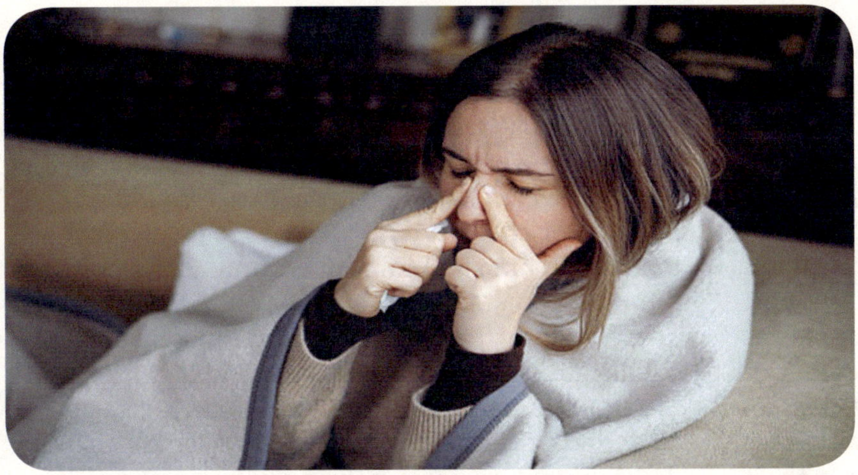

LEARNING OBJECTIVES

After studying this chapter, you will be able to:

1. Common nasal disorders.
2. Common sinus disorders.
3. Symptoms and diagnosis.
4. Treatment options.
5. Prevention strategies.

Introduction

The diagnosis of nasal and sinus conditions is a multifaceted interaction between physiological, anatomical, and pathological factors that profoundly affect an individual's overall health and well-being. They manifest as common conditions, such as allergic rhinitis and sinusitis, to less frequent conditions, such as nasal polyps and chronic rhinosinusitis, all of which are challenging to diagnose and treat. Knowledge of the pathophysiological mechanisms underlying such disorders is essential in an effort to design effective therapeutic protocols. For instance, chronic rhinosinusitis has the potential to lead to significant impairment of the quality of life, and thus, a multidisciplinary approach combining medical and surgical intervention is warranted. This introduction is background for a detailed discussion of most nasal and sinus diseases with a specific focus on their incidence and requirement for effective treatment protocols. The multifactorial pathogenesis of nasal and sinus diseases poses a big challenge to clinicians and researchers alike. Environmental allergens, anatomical variation, and infectious etiologies all have roles in the development and exacerbation of such diseases. For example, studies have established that patients with nasal polyps often experience concomitant loss of olfactory function, thus further restricting treatment and quality of life for the patients. Increasing recognition of the value of standardized definitions and measurement procedures in this area has created a need for improved methodological accuracy in studies, as proposed in the guidelines for the assessment of olfactory dysfunction (Altundag et al., 2017). Such standardization is central to the assurance that new treatments not only function but are also translatable from trial to trial, and therefore, the practice of nasal and sinus disease care is enhanced. The economic burden of nasal and sinus disorders is widespread, encompassing healthcare systems and affecting patient productivity. As underscored in the pharmacoeconomic analysis of Cyclamen europium in the management of acute rhinosinusitis, the cost-effectiveness of different treatment approaches is an important aspect to be viewed by healthcare policymakers and professionals (Anzai et al., 2013). Following the growing rate of chronic nasal conditions, evaluation of the treatment options in terms of their economic and clinical success is more essential than ever. Effective management approaches not only attempt to relieve symptoms but also reduce healthcare expenditures associated with prolonged treatments and lost efficiency. In this introduction, a premise is established for a critical discussion of treatment effectiveness and economic consequences that ultimately gives rise to an understanding of nasal and sinus conditions and their management in practice.

Definition of Nasal and Sinus Disorders

Nasal and sinus disease is a general term for the wide range of conditions that involve the upper airway, primarily the nasal passages and paranasal sinuses. Nasal and sinus disease may be caused by many factors, such as infectious agents, allergy, and anatomic abnormalities. Finally, nasal and sinus disease is most often manifested by inflammation, with symptoms ranging from nasal obstruction to sinus pain to impaired olfactory function. For example, allergic rhinitis, a common disorder, greatly influences quality of life in patients by causing a range of symptoms and frequently recurring with infections and structural problems, for example, nasal polyps (Hardjojo et al., 2012). Such disorders are made even more complicated by their possibility to be worsened by the environment, and hence both their diagnosis and treatment are also especially hard. Nasal and sinus conditions are commonly classified as acute or chronic, with chronic rhinosinusitis being the most common chronic disorder. Chronic rhinosinusitis is a chronic inflammation of the sinuses for more than 12 weeks, causing significant discomfort and decreased quality of life in patients. In addition to this, the disease also leads to other complications such as the development of nasal polyps or long-standing sinus infection (Hardjojo et al., 2012). The interplay between anatomical, environmental, and immunological conditions is crucial in the pathophysiology of chronic disease of the nasal and sinus regions, treatment needs to be holistic with both medical and surgical treatment modalities. Anosmia or olfactory impairment is another essential aspect of nasal and sinus disorders that is underappreciated in spite of its important consequences for patients. It can arise from illness, such as chronic rhinosinusitis or structural obstructions, which impede normal smell capability. Clinicians should include holistic practice that evaluates not only nasal and sinus symptoms but also sensory perception in the diagnosis and management of these disorders. Such patients with known olfactory loss must be subjected to rigorous workups to determine the etiology and systematic evaluation of their olfactory function. An overview of regularly employed diagnostic tests and treatment strategies is aimed at providing the highest level of effectiveness of treatment and the best results for patients in the event of olfactory disorders, and to aid in a comprehensive understanding of nasal and sinus disease (Figure 8.1).

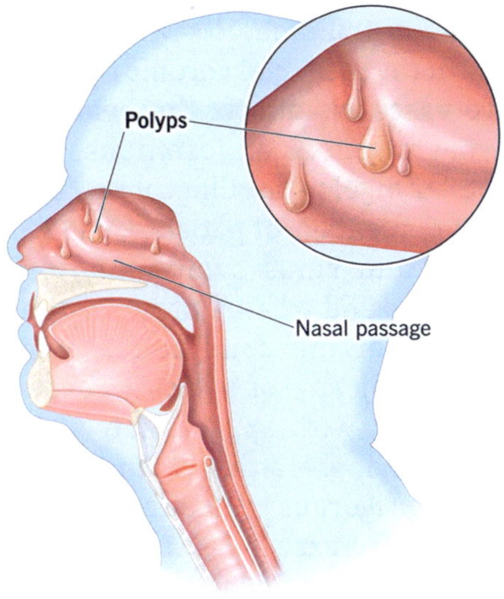

Figure 8.1. The nasal and sinus disorders.

Source: https://my.clevelandclinic.org/-/scassets/images/org/health/articles/nasal-polyps.

Importance of Understanding These Disorders

Nasal and sinus disease significantly impacts the quality of life in millions of individuals, and therefore, the understanding of such diseases is critical in treatment as well as management. Information about the pathophysiology of conditions such as chronic sinusitis and nasal polyposis will allow clinicians to design personalized therapeutic regimens for the management of symptoms and improvement in outcomes. Also, the determination of the genetic and environmental factors of such diseases will lead to more effective predictive models and screening strategies. For instance, research into genetic modifiers like the T2R38 gene highlights the complexity of conditions like cystic fibrosis (CF) and its association with the severity of sinonasal disease. The discovery of such genetic markers provides valuable information to clinicians in disease progression prognosis and personalization of treatment plans for these patients, hence optimizing treatment and even reducing healthcare spending (Amato et al., 2020). Involvement of inflammatory cytokines, particularly interleukin-17A (IL-17A), in nasal and sinusitis only contributes to the importance of understanding more about such conditions. Elevated levels of IL-17A occur in sinonasal polyposis, suggesting an immediate correlation with inflammation and disease presentation. Not only does such information contribute to scientific recognition of sinonasal disease, but it also provides a foundation for therapeutic maneuvers against these inflammatory pathways. By appreciating distinctions between atopic and non-atopic patients, researchers are able to study IL-17A variability in expression and its prognostic and therapeutic implications. Such studies may reveal new intervention targets, ultimately facilitating improved patient treatment and relief from chronic nasal and sinus disease (Albanesi et al., 2013). Aside from individualized patient treatment, the broader effects of nasal and sinus disease involve public health. By making individuals aware of such conditions, health workers can enhance education at the community level and promote early intervention methods, hence possibly reducing the prevalence and severity of such disorders among populations. Such a proactive approach not only enhances better health outcomes but also leads to overall reduced healthcare expenditure in the long run. Furthermore, integration of evidence from research into clinical practice can lead to improved guidelines for the management of nasal and sinus disorders, informing policy through an evidence-based patient-centered approach. Ultimately, facilitating increased understanding of the disorders is vital to both advancing clinical practice and public health programs for the improvement of respiratory well-being (Albanesi et al., 2013).

8.1. Common Nasal Disorders

Learning Outcome

1. Allergic Rhinitis
2. Nasal Polyps
3. Deviated Septum

Nasal diseases constitute a heterogeneous spectrum of illnesses that have a broad impact on the quality of life of affected individuals. Amongst these, one of the most prevalent illnesses in an estimated one quarter of the global population is allergic rhinitis. Characterized by symptoms such as sneezing, nasal discharge, and nasal obstruction, allergic rhinitis is known to produce a significant impairment of daily activity and imposes enormous economic costs, with healthcare costs running into billions yearly. Patients typically experience the symptom of nasal congestion, fullness, or blockage that affects the passage of air and results in lost productivity at school and in the workplace. This undue burden underscores the significance of holistic treatment methods to alleviate the symptoms and promote the overall health of individuals affected by this disorder. Non-allergic rhinitis is another nasal condition characterized by symptoms that mimic allergic rhinitis but in the absence of an identifiable allergenic etiology. The etiology of the disorder is heterogeneous and may include environmental irritants, infections, or vascular disorders of the nasal mucosa. Treatment for non-allergic rhinitis differs from that of allergic rhinitis and emphasizes the importance of accurate diagnosis. The disorder can be widespread and result in chronic congestion with sleep impairment. When patients struggle with such chronic symptoms, clinicians are required to provide individualized treatment regimens that combat the etiologies, rather than merely suppress the symptoms. Such fine-tuned intervention can enhance patient outcomes and reveal the imperative of comprehending the intricate nature of disease in the nose (Basnyat et al., 2016). Another notable condition impacting nasal function is eosinophilic granulomatosis with polyangiitis, especially in the setting of chronic rhinosinusitis. This rare vasculitis affects the head and neck with a wide range of manifestations recognized first by otolaryngologists. Clinical practice shows that a high percentage of patients manifest nasal obstruction and sinus symptoms, for which early diagnosis and treatment are crucial. Early identification of the condition is warranted because the majority of patients recover with steroid therapy, with approximately 95.8% of patients improving. Multidisciplinary approach, incorporating rigorous evaluations and targeted therapies, can decrease long-term complications, warranting the engagement of otolaryngologists in the management of this complex disorder (Basnyat et al., 2016) (Figure 8.2).

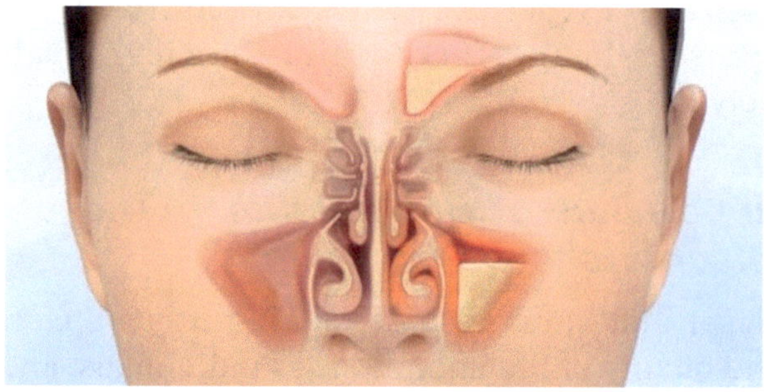

Figure 8.2. Nasal disorders represent a diverse range of conditions.

Source: https://fadlullahaksoy.com/en/wp-content/uploads/2019/12/Nasal-Diseases-Rhinology.jpg.

8.1.1. Allergic Rhinitis

Allergic rhinitis's prevalence serves to underscore its role as a major cause of nasal and sinus disease. Widespread in nearly a quarter of the global population, the chronic condition manifests as an intricate spectrum of symptoms with sneezing, itching, and nasal congestion. The latter is of particular significance in terms of its impact on the quality of life of affected individuals. Patients will often present with complaints of considerable disruption of daily activities and sleep that result from continuous congestion, a characteristic of allergic rhinitis. This symptom not only affects physical well-being but also reduces productivity in schools and workplaces, resulting in an economic burden of billions of dollars in healthcare costs annually. The dynamic relationship between allergic rhinitis and other rhinologic spectrum disorders demands integrated treatment, as this has significant implications for both public health and patient experience (Ferguson et al., 2010). As allergic rhinitis may occur concomitantly with other respiratory illnesses, it is essential for both patients and health care providers to understand its management. Relief through over-the-counter antihistamines or nasal corticosteroids is most desired by most patients, but efficacy can be significantly unpredictable. Underlying illness, the occurrence of comorbidities like asthma, and reactions to drugs increase the complexity of the treatment regimens. The patients also have worries about symptom control, such as the timing of referral and the adequacy of treatment. This dissatisfaction may lead to recurrent visits to medical practitioners and to alternative practitioners, underscoring the critical need for additional research and the development of targeted interventions to streamline guidelines for treating allergic rhinitis and improve patient outcomes (Ah-See et al., 2015). The overlap between allergic rhinitis and concomitant diseases such as chronic rhinosinusitis (CRS) highlights the relevance of a comprehensive understanding of such diseases. The link between CRS and allergic rhinitis illustrates how, left untreated or poorly treated, symptoms are able to produce more health sequelae in the form of nasal polyps and sinusitis. Both conditions have people who are often described as having high psychosocial burden, anxiety, and frustration of managing symptoms that might be brought about by an inability to access effective treatment. Besides individualized health costs, the economic impact extends to work productivity and health expenditure. Enhanced compliance with management guidelines is essential, as this may lead to a reduction in symptom burden and improved patient satisfaction with rhinitis and CRS. Both these need a multidisciplinary management style, with medical and lifestyle interventions combined to minimize the societal burden of these common disorders (Ah-See et al., 2015).

8.1.2. Nasal Polyps

While nasal polyps are common presentations in most nasal and sinus conditions, they are extremely common in patients with chronic rhinosinusitis (CRS). They are benign tumors secondary to an inflammatory process that most often stems from chronic nasal mucosal inflammation, often associated with asthma, allergic rhinitis, or cystic fibrosis. Their clinical relevance goes beyond simple physical blockage; they may also play a part in a variety of symptoms such as nasal stuffiness, impaired olfactory function, and facial pressure. It is critical to appreciate the pathophysiological mechanisms behind them, especially since treatment plans are largely contingent on proper diagnosis of the associated conditions. For instance, their identification as eosinophilic inflammatory pathways with nasal polyps highlights their potential for involvement in more systemic disease processes to allow for a more directed approach in intervention (Basnyat et al., 2016). Treatment of nasal polyps can be challenging, as it must target a multifaceted process that requires both pharmacologic and surgical interventions. Intranasal corticosteroids are administered daily to reduce inflammation and reduce polyp size, and several studies have found them effective in the relief of nasal symptoms and quality of life. Additionally, the addition of functional endoscopic sinus surgery (FESS) has also been found to be beneficial in treating recalcitrant cases, particularly in situations where polyps greatly block the nose or sinus complications resulting from chronic sinusitis. Evidence indicates that corticosteroids administered pre-operatively, combined with FESS, can lead to optimized operative outcomes, including reduced blood loss and improved quality of the surgical site, which may be of particular concern in the presence of chronic rhinosinusitis with polyps (Baer et al., 2016). These results justify the importance of a thorough evaluation that takes into account the worth of holistic surgical and medical treatment. Epidemiologically, nasal polyps are likely to show an impressive concordance with other atopic conditions, complicating their clinical presentation.

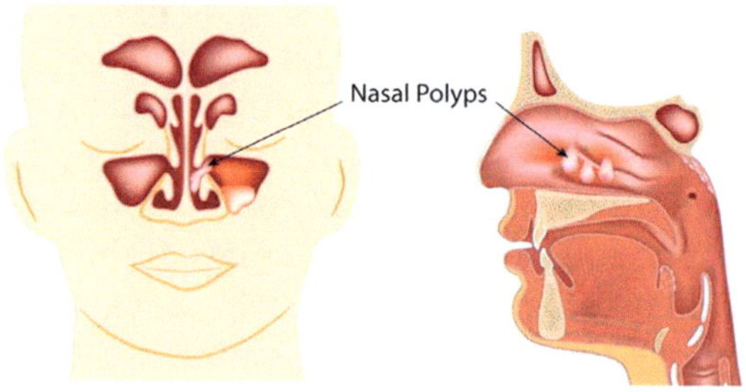

Figure 8.3. Nasal polyps are common manifestations of various nasal and sinus disorders.

Source: https://cdn2.hubspot.net/hubfs/3276300/blog%20images/what%20are%20nasal%20polyps%20houston%20ent%20and%20allergy.jpg.

The association not only requires careful investigation for the co-existence of such conditions as asthma and allergic rhinitis but also emphasizes the need to understand the immunological pathways leading to the formation of polyps. Given the ubiquitous nature of nasal polyps among patients with CRS, knowledge about such conditions will optimize diagnostic and therapeutic impact. Included is the risk of malignant transformation in nasal polyps, while rare, requiring vigilance and follow-up. Lastly, a common understanding of nasal polyps within the broader picture of nasal and sinus disease will be demanded of practitioners so that patients receive best, evidence-based care based on their individualized needs (Basnyat et al., 2016) (Figure 8.3).

8.1.3. Deviated Septum

The deviated septum is a common structural deformity wherein the nasal septum, the cartilage and bone that divides the nasal airway, becomes deviated to one side. It is either congenital or becomes acquired as a sequelae of trauma. Patients with a deviated septum typically present with severe nasal obstruction, leading to an inability to breathe through the nose. The effects of such obstruction can be more significant than simple discomfort, impacting sleep and leading to conditions such as chronic sinusitis, where the sinus cavities become swollen and inflamed. This indicates the intricate relationship between nasal anatomy and respiratory function as a whole, and highlights the importance of diagnosis and treatment of the condition in order to improve patient quality of life. Treatment of a deviated septum is usually through the implementation of a surgical procedure known as septoplasty to realign the septum. This has proved to be effective, particularly among patients with chronic rhinosinusitis. A comparative study clarifies the advantages of performing functional endoscopic sinus surgery (FESS) in conjunction with septoplasty, reporting that patients who underwent both procedures experienced greater symptom relief from facial pain and nasal blockage than those who underwent FESS alone. The evidence shows that correction of obstructive potential due to a deviated septum might additively influence the efficacy of sinus treatment, emphasizing the significance of detailed assessment and management in patients with nasal disorders (Ahluwalia et al., 2017). Moreover, incidental findings of underlying pathology during septoplasty emphasize the significance of adequate preoperative assessment and postoperative pathology review. In one case series, two septoplasty patients were diagnosed with unsuspected lymphoma, demonstrating that routine debridements of the nose may uncover serious disease that would be otherwise asymptomatic. This correlation underscores the need for greater surgeon vigilance during nasal surgery, as early detection of malignancy would enable earlier treatment and improve patient outcomes. As highlighted in the literature, identification of the nasal and sinus conditions' complexities, like the deviated septum, not only offers relief from the symptoms at the moment but also gains wider knowledge on the patient's health status at large (Bhuta et al., 2016).

Test Your Knowledge

1. What are the most common nasal disorders, such as rhinitis, nasal polyps, and deviated nasal septum, and what are their typical causes and clinical features?
2. Describe the diagnosis and management strategies for common nasal disorders, including medical and surgical treatment options.

8.2. Common Sinus Disorders

Learning Outcome

1. Sinusitis (Acute and Chronic)
2. Fungal Sinus Infections
3. Barometric Sinusitis

Sinus disorders are common conditions that can severely impair the quality of life of patients, with a variety of symptoms ranging from nasal obstruction to chronic facial pain. Sinusitis is one of the most widespread forms and is an inflammation of the sinus cavities that is either acute or chronic in character. Acute sinusitis typically results from an upper respiratory viral infection and resolves within a few weeks; however, if the condition persists beyond 12 weeks, it is chronic. The chronic inflammation typically causes further complications, so proper diagnosis and tailor-made treatment protocols are essential. In the majority of situations, sinus headaches are also associated with facial pressure and pain, and therefore differentiation among various head pain etiologies during evaluation must be made (Kaur et al., 2013). Nasal blockage and drainage issues are commonly associated with sinus disease, and this may result in significant disruption of daily functioning. Allergic rhinitis is another common condition that exacerbates sinus conditions by inducing inflammation and increased mucus production, hence clogging sinus drainage pathways. Interaction between the two conditions supports the use of an integrated therapeutic regimen that includes environmental modification to reduce exposure to allergens and drug therapy. Physical examination complemented by investigative radiological techniques, such as CT scans, is also crucial to establish the etiology and determine management. In some cases, surgical treatment, for example, endoscopic sinus surgery, will be required in order to restore sinus ventilation (Kaur et al., 2013). Significantly, some pathological and anatomical conditions also complicate the clinical condition of sinus disorders. For instance, a deviated septum may lead to chronic nasal obstructions and recurrent sinus infections. Surgical interventions like septoplasty can repair such anatomical aberrations, but they are at risk of incidental findings, such as malignancies, that are overlooked until postoperative pathology reveals them. Incidental diagnosis of lymphomas in otherwise unremarkable sinus operations points to the value of careful histopathologic examination of resected tissue. Such results not only depict the complexities of diagnosing sinus disease but also highlight the importance of close follow-up after surgery to detect any underlying issues that will alter patient management strategies (Figure 8.4).

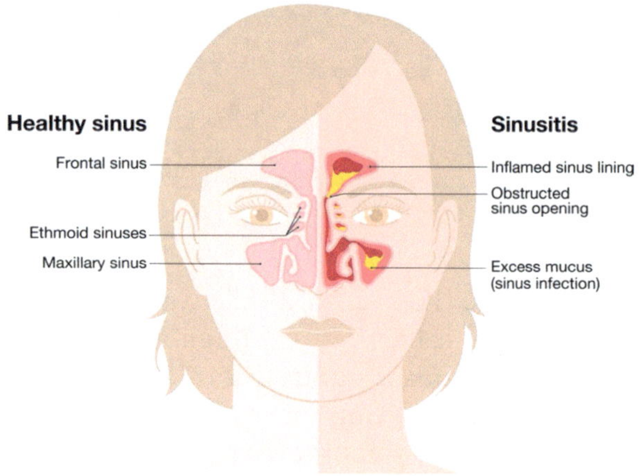

Figure 8.4. Common sinus disorders.

Source: https://www.addmoretolives.com/wp-content/uploads/2023/10/Image-AMTL-Sep-23-Blog5-Understanding-Sinus-Health-Debunking-Common-Myths-scaled.jpeg.

8.2.1. Sinusitis (Acute and Chronic)

Both acute and chronic sinusitis are significant health issues due to their impact and prevalence. Acute sinusitis is most commonly a sequel to an upper respiratory tract infection caused by viruses, leading to inflammation of the sinus mucosa. The symptoms are usually nasal discharge with a purulent character, facial pain, and nasal congestion. Chronic sinusitis is at least 12 weeks' duration and may be accompanied by repeated episodes of acute sinusitis. This long-term condition may be triggered by anatomical defects, allergic rhinitis, or chronic infection. Proper diagnosis is thus essential for the direction of appropriate treatment measures that may include antibiotics, corticosteroids, and even surgery to increase sinus ventilation and drainage in some patients. Sinusitis diagnosis is based on careful examination of signs and conditions. The patients usually present with facial pain and headache and are then referred to otolaryngologists for evaluation. Interestingly, patients may develop rhinogenic headaches wherein complaints of sinus origin are the predominant symptoms but without actual nasal or sinus disease. In this scenario, careful history and examination complemented by nasal endoscopy and imaging studies—like coronal CT scans—are required for proper diagnosis. Headaches associated with sinus disease typically present with symptoms such as nasal pressure or congestion, which can help differentiate them from other headache conditions and guide appropriate treatment (Kaur et al., 2013). Diagnosis of chronic rhinosinusitis is even more complex if the facial pain is considered. New evidence suggests that many patients with chronic rhinosinusitis may not have objective findings of sinonasal inflammation, thus questioning overdiagnosis on the basis of subjective symptom reports. As an example, a retrospective cohort study evaluated diagnostic criteria by excluding consideration of dental and facial pain and resulted in higher specificity at the expense of limited loss in sensitivity (DiNardo et al., 2017). This shift in diagnostic criteria is significant because it can enable clinicians to make more accurate predictions regarding the development of sinus inflammation. Therefore, this could in turn reduce avoidable antibiotic use and help patients referred to proper therapeutic regimens, minimizing the anguish of misdiagnosis and undertreatment.

8.2.2. Fungal Sinus Infections

Fungal sinus infections, a subset of the broader category of sinusitis, are a serious and complex subset of nasal and sinus disorders. Fungal sinusitis is a relatively infrequent condition that occurs in individuals with underlying conditions that compromise their immune systems, including diabetes or chronic respiratory illness. The distinction between chronic and acute fungal sinus infection is paramount; acute infection may arise after exposure to fungal spores in the environment, while chronic infections, such as allergic fungal sinusitis, are related to persistent inflammation and morbidity. Traditionally, the symptoms may encompass nasal congestion, facial pain, and, in advanced presentations, orbital complications due to sinuses being anatomically situated near ocular structures. Understanding of such nuances is crucial in effective intervention and management strategies among affected patients. The epidemiologic profile of fungal sinus infections is multifaceted, offering important insights into concurrent medical diseases and quality of life outcomes. Research has established that chronic rhinosinusitis (CRS) and, by extension, its allergic subtype is often accompanied by comorbidities such as asthma and allergic rhinitis (all termed collectively as allergic fungal rhinosinusitis, AFRS) (Anari et al., 2016). The chronic inflammation of these conditions heightens the patient's experience, and a number of studies have reported severe decrements in quality of life among those with CRS relative to healthy controls. The psychological impact of enduring nasal obstruction and repeated infections further heightens this burden, producing a cycle of worsening and distress that requires an integrative approach to treatment addressing both the medical and psychological aspects. Treatment for fungal sinus infections is usually a multidimensional approach that includes the use of corticosteroids to reverse inflammation to enable surgical intervention where necessary. Recent meta-analyses indicate that preoperative use of corticosteroids not only lowers estimated blood loss during functional endoscopic sinus surgery (FESS) but also decreases operative time and improves postoperative recovery for individuals with chronic rhinosinusitis (Baer et al., 2016). This evidence validates the necessity of an aggressive management strategy in the prevention of chronic recurrence of fungal sinus infections, particularly for CRS with nasal polyps, which represents a unique set of challenges. Moreover, ongoing investigation on the efficacy of many therapeutic modalities continues to guide clinical practices, ultimately to better patient outcomes in the treatment of nasal and sinus disease (Figure 8.5).

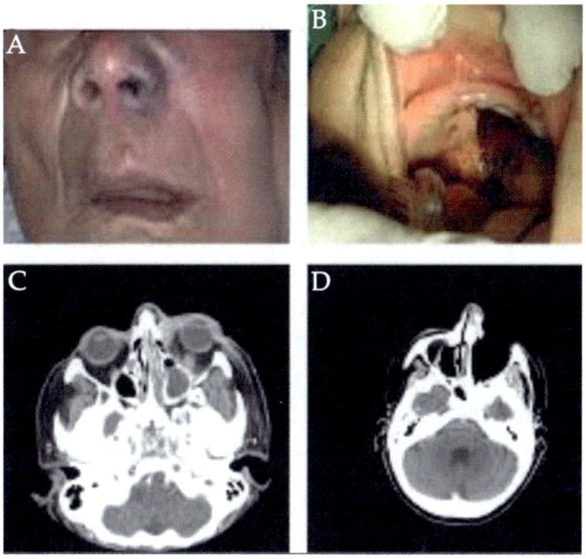

Figure 8.5. Fungal sinus infections, classified under the broader spectrum of sinusitis.

Source: https://encrypted-tbn0.gstatic.com/images?q=tbn:ANd9GcT_sIqRrk19CL0Sb7rTRMLe0HZWoYgleMHAWA&s.

8.2.3. Barometric Sinusitis

Sinusitis barometric or sinus barotrauma is a major concern for individuals who are subjected to abrupt changes in environmental pressure, including those who travel by plane or scuba dive. The pathophysiology of this condition lies in the reality that the paranasal sinuses cannot equalize pressure in a manner that leads to pain and potential inflammation.

Barometric shifts thus made will vacuum or apply additional pressure over the sinus cavities, causing pain and malfunction. The condition, in most cases, can lead to other sinus illnesses being incorrectly diagnosed due to its identical symptoms. Barometric sinusitis understanding needs an intensive analysis of its multiplicity of presentations that may range from singular acute presentations to recurrent or chronic cases, each requiring peculiar management patterns to alleviate the sufferings of the patients (Nayak et al., 2017). Barometric sinusitis commonly presents clinically similar to more common sinus conditions, thereby making diagnosis challenging. Symptoms may involve severe pain and pressure in the face, as well as, on some occasions, nasal stuffiness that most seriously occurs with the take-off and landing phases of air travel. Perhaps amazingly, recent studies have found that airplane headache, a headache attributed to airplane flight, is frequently related to sinus barotrauma. Sinus barotrauma is an unpredictable affliction for both those who experience it and physicians who must differentiate it from other headache-causing entities. Since, as has been emphasized in recent research, such as a systematic review on airplane headache, sinus barotrauma is a supraordinate causative factor, the imperative of specific training and sensitization among medical professionals for proper diagnosis and treatment is essential (Bui, S. B. D., & Gazerani, P., 2017). Treatment of barometric sinusitis is crucial for symptom alleviation and prevention of recurrence, particularly in chronic travelers. Treatment may include decongestants, nasal saline lavage, and, in certain cases, nonsteroidal anti-inflammatory drugs to alleviate pain and inflammation. Prophylactic measures, including the administration of nasal sprays before flights or the use of proper respiratory maneuvers with changes in altitude, have been effective in reducing the incidence of barometric sinusitis. With continued research in this topic, progressively more detailed classification systems for sinus barotrauma have been proposed, an indicator of the heterogeneity and complexity of this illness (Nayak et al., 2017). Increased awareness and a tailored treatment strategy are critical to maximizing patient outcomes, particularly among those individuals who might be susceptible to the pathologic effects of pressure change.

Test Your Knowledge

1. What are the most common disorders of the paranasal sinuses, such as sinusitis and mucocele, and what are their typical causes and clinical features?
2. Explain the diagnosis and management of common sinus disorders, including medical therapy, surgical intervention, and preventive measures.

8.3. Symptoms and Diagnosis

Learning Outcome

1. Common Symptoms of Nasal and Sinus Disorders
2. Diagnostic Methods (e.g., Imaging, Endoscopy)
3. Importance of Accurate Diagnosis

Understanding the symptomatology of nasal and sinus disease is key to guiding appropriate investigative measures. The symptomatology reported by patients is often extremely diverse, like nasal congestion, facial pressure or pain, and alteration in the sense of smell, and can render the clinical presentation complicated. These complaints can be related to a range of underlying pathologies, including acute sinusitis, chronic rhinosinusitis, or even more intricate pathologies like neoplasms. For example, an apparently simple case of nasal blockage can actually present a more complicated problem and needs careful assessment. These types of assessments can involve taking a thorough history from the patient and performing a thorough physical examination to determine the precise features of the symptoms. This initial step provides the foundation for proper diagnosis, as understanding symptomatology in its totality is necessary before one can progress to other investigative modalities like nasal endoscopy and imaging studies when indicated. Diagnostic evaluation of nasal and sinus diseases often requires a multidisciplinary approach, particularly when symptoms are nonspecific or overlap with other conditions. Rhinogenic headaches, in turn, may be inseparable from primary headaches and can only be misdiagnosed if concomitant manifestations are not stringently assessed. As highlighted in recent reports, diligent history and ENT examination with nasal endoscopy and, where required, coronal CT scans form crucial keys to the discovery of the underlying cause of headaches secondary to nasal or paranasal sinus disease (Kaur et al., 2013). The clinical profile of headache with sinus pathology will, in many cases, feature other presenting signs and symptoms, including nasal discharge and congestion, which can prove helpful in diagnosis. However, in some cases, sinus-related headaches may occur without classic symptoms, underscoring the need for careful, comprehensive assessment to avoid unnecessary interventions or undue delay in management of the underlying pathology. Incidental findings during surgery, such as septoplasty, also point towards the challenges of nasal and sinus disease diagnosis. In certain cases, pathological examination of the resected tissues can identify unexpected malignancies, as evidenced in a case study of two patients in whom lymphoma was diagnosed after surgery (Bhuta et al., 2016). These illustrations demonstrate that symptoms, as useful as they are, are not necessarily adequate to completely grasp a patient's status, and histopathologic evaluation might be needed. Hence, the standard procedure of submitting resected tissue for pathologic evaluation must be reserved for case-by-case determination, especially for patients who present with atypical presentation or failure of treatment. This degree of diagnostic vigilance not only has the potential to enhance patient outcomes but also underscores the importance of being vigilant in evaluating and treating nasal and sinus illness (Figure 8.6).

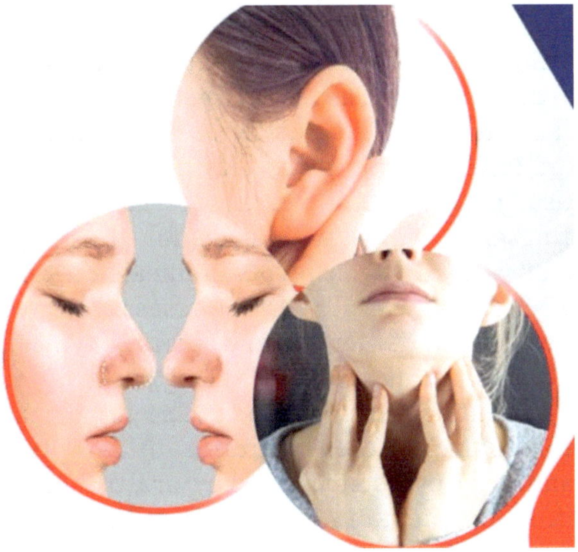

Figure 8.6. The symptoms associated with nasal and sinus disorders.

Source: https://amandeephospital.org/wp-content/uploads/2023/10/Top-ENT.jpeg.

8.3.1. Common Symptoms of Nasal and Sinus Disorders

It requires knowledge of the overall signs and symptoms of nasal and sinus disease to enable correct diagnosis and treatment. Nasal blockage is among the primary complaints that prompt individuals to seek medical attention. The symptom often presents as an obstructed nasal airway caused by swelling of the nasal mucosa and other underlying factors, ranging from infection to structural abnormalities. Concomitant nasal obstruction, patients will generally describe the sensation of facial pain or pressure, particularly localized about the sinuses. The pain is inconstant in nature and will tend to be exacerbated by motion, such as leaning forward or lying down, highlighting its probable connection with sinus inflammatory disease. The combination of these symptoms is also usually suggestive of disorders like rhinitis or sinusitis, which need appropriate evaluation to devise the proper course of treatment. Nasal discharge is another frequently encountered symptom of nasal and sinus patients, which may be thin, watery, or thick and purulent according to the etiology. This discharge, naturally, can take a toll on one's quality of life, as it could lead to persistent throat clearing or persistent nasal blowing. One significant characteristic of nasal discharge in sinusitis, for instance, is color variation, which would indicate bacterial infection and call for further assessment. And allergic rhinitis, for instance, comes typically with itching and sneezing, adding to the misery of patients suffering from it. The importance of recognizing these patterns of symptoms cannot be overstated, as they are the key to being diagnostic and guiding clinicians in the selection of appropriate treatment with medication or surgery where needed. Yet another less commonly discussed symptom, though similarly important, is the alteration in sense of smell, or anosmia, which can severely affect a patient's overall quality of life. Nasal and sinus disorders can lead to inflammation and blockage of the olfactory receptors, resulting in loss or reduction of the sense of smell. This is very distressing and can lead to loss of taste as well as affect one's appetite and enjoyment of food. Patients would have had these changes for a long period if they had the chronic forms, and this can have psychological repercussions, for example, increased anxiety or depression. Besides being troublesome, anosmia may be a symptom of serious underlying disorders like neoplasms like lymphoma, which, though rare, may be incidentally discovered during procedures like septoplasty, stressing the importance of vigilance in symptom assessment (Bhuta et al., 2016) and anatomical blockade and pathogenesis of chronic sinusitis (Basith et al., 2012).

8.3.2. Diagnostic Methods (e.g., Imaging, Endoscopy)

Diagnostic procedures are significant when diagnosing and treating nasal and sinus diseases to enable the recognition of targeted diseases. Among all the methods available, endoscopy is a frontline technique used for direct observation of the nasal and sinus cavities. It is a non-surgical procedure that enables one to see pathology such as polyps, tumors, and chronic rhinosinusitis findings. Endoscopic techniques can be used not only for diagnosis but also for treatment, to allow intervention such as retrieval of biopsy or removal of polyps. The data from endoscopic procedures are often crucial in the planning of effective treatment regimens, particularly for refractory cases, for routine medical therapy. Imaging modalities such as CT and MRI have further widened the diagnostic means for nasal and sinus disease beyond endoscopy. CT scanning is nevertheless regarded as the gold standard for paranasal sinus evaluation due to its ability to generate high-quality cross-sectional images. Such imaging allows one to detect anatomical abnormalities, as well as pathologies such as sinus obstructions, mucosal thickening, and neoplastic changes. MRI is not routinely used in diagnosis, but it may be utilized in certain situations, particularly when an assessment of soft tissues is indicated. The integration of these imaging modalities helps in preoperative planning as well as the prediction of surgical-related complications. Historically, histopathological analysis of tissue removed during surgeries such as septoplasty has not been fully exploited. Recent developments underscore the importance of this practice, with incidental findings playing a vital role in patient management. For instance, incidentally discovered lymphoma during routine surgeries on otherwise healthy individuals emphasizes the value of careful histopathological examination of biopsies. These findings emphasize that the diagnostic process in sinus and nasal surgery should extend beyond an immediate clinical evaluation, as the silent appearance of occult malignancy is possible. As noted by the reporting on these occurrences, making histopathologic examination a standard will have the ability to lead to an earlier diagnosis and improved patient outcomes, displaying the important amalgamation of diagnosis methods and optimal patient care (Bhuta et al., 2016; Durand et al., 2016) (Figure 8.7).

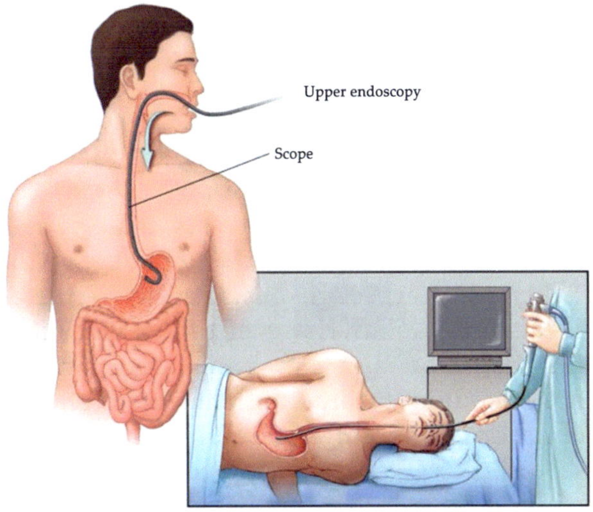

Figure 8.7. Diagnostic methods play a crucial role in the assessment and management of nasal and sinus disorders.

Source: https://gastroclinic.com.sg/wp-content/uploads/2023/07/endoscopy.jpg.

8.3.3. Importance of Accurate Diagnosis

An accurate diagnosis is the pillar in effective control of nasal and sinus illnesses since it plays a significant role in treatment outcomes and the quality of the patient's life. Nasal and sinus illnesses have a wide array of symptoms, ranging from nasal congestion and facial pain to disorders of smell that might have more than one cause. Misdiagnosis can lead to the use of inappropriate treatments—such as unwarranted surgery or ineffective medication—that not only fail to address the patients' conditions but may even further complicate the latter. It is thus important to be able to differentiate among conditions such as allergic rhinitis, chronic rhinosinusitis, or infections. Furthermore, enabling timely and correct diagnoses can minimize healthcare spending and ease the burden on healthcare systems by preventing prolonged pain and potential complications of undiagnosed disorders.

The clinical appropriateness of correct diagnoses transcends treatment protocols and economic considerations; it is also linked with patient satisfaction and health-related quality of life. For instance, smell disorder patients, like anosmia or hyposmia patients, can complain of excessive anxiety and compromised quality of life due to the deprivation of experienced sensation. Neglect of proper care for such disorders can lead to stigmatization and emotional distress, further complicating the medical situation. An otolaryngologist's recognition of such disorder intricacies is able to instill a more empathetic and effective treatment pattern. Additionally, recognition of the psychosocial implications of nasal disease makes the clinician adopt a multidisciplinary strategy for patient management, and thus overall outcomes as well as adherence to treatment plans are promoted. Evidence reveals that an accurate diagnosis is most important for the provision of effective treatment protocols in nose and sinus diseases. Deceptive presentations and superimposed symptoms are most frequently used to conceal underlying disorders and necessitate a thorough diagnostic workup that may involve imaging, allergy testing, and patient interviews to identify the clinical profile in precise terms. A study of patients with olfactory disorders noted, for example, that a significant number of cases were idiopathic, while others were secondary to chronic rhinosinusitis with polyps or allergic rhinitis (Ameur et al., 2017). This diversity calls for rigorous evaluation. More so, enhanced diagnostic techniques bolster clinicians' ability to make precise diagnoses, therefore reducing unjustified interventions and enhancing favorable patient outcomes (Ameur et al., 2017). In the end, the importance of accurate and cautious diagnosis in nasal and sinus diseases cannot be overstated, as it is the cornerstone of efficient, patient-focused care.

Test Your Knowledge

1. What are the common symptoms of ENT and head & neck disorders, and how do they help in guiding the diagnostic process?
2. Explain the diagnostic approach, including history taking, physical examination, and the use of investigations such as endoscopy, imaging, and laboratory tests, in ENT practice.

8.4. Treatment Options

Learning Outcome

1. Medications (e.g., Antihistamines, Decongestants)
2. Surgical Interventions (e.g., Endoscopic sinus Surgery)
3. Home Remedies and Lifestyle Changes

The therapy for nasal and sinus disorders encompasses various therapeutic interventions, namely for managing acute rhinosinusitis (ARS) and chronic rhinosinusitis. Among all such interventions, pharmacotherapy is the most primitive. Cyclamen europaeum (CE), a herbal therapy, has also gained limelight in recent studies as a treatment for ARS. A pharmacoeconomic analysis noted that CE, when used as a monotherapy, was 15.3% more efficient compared to other monotherapies, and it was also demonstrated to be more effective when used in combination with two-drug regimens (Anzai et al., 2013). This new evidence supports the use of CE as a cost-effective and potentially effective intervention in therapeutic regimens, particularly if standard therapy is not yielding maximum effect. Beyond the use of pharmacologic treatments, surgery may be required in patients with ongoing symptoms in spite of aggressive medical therapy. Functional endoscopic sinus surgery (FESS) is now more widely accepted as a means of restoring sinus ventilation and drainage in chronic rhinosinusitis. The surgery can help the patient by alleviating symptoms and enhancing the quality of life through obstruction release at the level of anatomy. However, the complications and risks of surgery and postoperative care mandate careful patient selection and counseling. Therefore, careful assessment of the disorder's severity and scope is required before surgical treatment is recommended, so that case-specific management that optimizes patient benefit, with an eye to the potential for improved nasal and sinus function, can be planned. More advanced therapies are also being used more commonly in the management of olfactory dysfunction, a generally associated condition in various nasal and sinus disorders. Platelet-rich plasma (PRP) therapy is one of the new therapies that has been highly promising for stimulating olfactory neurodegeneration. The patients with chronic olfactory loss experienced subjective improvement following PRP injection in early trials, particularly those with moderate impairment. While results indicate potential for efficacy—evinced by a significant number of participants achieving normosmia—further research is needed to outline treatment protocols and long-term results (Mundy et al., 2020). Such breakthroughs highlight the need for ongoing research into alternative treatments, which can supplement or even replace standard treatment protocols for nasal and sinus disorders, as they serve to meet the diverse needs of concerned patients (Figure 8.8).

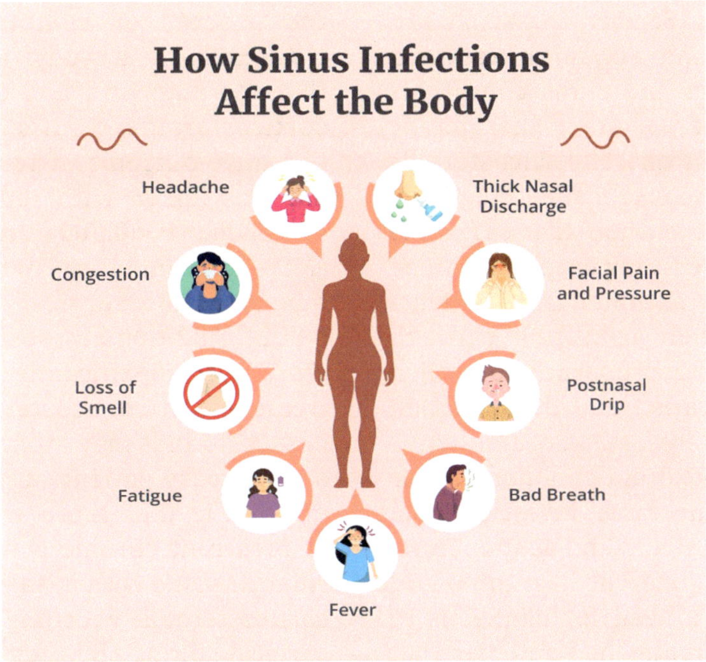

Figure 8.8. The management of nasal and sinus disorders encompasses a variety of treatment options.

Source: https://images.everydayhealth.com/images/seo-graphic-content-initiative/eh-how-sinus-infections-affect-the-body--seo-graphics.png?sfvrsn=e3f1ca27_3.

8.4.1. Medications (e.g., Antihistamines, Decongestants)

Medications have a strong role to play in managing nasal and sinus infections, more so for patients with rhinitis. Antihistamines and decongestants are most commonly the first-line drugs to be used in order to treat symptoms. Antihistamines work by preventing the action of histamine, a substance that is released during an allergy, thereby reducing symptoms of sneezing, itching, and nasal congestion. Allergic rhinitis patients usually find intranasal as well as oral antihistamines helpful because they reduce inflammation in the nasal passages easily. For the geriatric population, rhinitis prevalence will most probably increase, thus reinforcing the need to identify the contribution of these drugs towards symptom management and also towards overall quality of life, as depicted by the increasing incidence of rhinitis among elderly individuals (Apter et al., 2010). Decongestants, whether systemic or local, are second-line or adjunctive therapies for the management of nasal congestion in rhinitis. They act by inducing vasoconstriction of the widened nasal mucosal vessels, thereby reducing edema and allowing free passage of air through the nasal airways. While decongestants are effective for immediate relief, their administration has to be exercised with caution, particularly in elderly patients or those with comorbid conditions, as the side effects of hypertension and insomnia can further complicate existing ailments. The decision to use antihistamines or decongestants usually relies on the individual symptoms manifested and the etiology of nasal congestion, such that case-specific treatment modalities are adopted (Samarrae et al., 2011). Apart from decongestants and antihistamines, the treatment of nasal and sinus conditions encompasses a number of other therapeutic agents. For instance, intranasal corticosteroids are well-known to be an established long-term therapy for both allergic and non-allergic rhinitis that serves the role of reducing nasal membrane inflammation. Severely uncomfortable patients may also alleviate their condition through the use of nasal saline preparations, which can result in the hydration and decongestion of nasal passages. There are also adjunctive therapies such as topical anticholinergics for rhinorrhea and, in some cases, investigational treatments such as capsicum and acupuncture. With the complexities inherent in rhinitis and its subtypes, there is a need for clinicians to keep abreast of new treatment strategies that account for the wide variability of symptomatic profiles typical of nasal and sinus conditions (Samarrae et al., 2011).

8.4.2. Surgical Interventions (e.g., Endoscopic Sinus Surgery)

The increasing prevalence of nasal and sinus disease requires expanding knowledge of surgery, especially endoscopic sinus surgery (ESS), now a standard therapeutic option. ESS provides a minimally invasive approach to treating conditions such as chronic rhinosinusitis and nasal polyps by restoring sinus drainage and ventilation. ESS employs endoscopes to visualize the nasal passages and sinus openings, allowing selective excision of obstructive tissue with minimal external incisions. The benefits of ESS extend beyond its cosmetic advantages; it also reduces postoperative complications and healing time compared with traditional surgery. As a result, ESS has been of interest to medical professionals as an alternative treatment for nonresponsive patients when combined with medical therapy, validating its application in the management of many nasal and sinus disorders. Recent meta-analyses have indicated the success of combining corticosteroids with ESS. In a study, it was demonstrated that the augmentation of local and systemic corticosteroids results in greatly improved operative outcomes. Specifically, corticosteroid use was linked with reduced blood loss (MD −28.32 mls; $P < 0.0001$), reduced operating time (MD −10.70 minutes; $P < 0.0001$), and enhanced quality of the surgical field (MD −0.81; $P = 0.002$). Additionally, postoperative endoscopic scores were significantly higher among patients treated with corticosteroids, suggesting that corticosteroids may optimize surgical outcomes and increase patient satisfaction. Of particular interest is that there was no increased risk of recurrent chronic rhinosinusitis or chronic rhinosinusitis with nasal polyps with the use of corticosteroids, vouching for their safety in the surgical setting (Baer et al., 2016).

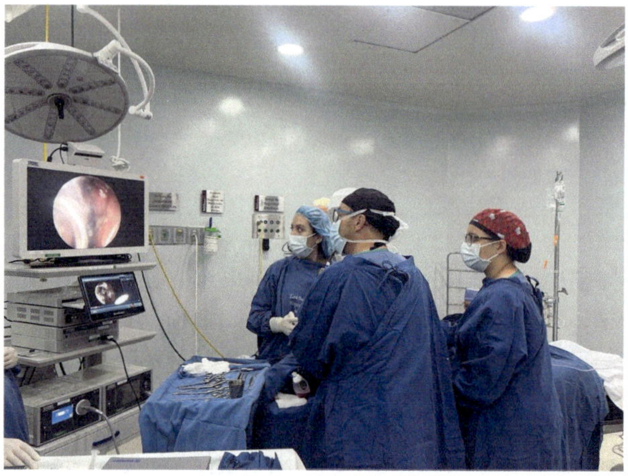

Figure 8.9. Surgical interventions (e.g., endoscopic sinus surgery).

Source: https://centrodeorl.com/wp-content/uploads/2024/06/Cirugia-Endoscopica.webp

Apart from chronic rhinosinusitis, endoscopic techniques have also revolutionized the treatment of seller tumors. Previously, a neurosurgeon procedure, the trans nasal endoscopic approach allows direct access to the sphenoidal sinus without destruction of essential nasal structures, thus lessening postoperative pain and complications. The results of 91 cases in clinical studies highlighted the feasibility and safety of this approach, as no extensive septal dissection was required. The most important issue was potential cerebrospinal fluid (CSF) leaks; however, the overall procedure-related morbidity was minimized. This illustrates the flexibility of endoscopic procedures as well as their potential to enhance patient outcomes in various nasal and sinus disorders with ongoing focus on preserving anatomical integrity (Abucham et al., 2007) (Figure 8.9).

8.4.3. Home Remedies and Lifestyle Changes

In the treatment of nasal and sinus disease, lifestyle changes and home remedies cannot be overstressed. These are adjunctive measures that the patient can employ to limit symptoms and optimize comfort overall. Saline nasal lavage and inhalation of steam are commonly recommended to relieve obstruction and allow drainage from the sinuses, respectively. They are easy, effective maneuvers that may relieve pain associated with nasal and sinus disease. In addition, staying hydrated promotes the production of thinner mucus, which, in turn, helps alleviate nasal congestion. Small modifications, such as maintaining the house somewhat humid, can be extremely beneficial. By creating a comfortable setting that facilitates easier breathing, individuals who experience long-term symptoms can find exemplary improvement. Additionally, lifestyle adjustments have to be made in the management of sinus disorders. Consuming anti-inflammatory foods, such as omega-3 fatty acid-containing fish and green vegetables, may reduce inflammation in the nasal passages and strengthen the immune system. Spicy meals, by thinning mucus, may also aid in clearing the sinuses. Emphasis on a healthy diet for overall wellness may reduce the frequency and severity of sinus infections. Adopting these lifestyle changes allows individuals to take control of their health. Moreover, knowledge of food intolerance, such as dairy or gluten, can allow individuals to implement particular dietary adjustments that restrict nasal congestion, hence encouraging an active solution in the management of health. Finally, the integration of holistic interventions such as mindfulness and stress-reduction practices can further encourage symptom improvement. Stress has been linked with the deterioration of many health ailments, including sinus illnesses. For individuals who are coping with chronic nasal diseases, practices such as yoga, meditation, and regulated breathing can result in relaxation as well as improved respiratory patterns. Elements of lifestyle that are likely to favor healthy sleep, as well as regular physical exercise, are likely to have significant impacts on the immune function of the body. These practices have been shown to decrease inflammation and total lung function. These home remedies and lifestyle modifications complement one another, facilitating recovery from nasal and sinus disorders and ultimately enhancing patients' quality of life and empowering them to manage their health (Pataka, A., & Riha, R. L., 2009; Izu et al., 2011).

Test Your Knowledge

1. What are the indications, principles, and steps of endoscopic sinus surgery in the management of sinus disorders?
2. Discuss the advantages, potential complications, and postoperative care associated with surgical interventions in ENT, particularly sinus surgery.

8.5. Prevention Strategies

Learning Outcome

1. Medications (e.g., Antihistamines, Decongestants)
2. Surgical Interventions (e.g., Endoscopic sinus Surgery)
3. Home Remedies and Lifestyle Changes

Effective prevention strategies for nasal and sinus diseases play an important role in reducing the occurrence and severity of the diseases. Effective prevention strategies typically begin with the identification of environmental triggers of symptoms, such as allergens and irritants. Individuals can assist themselves by maintaining a clean environment through the use of air purifiers and surface cleanliness to limit dust, mold, and pet dander. Moreover, the use of saline nasal sprays has the benefit of keeping the nasal passage moistened, which is vital in the maintenance of the mucosal barrier to infection. The preventive measure, besides alleviating already present symptoms, plays a significant role in the prevention of the development of future, more severe nasal and sinus afflictions, thus improving the overall respiratory condition. Vaccination is a second mainstay of prevention against nasal and sinus disease among groups at higher risk for respiratory illness. The influenza and pneumococcal vaccines have been shown to reduce the occurrence and severity of upper respiratory tract illness, which causes sinusitis. On top of that, educating the patients about the importance of treating upper respiratory infections early on may also help minimize the risk of acquiring more serious complications, such as chronic sinusitis. Prophylactic antibiotic treatment in some high-risk patients is still another strategy that may be implemented. All of these preventions blend synergistically to boost the immune system's function, thereby reducing susceptibility to pathogens that exacerbate nasal and sinus issues. The integration of multidisciplinary management is essential in managing the multifaceted nature of sinonasal disorders. This includes co-management among healthcare professionals such as allergists, otolaryngologists, and primary care physicians to ensure proper patient care. Management of existing co-morbid conditions, such as allergic rhinitis or 22q11.2 deletion syndrome, at the initial stages can have a tremendous impact on patient outcomes. For instance, correction of underlying anatomical abnormalities or immunodeficiencies can prevent recurrent infections or secondary complications due to untreated sinus and nasal conditions. Comprehensive education of the patient towards lifestyle modifications, follow-ups, and adherence to treatment plans additionally strengthens the effectiveness of prevention strategies (Bassett et al., 2015; Abita et al., 2019). In short, an aggressive, multi-modal strategy is required in minimizing the burden of sinus and nasal disorders (Figure 8.10).

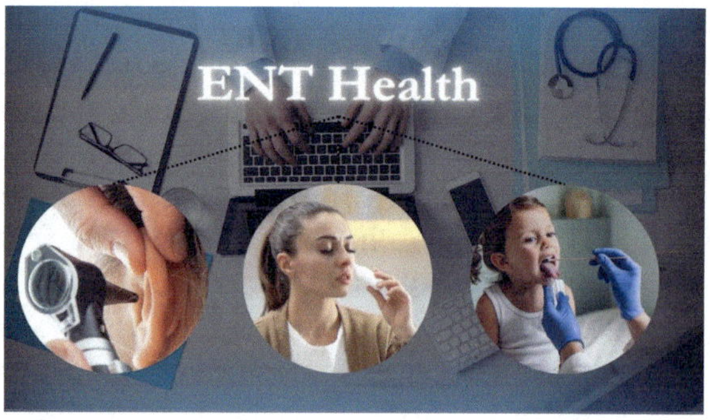

Figure 8.10. The prevention strategies for nasal and sinus disorders.

Source: https://www.sakethospital.in/wp-content/uploads/2023/12/Saket-Hospital-3.jpg.

8.5.1. Avoiding Allergens and Irritants

Nose and sinus disorders exhibit a complex interplay between patient susceptibility and environmental exposures, particularly to allergens and irritants. Avoiding exposure is of utmost significance to patients with diseases such as allergic rhinitis and chronic sinusitis. Treatment is successful not only because of drugs but also due to an integrative process that maximizes allergen avoidance steps. Environmental allergens such as pollen, mold, dust mites, and pet dander can exacerbate symptoms and contribute to related morbidity. Adequate education regarding how to identify and avoid these irritants is essential. For instance, maintenance of clean living spaces and installation of air purifiers can significantly reduce the concentration of allergens and thereby alleviate suffering for afflicted persons, as demonstrated in current studies vindicating the role of management strategies integrated together (Waal et al., 2023). In addition, one cannot overstate the role of lifestyle modification in efforts to reduce irritants and allergens in daily life. Daily hygiene and hypoallergenic material utilization for bedding and upholstery may lower the amount of dust mites, a potent inducer of nasal inflammation. Patients are also urged to monitor pollen levels in their region and minimize outdoor activity when pollen is most heavy, especially during high-pollen periods. The use of nasal saline lavage can also serve as a helpful adjunct, cleaning allergens and mucus from the nasal passages. By enforcing these preventive measures, patients not only improve their overall lifestyle but can even minimize the need for medical treatments, aiding in a holistic control of nasal and sinus illness (Vykhrystenka, L. R., & Yanchanka, U. V., 2008). Further, increasing the importance of customized care programs with reference to patient sensitivities accentuates the complexity in efficiently handling nasal and sinus illnesses. Health professionals are encouraged to complete patient histories to identify specific allergens responsible for symptoms. This history will enable more specific intervention planning, which usually involves allergen immunotherapy for long-term management. Regular follow-up and evaluation of the effectiveness of such interventions should be included in the management plan, as recommended by the South African Allergic Rhinitis Working Group. Active follow-ups and tailoring changes will bring about an active response to environmental stimulation, integrating pharmacological control and modification of lifestyle. Ultimately, treatment of both the dual roles of allergen avoidance and symptom relief is most important in reducing the overall impact of nasal and sinus conditions (Waal et al., 2023).

8.5.2. Maintaining Nasal Hygiene

Nasal cleanliness plays an important role in the prevention of the majority of nasal and sinus ailments, particularly given the dynamic nature of nasal anatomical and physiological structures. The nasal airway and paranasal sinuses are lined with mucosa, which plays a crucial role in trapping the pathogens and irritants that are inhaled. Effective mucociliary clearance enables the mucus to be cleared from the airways on a regular basis, hence preventing chronic infection and other sequelae related to it, such as fungal rhinosinusitis. This infection is often seen in immunocompromised individuals, meaning there is a need to come up with hygiene practices that improve the immune system within the nasal cavity. Studies have established that understanding the immunological profile of nasal tissues can guide nasal hygiene practices in ways that substantially enhance overall respiratory health and prevent the progression of serious disease, as evidenced by increasing reports of fungal infections (Cojocari et al., 2018). Introducing nasal irrigation and humidification practices into standard care can immensely enhance nasal hygiene. Saline sprays and nasal rinses allow cleaning out of allergens and irritants and maintenance of proper moisture levels within the nasal mucosa. These procedures may also be beneficial in easing the symptoms of chronic rhinosinusitis and other sinus disorders by allowing freer flow of air and reduced discomfort. Such methods may be particularly beneficial for people with allergic rhinitis, since mucus clogging is avoided and mucociliary function is increased. Through frequent nasal passage cleaning, it becomes possible to prevent the risk of getting complications such as fungal or bacterial infection. Acceptance of all these practices is not just preventive but also an integral part of treating the existing conditions that have adverse effects on nasal and sinus hygiene (Anesi et al., 2014). Furthermore, an understanding of environmental issues is also a determining factor in maintaining healthy nasal hygiene. Exposure to allergens, irritants, and pollutants could aggravate the status, and therefore, proactive intervention is needed. City residents or individuals with high exposure to allergens should consider establishing a clean indoor environment, using air cleaners, and practicing rigorous hygiene. Enabling individuals to know the risks of poor nasal hygiene can educate them to look after their health. Because the nasal cavity is a first line of defense against respiratory infections, comprehending its complexity further underscores the necessity of adhering to holistic disciplines of hygiene. Ultimately, the combination of body cleaning, environmental awareness, and good medical guidelines can yield favorable outcomes in combating nasal and sinus diseases, further underscoring the necessity of nasal hygiene (Cojocari et al., 2018) (Figure 8.11).

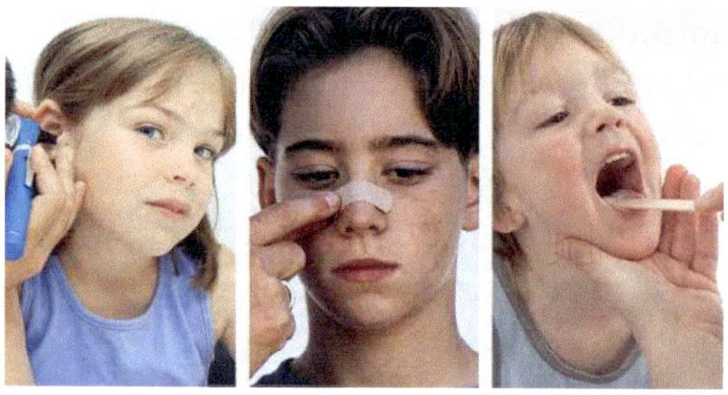

Figure 8.11. Maintaining nasal hygiene is essential in preventing various nasal and sinus disorders.

Source: https://images.jdmagicbox.com/comp/temp/catalogue/-hdr9g4ukj9.jpg.

8.5.3. Importance of Regular Medical Check-Ups

Regular medical check-ups are a critical aspect of proactive health care, particularly when it comes to nasal and sinus issues. Regular check-ups allow physicians to detect likely problems early enough that they may develop into more intricate issues. For instance, diseases such as chronic sinusitis or allergic rhinitis tend to begin with mild symptoms that patients do not notice. By regular screening, clinicians can pick up early warning signs for such disorders and can suggest the right interventions or lifestyle changes. Furthermore, periodic reviews ensure that patients are well informed about their health status and can readily participate in joint decision-making regarding any required interventions, thereby encouraging collaborative management of healthcare. In addition to early detection, regular medical check-ups are also essential to facilitate monitoring of existing conditions, especially for those patients with histories of nasal and sinus diseases.

The long-term management of these conditions usually consists of ongoing assessment and revision of care plans to fit the patient's evolving requirements. For instance, improved diagnostic instruments and modality treatment imply that patients need to remain responsive to their well-being. Regular check-ups are not only useful for following the course of disease but also allow practitioners to modify therapy in accordance with the patient's response. Such continuity of care is vital in averting complications and enhancing overall health outcomes, check-ups bringing to the fore the significant role in the management of chronic illness of nasal and sinus disease. But the benefits of regular medical check-ups extend beyond the individual; wider public health schemes are also impacted. Epidemiological studies demonstrate that regular consultations with a doctor have the ability to enhance patients' health literacy, which enables them to understand their risks as well as the importance of disease prevention better. When individuals give due attention to health check-ups, this helps bring higher rates of early diagnosis and treatment of nasal and sinus conditions, thus relieving the health system. This proactive style not only increases individual quality of life but also maintains the total health of the population by lowering the prevalence of chronic respiratory disease. Thus, the practice of regular medical check-ups becomes unavoidable in shaping individual health courses and public health strategies.

Test Your Knowledge

1. What home remedies and lifestyle modifications can help prevent or alleviate common ENT conditions such as rhinitis, sinusitis, and mild ear infections?
2. Explain the role of environmental control, diet, hydration, and hygiene practices in maintaining ENT and head & neck health.

SUMMARY

The complex interaction among anatomical, pathological, and environmental factors underscores the multifactorial etiology of nasal and sinus disease. Chronic obstruction of the nose, typically from a structural abnormality such as a deviated septum, can lead to serious effects, one of which is chronic sinusitis. With the observation of anatomical variations and their contribution to airway obstruction, clinicians can gain better insight into the etiology of these diseases. For instance, Basith et al. (2012) highlight how anatomical occlusion can lead to chronic rhinosinusitis and advise that complete assessment of each patient's nasal architecture is critical in effective treatment. This appreciation of anatomical patterns is a critical component of patient management practices. Moreover, the unforeseen discovery of malignancies after apparently uncomplicated surgical interventions, as demonstrated in the case studies, underscores the potential for underlying complexity in seemingly benign presentations of nasal afflictions. Accordingly, the discovery by Bhuta et al. (2016) of the diagnosis of lymphoma among septoplasty patients serves to underpin the significance of pathological examination despite the absence of overt symptoms of malignancy. Such a policy not only allows for early diagnosis of cancer but also enhances the overall quality of patient care through addressing unanticipated medical issues that may arise in conjunction with what are otherwise elective procedures. Lastly, these implications extend beyond individual cases, and the conclusion emphasizes the applicability of integrating both surgical and clinical approaches in treating nasal and sinus disease. Understanding of underlying anatomical variation and the possibility of incidental diagnosis can transform patterns of treatment, teaching surgeons to move forward with greater sensitivity. This wider appreciation underscores the importance of continued study and education in rhinology, supporting a model of care that treats patients holistically but is alert to the innumerable possibilities presented by nasal disease, as informed by current investigation in the field.

In investigating the co-morbidities of nasal and sinus illness, namely eosinophilic CRS with nasal polyps (CRSwNP), research has revealed the efficacy of budesonide transnasal nebulization therapy. This novel treatment was subjected to rigorous investigation, revealing its capacity to significantly reduce polyp size, in addition to its efficacy in treating nasal symptoms in affected patients. The 60-patient trial demonstrated that budesonide-treated patients had reductions in inflammatory cytokines and eosinophilic infiltrates, indicating that the therapy effectively modulates resident immunologic processes in CRSwNP. Secondly, the regulation of T-cell subset distribution highlights the therapeutic value of budesonide to not just alleviate the symptoms but also reverse the pathological mechanisms of the disorder, making it a therapeutic choice in treating this chronic disorder (Bachert et al., 2015). In addition, corticosteroid use in functional endoscopic sinus surgery (FESS) has been of particular interest as a predictive factor for surgical success in patients with nasal and sinus disease. The analysis of various studies revealed that pre-operative corticosteroid was associated with reduced operating time and reduced blood loss, hence an overall improved quality of the operating field. Evidence incorporating eighteen randomized controlled trials established that corticosteroid use presents no greater risk of developing postoperative complications such as sinusitis, but improves endoscopic scores after surgery. Most notable is the reduction in rates of recurrence of chronic rhinosinusitis among patients with polyps, establishing the relevance of corticosteroids in improving outcomes of patient care following surgical interventions (Baer et al., 2016). Lastly, these findings of the management of sinus and nasal diseases show the immense progress that has been made in the knowledge and management of conditions like CRSwNP. Budesonide's anti-inflammatory action via transnasal nebulization presents a highly promising non-surgical therapy, and corticosteroids complement the surgical treatment of chronic rhinosinusitis with FESS. The findings reiterate the continuous need for research into new treatments and approaches, reaffirming the commitment towards improved patient care in otolaryngology. With the shifting landscape in treatment, these key points, fully understood, not only guide clinical practice but also serve as a basis for future research on addressing the challenging issues posed by sinus and nasal disease.

KEY TERMS FROM THIS CHAPTER

- Rhinitis
- Vasomotor Rhinitis
- Sinusitis
- Chronic Sinusitis
- Nasal Polyps
- Epistaxis
- Hypertrophic Rhinitis
- Turbinate Hypertrophy
- Furunculosis
- Allergic Rhinitis
- Infective Rhinitis
- Acute Sinusitis
- Rhinosinusitis
- Deviated Nasal Septum (DNS)
- Atrophic Rhinitis
- Concha Bullosa
- Nasal Vestibulitis
- Septal Hematoma

CRITICAL THINKING QUESTIONS

1. **Inflammation of the nasal mucosa is called:**
   a) Rhinitis
   b) Sinusitis
   c) Nasopharyngitis
   d) Tonsillitis
2. **Allergic rhinitis is commonly associated with:**
   a) Fever
   b) Sneezing, nasal congestion, and itching
   c) Ear discharge
   d) Hearing loss
3. **The commonest type of sinusitis is:**
   a) Acute frontal sinusitis
   b) Maxillary sinusitis
   c) Sphenoid sinusitis
   d) Ethmoid sinusitis
4. **Acute bacterial sinusitis usually lasts:**
   a) <4 weeks
   b) 4–12 weeks
   c) >12 weeks
   d) 6 months
5. **Chronic sinusitis lasts for:**
   a) <2 weeks
   b) 4–12 weeks
   c) >12 weeks
   d) 1 month

Short Answer Questions

1. What are the common disorders of the nose and paranasal sinuses, and how are they classified?
2. Describe the clinical features, causes, and management of acute and chronic rhinitis.
3. Explain the etiology, signs, and treatment of sinusitis.
4. What are nasal polyps? Discuss their pathophysiology, symptoms, and management.
5. Explain the causes, clinical presentation, and treatment of a deviated nasal septum.

Answers to Critical Thinking Questions

1. (a) 2. (b) 3. (b) 4. (a) 5. (c)

REFERENCES

1. Abita, P., Bruno, R., Freni, F., Galletti, C., et al. (2019). *Multidisciplinary approach in the removal of post-trauma foreign bodies in the head and neck district: , case report, and review of literature.* https://core.ac.uk/download/196288470.pdf (accessed on 7th August 2025).
2. De Paula Santos, R., Zymberg, S. T., Filho, J. Z. A., Gregório, L. C., & Weckx, L. L. M. (2007). Endoscopic transnasal approach to sellar tumors. *Brazilian Journal of Otorhinolaryngology, 73*(4), 463–475. https://doi.org/10.1016/s1808-8694(15)30098-7Ahluwalia, A., Gupta, V. D., Surya, M., Thakur, A., et al. (2017). *Comparative evaluation of FESS and septoplasty with FESS in cases of DNS with chronic maxillary sinusitis.* https://core.ac.uk/download/551598832.pdf (accessed on 7th August 2025).
3. Ah-See, K. W., Akkerman, A. E., Angier, E., Benninger, M. S., Bhattacharyya, N., Blanc, F., Braun, H., et al. (2015). *Chronic rhinosinusitis: Patient experiences of primary and secondary care – A qualitative study.* https://core.ac.uk/download/41992230.pdf (accessed on 7th August 2025).
4. Akgoz, A., Bulut, E., Gocmen, R., Gunes, A., et al. (2018). *Trigeminal nerve and pathologies in magnetic resonance imaging: A pictorial review.* https://core.ac.uk/download/160736722.pdf (accessed on 7th August 2025).
5. Albanesi, A. P. L. L., Bernstein, J. M., Bernstein, I. L., Fokkens, W. J., Gliklich, R. E., Wastowski, I. J., et al. (2013). *Interleukin-17A Expression in Patients Presenting with Nasal Polyposis.* https://core.ac.uk/download/37711269.pdf (accessed on 7th August 2025).
6. Al-Samarrae, A., Banov, C., Benninger, M. S., Bernstein, J., Bhargava, V., Blaiss, M. S., Blom, H. M., et al. (2011). *Management of Rhinitis: Allergic and Non-Allergic.* https://core.ac.uk/download/pdf/8583828.pdf (accessed on 7th August 2025).
7. Altundag, A., Andrews, P., Cinghi, C., Costanzo, R. M., et al. (2017). *Position Paper on Olfactory Dysfunction.* https://core.ac.uk/download/77029518.pdf (accessed on 7th August 2025).
8. Amato, F., Carnovale, V., Castaldo, A., Cernera, A., et al. (2020). *TAS2R38 is a Novel Modifier Gene in Patients with Cystic Fibrosis.* https://core.ac.uk/download/pdf/323187684.pdf (accessed on 7th August 2025).
9. Ameur, A., Coxon, F. P., Dahl, N., Hallmans, G., et al. (2017). *SNX10 gene mutation leading to osteopetrosis with dysfunctional osteoclasts.* https://core.ac.uk/download/131023916.pdf (accessed on 7th August 2025).
10. Anari, S., Clark, A., Coombes, E., Erskine, S., et al. (2016). *A case-control study of medical, psychological and socio-economic factors influencing the severity of chronic rhinosinusitis.* https://core.ac.uk/download/41990799.pdf (accessed on 7th August 2025).
11. Anesi, A., Cavani, F., Chiarini, L., Ferretti, C., et al. (2014). *Preliminary findings of a potenziated piezosurgical device at the rabbit skull.* https://core.ac.uk/download/80171725.pdf (accessed on 7th August 2025).
12. Anzai, Y., Barberan, T. S., Bhattacharyya, N., Burton, M. J., Demoly, P., Fokkens, W. J., et al. (2013). *Pharmacoeconomics of Cyclamen europaeum in the management of acute rhinosinusitis.* https://core.ac.uk/download/18618191.pdf (accessed on 7th August 2025).
13. Apter, A., Cervin, A., Greiner, A., Gruver, A., Kalpaklioglu, A., Mediaty, A., Rogkakou, A., et al. (2010). *Rhinitis in the Geriatric Population.* https://core.ac.uk/download/pdf/8419413.pdf (accessed on 7th August 2025).

14. Aubert, G., Cottier, M., Durand, M., Forest, N., et al. (2011). *Impact of acoustic airflow nebulization on intrasinus drug deposition of a human plastinated nasal cast: New insights into the mechanisms involved.* https://core.ac.uk/download/52621186.pdf (accessed on 7th August 2025).

15. Bachert, C., Fan, E., Li, Y., Lou, H., et al. (2015). *Effect of budesonide transnasal nebulization in patients with eosinophilic chronic rhinosinusitis with nasal polyps.* https://core.ac.uk/download/55846522.pdf (accessed on 7th August 2025).

16. Baer, S., Cornet, M., Fokkens, W. J., Gerogalas, E., et al. (2016). *Role of corticosteroids in functional endoscopic sinus surgery – A systematic review and meta-analysis.* https://core.ac.uk/download/42416368.pdf (accessed on 7th August 2025).

17. Basith, Y. A., & Thiagarajan, B. (2012). *Role of Anatomical Obstruction in the Pathogenesis of Chronic Sinusitis.* https://core.ac.uk/download/pdf/9634114.pdf (accessed on 7th August 2025).

18. Basnyat, S., Goldfarb, J. M., Nyquist, G. G., Rabinowitz, M. R., et al. (2016). *Head and neck manifestations of eosinophilic granulomatosis with polyangiitis: A systematic review.* https://core.ac.uk/download/83049399.pdf (accessed on 7th August 2025).

19. Bassett, A. S., Emanuel, B. S., Marino, B., McDonald-McGinn, D. M., et al. (2015). *22q11.2 Deletion Syndrome.* https://core.ac.uk/download/188828218.pdf (accessed on 7th August 2025).

20. Baumann, U., Jolles, S., Routes, J. M., Soler-Palacín, P., et al. (2018). *The Lung in Primary Immunodeficiencies: New Concepts in Infection and Inflammation.* https://core.ac.uk/download/160275976.pdf (accessed on 7th August 2025).

21. Beahm, D. D., Evans, J. J., Farrell, C. J., et al. (2014). *Comprehensive management of the paranasal sinuses in patients undergoing endoscopic endonasal skull base surgery.* https://core.ac.uk/download/46973719.pdf (accessed on 7th August 2025).

22. Bhuta, S. M., Kedeshian, P. A., Kuan, E. C., Palma Diaz, M., et al. (2016). *Incidental Finding of Lymphoma After Septoplasty.* https://core.ac.uk/download/305124586.pdf (accessed on 7th August 2025).

23. Bui, S. B. D., & Gazerani, P. (2017). *Headache attributed to airplane travel: Diagnosis, pathophysiology, and treatment: A systematic review.* https://core.ac.uk/download/94572625.pdf (accessed on 7th August 2025).

24. Cantone, E., Capriglione, P., Catalano, L., Di Lullo, A., et al. (2017). *Strategy for the treatment and follow-up of sinonasal solitary extramedullary plasmacytoma: A case series.* https://core.ac.uk/download/pdf/90979536.pdf (accessed on 7th August 2025).

25. Caparroz, F. de A. [UNIFESP], Gregorio, L. L. [UNIFESP], Kosugi, E. M. [UNIFESP], Neves, M. C., et al. (2014). *Olfaction Disorders: Retrospective Study.* https://core.ac.uk/download/37711504.pdf (accessed on 7th August 2025).

26. Carafa, M., Di Marzio, L., Hanieh, P. N., Marianecci, C., et al. (2017). *Drug delivery in overcoming the blood-brain barrier: Role of nasal mucosal grafting.* https://core.ac.uk/download/80314980.pdf (accessed on 7th August 2025).

27. Cascino, F., Cavati, G., Gennari, L., Gennaro, P., Giovannetti, F., Latini, L., & Vannucchi, M. (2024). *Maxillofacial bone involvement in fibro-osseous lesions: Emphasizing the significance of*

differential diagnosis. https://core.ac.uk/download/643630194.pdf (accessed on 7th August 2025).

28. Cojocari, L., & Sandul, A. (2018). *Fungal Rhinosinusitis: Pathophysiology, Diagnosis and Treatment.* https://core.ac.uk/download/337304486.pdf (accessed on 7th August 2025).
29. De Waal, P., Feldman, C., Friedman, R., Gray, C., et al. (2023). *Allergic rhinitis: Review of the diagnosis and management: South African Allergic Rhinitis Working Group.* https://core.ac.uk/download/613869970.pdf (accessed on 7th August 2025).
30. DiNardo, L. J., Hirsch, S. D., Reiter, E. R., Schuman, T. A., et al. (2017). *Elimination of pain improves specificity of clinical diagnostic criteria for adult chronic rhinosinusitis.* https://core.ac.uk/download/130355229.pdf (accessed on 7th August 2025).
31. Durand, A., Finck, M., Hammond, G., & Sullivan, M., et al. (2016). *Computed tomography and magnetic resonance diagnosis of variations in the anatomical location of the major salivary glands in 1680 dogs and 187 cats.* https://core.ac.uk/download/42370872.pdf (accessed on 7th August 2025).
32. Ferguson, B. J., Fromer, L., & Stewart, M. (2010). *Epidemiology and Burden of Nasal Congestion.* https://core.ac.uk/download/12213834.pdf (accessed on 7th August 2025).
33. Gallimore, A., Lund, V. J., & Paun, S. (2005). *Nasal fibrosis: Long-term follow-up of four cases of eosinophilic angiocentric fibrosis.* https://core.ac.uk/download/1669284.pdf (accessed on 7th August 2025).
34. Hardjojo, A., Shedden, A., Stuck, A., Cruz, A. A., Stevenson, A. N., Chauhan, B., Engel-Yeger, B., et al. (2012). *Allergic rhinitis and its associated co-morbidities at Bugando Medical Centre in Northwestern Tanzania: A prospective review of 190 cases.* https://core.ac.uk/download/pdf/11307799.pdf (accessed on 7th August 2025).
35. Kaur, A., & Singh, A. (2013). *Headache—A Sinonasal Symptom and More... A Review Article.* https://core.ac.uk/download/201677922.pdf (accessed on 7th August 2025).
36. Mundy, D. C., Patel, Z. M., & Yan, C. H. (2020). *The use of platelet-rich plasma in the treatment of olfactory dysfunction: A pilot study.* https://core.ac.uk/download/323064387.pdf (accessed on 7th August 2025).
37. Nayak, J. V., Patel, Z. M., Psaltis, A. J., Rao, A. S., et al. (2017). *Barosinusitis: Comprehensive Review and Proposed New Classification System.* https://core.ac.uk/download/482268354.pdf (accessed on 7th August 2025).
38. Pataka, A., & Riha, R. L. (2009). *The Obstructive Sleep Apnoea/Hypopnoea Syndrome – An Overview.* https://core.ac.uk/download/pdf/82646289.pdf (accessed on 7th August 2025).
39. Sacco Izu, R. A. (2011). *Fibromyalgia Self-Care Management: Use of Essential Oils.* https://core.ac.uk/download/477679542.pdf (accessed on 7th August 2025).
40. Vykhrystenka, L. R., & Yanchanka, U. V. (2008). *Handbook of Clinical Allergology.* https://core.ac.uk/download/80149814.pdf (accessed on 7th August 2025).

DISORDERS OF THE NASOPHARYNX

9

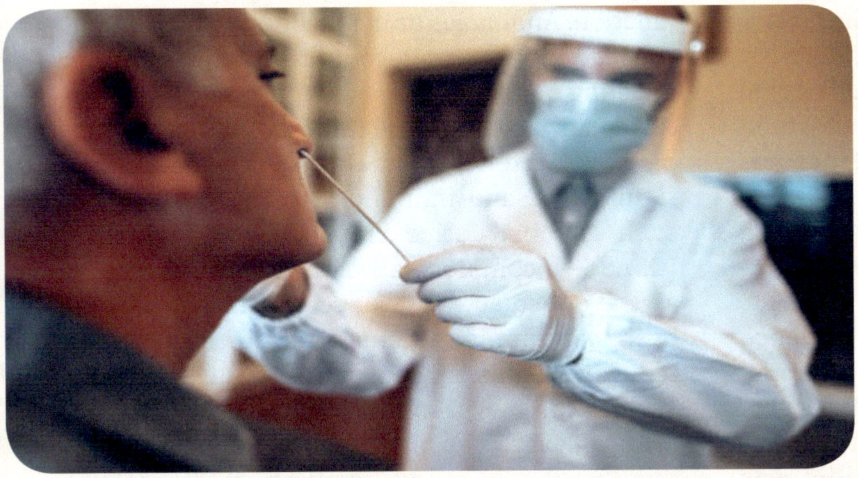

LEARNING OBJECTIVES

After studying this chapter, you will be able to:

1. Anatomy and physiology of the nasopharynx.
2. Common disorders of the nasopharynx.
3. Symptoms and diagnosis of the nasopharynx.
4. Treatment options for the nasopharynx.
5. Complications of nasopharyngeal disorders.
6. Preventive measures of the nasopharynx.

Introduction

The nasopharynx, located at the very top of the throat behind the nose, is a critical organ in breathing and hearing functions. The physical structure is a crucial air passageway to the lungs, and it also connects the middle ear with the nasal passages via the Eustachian tube. Nasopharyngeal diseases encompass a wide range of conditions, ranging from infections to obstruction and structural deformities, and mainly affect the quality of life. Prevalence of nasopharyngeal diseases such as otitis media (OM) among children highlights the importance of being well-versed with their pathophysiology and treatment regimens. The association between these disorders and the developmental anatomy of the nasopharynx can yield important clinical information used to guide treatment algorithms and prevention strategies in clinical and public health practice. Perhaps the most prevalent disorder affecting the nasopharynx is otitis media, a disease continuum that imitates unrelated symptoms and complications, particularly in children. The most common presentations are acute otitis media (AOM) and otitis media with effusion (OME), and are often caused by viral or bacterial infection. Upper respiratory infections, particularly those that produce nasal congestion, have been found to be associated with OM; the virus can predispose to bacterial colonization by ascending from the nasopharynx via the Eustachian tube to the middle ear (Casselbrant et al., 2016). Further, the sequelae of chronic OME are potential hearing impairment and developmental delay, and these bring further significance to early diagnosis and active treatment. Accordingly, there is a need to understand the pathologies underlying these conditions so that interventions can be developed that will mitigate their ill effects in vulnerable subjects. More recent evidence has unraveled high levels of interaction between nasopharyngeal pathology and more widespread syndromic disease. For instance, children with craniofacial abnormalities, such as 22q11.2 Deletion Syndrome, have a higher incidence of otitis media due to differences in anatomy affecting the functioning of the Eustachian tube. Research suggests that levator veli palatini muscle hypoplasia can impair middle ear ventilation capacity appropriately and therefore render them susceptible to OM (Baldini et al., 2014). Identification of these correlations not only clarifies the complexity of nasopharynx disorders but also indicates therapeutic directions for management. Interventions for muscle function, combined with traditional methods of OM management, can reveal new therapies reducing recurrence and improving overall prognosis in affected populations. These efforts emphasize the mandates for continued research and education on the multifaceted nature of nasopharyngeal disorders.

Definition of the Nasopharynx

The nasopharynx is a significant anatomical structure, the most superior portion of the pharynx located posterior to the nasal cavity and superior to the oropharynx. Function-wise, it forms a passage to the respiratory and gastrointestinal tracts by allowing airway access from the nasal passages to the lower respiratory tract. This space is lined by mucosal tissue, important in pathogen and particulate trapping and thus in the body's immune response. Adenoids, lymphoid tissues that contribute to immune defenses, are also found within the nasopharynx. The functional and structural significance of the nasopharynx should be appreciated, for its health is valuable for normal respiratory mechanics and general upper airway function. Anomalies or dysfunction in this region can lead to a myriad of complications, negatively affecting quality of life and respiratory function. Nasopharyngeal disease can present in a myriad of ways, often secondary to its anatomical significance and immunological role. Diseases such as obstructive sleep apnea syndrome (OSAS)—a complex pathology related to upper airway obstruction — are primarily caused by hypertrophied adenoid tissue in children, resulting in disturbed airflow during sleep. Tastes Narrow nasopharynx dimensions may lead to severe consequences such as impaired quality of sleep and respiratory disorders. The prevalence of such diseases reinforces that nasopharyngeal complications should be diagnosed and treated in time. While the present research continues to uncover the distinct etiologies of these disorders, medical professionals remain more vigilant than ever to track the nasopharyngeal status of individuals. This vigilance is most needed, as a result of the long-term sequelae of untreated disease, including developmental delay in pediatric patients. A second very prevalent condition of the nasopharynx is otitis media (OM), a middle ear infection occurring most frequently in young children. The proximity of the nasopharynx to the Eustachian tube allows for a pathway in which infections can migrate upwards, especially when respiratory infections like colds are present. This interaction between the nasopharynx and the middle ear is of importance as pathogens in the nasopharyngeal space can easily infect the middle ear with complications such as loss of hearing and recurrent infections. Implications of OM dictate that nasopharyngeal health should be taken into account in pediatric practice. Effective diagnosis and treatment interventions, including observation and potential surgeries, are crucial in avoiding the complications of this condition. Developing the pathophysiology of the conditions continues to grow, and it will help develop improved treatment policies and enhance the outcome of patients with nasopharyngeal conditions (Figure 9.1).

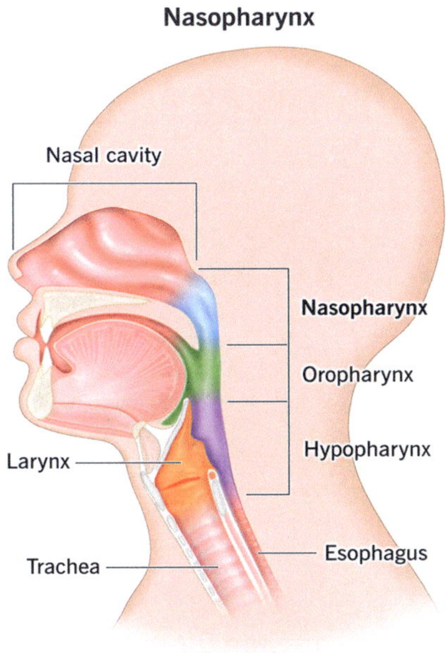

Figure 9.1. The nasopharynx.

Source: https://my.clevelandclinic.org/-/scassets/images/org/health/articles/22376-nasopharynx.

Importance of the Nasopharynx in Respiratory Health

The nasopharynx is a critical nexus of the respiratory system, having a real influence on respiratory well-being. It serves as a passageway for air entering the lungs, purifying and humidifying it, as well as serving as an immune defense to protect against invading disease-causing organisms. Adenoids, lymphoid tissues present in the nasopharyngeal region, play a pivotal role in this defense mechanism. They can filter airborne pathogens so that they do not reach the lower respiratory tract. Nasopharyngeal impairment can significantly affect overall respiratory efficiency, particularly in children, with hypertrophied adenoids often causing obstructive sleep apnea and recurrent chronic upper respiratory tract infections. These disorders not only affect the airflow but may even result in further complications, such as chronic otitis media, which proves the interdependence of nasopharyngeal health and the entire integrity of the respiratory system, as theorized in studies about middle ear inflammation and nasopharyngeal correspondence (Casselbrant et al., 2016). Control of airflow in the nasopharynx is also most important for effective breathing, especially during sleep. Diseases such as obstructive sleep apnea syndrome (OSAS) are based so much on the condition of the nasopharynx. In children, adenotonsillar hypertrophy can lead to partial or complete upper airway obstruction and result in sleep disorders and subsequent neurocognitive consequences. That obesity-induced OSAS occurs in up to 78% of children is proof of the severity of maintaining the anatomical status and function of the nasopharynx. The systemic risks of untreated OSAS, including systemic arterial blood pressure and potential growth retardation, also place an added importance on the nasopharynx's vital role in healthy respiration and long-term health of the infected (Giuliana et al., 2019). Thus, it can be said that the safeguard of the nasopharynx is imperative for preventing various respiratory diseases. The nasopharynx is not only a vital air pathway but also an important component of the immune system response against airborne infections, hence its significance in respiratory efficiency. Treatment of conditions such as adenoid hypertrophy and awareness of their potential effect on sleep and overall well-being remain very important to healthcare workers. Relative frequencies of conditions like otitis media and obstructive sleep apnea underscore the need for caution and proactive management strategies, particularly in vulnerable populations like children. The upkeep of ideal nasopharyngeal status ultimately prevents a host of respiratory conditions, consequently enhancing the quality of life and overall health condition in patients.

Overview of Common Disorders Affecting the Nasopharynx

The nasopharynx is a critical anatomical structure that connects the nasal cavity to the oropharynx, and certain diseases can affect its function and overall health. The most frequent condition of the nasopharynx is otitis media (OM), which encompasses different forms such as acute otitis media (AOM) and chronic suppurative otitis media (CSOM). OM is commonly caused by ascent of pathogens from the nasopharynx through the Eustachian tube, particularly in the setting of upper respiratory tract infections. The condition is most common in young children, and it will resolve spontaneously in most cases, although in severe instances, it has been known to lead to complications such as permanent hearing loss. Diagnosis tends to be clinical in nature and can include otoscopic examination in assessing the integrity of the tympanic membrane. Furthermore, OM management tends to be symptomatic, whereas in chronic cases, surgical interventions such as tympanostomy tubes are also used (Casselbrant et al., 2016). Obstructive sleep apnea syndrome (OSAS) is yet another well-known nasopharyngeal disorder, which arises during obstruction of the airway during sleep and leads to respiratory abnormalities. OSAS in children has a prevalence rate of about 2%, which may accompany hypertrophied adenoid tissue in the upper respiratory tract. This condition also causes inappropriate sleep habits, behavioral issues, and growth and developmental issues. Pediatric OSAS has a multifactorial etiology that makes it difficult to manage, considering that it is associated with conditions such as obesity and craniofacial malformations. Diagnosis is based on clinical assessment and may also involve sleep testing to evaluate nocturnal breathing patterns. In the management of OSAS, interventions can range from adenoidectomy to lifestyle modification, underlining the importance of early detection and treatment to prevent long-term sequelae (Bellini et al., 2019). Moreover, allergic rhinitis is a frequent nasopharyngeal condition characterized by an inflammatory response to allergens and symptoms like nasal congestion, sneezing, and postnasal drip.

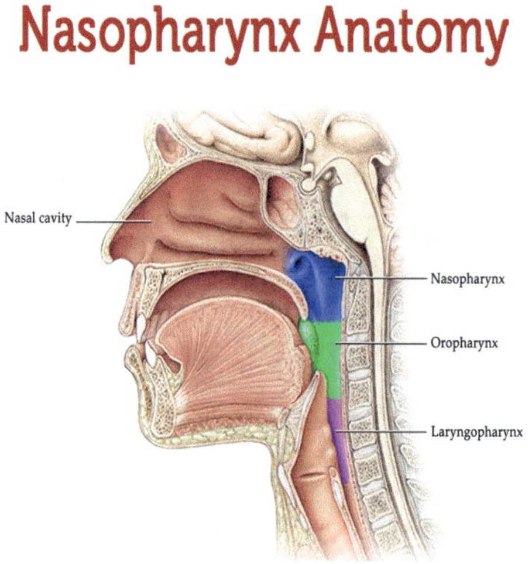

Figure 9.2. The common disorders affecting the nasopharynx.

Source: https://assets.lybrate.com/imgs/tic/enadp/image-of-the-nasopharynx.jpg.

This syndrome can be induced by a variety of environmental stimuli such as pollen, dust mites, and pet dander, resulting in a considerable morbidity load among affected individuals. Pathophysiology of allergic rhinitis relies on immunoglobulin E-mediated responses, and hence, normal treatment protocols become challenging. Treatment is typically with avoidance of allergens, pharmacotherapy with antihistamines and nasal corticosteroids, and in some cases, immunotherapy. Understanding of how allergic rhinitis coexists with other nasopharyngeal disorders, such as sinusitis and asthma, is crucial in providing comprehensive care and enhancing patient quality of life. A careful diagnostic and management strategy thus becomes essential in addressing the multifaceted collection of conditions that affect the nasopharynx (Figure 9.2).

9.1. Anatomy and Physiology of the Nasopharynx

Learning Outcome

1. Structure and Location of the Nasopharynx
2. Functions of the Nasopharynx in the Respiratory System
3. Relationship Between the Nasopharynx and Other Anatomical Structures

The nasopharynx is a significant anatomical channel that is involved in a multiplicity of physiological processes, most critically linked to the auditory and respiratory systems. Located posterior to the nasal cavity and above the soft palate, the nasopharynx is an airway that also encompasses the general function of the upper respiratory system. This region is bounded by a mucosal membrane containing ciliated epithelial cells that assist in moving mucus and pathogens away from the airway. The nasopharynx is also important in equalizing middle ear air pressure through the Eustachian tubes that run between this area and the tympanic cavity. Dysfunction in this anatomical region may contribute to numerous disorders, emphasizing its importance in ensuring respiratory well-being and auditory function. The nasopharyngeal anatomy is intimately associated with a number of common disorders, with obstructive sleep apnea (OSA) emerging as one of the most common conditions involving this region. OSA is defined by recurrent interruptions in breathing, usually caused by an obstruction in the upper airway, which encompasses the nasopharynx. This condition can lead to severe health complications, including cardiovascular disease and impairment of cognitive function due to sleep deprivation. The anatomical alignment of the soft palate and structures above it can influence the severity of OSA. The realization of the connection between the anatomical framework of the nasopharynx and such sleep disorders highlights the relevance of the area in medical practice because of its role in successful diagnosis and intervention, leading to better patient outcomes. Apart from its structural anatomy, the function of the nasopharynx also lies in its connection with conditions like otitis media (OM) in children. Anatomy of the Eustachian tubes, in infants, is more horizontal, hindering drainage, and is one of the causes of a high prevalence of OMs. Chronic otitis media with effusion conductive hearing loss affects the developmental milestones of children. The condition may also be associated with other conditions of various craniofacial syndromes, for example, 22q11.2 Deletion Syndrome (22q11.2DS). Results from animal models suggest that hypoplasia of the muscles regulating the Eustachian tube could worsen OM, a novel mechanism in nasopharyngeal disease. These findings lean towards an enhanced understanding of nasopharyngeal anatomy and physiology for instituting advanced treatments to correct these dysregulations effectively.

9.1.1. Structure and Location of the Nasopharynx

The nasopharynx holds a significant structural and functional role in the upper respiratory system and acts as a pivotal passageway between the nasal cavity and oropharynx. It is anatomically positioned behind the nasal cavity and above the soft palate and continues from the skull base to the level of the soft palate. The nasopharynx is bordered laterally by the Eustachian tubes, regulating middle ear air pressure and drainage. Because of the location, such structural deformities or obstructive conditions here have serious implications for respiratory functions and general well-being. The nasopharynx's intricate structure also includes lymphoid tissues such as the adenoids, which are active in immune processes. Therefore, a thorough understanding of its anatomy and location is essential in handling disorders starting from or affecting the nasopharynx. Recent research has highlighted the interplay between nasopharyngeal anatomy and respiratory conditions. In studies, it has been observed that the severity of obstructive sleep apnea (OSA) may be directly proportional to the anatomical dimensions of the upper airways, including the nasopharynx. Computational fluid dynamics (CFD) models constructed from three-dimensional (3D) CT scans provide valuable insights into air flow patterns through such tissues. Evidence attests that nasopharyngeal measurements have a direct effect on pressure dynamics of the airway, as seen in the strong correlation of a CFD-derived parameter with the apnea-hypopnea index (Jafari et al., 2019). Thus, understanding the nasal subanatomy of the nasopharynx is critical in the diagnosis and treatment of concurrent respiratory diseases. The implications of alterations in the anatomy of the nasopharynx extend beyond respiratory illnesses. Changes in jaw relationship, for example, have been discovered to have significant effects on the volume of the nasopharynx, demonstrating the dynamic nature of this anatomical region. In a more recent work, researchers pointed out that movement from an open to a closed position of the mandible resulted in measurable changes in airway dimensions, both the volume of the nasopharynx and the total constriction of the airway (Babler et al., 2015). The findings emphasize the intricate relationship between craniofacial structure and function of the nasopharynx and that positional variation as well as structural integrity can trigger and sustain disorders. This variability will require a cautious approach to the treatment and management of nasopharyngeal conditions, indicating the importance of proper anatomical assessment in clinical practice (Figure 9.3).

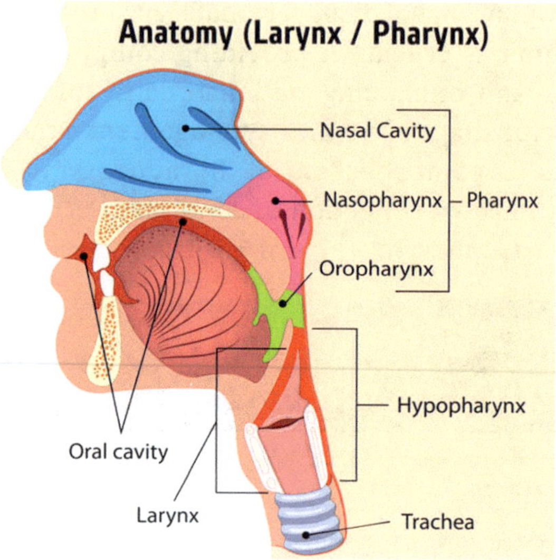

Figure 9.3. The nasopharynx serves a crucial structural and functional.

Source: https://www.vedantu.com/question-sets/fb97e62b-26fe-4309-bdc6-57f15c3f3c8067979276118795460 59.png.

9.1.2. Functions of the Nasopharynx in the Respiratory System

The nasopharynx is of the highest significance in the respiratory process, as it is a necessary route from the nasal cavity to the oropharynx. The anatomy provides an air passage, facilitating proper respiration and the first point of filtration for airborne matter. The mucosa lining the nasopharynx has cilia and mucous glands and traps dust, disease, and other foreign particles. This role is important to respiratory health since it defends against the entry of harmful agents into the lower airways. Moreover, adenoid tissue in the nasopharynx contributes to the immune role by secreting antibodies to invading pathogens in the airway. Appreciating these roles brings out the importance of the nasopharynx to respiratory health and demonstrates how its failure causes nasopharyngeal diseases, including infections and blockages. Other than air passing through and filtration, the nasopharynx plays a vital regulatory function in controlling the rate of flow and pressure of air during breathing. Its pressure-equalizing mechanism plays a crucial role, particularly when one is engaged in activities such as swallowing or yawning, during which air pressure changes may occur. This equalization is important for maintaining maximum functioning of the eustachian tubes, which are tubes that connect the middle ear and the nasopharynx and serve to keep diseases like otitis media at bay. This connection between the nasopharynx and the eustachian tubes illustrates the interconnected nature of anatomical structures in the respiratory system. Conditions such as obstructive sleep apnea (OSA), which consist of repeated pauses in breathing when sleeping, could be a consequence of nasopharyngeal dysfunction abnormalities, further solidifying its role in respiratory health and overall well-being (Mohammed, 2005). Moreover, the nasopharynx plays a significant role in immune protection against environment-borne pathogens. It is a point of colonization by bacteria such as *Streptococcus pneumoniae*, which may exist asymptomatically in the nasopharyngeal mucosa until conditions permit pathological proliferation, leading to life-threatening illness such as pneumonia or meningitis (Olliver, 2012). Immune response within the nasopharynx is critically balanced so that, although it can protect against infection, its disruption can lead to inappropriate inflammatory responses and immunopathology. This twofold role — both protecting the host and causing injury when dysregulated — mirrors the complex nature of the nasopharynx in the respiratory tract. Such immune interactions are critical to understand in order to value the nasopharynx disorders as well as devise specific therapeutic approaches.

9.1.3. Relationship Between the Nasopharynx and Other Anatomical Structures

The nasopharynx is a critical intersection between the nasal cavity and pharynx, bridging the respiratory system to the auditory system and the gastrointestinal system. Anatomically posterior to the nose and superior to the oropharynx, this structure stands in a critical position to regulate a multitude of functions. Significantly, the eustachian tubes that connect the nasopharynx to the middle ear are used for equilibration of air pressure and drainage, reflecting the connection of the nasopharynx with the auditory apparatus. Consequently, any inflammation or blockage of the nasopharynx is bound to lead to hearing complications, some of which include otitis media. These relationships place the need to take into account disorders that affect the nasopharynx in prominence, as these secondarily affect neighboring structures and also cause a chain of disorders attributed to hearing and respiration. Aside from being related to the auditory apparatus, the nasopharynx is closely related to the processes of the oropharynx and larynx. The nasopharynx is an air passageway for respiration, running smoothly into the oropharynx and then continuing on to the larynx and finally the trachea. This functional connection plays a significant role in both unobstructed respiration and phonation. Furthermore, nasopharyngeal illness, such as chronic rhinitis or adenoidal hypertrophy, may lead to obstruction, thus providing abnormal airflow dynamics. Therefore, patients may exhibit symptoms such as breathing complications or obstructive sleep apnea, a disease characterized by repeated interruptions of breathing (apneas) lasting at least 10 seconds or longer while sleeping (Mohammed, 2005). It is worth noting these associations when it comes to understanding the manner in which nasopharyngeal conditions provoke broader respiratory and vocal issues. Nasopharyngeal conditions also have a significant impact on overall health and wellbeing. Research has indicated that anatomical defects in the nasopharynx have been linked with obstructive sleep apnea (OSA), whereby periodic breathing disturbances are responsible for lowered quality of sleep and a raised risk of systemic health-related complications. For instance, a piece of research that utilized three-dimensional models together with computational fluid dynamics (CFD) simulations revealed a strong degree of correlation between anatomical measurements of the upper airway and the severity of OSA. In particular, the pressure coefficient (Cp*) estimated using CFD modeling showed a high correlation with the apnea-hypopnea index, highlighting the manner in which anatomical alterations of the nasopharynx influence the air flow patterns and, consequently, the quality of sleep (Jafari et al., 2019). Such evidence verifies the high correlation between the nasopharynx and other anatomical sites, necessitating vigilant assessment and management of patients with nasopharyngeal disease (Figure 9.4).

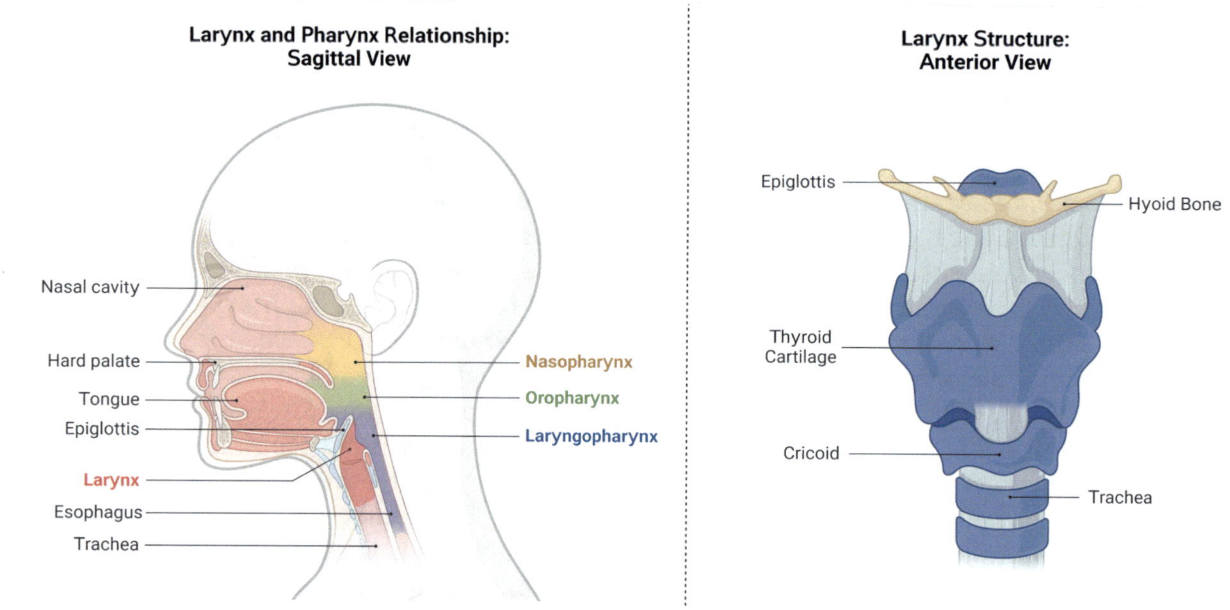

Figure 9.4. Relationship between the nasopharynx and other anatomical structures.

Source: https://upload.wikimedia.org/wikipedia/commons/2/2a/Larynx_and_Pharynx_Anatomical_Relationship.png.

Test Your Knowledge

1. Describe the anatomical boundaries and key structures of the nasopharynx, including the pharyngeal tonsils and openings of the Eustachian tubes.
2. Explain the physiological functions of the nasopharynx, including its role in respiration, immune defense, and connection between the nasal cavity and middle ear.

9.2. Common Disorders of the Nasopharynx

Learning Outcome

1. Allergic Rhinitis
2. Nasopharyngeal Carcinoma
3. Adenoid Hypertrophy

Nasopharyngeal conditions encompass several different conditions that impact the respiratory system significantly. One of the most prevalent conditions is epistaxis (nosebleeds), which occurs in nearly 60% of the population at least once in their lifetime. The pathophysiology of this condition might be related to trauma, hypertension, or even an idiopathic etiology. It has been noted, in a recent study at the Bugando Medical Centre, that trauma was the cause of nearly 31% of epistaxis. Most patients presented with anterior nasal bleeding, and this highlights the importance of the frequent presentations and causes of the condition. Treatment ranges from conservative management in the form of observation and nasal packing to more complex surgical interventions, though the former are rarely needed. Effective control of epistaxis shifts focus back to preventive approaches, particularly in reducing trauma, which remains the dominant causative factor in emergency centers (Daudia et al., 2011). Another common disorder of the nasopharynx is otitis media, which is extremely common among children. Not only is the middle ear inflammation common, but it also has long-term implications on overall health, including hearing loss and retardation of speech in developing children. The susceptibility to otitis media has been attributed to environment and genetics, which impact the immune system as well as bacterial colonization. Recent research indicates that evolutionary forces can also play a role in the prevalence of this illness, particularly in certain native populations. For instance, previous exposure to new strains of bacteria as a result of colonization has disrupted stable host-pathogen interactions and thus exposed them more in these populations. Understanding the interplay among the environment, immunity, and genetics in the prevention and care of otitis media is critical, particularly for informing public health interventions (Bhutta, 2015). The conditions of the nasopharynx are also complicated by chronic sinusitis, which is an ongoing inflammation that leads to recurring nasal obstruction, facial pain, and loss of sense of smell. It typically results from chronic infections, allergies, or anatomical abnormalities of the nasal passages. Chronic sinusitis patients typically have recurring symptoms that can severely impair quality of life. Advances in treatment, including nasal corticosteroids, saline nasal irrigation, and surgery for structural issues, have been encouraging for controlling and reducing symptoms. Furthermore, understanding the pathophysiology of chronic sinusitis can inform the development of pathway-specific therapies that address not only the immediate symptoms but also the underlying chronic inflammatory processes themselves. Because of its multifactorial pathogenesis, treatment of chronic sinusitis must be a worldwide approach, individualized according to the etiologies in each patient (Daudia et al., 2011).

9.2.1. Allergic Rhinitis

Allergic rhinitis presents itself as a significant clinical problem among the nasopharyngeal disorders and is characterized primarily by an overactive immune response to allergens. The disease exists as a group of symptoms, including sneezing, nasal congestion, and rhinorrhea, that thoroughly impacts quality of life in patients. Studies have established that the prevalence of allergic rhinitis can be as high as alarming figures, such as in a study at Bugando Medical Centre, which had 14.7% prevalence among patients who reported otorhinolaryngology symptoms, especially commenting on its frequent presentation in children and adolescents. The relevance of these results underscores the significance of elevated awareness and early identification of allergic rhinitis, particularly in children, since their failure to do this has dire consequences in the form of severe comorbidities like sleep disorders and other respiratory diseases, making their treatment outcomes more complicated. The linkage between allergic rhinitis and comorbidities establishes the multicenter nature of the condition and the complex relationship between physical health and quality of life. Of specific interest was the study carried out at Bugando Medical Centre, which identified that 92.6% of patients were found to have comorbidities, including adenoid hypertrophy, sinusitis, and otitis media, which explains the huge healthcare burden of allergic rhinitis. In children, the relationship between enlarged adenoidal tissue and breathing diseases, with a result including obstructive sleep apnea syndrome (OSAS), is worthy of note. OSAS, which affects about 2% of children aged between two and eight years, is often accompanied by allergic rhinitis and adenoid enlargement and implies that uncorrected allergic reactions will continue to cause airway obstruction during sleep, ultimately leading to worsening sleep and cognitive impairment affecting a child's school functioning and growth. Allergic rhinitis demands a complete management plan with both medical and surgical interventions, particularly in complicated cases where comorbidities present serious issues. In the previous study, it was astounding to see that 68.8% of patients had actually undergone surgery for treating accompanying complications, emphasizing the possibility that symptomatic treatment alone might not be sufficient. Moreover, early identification of the allergic causes—such as dust and strong odors, as was elicited in the study—can inform prevention and targeted treatment strategies. Relief of symptoms is desired alongside concurrent treatment of the high burden of comorbidities to enhance patient outcomes overall. It is thus the existence of a multidisciplinary treatment protocol of allergy testing, environmental factor modification, and therapeutic management that is required for effective management of allergic rhinitis and its associated disorders, encouraging an interdisciplinary health care approach to nasopharyngeal disease (Figure 9.5).

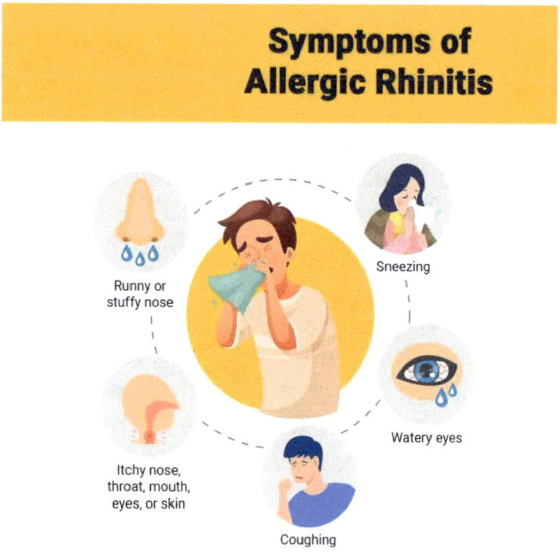

Figure 9.5. Allergic rhinitis emerges as a significant clinical concern within the spectrum of nasopharyngeal disorders.

Source: https://entspecialistsingapore.com/wp-content/uploads/2024/03/ENT-Specialist-ENT-Surgeons-Medical-Centre-Symptoms-of-Allergic-Rhinitis-1024x1007.jpg.

9.2.2. Nasopharyngeal Carcinoma

Nasopharyngeal carcinoma (NPC) is a significant medical condition among otolaryngologic diseases, characterized by distinctive etiology and clinical presentation. The type of cancer, characterized by malignancies within the nasopharynx, accounts for approximately 4% of malignant ear, nose, and throat tumors and 1% of all cancers in total. Anatomical location of the nasopharynx hinders early diagnosis, and thus usually results in delayed diagnoses, which can deteriorate patients' outcome. Presentation in the late stage is also prevalent, as nearly 70% of patients with NPC are already in a late local stage upon diagnosis, which calls for greater awareness and screening practice on both the part of healthcare providers and patients (Alexe et al., 2024). Knowledge about the exceptional interaction of geographic, genetic, and environmental forces in the disease pathology of NPC is required for effective management and treatment. The pathogenesis of nasopharyngeal carcinoma is strongly related to the EBV latent infection, which is a key risk factor for NPC. The virus is implicated in a number of malignancies, and the malignancy has a well-established correlation, particularly in the Southeast Asian and North African populations. In addition, the clinical presentation of NPC can be atypical, presenting with symptoms such as nasal obstruction, unilateral hearing loss, and ear pain, which are often attributed to more common causes. Thus, initial symptoms are often overlooked, so most patients are seen with advanced disease. Treatment of these early signs is essential for enhancing outcomes in patients since early intervention can greatly improve therapeutic chances and survival rates (Alexe et al., 2024). In addition to the biological and epidemiological dimensions, the psychological and social ramifications of a diagnosis of nasopharyngeal carcinoma also make treatment paradigms more complex. Patients typically go through a lot of difficulty through the invasive treatment process itself, which may include such interventions as chemotherapy and radiation, with side effects leading to a notable reduction in their quality of life. As testified to in studies, NPC's multifactorial etiology necessitates the incorporation of a holistic care model that addresses not only their physical well-being but also their emotional well-being. Comprehensive treatment plans should therefore incorporate supportive therapies to deal with pain, anxiety, and the psychosocial implications of having cancer. Once these issues have been handled, the medical team is in a position to offer a more supportive environment, enabling patients to navigate their treatment with a greater sense of control and hope (Alexe et al., 2024).

9.2.3. Adenoid Hypertrophy

Adenoid hypertrophy is a severe pathological condition in the field of nasopharyngeal pathology, particularly in children. It is a disease where adenoid tissue at the posterior end of the nasopharynx becomes hypertrophic and can lead to a variety of complications, notably obstructive sleep apnea (OSA) and chronic respiratory disease. Adenoid hypertrophy is highly prevalent among children, especially those two to eight years old, as they are at risk of obstructive sleep apnea syndrome (OSAS). The etiology is multidimensional in nature, encompassing both genetic variables and environmental factors, such as recurrent respiratory infections, which lead to hypertrophy of adenoid tissue. Accurate identification and diagnosis of adenoid hypertrophy is important, as left untreated, the condition can greatly affect the quality of a child's life, including respiratory function and sleep patterns. When noting symptoms that are associated with adenoid hypertrophy, one must consider its pervasive impact on a child's normal functioning and overall well-being. Children with hypertrophied adenoids have nasal congestion that results in breathing difficulties, altered speech, and persistent mouth breathing. Additionally, there are also complications that can follow, such as recurrent ear infections and sinusitis, due to the anatomical connection of the adenoids with the Eustachian tube and sinus drainage pathways. The correlation with allergic rhinitis conditions is also notable; patients typically present with similar symptoms. In a descriptive study on allergic rhinitis at Bugando Medical Centre, adenoid hypertrophy was identified as one of the prevalent comorbidities that affected a staggering 92.6% of the cases. This correlation is indicative of the necessity for a comprehensive management plan that incorporates both surgical and medical interventions to adequately alleviate symptoms and prevent future complications, such as sleep disorders and repeated infections. Surgery, through adenoidectomy, is typically recommended for kids with recurrent instances of adenoid hypertrophy, particularly in combination with symptoms typical of obstructive sleep apnea. The operation has been shown to produce a significant improvement in respiratory function and quality of life, with improved sleep patterns and enhanced daytime functioning. Postoperative assessments report a high level of patient satisfaction, along with considerable reductions in obstructive upper airway complications. It is, however, worth mentioning that adenoid hypertrophy should not be treated with surgery alone. Medical management, including relief of co-morbid conditions such as allergic rhinitis, is essential to best outcomes. Early diagnosis and intervention are essential, since sequelae of undiagnosed adenoid hypertrophy can be long-lasting, including OSA and concomitant difficulty with cognitive development and social interaction, justifying ongoing research and clinical attention to this common condition (Hardjojo et al., 2012; Bellini et al., 2019) (Figure 9.6).

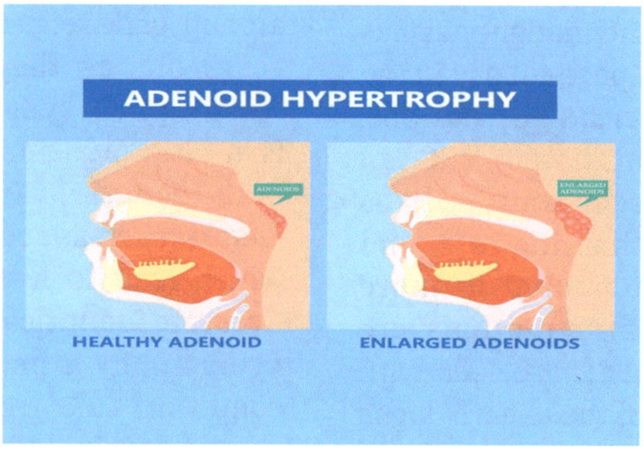

Figure 9.6. Adenoid hypertrophy represents a significant pathological condition

Source: https://www.sakraworldhospital.com/assets/spl_splimgs/adenoid-hypertrophy-01.webp.

Test Your Knowledge

1. What are the common disorders of the nasopharynx, such as adenoid hypertrophy, nasopharyngitis, and nasopharyngeal carcinoma, and what are their typical causes and clinical features?
2. Explain the diagnosis and management strategies for nasopharyngeal disorders, including medical treatment, surgical intervention, and preventive measures.

9.3. Symptoms and Diagnosis

Learning Outcome

1. Common Symptoms Associated with Nasopharyngeal Disorders
2. Diagnostic Techniques Used in Evaluating Nasopharyngeal Conditions
3. Importance of Early Diagnosis in Treatment Outcomes

Symptoms of nasopharyngeal diseases are also very varied, with a tendency to display nonspecific signs that complicate diagnosis. Nasal congestion, postnasal drip, and recurrent sinusitis, among other symptoms, are common to induce patients to seek treatment. More severe symptoms of snoring, sleep apnea, and dysphagia may also ensue, especially if there is a structural defect. In such cases where a mass has been described in the literature, malignancy cannot be ruled out. For instance, an 86-year-old male with chronic postnasal drip had a large nasopharyngeal bulge, which was diagnosed by biopsy as amyloidosis (Abrams et al., 2010). This underlines the importance of careful clinical evaluation because early recognition of signs can have a dramatic effect on patient outcomes for nasopharyngeal disease. Nasopharyngeal disorders are typically diagnosed using a multidisciplinary approach that includes detailed history-taking, clinical examination, and high-resolution imaging. Nasal endoscopy is often utilized to demonstrate structural anomalies within the nasopharynx. This prompt response can enable the identification of masses or lesions, like in the case above, where a swelling prompted examination (Abrams et al., 2010).

Imaging examinations, such as magnetic resonance imaging (MRI) or computed tomography (CT), become relevant in identifying the extent of the disorder and arriving at a differential diagnosis. For example, differences in airway dimensions might provide additional insight, with studies demonstrating clearly different changes in nasopharyngeal volume with jaw position. Such findings can be used to inform future therapy as well as enhance the overall diagnostic framework. In general, recognition of the symptoms and diagnostic processes that take place in nasopharyngeal disorders is critical to facilitate effective management. The heterogeneity of symptoms, ranging from general nasal issues to more complicated afflictions, renders it a comprehensive evaluation scheme. As noted in clinical literature, early diagnosis correlates with better prognoses, particularly when malignancy is a concern (Abrams et al., 2010). In addition, the use of imaging studies in addition to normal examination techniques is able to shed light on more internal anatomical alterations, further guiding the treatment plan. Hence, a well-educated grasp of symptomatology and diagnostic approaches is needed on the part of healthcare professionals involved in managing nasopharyngeal conditions to allow the patient suitable treatment and intervention.

9.3.1. Common Symptoms Associated with Nasopharyngeal Disorders

The nasopharynx, being posterior to the nasal cavity and above the oropharynx, is susceptible to a number of disorders and can present with a wide range of common symptoms that may significantly impact the quality of life. The most frequent of these symptoms are nasal obstruction and congestion, which can be precipitated by conditions such as rhinitis, sinusitis, or adenoid hypertrophy. Patients will complain of not being able to breathe through the nose, and this has implications such as problems with sleep and loss of voice resonance. These obstructive symptoms can also lead to complications such as secondary sinusitis, which further highlights the need for early medical assessment and treatment. How these symptoms relate to nasopharyngeal disorders must be appreciated in order to develop adequate treatment methods that decrease patient discomfort and restore normal function. Another significant symptom of nasopharyngeal conditions is that of pain or discomfort, which is localized in the area of the ear or throat. Pain can result from inflammation or infection, with conditions like acute pharyngitis and otitis media routinely found to be associated with nasopharyngeal conditions. Acute pain with fever, swelling, or purulent drainage may raise the suspicion of a more severe underlying condition, such as a peritonsillar abscess or malignancy, that should be immediately evaluated. Most important is the presence of ear referral, typically secondary to the close relationship between the nasopharynx and the auditory apparatus. Severe discomfort and precise diagnostic evaluation are important in the care of these symptoms and etiology so that therapy can be instituted appropriately. Neurological symptomatology is also presented within the context of nasopharyngeal illness, including viral illnesses such as COVID-19. Recent literature indicates that cranial nerve abnormalities, including olfactory and gustatory dysfunction, are frequent in patients, highlighting the interconnection between neurological function and nasopharyngeal health. These symptoms may occur even with minimal nasal findings, demonstrating how viral infections overcome respiratory limitations and profoundly affect sensory perception. Moreover, these dysfunctions may be present at early phases of viral illness, necessitating vigilance by physicians to facilitate early detection and treatment. This encounter highlights the subtlety of nasopharyngeal conditions and the importance of comprehensive approaches that encompass both anatomical and neurological aspects of these conditions (Akgoz et al., 2018; Boon et al., 2020) (Figure 9.7).

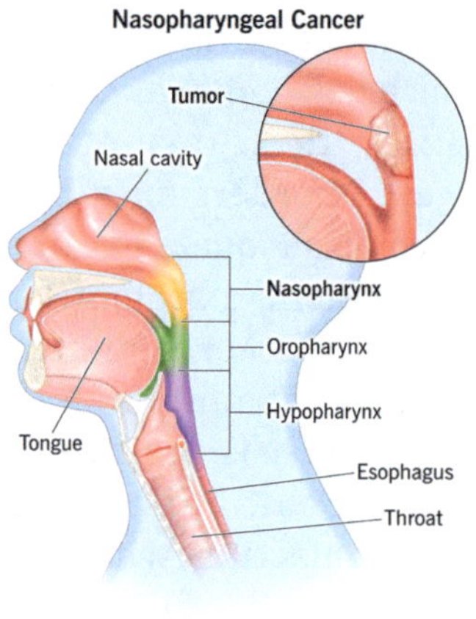

Figure 9.7. Common symptoms associated with nasopharyngeal disorders.

Source: https://my.clevelandclinic.org/-/scassets/images/org/health/articles/21661-nasopharyngeal-cancer.

9.3.2. Diagnostic Techniques Used in Evaluating Nasopharyngeal Conditions

Nasopharyngeal evaluation is of extreme significance for accurate diagnosis and treatment planning. Nasopharyngeal evaluation is performed by utilizing a number of diagnostic techniques to analyze structural as well as functional aspects of the nasopharynx. Acoustic rhinometry is one of these techniques, which estimates nasal patency in a quantitative manner and is able to identify velopharyngeal insufficiency (VPI). Area-distance curves are obtained from acoustic reflections, and volume changes during speech tasks are measured. Studies have demonstrated that acoustic rhinometry is of high discriminatory power in distinguishing patients with impaired velopharyngeal function from those with intact function. The technique is thus of great value in clinical assessments, particularly in those with histories of cleft palate repair, where effective treatment of VPI becomes crucial for optimal communicative outcomes (Araújo et al., 2014). Another advanced diagnostic modality is Positron Emission Tomography (PET), a significant advancement in imaging technology. PET employs the radioactive tracer 18F-Fluorodeoxyglucose (18F-FDG) to provide functional information as well as the structural information that can be gained using computed tomography (CT). PET imaging is particularly valuable in oncology since it allows the assessment of neoplastic lesions of the nasopharynx. 18F-FDG PET is supported by evidence to be superior in delineating the tumor margins caused by highly vascularized tissues, in greater accuracy for surgical planning. Also, its sensitivity in detecting lymph node metastasis underscores its role in nasopharyngeal cancer staging. Application of PET in diagnostic protocols suggests a promising line for enhanced accuracy of nasopharyngeal condition evaluation (Culp et al., 2019). In addition to these techniques, endoscopic assessment remains a cornerstone in the diagnosis of various nasopharyngeal diseases. Rigid and flexible endoscopy allows the observer to visualize mucosal surfaces, assess anatomical relationships, and biopsy suspicious lesions in the nasopharyngeal region. This technique is extremely helpful in the identification and diagnosis of infectious illness, tumors, and structural anomalies. Endoscopy not only facilitates direct visualization but also can be coupled with therapeutic intervention, for example, therapeutic biopsies or therapy of obstructive lesions. Interactive evaluation of the nasopharynx in diagnostic examinations enhances clinical decision-making and patient care protocols and further establishes the role of endoscopy in contemporary evaluation of nasopharyngeal illness.

9.3.3. Importance of Early Diagnosis in Treatment Outcomes

The value of early diagnosis in the treatment outcome of nasopharyngeal disease cannot be overemphasized. Early diagnosis of such conditions as otitis media and allergic rhinitis has a clear consequence on the effectiveness of treatment, as well as avoiding future damage. For instance, excessive delay in diagnosing otitis media leads to chronic effusion or chronic infection, which increases the risk of permanent hearing loss and intellectual delay among children.

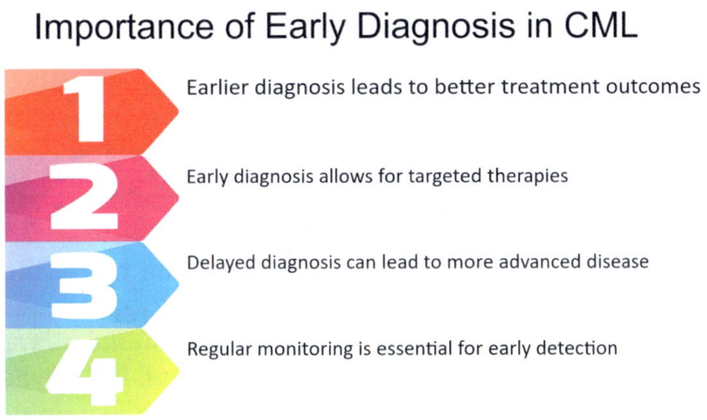

Figure 9.8. Importance of early diagnosis in treatment outcomes.

Source: https://fastercapital.co/i/CML-Diagnosis--Tests-and-Techniques-Explored--Importance-of-Early-Diagnosis-in-CML.webp.

As acute otitis media (AOM) and its variations are prevalent in pediatrics, the recognition of symptoms like earache or fever at an early stage might assist in ensuring the right intervention, thereby improving the chances of good outcomes. Secondly, the advancement in technology associated with diagnostic methods such as tympanometry and otoscopy has enabled experts to accurately diagnose the type of these conditions, hence the focus on the principles of early detection guidelines in maximization of care strategies (Casselbrant et al., 2016). Allergic rhinitis is another prevalent condition that underscores the importance of early diagnosis and treatment. Many patients who have allergic rhinitis also develop co-morbid conditions like adenoid hypertrophy, otitis media, and sinusitis that can aggravate their overall health conditions. Early diagnosis of allergic rhinitis allows physicians to initiate necessary treatment protocols that not only control the nasal manifestations but also take care of the complications. A study at Bugando Medical Centre revealed that the majority of the patients required surgery due to underlying complications, thus emphasizing the importance of early intervention in a bid to successfully manage these interdependent illnesses. Early detection of allergic rhinitis by healthcare providers can significantly enhance patient outcomes, minimizing the chances for secondary complications and improving the quality of life for the affected population (Hardjojo et al., 2012). Besides, early diagnosis also plays a significant role in the definition of appropriate therapeutic strategies toward nasopharyngeal disease patients. The application of certain interventions following an accurate diagnosis not only alleviates temporary symptoms but also affects the patient's long-term health trajectory. In chronic diseases, for instance, those due to repeated otitis media or chronic allergic rhinitis, early intervention averts worsening of the disease. Early treatment can prevent more invasive procedures later and thus reduce healthcare costs as well as improve patient satisfaction. By creating the imperative of early diagnosis in the treatment of nasopharyngeal conditions, medical professionals can optimize treatment efficacy and lay the ground for better future health for their patients (Hardjojo et al., 2012; Casselbrant et al., 2016) (Figure 9.8).

Test Your Knowledge

1. What are the common symptoms of nasopharyngeal disorders, such as nasal obstruction, snoring, epistaxis, and ear-related complaints, and how can they guide diagnosis?
2. Describe the diagnostic approach for nasopharyngeal conditions, including physical examination, nasopharyngoscopy, imaging, and biopsy when indicated.

9.4. Treatment Options of the Nasopharynx

Learning Outcome

1. Medical Management of Nasopharyngeal Disorders
2. Surgical Interventions for Severe Cases
3. Role of Lifestyle Changes in Managing Symptoms

Treatment modalities for nasopharyngeal conditions are diverse and tailored to the condition at hand. The majority of problems, including recurrent infection or allergic rhinitis, can be addressed initially with conservative measures, including antihistamines and nasal corticosteroids. Pharmacologic treatment is aimed at reducing inflammation and resolving symptoms. For those with obstructive sleep apnea (OSA), a more intense intervention may be required. Current studies have also shown a correlation between OSA severity and the shape of the upper airway anatomy, showing how treatment can be maximized by implementing customized approaches through the use of three-dimensional airway models infused with computational fluid dynamics (CFD) analysis to provide additional information regarding the nature of airflow and aid in the creation of more specific treatment modalities for victims (Jafari et al., 2019). Patients with acute and severe conditions, such as epistaxis, primarily require immediate treatment. Conservative treatments such as anterior nasal packing or cauterization are often used initially and can effectively control bleeding in the majority of cases. As quoted in key studies, non-surgical interventions comprise the majority of treatment interventions, and approximately 98% of cases could be addressed without employing invasive methods (Daudia et al., 2011). Yet, when conservative treatment fails, or in instances of severe trauma with massive hemorrhage, surgical intervention may become necessary. While these are a small minority of epistaxis, surgical options like arterial ligation can be life-saving, and again, there is the importance of considering the individual patient's requirement and clinical presentation. In the field of therapeutic modalities for nasopharyngeal disease, the multidisciplinary management approach is more and more emphasized. Coordination between otolaryngologists, allergists, and primary care physicians is critical to optimize patient outcomes. This multidisciplinary approach enables identification of the underlying etiology and the formulation of a comprehensive management plan that may include both medical and surgical interventions as necessary. Further, education regarding the use of preventative maneuvers, particularly trauma, can significantly minimize the incidence of epistaxis and other conditions within the nasopharynx. Finally, knowing the details of each case, risk factors, and treatment effectiveness guarantees that the interventions selected match closely with the patient's overall well-being objectives and quality of life.

9.4.1. Medical Management of Nasopharyngeal Disorders

Treatment of nasopharyngeal disease encompasses a vast array of methods suitable to the specific pathologies that may present in this region of anatomy. Effective assessment begins with careful symptom assessment, with epistaxis presenting as particularly common. For instance, a Buganda Medical Centre study identified traumatic injury as a significant source of cases of epistaxis, and medical staff should thus use a conservative management approach that minimizes surgical intervention. Non-surgical management options like anterior nasal packing and observation were effectively used in nearly all patients assessed, and surgery was reserved for the most complex cases. This accounts for the importance of having tailored treatment regimens that ensure patient safety and comfort, with particular respect for risks of complications of more invasive interventions (Daudia et al., 2011). For nasopharyngeal malignancies, medical management is also multidisciplinary in approach, bringing together oncological, radiological, and surgical expertise. It is recognition of the endemicity of Epstein-Barr virus-associated malignancies in these areas that requires accurate screening and early detection measures. Careful diagnostic techniques, such as endoscopic examinations and biopsies, are key to delineating the etiology of nasopharyngeal enlargements. For example, in a case of amyloidosis, it was demonstrated that not all nasopharyngeal enlargements are malignancies; careful pathological examination confirmed an alternative diagnosis, and the need for accurate differentiation was made evident.

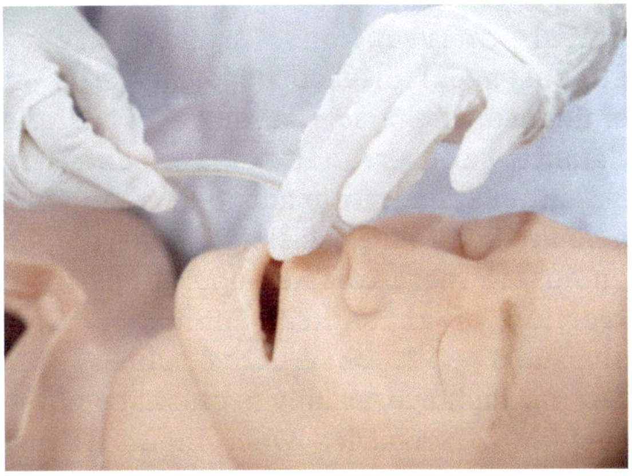

Figure 9.9. Medical management of nasopharyngeal disorders.

Source: https://blog.sscor.com/hubfs/Nasopharyngeal%20Airway%20Complications.png.

The treatment may range from observation monitoring to radiotherapy and chemotherapy, based on the underlying diagnosis and extent of disease progression (Abrams et al., 2010). Efforts should also be made to include educational interventions for avoiding the occurrence of nasopharyngeal disorders by addressing risk factors associated with them. Preventive public health measures, such as anti-smoking campaigns and education on the consequences of trauma, can efficiently influence the overall prevalence of conditions like epistaxis or nasopharyngeal cancer. Knowing that disorders like trauma or viral infections have a massive effect on the burden of nasopharyngeal disease assists healthcare workers in establishing effective intervention tactics. Lastly, the clinical care of nasopharyngeal illness should be a compromise among early diagnosis, effective patient-centered treatment, and aggressive public health intervention in order to lower risk, thus maximizing overall patient outcomes (Figure 9.9).

9.4.2. Surgical Interventions for Severe Cases

Surgical interventions in the area of nasopharyngeal disease generally step into prominence as the sole recourse in instances resistant to conservative management. These interventions range from adenoidectomy, which can be defined as the excision of hypertrophied adenoids, to more complex operations for the correction of anatomical anomalies. Those individuals with obstructive sleep apnea (OSA), for instance, usually necessitate surgery, especially in scenarios wherein the severity of involvement is linked with upper airway anatomy. Recent studies using advanced imaging techniques, such as CT scans, and computational fluid dynamics have highlighted the importance of understanding these anatomical variations. Finding a correlation between airway occlusion and apnea-hypopnea index, doctors can tailor surgical interventions based on the individual patient, thereby delivering an increased rate of success in alleviating OSA symptoms and overall quality of life improvement (Jafari et al., 2019). Aside from sleep apnea, allergic rhinitis is also the most severe of which intervention is via surgery due to co-morbid conditions such as adenoid hypertrophy, nasal polyps, and sinusitis. Research conducted at Bugando Medical Centre noted that almost 68.8% of patients with allergic rhinitis had surgical procedures to manage concomitant complications. Conditions such as adenoidal hypertrophy are easily added to obstructive symptoms and sleep disturbances, hence making it a more challenging task in managing such patients. Not only does the surgery procedure address such physical obstructions, but symptomatic burdens such as nasal congestion and chronic infection are eliminated, which can easily disrupt a patient's daily life. These interventions emphasize the clinical importance of managing both direct and indirect effects of allergic rhinitis as integral parts of integrative treatment protocols (Hardjojo et al., 2012). Lastly, successful surgical intervention for severe nasopharyngeal abnormalities relies on a multifaceted approach through meticulous preoperative assessment and postoperative care. The most important aspect is to make sure that the chosen operation effectively alleviates the underlying pathophysiology without incurring too many complications. Postoperative outcomes, such as satisfaction and symptom resolution rates, are important indicators of the efficacy of such treatments. As our understanding of the subtleties of the nasopharynx continues to expand with research, surgical techniques will evolve to meet individual patient needs. This commitment towards the improvement of surgical processes ensures that patients receive optimum care, fostering improved health status and enhanced living standards for patients suffering from serious nasopharyngeal illness.

9.4.3. Role of Lifestyle Changes in Managing Symptoms

Lifestyle modifications are needed in symptom management of nasopharyngeal disorders, particularly in conditions such as obstructive sleep apnea (OSA) and chronic rhinosinusitis. Data indicate that habit change is a good strategy to reduce the severity of symptoms experienced by patients. One such example is weight reduction for OSA patients because obesity is responsible for airway obstruction during sleep. Employment of a balanced diet with intensive intake of anti-inflammatory foods in addition to the elimination of processed foods can also contribute positively. The patients, by focusing on dietary alteration, not only relieve symptoms but also get better generally, paving the way for a holistic approach to nasopharyngeal disorder management. Exercise is also an essential factor in symptom alleviation related to nasopharyngeal disorders.

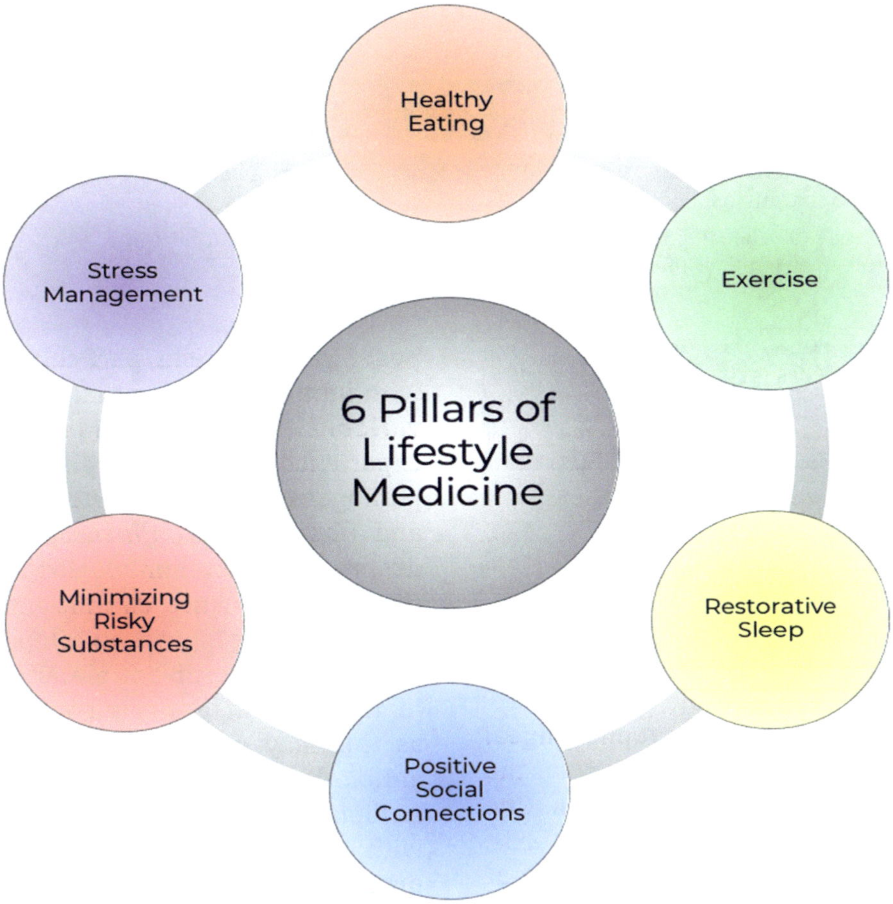

Figure 9.10. Role of lifestyle changes in managing symptoms.

Source: https://upload.wikimedia.org/wikipedia/commons/thumb/c/cf/Lifestyle_Medicine_Pillars.png/640px-Lifestyle_Medicine_Pillars.png.

Exercise can improve respiratory function, assist with weight reduction, and enhance overall health. Aerobic conditioning exercise, such as swimming or a brisk walk, can directly benefit the patient by improving oxygenation and reducing the severity and frequency of apnea during sleep. Stress reduction with yoga or mindfulness exercises may also decrease the severity and frequency of flare-ups of chronic rhinosinusitis. Therefore, the addition of physical activity to daily life not only controls symptoms but also encourages an active strategy toward health-related problems with nasopharyngeal disorders. Lastly, sleep hygiene practices can efficiently control symptoms of nasopharyngeal disorders, particularly in maintaining sleep. Establishing a regular sleep schedule, a good sleeping place, and minimizing exposure to allergens in the sleeping room can improve sleep quality. For patients with disorders like OSA, positional therapy, that is, sleeping on one side, can also prove beneficial by preventing airway collapse while asleep. Further, avoiding alcohol and sedatives at night enhances sleep's restorative quality, hence reducing the severity of symptoms. Taken together, these lifestyle changes provide patients with the means to control their condition, hence showing how non-pharmacological treatments can control nasopharyngeal disorders as well as improve overall quality of life (Figure 9.10).

Test Your Knowledge

1. What are the medical and surgical treatment options for common nasopharyngeal disorders such as adenoid hypertrophy, nasopharyngitis, and nasopharyngeal carcinoma?
2. Explain the criteria for choosing between conservative management and surgical intervention, and describe the post-treatment care and follow-up for nasopharyngeal conditions.

9.5. Complications of Nasopharyngeal Disorders

Learning Outcome

1. Potential for Airway Obstruction
2. Impact on Hearing and Speech
3. Risk of Systemic Infections

Complications arising from nasopharyngeal pathology can have serious implications for the overall health and well-being of a person. One of the most common complications is epistaxis, or nosebleed, and it may be brought about by several etiologic factors such as trauma, hypertension, or idiopathic origin. In studies, epistaxis has been reported to be present in up to 60% of the population at some point in their lives, necessitating medical care in approximately 6% of presentations, highlighting the actual prevalence of this condition. Most treatment is non-surgical, including observation and anterior nasal packing, but surgery is rarely necessary. However, the morbidity of such disorders, say, a rate of 3.8%, reveals that even simple procedures have risks. Thus, awareness of such potential complications is important in successful management and preventive measures in clinical practice (Daudia et al., 2011). Chronic infections of the nasopharynx also pose significant risks, particularly in individuals with immunodeficiency. Patients with common variable immune deficiency (CVID) mostly experience repetitive respiratory infections by pathogens such as *Streptococcus pneumoniae* and *Haemophilus influenzae*. These patients, despite being on immunoglobulin replacement therapy, experience chronic infection, leading to chronic lung injury and compromised quality of life. Overuse of antibiotics as prophylaxis in this patient group also poses a problem, as this may contribute to airway microbiota antibiotic resistance. Therefore, infection risks of nasopharyngeal diseases, particularly in patients with underlying immunological conditions, are urgently needed in terms of disease-specific studies (Camilli et al., 2018). Untreated or poorly treated nasopharyngeal diseases may also lead to more severe complications, including the development of nasopharyngeal tumors or chronic sinusitis. These conditions may result from prolonged inflammation or chronic infection in the nasopharyngeal region. Nasopharyngeal masses may lead to obstructive symptoms and, if left untreated early, may also metastasize, emphasis is laid on early diagnosis and treatment. Chronic sinusitis has fewer complications beyond the nasal passages and can lead to secondary infection or even intracranial and orbital complications. The complexity of nasopharyngeal conditions confirms the necessity of watchfulness on the part of healthcare providers to observe and deal with potential complications in the provision of comprehensive patient care.

9.5.1. Potential for Airway Obstruction

The danger of airway obstruction is a daunting challenge in nasopharyngeal disorders research. The disorders commonly result from anatomical or functional defects, which jeopardize the airway patency and lead to severe health consequences. For instance, enlarged adenoids or tonsils may physically intrude into the airway, particularly when muscles are relaxed during sleep. This reduction could result in obstructive sleep apnea (OSA), a state where there are repeated intervals of absence of breathing lasting at least 10 seconds, according to Mohammed (2005).

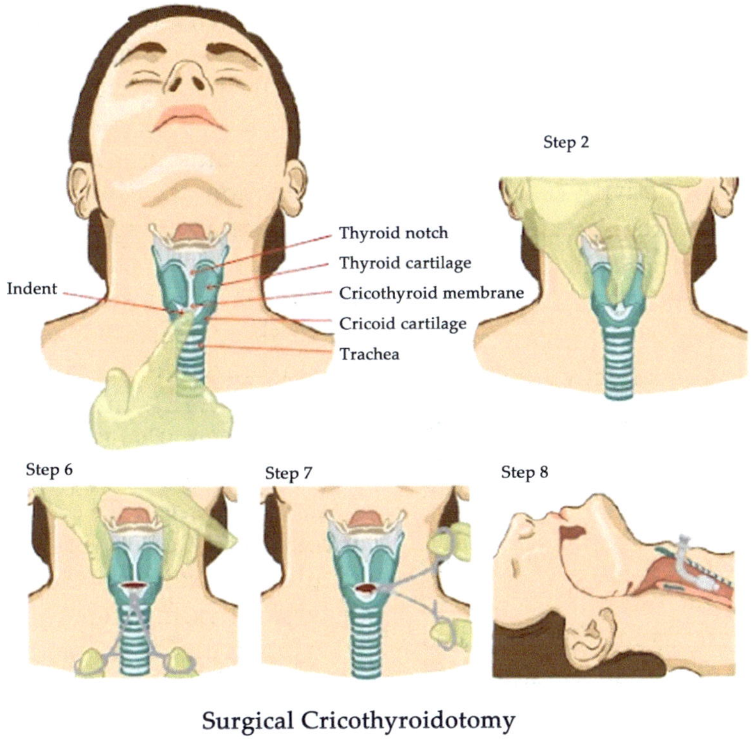

Figure 9.11. The potential for airway obstruction.

Source: https://image.prepladder.com/prepladder/2024/08/06100105/Crico-Thyroidotomy.webp.

The relationship between anatomical abnormalities and behavioral airways must be carefully evaluated to accurately diagnose underlying factors and potential obstructive sites, which is vital for proper management and treatment of patients who present with these signs. The incorporation of advanced diagnostic devices is increasingly important to assess the dangers of airway obstruction for patients with nasopharyngeal conditions. Computational fluid dynamics (CFD) simulation and three-dimensional (3D) modeling have become good tools for the airflow characterization in the upper airway. There is now established evidence of an association between CFD parameters, such as the adjusted pressure coefficient (Cp*), and the severity of OSA, indicating that these models can supply significant information about regions of obstruction. By expanding our understanding of airflow properties, clinicians are able to more precisely design interventions, thereby improving outcomes. This new approach allows for a better identification and management of the multifaceted nature of airway obstruction in the context of nasopharyngeal disease, as illustrated by findings that incorporate quantitative assessment of airway function. The clinical implications of uncontrolled airway obstruction extend far beyond mere annoyance, as it can generate substantial systemic effects. In patients with OSA, the repetitive sleep obstruction may precipitate a cascade of physiologic reactions like hypoxemia and increased sympathetic activity, resulting in an elevated risk of cardiovascular disease. The recognition of obstructive sleep apnea as a sleep disorder but also as a multifactorial condition with complications lasting for many years underscores the necessity of effective diagnosis and treatment processes. With emerging research, a more complex understanding of the interactive functions of anatomical variation and functional dynamics of airflow will allow the development of targeted therapies correcting the primary causes of airway obstruction in the context of nasopharyngeal disease, thus potentially reducing associated morbidities and enhancing overall quality of life (Figure 9.11).

9.5.2. Impact on Hearing and Speech

The impacts of nasopharyngeal pathologies on hearing and speech are substantial, particularly among toddlers. Otitis media (OM) is typical and typically leads to conductive hearing loss due to the accumulation of fluid in the middle ear, which interrupts sound conduction. Once OM has established, particularly if it is long-standing, it can significantly impede the processing of sound and linguistic acquisition. Research establishes that if OM is left untreated, it will result in delayed speech and language development in the long term, thus the need for intervention at an early stage. Children with chronic or frequent hearing loss struggle to speak, expand their vocabulary, and communicate. Recognition of the complex relationship between nasopharyngeal pathology and auditory function is important for developing effective treatment strategies and preventive measures to reduce adverse outcomes in young patients. The anatomical and physiologic features of the nasopharynx play a crucial role in otitis media formation, affecting hearing in turn. The Eustachian tube, an opening from the nasopharynx to the middle ear, is more sloping and narrower in children, thus predisposing them to infection. Dysfunction of this tube can lead to fluid build-up and thus impairment of hearing. Studies have shown that children with nasopharyngeal disease largely experience bouts of OM, which affect their hearing as well as communication. For instance, during chronic otitis media with effusion (OME), the conductive hearing loss that subsequently occurs may lead to significant auditory deprivation that affects the neural pathways essential to speech development. Intervening on this dysfunction through medical or surgical therapy is important for reversing hearing and promoting optimal speech development, and in the process highlights the significance of proactive intervention within pediatric populations. Finally, the relationship of nasopharyngeal disease to speech acquisition extends beyond sensory influence. Children with chronic diseases like OME will have difficulty making sounds in appropriate contexts since their hearing is compromised. The critical period for speech acquisition occurs early in life, when exposure to auditory stimuli is a requirement. Hearing loss during this critical window will lead to compensatory mechanisms that will not fully substitute for normal auditory input, resulting in speech delays or abnormalities. Additionally, children with craniofacial syndromes, which also involve nasopharyngeal dysfunction, commonly have a heightened frequency of OM, further complicating speech and hearing. Understanding these correlations reinforces the necessity of proper monitoring and management of nasopharyngeal disease to set the stage for healthy speech and hearing development for affected children, as these diseases have implications for communication skills throughout life.

9.5.3. Risk of Systemic Infections

Nasopharyngeal conditions, particularly otitis media, are highly predisposed to the development of systemic infections, most commonly in children. Acute otitis media (AOM) is characterized by middle ear inflammation, most commonly due to bacterial or viral infection spreading up from the nasopharynx. In respiratory infections such as the common cold, the viral pathogens will permit the ascent of bacteria from the nasopharynx to the middle ear and lead to AOM.

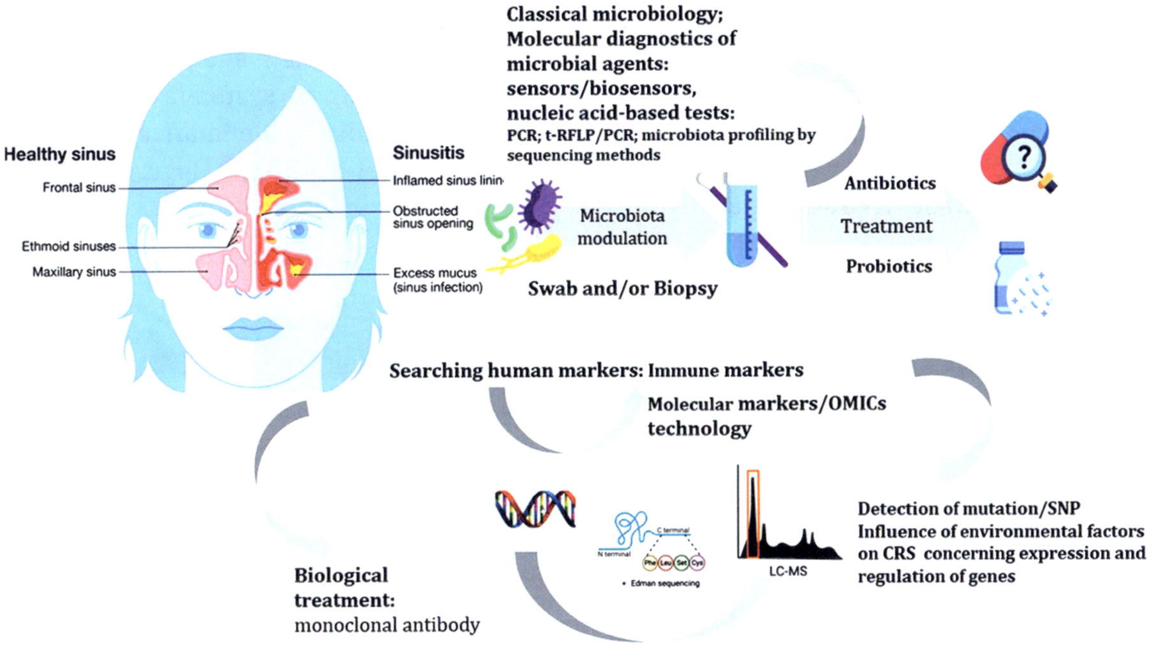

Figure 9.12. Nasopharyngeal disorders, particularly otitis media, pose a significant risk of systemic infection.

Source: https://pub.mdpi-res.com/ijms/ijms-25-03201/article_deploy/html/images/ijms-25-03201-ag.png?1710151165.

This diagnosis needs to be treated medically because uncontrolled or recurrent AOM can lead not only to chronic inflammatory processes but also systemic complications, including hearing loss and potential dissemination of pathogens to more serious sites, such as the blood. An understanding of the anatomical and functional interactions between the nasopharynx and middle ear is important in realizing how seemingly localized infections become systemic disease (Casselbrant et al., 2016). Aside from that, evidence-based systematic review of treatment for AOM further highlights the complexities of management as well as implications of systemic infection risks. While antibiotics are typically administered to control symptoms and reduce infection duration, their efficacy has been challenged by limited symptom and pain relief. Systemic corticosteroids with anti-inflammatory effects, in trials designed to assess their activity with antibiotic treatment, have given inconclusive results (Beller et al., 2018). Such vagueness can encourage irresponsible prescribing or antibiotic dependence, thereby increasing the risk of the emergence of antibiotic-resistant organisms. Clinicians must thus be careful to diagnose and treat AOM so as to avoid not just local complications, but also the risk of systemic infections from untreated or inadequately treated nasopharyngeal conditions. In addition to the implication in systemic infections, nasopharyngeal disorders must also be well-equipped with a comprehensive understanding of preventive actions and long-term management. Immunization against frequent pathogens, for example, Streptococcus pneumoniae, has effectively minimized the occurrence of AOM and associated complications. In addition, intervention like addressing environmental determinants for the occurrence of upper respiratory infections—such as exposure to tobacco smoke and allergens—can also reduce risks related to systemic infections. Routine monitoring and follow-up must be used to identify individuals at risk of recurrent AOM, and these children may require surgical interventions such as tympanostomy tube placement for ventilation. These interventions can maintain ear health and prevent the cascade of events leading to systemic infection, hence improving quality of life in affected individuals (Casselbrant et al., 2016) (Figure 9.12).

Test Your Knowledge

1. What are the common complications of nasopharyngeal disorders, such as adenoid hypertrophy, chronic nasopharyngitis, or nasopharyngeal tumors, including otitis media, sleep disturbances, and airway obstruction?
2. Explain the potential systemic and local complications of untreated nasopharyngeal disorders and how early diagnosis and management can prevent them.

9.6. Preventive Measures of the Nasopharynx

Learning Outcome

1. Importance of Regular Medical Check-Ups
2. Strategies for Reducing Exposure to Allergens
3. Vaccination and Its Role in Preventing Infections

Good preventive care is important in the management of nasopharyngeal disorders, in that it significantly reduces the incidence and severity of acute otitis media and related diseases. At the center of such prevention care is the promotion of good hygiene among children who are especially susceptible to nasopharyngeal infections. Regular cleaning of the environment and regular hand washing may decrease the spread of pathogens that cause these diseases. In addition, vaccination against prevalent viral and bacterial causes of infections such as influenza and *Streptococcus pneumoniae* is an important ingredient in these strategies. Immunization of children decreases the odds of contracting both otitis media and its resultant complications, leading to improved health outcomes and reduced healthcare utilization. Thus, the inclusion of hygiene and immunization as prophylactic factors occupies a central role in the preservation of nasopharyngeal health. The role of the environment to the pathogenesis of nasopharyngeal pathology cannot be overstressed. Poor quality air, exposure to tobacco smoke, and high concentrations of environmental allergens have been implicated in extremely high frequencies of disease conditions like otitis media and respiratory infection. Thus, implementing community-level programs to improve air quality and restrict exposure to harmful pollutants is significant for preventive health. Secondly, informing parents and caregivers regarding the health effects of secondhand smoke can allow them to offer healthier home environments for children. For instance, establishing smoke-free home environments, particularly where children stay most of the time, can be crucial in protecting their respiratory health. By intervening through environmental determinants, public health programs can induce an environment that is less conducive to the etiology of nasopharyngeal disorder. Nutrition is also an important aspect in preventing nasopharyngeal disorders, particularly among children. The intake of appropriate nutrients plays a vital role in ensuring good immune function, which in turn helps the body to resist infection of the nasopharynx. For instance, high vitamin A, C, D, and zinc dietary intake is associated with augmented mucosal immunity, and thus with lower infection risk, such as acute otitis media. In addition to dietary interventions, breastfeeding should also be promoted as a significant preventive strategy because it provides infants with essential antibodies and nutrients that augment their immunity. The parents must be educated on the benefits of unilateral breastfeeding throughout the first six months of life, as it not only nourishes but also protects against a host of infections. Through a combination of dietary management and nutrition counseling, health professionals can provide an environment conducive to healthy ear and throat function, thereby lightening the burden of nasopharyngeal disorders.

9.6.1. Importance of Regular Medical Check-Ups

Regular medical check-ups play a very important role in early detection and avoidance of nasopharyngeal disorders since early intervention of all types of illnesses is made possible. A complete physical examination by a physician can identify symptoms such as persistent sore throat, nasal obstruction, and frequent infections which may be symptoms of underlying conditions such as allergies, infection, or complicated diagnosis such as cancers. For instance, a case report emphasized the need to consider atypical sore throat presentations, in which a detailed examination following prolonged assessment revealed that the diagnosis could have been overlooked, underscoring the importance of vigilance in the differential diagnosis (Carney et al., 2020). Routine follow-ups enable health practitioners to monitor variation in patient nasopharyngeal health, informing proactive management guidelines that can significantly improve health outcomes. Also, regular check-ups can facilitate more patient-healthcare provider interaction, which is crucial in addressing some nasopharyngeal disorder-related problems. Dysphagia or chronic nasal congestion are two frequent complaints that are typically underreported by patients, which may lead to their misdiagnosis or untreated conditions. This region of preventive treatment is particularly crucial in cases involving individuals who are not likely to accept medical advice, such as men with symptoms of nasopharyngeal diseases and possible stigmatization due to these issues. Research emphasizes that primary care providers should actively refer for health check-ups, particularly among male patients who are less likely seek consultations for men's health issues (Tong, 2012). Through such discussions, becoming a standard part of periodic visits, healthcare providers are able to de-emotionalize them and promote a health sentinel culture, guaranteeing patient engagement. In addition to improving initial diagnosis and doctor-patient interaction, frequent medical check-ups may also play a vital role in managing nasopharyngeal illnesses in the long term. For recurrent diseases such as allergic rhinitis or chronic sinusitis, a pattern of follow-up visits enables adjustment of treatment regimens based on evolving symptoms and therapeutic responses. Such continuity of care not only allows for the delivery of treatment for immediate requirements but also education regarding probable complications and lifestyle modifications that might alleviate symptoms. Early detection of complications or exacerbations, through regular check-ups, can prevent serious health issues from arising, thus enhancing general quality of life. Maintenance in an active lifestyle through hospital visits ensures overall health consciousness, making check-ups a necessary component in the proper management of nasopharynx conditions (Figure 9.13).

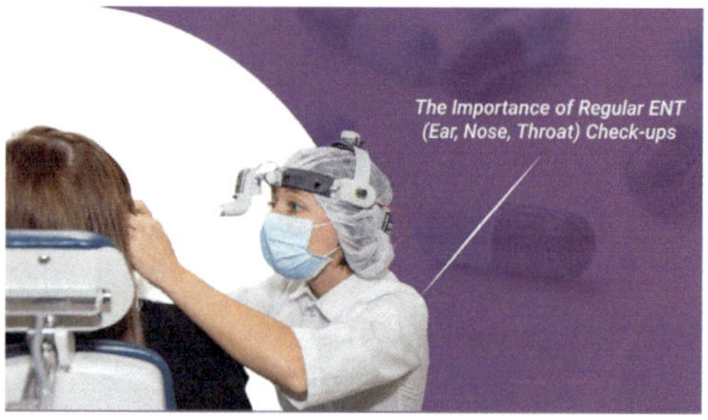

Figure 9.13. Importance of regular medical check-ups.

Source: https://www.aceneuroenthospital.com/wp-content/uploads/2024/01/Importance-of-Regular-ENT-Check-up.png.

9.6.2. Strategies for Reducing Exposure to Allergens

In the treatment of the nasopharyngeal conditions, particularly those exacerbated by allergic response, gaining access to meaningful means of reducing exposure to allergens becomes increasingly significant. One of the components is the careful control of environmental conditions. Persons with nasal allergies need to incorporate practices such as meticulous cleaning and disinfection of living spaces to prevent exposure to dust mites and mold – two of the most common allergens. Additionally, home use of high-efficiency particulate air (HEPA) filters will reduce airborne allergens considerably. This is significant since aerosolized particles are typically responsible for nasopharyngeal tissue inflammation that leads to secondary complications such as sinusitis and chronic rhinitis. By working to prevent exposure to allergens in the home environment, patients can effectively improve the quality of life while reducing the severity and frequency of acute exacerbations associated with allergic diseases. The other crucial strategy includes the modification of lifestyle elements that predispose to allergen sensitization. Cigarette smoking and exposure to secondhand smoke are proven instigators of nasopharyngeal inflammation. An example is the secondhand exposure to cigarette smoke, which was observed to influence the immune system in children with adenoid hypertrophy, a clear sign of the importance of having a smoke-free environment. Protection from in-home exposure to toxic substances not only keeps one individual healthy but can also contribute to the better functioning of immunological protection. Creating a smoke-free indoor environment is particularly important in children, whose immune systems are developing and are thus more susceptible to toxic impacts, which in turn can exacerbate diseases such as adenoid hypertrophy—leading to surgical interventions in the case of no treatment (Brambilla, 2019). In addition, it is important to consider the role of systemic exposure in the management of nasopharyngeal allergies. Implementing dietary adjustment can also offer a useful approach because certain food allergens can have the ability to cause nasal congestion and inflammation. An anti-inflammatory diet that includes agents such as omega-3 fatty acids in fish and nuts has the ability to modulate the inflammatory response that occurs with allergens. Furthermore, it is important to recognize the history of atopic conditions; patients with a history of atopy may need certain steps taken to decrease exposure risk to future allergens. An integrative measure involving environmental control measures along with dietary interventions offers an effective method in handling the interactive mechanism between allergens and nasopharyngeal well-being (Aasand et al., 1989). Emphasis on these interactive measures may enable individuals to increase overall resistance to allergic disorders and improve respiratory health.

9.6.3. Vaccination and Its Role in Preventing Infections

Vaccination is a key to preventing nasopharyngeal-associated infections, reducing the incidence of many respiratory illnesses by a significant amount. Otitis media, or inflammation of the middle ear, is one of the most common pediatric disorders and is often caused by nasopharyngeal infection. Both bacterial and viral nasopharyngeal pathogens can ascend up the Eustachian tube to infect the middle ear. The use of pneumococcal conjugate vaccines has played a critical role in reducing the spread of such infections, demonstrating that targeted immunization not just protects individuals but also aids in creating herd immunity within the population. By selectively removing the disease burden from pathogens such as *Streptococcus pneumoniae*, vaccines are most significant for the prevention of sequelae of infection from these pathogens, including hearing loss and developmental delay, and therefore healthier developmental trajectories among children. Furthermore, the role of vaccination is evident in the prevention of other nasopharyngeal diseases such as acute sinusitis and pharyngitis, illnesses that also contribute to significant morbidity in infected individuals. Evidence indicates a marked decline in the incidence of acute otitis media due to vaccine utilization, with a contribution to public health. Through its ability to reduce nasopharyngeal colonization of disease-causing microorganisms, vaccination indirectly but strongly acts against the reduced incidence of secondary infection, as evidenced from various studies on children. As the relationship between nasopharyngeal infection and secondary complications becomes increasingly evident, continued efforts at vaccination are crucial to limiting the overall morbidity of respiratory disease, highlighting the necessity for ongoing public health efforts against vaccine-preventable disease. In addition to avoiding acute infection, vaccinations also confer long-term health benefits by attacking the virulence of individual pathogens. For instance, vaccines that stimulate immune responses to polysaccharides of biofilm-producing pathogens like *Staphylococcus aureus* and *Streptococcus pneumoniae* are especially relevant. Research demonstrates the function of PNAG, a polysaccharide subunit, in biofilm formation, making treatment difficult through chronic colonization (Jiang, 2016). By decreasing the frequency of infections from these pathogens, vaccinations decrease the risk factors for chronic nasopharyngeal conditions. Besides, clinical guidelines with a focus on vaccination have fewer cases of serious disease, ultimately decreasing healthcare costs and improving the quality of life. Combined, vaccinations not only prevent a myriad of nasopharyngeal diseases but also support a broader understanding of community health, reaffirming their fundamental role in infectious disease management in the current world.

Test Your Knowledge

1. What preventive measures and lifestyle practices can reduce the risk of nasopharyngeal disorders, including maintaining nasal hygiene, avoiding allergens, and proper ventilation?
2. Explain the role of vaccination, early treatment of upper respiratory infections, and regular medical check-ups in preventing complications of nasopharyngeal diseases.

SUMMARY

It should be kept in mind that these conditions are very multifaceted and have effects on people from different populations. Nasopharynx, as an important crossroad for respiratory and digestive systems, can be involved in a range of disorders, from allergic rhinitis to more complicated forms of obstructive sleep apnea syndrome (OSAS). The prevalence of OSAS among children, and in particular that with hyperplastic adenoid tissue, is a concern for pediatric healthcare workers because untreated conditions lead to recurrent respiratory illnesses and retardation in development. More epidemiology and etiology studies, as well as awareness, are, therefore, important, highlighting the need for tailored patterns in treatment and diagnosis, particularly among at-risk populations with individualized health profiles (Bellini et al., 2019). Furthermore, the overall relevance of nasopharyngeal pathology extends to general public health and clinical practice. The overlap between respiratory pathology and systemic diseases underscores the necessity of an integrated approach to the nasopharynx in medical education and practice. Pathologies like OSAS not only disrupt sleep but may also exacerbate or lead to cardiovascular disease, hence impacting long-term health outcomes. With the identification of such disorders' bases, doctors can have an integrated view, blending diagnostic information with life conditions in order to design more efficacious interventions. This requires interdisciplinary coordination, where professionals in every field have to work together to counteract the challenges posed by nasopharyngeal disorders (Bellini et al., 2019). Lastly, ongoing research and development of treatment methods are essential to enhance patient outcomes in nasopharyngeal disease. Current research still strives to seek out new therapy options, including new surgical methods and the development of targeted pharmacotherapies tailored specifically to address separate symptoms as well as underlying etiologies of the diseases. Furthermore, the potential to link chronic inflammatory diseases with bacterial pathogens, such as the relationship between *Mycobacterium avium* subspecies paratuberculosis and gastrointestinal disease, is but an example of the necessity for greater wholeness in thought in the understanding of how infection leads to nasopharyngeal impacts on health. Hence, the evolution of clinical practices for the treatment of nasopharyngeal illnesses will increasingly depend on the integration of research findings and clinical expertise, resulting in improved treatment practices.

The disorders of the nasopharynx encompass a wide range of diseases that have a serious impact on patient health and well-being. Of the disorders of the nasopharynx, chronic rhinosinusitis is a prevalent disorder, characterized by persistent sinus tissue inflammation, with accompanying symptoms of nasal blockage, facial pain, and decreased sense of smell. Other than chronic rhinosinusitis, adenoid hypertrophy and nasopharyngeal carcinoma are diseases that present special diagnostic and therapeutic challenges. The former primarily occurs in children and may present as obstructive sleep apnea, whereas the latter, a nasopharyngeal cancer, calls for a thorough understanding of the anatomical structures involved and etiologic risk factors for its occurrence. As such, a multidisciplinary approach that considers the multifaceted nature of these conditions is required for successful treatment intervention. Contributing to the difficulty in the landscape of nasopharyngeal conditions is also the fact that some patients have varied experiences with these conditions. As an illustration, it has been established that older populations may experience special challenges with adherence and prevalence with respect to treatment compared to younger age populations. Such circumstances as polypharmacy, cognitive impairment, and an absolute general rise in comorbidities can complicate effective treatment of such disorders as chronic rhinosinusitis in this group of patients. Furthermore, evidence suggests a need for treatment approaches suitable for the age group that are capable of intervening in obstacles to accessing healthcare services for older adults. With interventions that consider these unique factors, healthcare providers are able to maximize the overall efficacy of treatments for nasopharyngeal conditions, thereby achieving improved patient outcomes. In considering the treatment of nasopharyngeal conditions, it is evident that a multidisciplinary approach is paramount. The integration of otolaryngologists, allergists, and primary care physicians can enable whole-person care to have a more profound effect on the varied factors of such conditions. Moreover, the education of the patients is at the heart of enabling individuals to seek early intervention and adhere to treatment protocols. Current research underscores the importance of elucidating the interaction between environmental exposures, for example, allergens and pollutants, and the precipitating factor in the exacerbation of nasopharyngeal disease. By raising awareness of such connections, healthcare professionals can enable patients with interventions that prevent them from exposing themselves, thereby reducing cases of associated complications. Lastly, sustained exploration of these areas is necessary to advance knowledge and treatment paradigms in nasopharyngeal disorders.

KEY TERMS FROM THIS CHAPTER

Adenoid Hypertrophy
Nasopharyngitis
Chronic Nasopharyngitis
Adenoid Cystic Carcinoma
Eustachian Tube Dysfunction
Choanal Atresia
Thornwaldt's Cyst
Postnasal Drip
Tubal Tonsil Hypertrophy
Adenoiditis
Acute Nasopharyngitis
Nasopharyngeal Carcinoma
Lymphoid Hyperplasia
Otitis Media with Effusion
Nasopharyngeal Stenosis
Tornwaldt's Disease
Epipharyngeal Catarrh
Retropharyngeal Abscess

CRITICAL THINKING QUESTIONS

1. **The most common cause of adenoid hypertrophy in children is:**
   a) Viral infection
   b) Bacterial infection
   c) Allergic reaction
   d) Trauma
2. **Adenoid hypertrophy can lead to:**
   a) Nasal obstruction
   b) Mouth breathing
   c) Recurrent otitis media
   d) All of the above
3. **Chronic nasopharyngitis is commonly associated with:**
   a) Allergies
   b) Smoking and pollution
   c) Viral infections
   d) Fungal infections
4. **The commonest malignant tumor of the nasopharynx is:**
   a) Squamous cell carcinoma
   b) Nasopharyngeal carcinoma
   c) Lymphoma
   d) Adenocarcinoma
5. **Eustachian tube dysfunction can result in:**
   a) Otitis media with effusion
   b) Otosclerosis
   c) Tinnitus
   d) Vertigo

Short Answer Questions

1. What are the common disorders of the nasopharynx, such as adenoid hypertrophy, nasopharyngitis, and nasopharyngeal carcinoma, and what are their typical causes?
2. Describe the clinical features and symptoms of nasopharyngeal disorders, including nasal obstruction, snoring, epistaxis, and ear-related complaints.
3. Explain the diagnostic methods used for nasopharyngeal conditions, including physical examination, nasopharyngoscopy, imaging, and biopsy.
4. Discuss the treatment options for nasopharyngeal disorders, including medical management, surgical intervention, and post-treatment care.
5. What are the possible complications of untreated nasopharyngeal disorders, and how can preventive measures help reduce their occurrence?

Answers to Critical Thinking Questions

1. (b) 2. (d) 3. (b) 4. (b) 5. (a)

REFERENCES

1. Dushay, M. E., & Johnson, C. E. (1989). Management of allergic rhinitis: focus on intranasal agents. *Pharmacotherapy the Journal of Human Pharmacology and Drug Therapy, 9*(6), 338–350. https://doi.org/10.1002/j.1875-9114.1989.tb04148.xAbrams, K., Andersson, M., Fox, T., McInnes, A., et al. (2010). *Localized Nasopharyngeal Amyloidosis.* https://core.ac.uk/download/pdf/82068919.pdf (accessed on 7th August 2025).
2. Akgoz, A., Bulut, E., Gocmen, R., Gunes, A., et al. (2018). *Trigeminal nerve and pathologies in magnetic resonance imaging: A pictorial review.* https://core.ac.uk/download/160736722.pdf (accessed on 7th August 2025).
3. Alexe, A. A., Cindea, I., Gherghina, V., Hainarosie, R., et al. (2024). *Challenges in Diagnosing Nasopharyngeal Tumors.* https://core.ac.uk/download/624145763.pdf (accessed on 7th August 2025).
4. Araújo, B. M. A. M., Silva, A. S. C. da, Suedam, I. K. T., Teixeira, A. R., et al. (2014). *Velar activity in individuals with velopharyngeal insufficiency assessed by acoustic rhinometry.* https://core.ac.uk/download/pdf/37522201.pdf (accessed on 7th August 2025).
5. Babler, W., Ghoniema, A., Glupker, L., Kula, K., et al. (2015). *Three-dimensional computed tomography analysis of airway volume changes between open and closed jaw positions.* https://core.ac.uk/download/81633706.pdf (accessed on 7th August 2025).
6. Baldini, A., Fuchs, J. C., Linden, J. F., Tucker, A. S., et al. (2014). *A defect in early myogenesis causes otitis media in two mouse models of 22q11.2 deletion syndrome.* https://core.ac.uk/download/29410931.pdf (accessed on 7th August 2025).
7. Belfield, K., Birchall, J. P., Daniel, M., Lee, A., et al. (2014). *Update on Otitis Media – Prevention and Treatment.* https://core.ac.uk/download/29029689.pdf (accessed on 7th August 2025).
8. Beller, E. M., Del Mar, C. B., Pitoyo, Y., Ranakusuma, A., et al. (2018). *Systemic Corticosteroids for Acute Otitis Media in Children.* https://core.ac.uk/download/196606193.pdf (accessed on 7th August 2025).
9. Bellini, C., Cammaroto, G., Colizza, A., de Vincentiis, M., et al. (2019). *Risk factors for obstructive sleep apnea syndrome in children: State of the art.* https://core.ac.uk/download/231747914.pdf (accessed on 7th August 2025).
10. Bhutta, M. F. (2015). *Evolution and otitis media: A review, and a model to explain high prevalence in indigenous populations.* https://core.ac.uk/download/56687765.pdf (accessed on 7th August 2025).
11. Boon, P., De Herdt, V., Garrez, I., Hemelsoet, D., et al. (2020). *Neurological manifestations and neuro-invasive mechanisms of the severe acute respiratory syndrome coronavirus type 2.* https://core.ac.uk/download/323232708.pdf (accessed on 7th August 2025).
12. Brambilla, I. (2019). *Adenoidal immunity in children: Is there a correlation with passive smoke, atopy, and "low dose medicine compound"?* https://core.ac.uk/download/567662873.pdf (accessed on 7th August 2025).
13. Camilli, R., Cardines, R., Cerquetti, M., Ciervo, A., et al. (2018). *Risk factors for Hemophilus influenzae and pneumococcal respiratory tract colonization in CVID.* https://core.ac.uk/download/188826783.pdf (accessed on 7th August 2025).

14. Carney, M. B., Glickman, A. A., Rodgers, B., Schander, J., et al. (2020). *A 45-year-old female with an atypical presentation of pharyngitis.* https://core.ac.uk/download/305124157.pdf (accessed on 7th August 2025).

15. Casselbrant, M. L., Chonmaitree, T., Cripps, A. W., Haggard, M., et al. (2016). *Otitis Media.* https://core.ac.uk/download/79536551.pdf (accessed on 7th August 2025).

16. Crean, S., Harding, A., Kesavalu, L., Robinson, C., et al. (2014). *Oral inflammation, tooth loss, risk factors, and association with progression of Alzheimer's disease.* https://core.ac.uk/download/42137086.pdf (accessed on 7th August 2025).

17. Culp, W. T. N., Spriet, M., & Willcox, J. L. (2019). *Role of positron emission tomography in imaging of non-neurologic disorders of the head, neck, and teeth in veterinary medicine.* https://core.ac.uk/download/323070037.pdf (accessed on 7th August 2025).

18. Daudia, A., Abhay-Gupta, A. K., Nemer, A., Feusi, B., Huang, C., Yueng-Hsiang, C., Nash, C. M., et al. (2011). *Etiological profile and treatment outcome of epistaxis at a tertiary care hospital in Northwestern Tanzania: A prospective review of 104 cases.* https://core.ac.uk/download/pdf/11307803.pdf (accessed on 7th August 2025).

19. Forrester, D., Galvani, S., Lapworth, K., Sullivan, M., et al. (2011). *Working with Older Drinkers.* https://core.ac.uk/download/30322076.pdf (accessed on 7th August 2025).

20. Giuliana, G., Militi, A., Nucera, R., Pizzo, G., Spinuzza, P., & Tersigni, U. (2019). *Laterolateral teleradiography of the skull as a screening method for OSA/OSAS in patients in orthodontic treatment.* https://core.ac.uk/download/287859063.pdf (accessed on 7th August 2025).

21. Hardjojo, A., Shedden, A., Stuck, A., Cruz, A. A., Stevenson, A. N., Chauhan, B., Engel-Yeger, B., et al. (2012). *Allergic rhinitis and its associated co-morbidities at Bugando Medical Centre in Northwestern Tanzania: A prospective review of 190 cases.* https://core.ac.uk/download/pdf/11307799.pdf (accessed on 7th August 2025).

22. Jafari, B., López, S., Rahai, H., Shin, H., et al. (2019). *Evaluation of human obstructive sleep apnea using computational fluid dynamics.* https://core.ac.uk/download/323075650.pdf (accessed on 7th August 2025).

23. Jiang, F. (2016). *Characterization of the role that bacterial surface polysaccharide poly N-acetyl glucosamine plays in nonvaccine serotypes of Streptococcus pneumoniae colonization and pathogenicity.* https://open.bu.edu/bitstream/2144/16107/1/Jiang_bu_0017N_11102.pdf (accessed on 7th August 2025).

24. Lundborg, K. (2004). *Housing, Management, and Health in Swedish Dairy Calves.* https://core.ac.uk/download/11694701.pdf (accessed on 7th August 2025).

25. Magalhães, M. C. M. M. (2020). *Impact of adenotonsillectomy and rapid maxillary expansion on the upper airways in children with obstructive sleep apnea syndrome (OSA): A randomized controlled clinical.* https://core.ac.uk/download/323561437.pdf (accessed on 7th August 2025).

26. Mohammed, O. B. (2005). *A craniofacial morphology study of patients with obstructive sleep apnea.* https://core.ac.uk/download/32600297.pdf (accessed on 7th August 2025).

27. Olliver, M. (2012). *Linking Innate and Adaptive Immunity to Streptococcus Pneumoniae.* https://core.ac.uk/download/70340300.pdf (accessed on 7th August 2025).

ANATOMY AND PHYSIOLOGY OF THE THROAT AND LARYNX

10

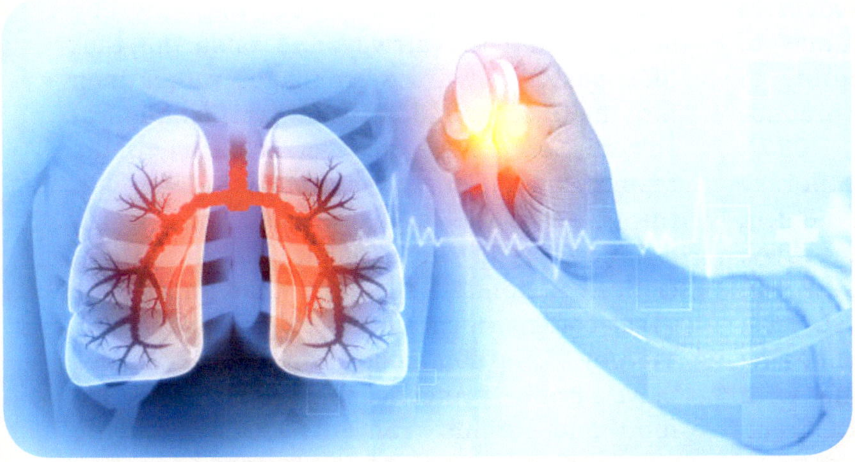

LEARNING OBJECTIVES

After studying this chapter, you will be able to:

1. Anatomy of the throat.
2. Anatomy of the larynx.
3. Physiology of the throat.
4. Physiology of the larynx.
5. Common disorders of the throat.
6. Common disorders of the larynx.

Introduction

The physiology and anatomy of the larynx and throat are essential topics in studying human disease and health. These structures work together in the digestive and respiratory systems to facilitate essential processes like breathing, swallowing, and voice production. As one of the initial fields of medical research, the throat has long intrigued clinicians, leading to a lot of research and development in treatment procedures. It is not only knowing the structural components but also the varying physiological functions that provide a picture of normal as well as pathological states. To quote an example, laryngeal diseases can significantly affect voice production and airway protection, emphasizing their value in otorhinolaryngology, a discipline that has gone a very long way in the decades, refining methods that supplement traditional practices with advanced technological incorporation (Américo et al., 2007). A close examination of the larynx and throat would reveal a complex interrelation of muscles, tissues, and nerve centers, all functioning their part towards their complete function. The larynx, popularly referred to as the voice box, harbors the vocal cords and is essential in forming sounds. It also functions as protective, as it prevents the aspiration entry during swallowing. Anatomically, the larynx sits at the juncture of the upper and lower respiratory tract, so its physiological integrity is central to general health. Historically, individuals have come a considerable distance in understanding laryngeal anatomy, as can be gleaned from various cultural healing strategies throughout antiquity. With new discoveries continually emerging, the importance of a sound understanding of the anatomy of these regions for advancing medical practice is increasingly evident (Ahn et al., 2017). In addition, the evolution of contemporary medical technology has revolutionized the field of otorhinolaryngology to ensure improved diagnostic and therapeutic processes. The convergence of minimally invasive surgical skill, endoscopy, and computerized imaging technologies has provided clinicians with unparalleled access to the larynx and throat, allowing them to make precise interventions. This increase in technology demonstrates the necessity of ongoing revision of anatomy to continue being relevant in clinical practice. Moreover, a sharp understanding of the anatomical and physiological realms directly impacts patient care, which in turn equals better outcomes in the treatment of voice disorders and respiratory illness. As this field continues to evolve, respect for historical thought and present-day progress that forms the basis of our understanding of the throat and larynx is critical to ensure professionals are suitably equipped to address emerging challenges in health care (Américo et al., 2007).

Definition of the Throat and Larynx

The throat, or in medical jargon, the pharynx, is a muscular tube whose function is critical as a passageway for both respiratory and digestive activities. It extends from the back of the nasal cavity to the larynx and esophagus and serves as a route for respiratory and digestive purposes. The pharynx, from an anatomical point of view, is further divided into three categories: the nasopharynx, oropharynx, and laryngopharynx, each structured to serve specific functions. Importantly, the nasopharynx is primarily committed to breathing, but the oropharynx and laryngopharynx are essential to swallowing. The intricate musculature and structure of the throat enable a variety of reflex actions, such as swallowing and coughing, thereby safeguarding the airway and ensuring that food passes down the esophagus rather than into the trachea. Understanding this anatomical structure emphasizes its pivotal role in both the respiratory and digestive systems. Along with the throat is the larynx, or voice box, which is found directly beneath the pharynx. It is a critical anatomical structure that houses the vocal cords, which vibrate to produce sound, thereby aiding communication. The larynx also plays a critical protective function by protecting food and liquids from the trachea during swallowing because of the epiglottis, a flap covering the airway. The larynx holds several cartilaginous elements, like the thyroid, cricoid, and arytenoid cartilages, which contribute to its rigidity and flexibility. Besides voice production, the larynx plays a significant role in the control of airflow during respiration and thus has an effect on vocal sound quality and resonance. The inconspicuous coordination between the larynx and throat underscores their mutual importance in airway strength and vocalization, both of which are paramount to human communication (Américo et al., 2007). The advancements in technology during the last few years have propelled the understanding of the throat and larynx, particularly concerning surgeries and treatment plans for a number of disorders, including obstructive sleep apnea and cancers of the larynx. Computational fluid dynamics (CFD) is, for instance, a promising approach to the prediction of surgical outcomes through airflow dynamics modeling of the upper airway.

These technologies allow clinicians to quantify preoperative and postoperative alterations. For instance, CFD analysis has demonstrated surgical maneuvers to modify the airflow patterns, leading to improved respiratory function (Dahl et al., 2017). These advancements not only enhance clinical practice but also bring into focus the intricate anatomy and physiology of the larynx and throat, and bring about better treatment plans and outcomes for the patients. With advancements in research and technology, the integration of technology and a greater knowledge of such anatomical aspects will bring dramatic advancements in otorhinolaryngology (Figure 10.1).

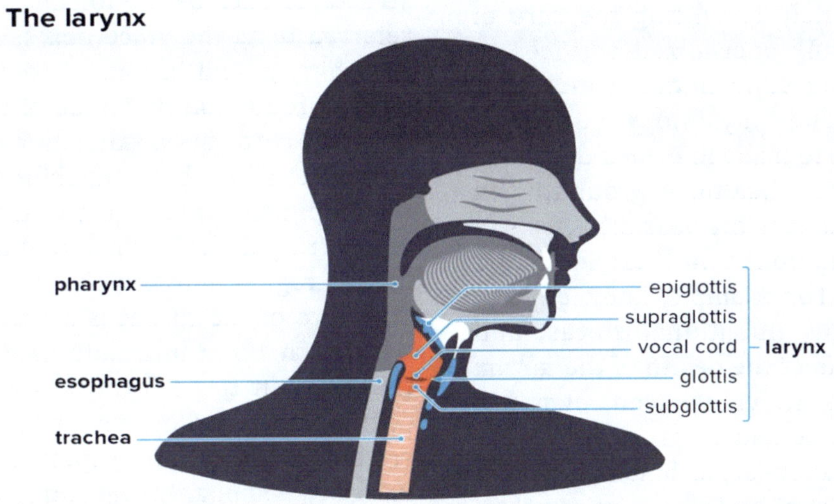

Figure 10.1. The throat and larynx.

Source: https://i0.wp.com/post.medicalnewstoday.com/wp-content/uploads/sites/3/2021/03/703850-the-larynx-1296x728-body-1024x712.jpg?w=1155&h=1894.

Importance of Studying Anatomy and Physiology

Anatomy and physiology are essential in understanding the intricate functions of the larynx and throat, as these areas are pivotal to both respiratory and voice functions. Understanding anatomical structures, such as the epiglottis, vocal folds, and musculature that accompany them, is not only significant for medical professionals but also for singers, actors, and individuals who need vocal timbre and power in their line of work. As Américo et al. (2007) explain, otorhinolaryngology development, encompassing the study of ears, nose, and throat, stems from early medical practices that laid the ground for contemporary surgical and clinical breakthroughs. By studying these structures and their function, learners are able to appreciate the relationship between structure and performance, and therefore improve care, rehabilitation techniques, and prevention strategies for voice health. Further, knowledge of anatomy and physiology facilitates interprofessional collaboration among healthcare providers, which enhances patients' outcomes. Programs such as Seeing Voices demonstrate the necessity of interdisciplinary education for acquiring a comprehensive vision of laryngeal health. As Andrade et al. (2023) demonstrate, the program was attended by students from various disciplines, where they could watch live laryngeal examination alongside learning the nuances of vocal production. Such exposure not just reinforces theoretical knowledge but also enhances practical skills necessary for assessing vocal health. The integration of interprofessional strategies emphasizes integration of anatomical knowledge from across different healthcare professions, ultimately enhancing the care of individuals requiring specialized services in voice disorders and concomitant conditions. Lastly, anatomy and physiology education teaches individuals to make informed decisions regarding their vocal health. A grounding in these disciplines informs the possible effects of environmental conditions and lifestyle factors on voice function. For example, knowledge of how hypohydration, nutritional status, and vocal misuse can affect the health of the larynx is essential for an individual who must use their voice to become successful at work. The background in the history of otorhinolaryngology, as stated in Américo et al. (2007), emphasizes the continued advances in techniques and treatments stemming from that fundamental knowledge. In the end, understanding the anatomy and physiology of the throat and larynx is advantageous not just for those who are pursuing careers in the related fields but also towards the ultimate goal of educating the public about vocal health and preventive care.

10.1. Anatomy of the Throat

Learning Outcome

1. Description of the Pharynx
2. Structure of the Esophagus
3. Relationship Between the Throat and Surrounding Structures

Throat anatomy plays a significant role in some physiological activities, including respiration, digestion, and speech. The complex region, involving the pharynx and larynx, serves as a channel through which air and food travel to their respective targets, that is, the trachea and esophagus. The pharynx, constituted by three components—the nasopharynx, oropharynx, and laryngopharynx—permits air from the nasal cavity and food from the oral cavity to pass through and also houses essential structures such as the tonsils. The larynx, also referred to as the voice box, is situated below the pharynx and has an important function of sound production by virtue of the vibration of the vocal cords upon exhalation. Together, these structures allow for optimal functioning of both the respiratory and digestive tracts, once more referencing the relationship of body structures in this region. Further, the overall anatomical structure of the throat is specifically designed with both bony and soft tissue frameworks that allow it to perform its various functions. Cartilaginous structures, such as thyroid and cricoid cartilages, are responsible for laryngeal integrity, and pharyngeal and laryngeal muscles enable modulation of airflow and vocalization. Understanding these interactions is crucial, as minor anatomical differences can lead to marked functional disparities in both voice and swallowing. Advances in imaging technologies, such as contrast-enhanced computed tomography, enable detailed examinations of these structures, as attested by continued research utilizing model organisms such as *Xenopus laevis*, which could further resolve the complexity of human throat anatomy and that of other organisms. The fusion of technology and anatomy provides a more meaningful background for studying the throat's function and significance in broader biological and medical contexts. The historical progression of otorhinolaryngology—studying the ear, nose, and throat—mirrors the major developments in comprehending the throat's anatomy over the years. The early physicians from various cultures did rudimentary treatment that prepared the way for contemporary practices, with the 20th century bringing a revolution in clinical and surgical methodology. Advancements in anesthesia and imaging technology transformed the specialty as less invasive techniques became an option, and the outcomes for patients were improved. Various prominent professionals in the development of otorhinolaryngology advocated the use of microscopes, local anesthesia, and endoscopic technologies, which enhanced the precision of surgeries. This richly colored history puts this ongoing interaction between surgery and anatomy into the foreground, as it emphasizes the value of considering historical things in shaping contemporary understanding of throat anatomy and physiology, as outlined in the surgical innovation literature on this specialty (Américo et al., 2007) (Figure 10.2).

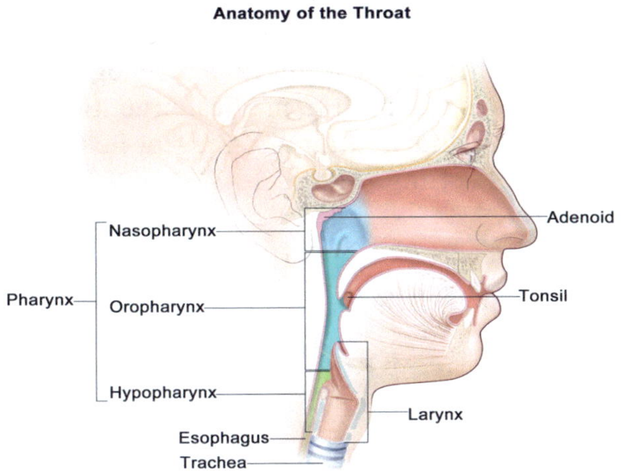

Figure 10.2. The anatomy of the throat.

Source: https://nci-media.cancer.gov/pdq/media/images/813315.jpg.

10.1.1. Description of the Pharynx

The pharynx is a significant anatomical structure in the anatomy and physiology of the larynx and throat, serving as a shared passage for both the respiratory and digestive tracts. It is located behind the nasal cavity and oral cavity and extends downward toward the larynx and esophagus. The pharynx consists of three anatomical components: the nasopharynx, oropharynx, and laryngopharynx. Each of these segments serves a special role in the process of respiration and swallowing. The nasopharynx transmits air, with adenoids to assist in immunological function, while the oropharynx transmits both air and food, interacting with the oral cavity. Lastly, the laryngopharynx is an airway to the larynx and esophagus, outlining its function as being multifunctional to the human respiratory and digestive systems. Its structural composition has a significant impact on its physical properties and functions. It is lined with stratified squamous epithelium in the oropharynx and laryngopharynx that is resistant to food and air wear and tear. The muscular walls of the pharynx are composed of circular and longitudinal muscle fibers and permit peristaltic movement that aids in swallowing. Moreover, the tonsils, which are components of the immune system and a first line of defense against infection, are located in the pharynx. Pharyngeal developmental variation in size and position from infancy through adulthood is a classic example of the dynamic nature of this structure, which not only is critical to understanding normal physiological function but also to predicting and interpreting possible pathologies of the airway, as with craniofacial and other abnormalities analysis (Akbudak, İ. H., & Mete, A., 2018). Additionally, the interaction of the pharynx and larynx is important in speech production and swallowing, which underscores the importance of this anatomical region. The pharyngeal muscles play a role in the elevation of the larynx during swallowing to prevent aspiration. Such an interaction is particularly important following surgical procedures, such as total laryngectomy. Understanding the normal anatomical and physiological characteristics of the pharynx is essential for evaluating the impact of such conditions on post-surgical speech production. Speech rehabilitation techniques, for instance, tracheoesophageal puncture, highlight the importance of pharyngeal and laryngeal anatomical knowledge in improving post-recovery outcomes of laryngectomized patients (Kerkhoff, 2013). Combined, these functions illustrate the pharynx's significant role not only in the throat and larynx but also in the human body at large.

10.1.2. Structure of the Esophagus

The esophagus is a critical component of the digestive tract that serves as a conduit for food and liquids from the pharynx to the stomach. It is a muscular tube, approximately 25 centimeters long in adults, that courses through the thoracic cavity to transfix the diaphragm. The esophagus is lined with a mucosa covering that permits smooth passage of materials, and deeper muscular layers, made up of circular as well as longitudinal muscles, permit peristalsis—involuntary movement that moves food into the stomach. The stratified squamous mucosa provides protection against mechanical damage from food particulates, which is necessary because of the varying textures of the materials being digested. Knowledge of this anatomy is key to knowledge of how disturbances in the functioning of the esophagus can lead to disease such as dysphagia or gastroesophageal reflux disease. Along its course, the esophagus has several significant anatomical landmarks, such as the upper and lower esophageal sphincters. The upper esophageal sphincter, composed of skeletal muscle, plays a significant role in preventing the entry of air into the esophagus through breathing and in the proper deflection of food into the esophagus. The lower esophageal sphincter, composed of smooth muscle, prevents gastric contents from refluxing back into the esophagus and thus provides a significant protective mechanism against acid reflux. These sphincters operate via complex neural and hormonal mechanisms and highlight the relationship between muscular structure and physiological function during homeostasis. These anatomical considerations are significant in the etiology of esophageal disease and in how they may be managed, since structural abnormalities will result in dysfunction. The structural integrity of the esophagus can be lost due to a wide range of disease processes, which highlights its importance in health in general. For instance, strictures and esophageal varices can be the result of underlying liver disease or inflammation that alters the caliber and function of the esophagus. Also, certain cancers, particularly laryngeal or upper respiratory ones, can affect the structure and functioning of the esophagus and thus the swallowing and speaking abilities—areas that are exhaustively evaluated when speech rehabilitation following laryngectomy is contemplated. Both Kerkhoff et al. (2013) and Ahn et al. (2017) discuss the interlinked nature of the esophagus with other anatomical structures and systems, reiterating the relevance of a good understanding of esophageal anatomy within the broader context of throat and laryngeal physiology. This knowledge is essential to medical practitioners in assessing and treating esophageal health in the clinical setting (Figure 10.3).

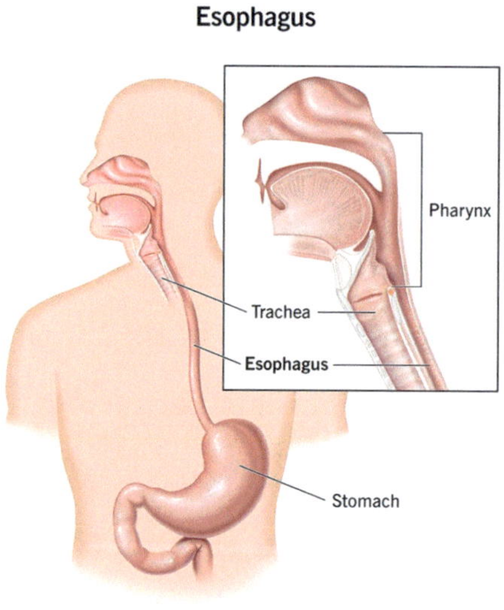

Figure 10.3. Structure of the esophagus.

Source: https://my.clevelandclinic.org/-/scassets/images/org/health/articles/21728-esophagus.

10.1.3. Relationship Between the Throat and Surrounding Structures

The relationship between the throat and the surrounding structures is a remarkable aspect of human anatomy, particularly due to its role in various physiological mechanisms such as respiration and digestion. The throat, anatomically, consists of the pharynx and the larynx and is connected to the nasal cavity and the oral cavity, respectively. This configuration creates an advanced interface along which air, food, and sound travel. The association among these structures is reciprocal, as the throat serves as a channel for both air to penetrate the respiratory system and food to enter the digestive system. Any defect or alteration in one of such correlated segments can lead to grave clinical implications with a tendency to engage other associated anatomical structures, thereby complicating diagnosis and treatment planning. Also, the functional anatomy of the upper airway is an important factor in its functioning within the realm of surrounding structures. The upper airway, including the mouth, nose, palate, and larynx, is not only an air conduit but is dynamically involved in optimizing the process of gas exchange. Changes in the anatomical configuration can change airflow dynamics, pressure, and resistance significantly. For instance, obstructions such as obstructive sleep apnea may happen due to changes in the structure of the upper airway, and hence a comprehensive understanding of such anatomical correlations is required. As the airways change and vary in shape when performing various activities, such as exercise or swallowing, it is clear that a thorough insight into the functional anatomy of the upper airway is necessary to address both routine physiological and pathological processes (Akbudak, İ. H., & Mete, A., 2018). From a clinical perspective, the linkage between the throat and structures associated with it is particularly significant in the understanding of conditions such as exercise-induced inspiratory symptoms (EIIS). Studies have demonstrated that laryngeal abnormalities can be the cause of symptoms usually mistakenly referred to as asthma, and thus, managing and treating patients is challenging. Because the throat has an important function in both respiration and digestion, laryngeal examination with caution in laryngoscopic procedures can yield useful indications of the cause of respiratory dysfunction. This, therefore, directs attention to the need for a thorough assessment of the entire upper airway system, with attention directed to how even minor disruptions in one part might affect overall function and cause systemic complications. Systemic clinical appraisal is crucial in mapping such relations and laying the groundwork for effective interventions (Clemm et al., 2016).

Test Your Knowledge

1. Describe the anatomical divisions of the throat (pharynx), including the nasopharynx, oropharynx, and laryngopharynx, and their boundaries.
2. What are the key structures of the throat, such as the tonsils, epiglottis, and laryngeal inlet, and what are their anatomical relationships?

10.2. Anatomy of the Larynx

Learning Outcome

1. Components of the Larynx
2. Location and Function of the Vocal Cords
3. Role of the Larynx in Respiration

The laryngeal anatomy, or voice box, plays a crucial role in several body functions, including phonation, respiration, and airway protection during swallowing. The larynx is located in the anterior part of the neck on top of the trachea and has different cartilages, like the thyroid, cricoid, and arytenoid cartilages. This intricate structure not only provides shape and structure but also facilitates the movement necessary for speech. The vocal folds, or vocal cords, bridge the laryngeal structure and are essential to produce sound as they vibrate when air flows through them to produce varying pitches depending upon tension and length. Anatomy of the larynx is necessary for health professionals who specialize in voice disorders, asphyxia, and respiratory diseases related to this vital organ (Américo et al., 2007). Aside from sound production, the larynx is an important protector of the respiratory system. The laryngeal framework is invested with intricate musculature, which allows manipulation of the vocal folds to enable sophisticated regulation of airflow on inspiration and expiration. The epiglottis, as a leaf-shaped structure, play a critical protective role in covering the trachea when swallowing to avoid food and liquids from entering the airway. This dynamic interaction between numerous elements of the larynx is crucial to facilitate unobstructed airflow without raising the risk of aspiration. The evolutionary significance of these adaptations underscores the duality of the functions of the larynx to produce sound and serve as an airway protector, underscoring its complexity and versatility as a critical organ in the human body (Américo et al., 2007). New developments in the area of medical technology have further improved our understanding of laryngeal anatomy. For instance, procedures such as high-resolution imaging and endoscopic examinations provide detailed information about the processes and structures of the larynx, thereby improving diagnostic accuracy. Computational dissection methods using contrast-enhanced imaging have been used to map out laryngeal anatomy, shedding light on intricate interactions between structural components. While newer technologies are crucial for clinical and research applications in academia, they are equally important in tailoring treatment to patients with conditions such as laryngeal cancer or dysphonia. Therefore, the study of the laryngeal anatomy continues to evolve, bearing testimony to its applicability in both the past and present eras in otorhinolaryngology.

10.2.1. Components of the Larynx

The larynx is primarily made up of several important elements, which are predominantly cartilage, ligaments, and muscles. Of its cartilaginous composition, the most important ones are thyroid, cricoid, and arytenoid cartilages, which play not only a supporting role to the structure but also the most important roles in sound-producing mechanisms and airway protection. The thyroid cartilage, commonly known as the Adam's apple, is especially prominent and protects the vocal cords. On the other hand, the cricoid cartilage, which encircles the airway in a complete ring, provides stability and patency to the larynx. The two pyramidal arytenoid cartilages control the opening and closure of the vocal folds and, therefore, the wide range of vocalizations, which form the basis of speech and communication tasks. In conjunction with the cartilages, the laryngeal muscles are also crucial for maintaining the tension and position of the vocal cords. These intrinsic and extrinsic muscles work together to alter the pitch and loudness of the voice by small movements of the cartilages and vocal folds.

Intrinsic muscles, such as cricothyroid and thyroarytenoid, control tension, affecting the frequency of sound produced, whereas extrinsic muscles are accountable for the positional stability of the larynx during activities such as swallowing. Correct functioning of these muscles is required; failure can disrupt the ability to produce intelligible speech or can lead to conditions such as dysphonia, thereby pointing out the sophistication of anatomical laryngeal structure to physiological function. Lastly, the mucosal tissue lining the larynx plays a crucial role in protecting the underlying tissues and facilitating sound production. This protective cover helps in the prevention of foreign particles from entering the trachea and lungs, as well as aiding in vocal fold hydration. The pattern of vibration of the vocal cords, which is used for voice modulation, relies heavily on this moist environment. Furthermore, alterations in this mucous lining can manifest as clinical complications in the form of laryngitis, an inflammation of the larynx with symptoms of hoarseness or loss of voice. Understanding the anatomy of the larynx, its components, and their actions is essential in comprehending the intricate physiology of the throat and the critical mechanisms of speech and swallowing, as described in dysphagia literature, highlighting the intricate relationships between the anatomy that participates in these activities (Gabriela et al., 2014) (Figure 10.4).

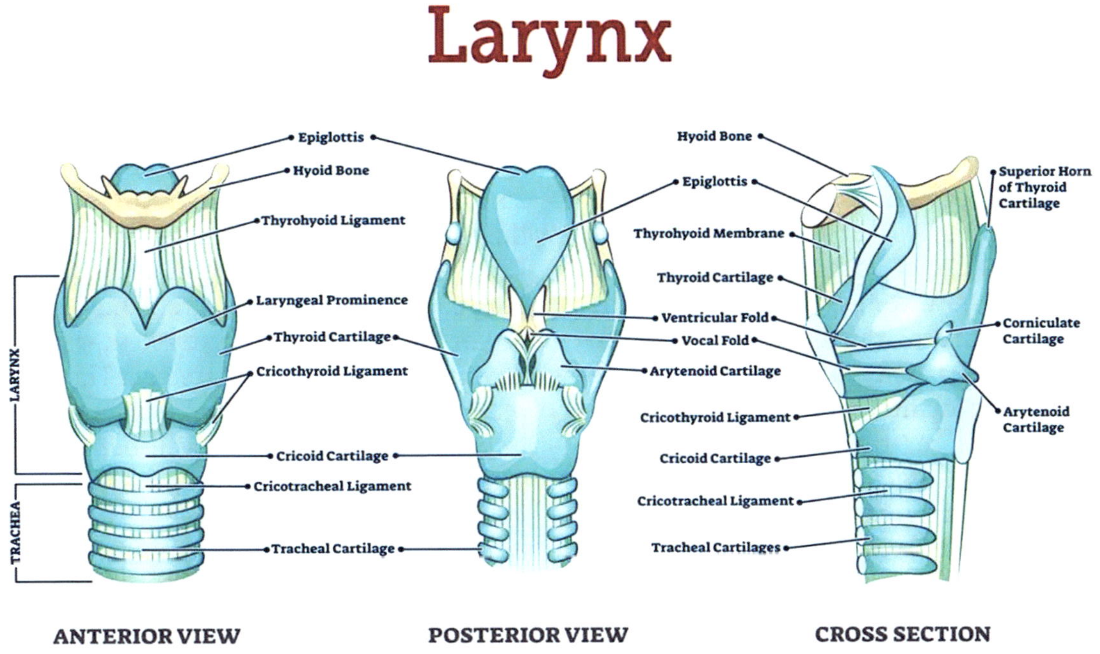

Figure 10.4. The larynx is predominantly constituted of several vital components.

Source: https://speechfit.io/_next/image?url=https%3A%2F%2Fimages.prismic.io%2Fspeechfit%2Fa76af431-7a6d-4588-8978-a060c6b23845_1675511253036%2B%25281%2529.jpeg%3Fauto%3Dcompress%2Cformat&w=3840&q=75.

10.2.2. Location and Function of the Vocal Cords

The vocal cords, or vocal folds, are located within the larynx, a highly significant structure in the neck. This anatomic positioning places the vocal folds directly in the center of the respiratory tract, allowing them to function effectively during breathing and phonation. The larynx itself is located anterior to the esophagus and extends from the base of the tongue to the trachea. Comprised of a series of cartilages, muscles, and ligaments, the larynx not only houses the vocal folds but also serves as an airway guard, preventing food and liquid from entering the trachea during swallowing. The location of the vocal cords within the laryngeal framework, thus, is of immense importance both in its function in speech production and in safeguarding the respiratory tracts. Functionally, the primary role of the vocal cords is to facilitate the production of sound through a process known as phonation. Since air from the lungs is directed through the closed vocal folds, they oscillate to produce sound waves. The voice can be modified in terms of pitch and loudness through variation of the tension, length, and mass of the vocal cords, which are controlled by the intrinsic laryngeal muscles. These muscles adjust the form and posture of the vocal folds, allowing for a range of vocal expressions from high-pitched to low tones. Furthermore, the quality and timbre of the voice also rely on factors such as elasticity and wetness of the vocal folds. A recognition of these functional elements underscores the fine line that must exist for successful vocal communication and the value in ensuring that the voice remains healthy in order to avoid disorders that can impair the production of the voice (Abdelal, 2013). Notably, the welfare of the vocal cords is essential for professional voice users as well as the general populace. Voice disorders are caused by misuse or overuse of the vocal folds and can be manifested in nodules, polyps, or laryngitis. These conditions have a critical impact on the process of communication and can necessitate speech-language pathology or medical treatment. Education materials for vocal health consist of good vocal technique, hydration, and rest to ensure optimal functioning of the vocal cords. With an integration of the understanding of anatomy and physiology, clinicians can design useful preventive interventions and strategies for voice disorders in a way that individuals can utilize their vocal abilities to the best of their capacity (Greene, 1968).

10.2.3. Role of the Larynx in Respiration

The larynx, or voice box, is responsible for respiration, serving as the passageway between the inlet of the larynx and the trachea. Its anatomical position is essential for adequate airflow, as it directs air from the pharynx into the lower respiratory tract. This control is achieved primarily by a process of vocal fold abduction and adduction, which opens and closes the respiratory air passage while breathing. In inhalation, the vocal folds abduct to allow maximum inflow of air into the trachea. Conversely, when exhaling, the vocal folds adduct entirely or in part, and in doing so, provide a function that creates an air trap during some activities such as coughing or heavy lifting—enhancing respiratory efficiency and lung condition. The larynx remains an important organ of the respiratory tract that ensures air flow is controlled and protected. The larynx also plays a role in protection mechanisms that are important to respiratory well-being. One of the primary functions is the prevention of aspiration, when foreign material may enter the trachea and lungs. The epiglottis, a spoon-shaped flap of cartilage, is vital to the swallowing process as it folds over the trachea to block food and liquid from entering the airway. The action serves to prevent aspiration pneumonia by ensuring that only air enters the lungs. Moreover, laryngeal resilience assists in sound production and maintains the airway patent during breathing. Through its intricate anatomy and functional dynamics, the larynx not only creates sound but is also a protective mechanism within the cycle of respiration, exposing its multifaceted role in human physiology. When explaining the relationship between the larynx and breathing, it is important to note the neurovascular interaction that governs laryngeal function. Laryngeal musculature is innervated by the vagus nerve and can vary in subtle movements during breathing. This interactive function ensures that the vocal folds respond appropriately to varying respiratory demands, such as rest or exercise. Additionally, the larynx participates in the respiratory process by accommodating changes in thoracic pressure and lung volume to facilitate smooth transition between inspiration and expiration. Disruption of laryngeal function has been shown to cause severe respiratory issues, impacting overall air exchange efficiency. Thus, valuing the larynx's function in respiration underscores its importance in supporting healthy homeostasis and enabling lung function, ultimately highlighting its role in both health and disease (Alip et al., 2011; Fón et al., 2018) (Figure 10.5).

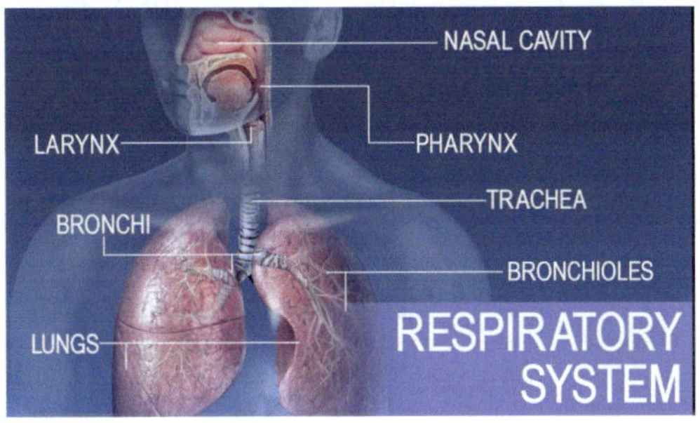

Figure 10.5. Role of the larynx in respiration.

Source: https://www.visiblebody.com/hs-fs/hub/189659/file-2545156127.jpg.

Test Your Knowledge

1. Describe the anatomical structure of the larynx, including its cartilages (thyroid, cricoid, arytenoid, epiglottis), muscles, and ligaments.
2. Explain the relationships of the larynx with surrounding structures, including the pharynx, trachea, and neurovascular supply, and their clinical significance.

10.3. Physiology of the Throat

Learning Outcome

1. Mechanisms of Swallowing
2. Role in Speech Production
3. Interaction with the Respiratory System

Throat physiology entails the complex processes of interaction between various anatomical structures, like the pharynx, larynx, and the muscles that encircle them. At the center of these mechanisms lies the action of the larynx, or voice box, which not only facilitates phonation but also has protective functions to fulfill during swallowing. The laryngeal skeleton comprises several cartilages, which harbor the vocal folds. These folds close and open rhythmically, and by this process, modulation of pitch and volume is accomplished in speech. Additionally, coordination of the laryngeal muscles is also crucial to successful vocal performance, as demonstrated by research on how knowledge of laryngeal anatomy is helpful in sustaining vocal health for students pursuing performing arts and speech-language pathology training, whereby instruments like nasendoscopic examination can play a very significant role in improving knowledge of functional vocal mechanisms (Andrade et al., 2023). Within the field of voice health, throat physiology is complemented by the requirement for proper vocal hygiene. Results studying vocal hygiene training among professional voice users have yielded significant improvement in self-rated vocal attributes following such therapy. Vocal hygiene training discusses strategies to reduce vocal strain, hydrate properly, and avoid abusive practices that may lead to voice disorders. Surprisingly, ratings of voice quality by listeners did not show a significant gain after training, but subjective observer reports of improved awareness and proficiency in producing the voice were recorded. This disparity shows the subtlety of vocal dynamics, where internal feelings about voice quality are not always related to external perception (Wait, 1999). Hence, it is essential to understand the physiological basis of the throat in order to ensure vocal health, most importantly among individuals who use their voice for occupational purposes. Moreover, the interplay between the throat's anatomical structures and their physiological functions is essential while considering the impact of various vocal practices. For instance, actors and singers can benefit from a finer understanding of how control of phonation is achieved through variations in laryngeal position and respiratory support. Courses like Seeing Voices illustrate how teamwork approaches to vocal instruction increase laryngeal function knowledge and enhance good technique. By observing true real-time laryngeal maneuvers and discussing their applications, students better understand the physiological processes that govern their art. This interdisciplinarity not only fosters more extensive vocal practice but also facilitates more extended interprofessional cooperation among individuals who are working with the throat and larynx in both clinical and artistic contexts (Andrade et al., 2023). Thus, ongoing research into throat physiology remains at the forefront of framing both educational and practical applications within the context of voice health and performance.

10.3.1. Mechanisms of Swallowing

The mechanisms of swallowing are extremely intricate, coordinated processes involving both voluntary and involuntary mechanisms, requiring the precise coordination of over 30 muscles and nerves. Swallowing is anatomically separated into three autonomous phases: oral, pharyngeal, and esophageal. During the oral phase, food is manipulated and directed onto the posterior part of the throat, where it passes into the pharyngeal phase. The bolus also triggers a series of reflex responses, such as elevation of the soft palate to prevent nasal regurgitation and closure of the vocal cords to protect the airway. This multistage process is important not only for the proper swallowing but also for safety, as it decreases the danger of aspiration, which can generate serious pulmonary complications, notably in risky groups such as the elderly or subjects affected by neurological impairments. Following the pharyngeal phase, the esophageal phase is activated, where peristaltic esophageal movements propel the bolus towards the stomach. This phenomenon is to a large degree involuntary, being controlled by intricate neuromuscular coordination between the lower and upper esophageal sphincters. Coordination between these sphincters ensures that the bolus glides smoothly without causing reflux from the stomach back into the esophagus. Dysphagia, or difficulty swallowing, arises when there is a structurally or functionally abnormal element somewhere in this timeframe, impairing the patient's ability to move food from the mouth, through the pharynx, and into the esophagus. Looking at the implications of dysphagia on health, such as malnutrition and increased rates of infection, understanding the mechanisms of swallowing becomes crucial with respect to the management and treatment of the disorder in affected individuals (Gabriela et al., 2014). Research currently indicates that the texture of food and its implications on swallowing mechanisms, with changes being important in respect to making it safer for dysphagic patients.

For instance, thickener addition, such as xanthan gum or starch, alters the liquid's viscosity and has the potential to modify oral transit time and swallowing bolus duration. Some research has shown that a higher concentration of thickeners results in a longer duration of swallowing, and that starch thickener shows significantly different properties compared to xanthan gum thickener (Cook et al., 2019). These findings are crucial to food development to provide both safe and acceptable dysphagia food, since food's mechanical properties directly influence swallowing effectiveness. Thus, an intimate knowledge of swallowing mechanisms not only contributes to clinical assessment but also informs dietary management to maximize patient safety without nutrient deprivation (Figure 10.6).

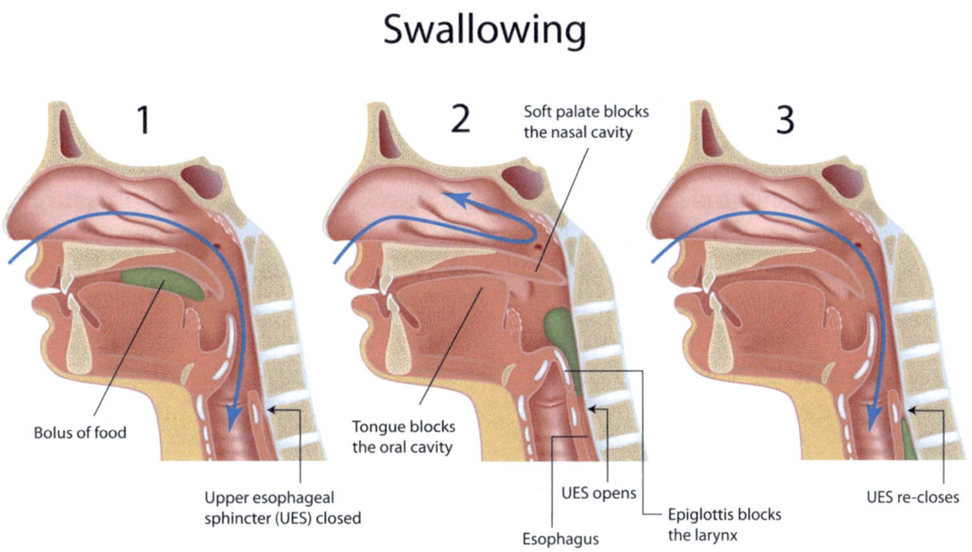

Figure 10.6. The mechanisms of swallowing.

Source: https://www.physio-pedia.com/images/9/9d/Swallow_2.png.

10.3.2. Role in Speech Production

The anatomy and physiology of the larynx and throat constitute the foundation of speech production, and the larynx, or voice box, houses the vocal cords whose vibration is the very foundation of making sound. When air passes through the glottis, the space between the vocal cords, it causes them to vibrate, and thus the sound waves are created. This sound is subsequently shaped into speech by articulators, including the tongue, lips, and palate. Moreover, tension and position of the vocal cords are controlled by intrinsic and extrinsic laryngeal muscles, thereby affecting pitch and tone. These physiological details mark the larynx's dual role as a source and a modulator of sound, enabling speech to be expressive and subtle. It is necessary to comprehend these functions for use in such fields as vocal training and speech-language pathology, where optimizing vocal performance and health is the goal. In the field of vocal health, the interaction between speech production and laryngeal anatomy is of primary importance. It is indicated in the literature that there must be an understanding of laryngeal function in order to maintain vocal quality and prevent disorders of vocal overuse and misuse. For instance, learning programs such as Seeing Voices emphasize the importance of integrating interprofessional knowledge into voice studies, thereby contributing to a more comprehensive understanding of laryngeal anatomy among performing arts and speech therapy students. In these environments, laryngostroboscopic examinations provide immediate feedback about the movement and functioning of the vocal cords, implying the necessity for healthy laryngeal habits. This meeting of knowledge is two-pronged: offering would-be vocalists and speech therapists the tools for effective communication and general voice health through practice guided by knowledge (Andrade et al., 2023). The dynamic relationship between the larynx and speech production is anatomical as well as behavioral. Vocalizations by other animals suggest a higher communication system based on anatomical constraints, similar to that of humans. Dogs, as observed in studies, possess a multitude of vocalizations corresponding to specific states or needs, and their vocal quality is generally determined by their physiology and affective states (Adachi et al., 2014). Such comparative analysis reveals that mechanisms involved in speech production are universal and move beyond human capabilities, further substantiating the basic entwining of anatomy and interspecies communication. Understanding the anatomical and physiological foundations of speech production reinforces our knowledge of these processes, providing depth to both human verbal communication and animal vocalization. It is ultimately needed to support effective interventions and practices in speech and communication disorders.

10.3.3. Interaction with the Respiratory System

The intricate relationship between the larynx and throat with the respiratory system is the foundation of learning their anatomy and physiology. The throat, or pharynx, is a conduit for both food and air, allowing for respiration and digestion as well as protection of the airway from aspiration during swallowing. The larynx, which takes up the upper portion of the trachea, plays a central role in the control of airways and speech production. When one inhales air, air flows through the laryngeal inlet, promoting gas exchange in the lungs. The coordination of muscle contractions between the structures of the larynx also regulates airflow and sound generation, illustrating the larynx's dual role in respiratory function and speech. In the case of obstructive sleep apnea syndrome (OSAS), coordination between the respiratory system and throat is of particular interest. Surgical treatments aimed at mitigating OSAS generally involve changes in upper airway anatomy to facilitate airflow. For instance, computational fluid dynamics models show marked alterations in airflow patterns and pressure distributions in the upper airway post-surgery and reveal how anatomical changes influence respiratory efficiency (Dahl et al., 2017). Such discoveries have wide-ranging implications for throat anatomy, airway obstructions, and respiratory health. Moreover, examination of these dynamics helps develop more effective treatment protocols tailored to the patient's individual anatomical variations and presentations. Integration of new technologies into the science of vocalization and communication behavior highlights the complex interactions between the respiratory mechanism and the throat/larynx. Quantitative and qualitative studies have begun to quantify the effect that voice recognition systems and artificial speech technology impose on respiratory function and the practice of communication (Fón et al., 2018). For instance, the emotional reaction of listeners to diverse aspects of voice illustrates how variation in voice production can be governed by respiratory mechanics. This communication between technology and human physiological responses offers potential directions for enhancing therapeutic practice in voice disorders and respiratory disease, highlighting the ongoing significance of studying the human throat and larynx in the broader context of respiratory well-being and communication (Figure 10.7).

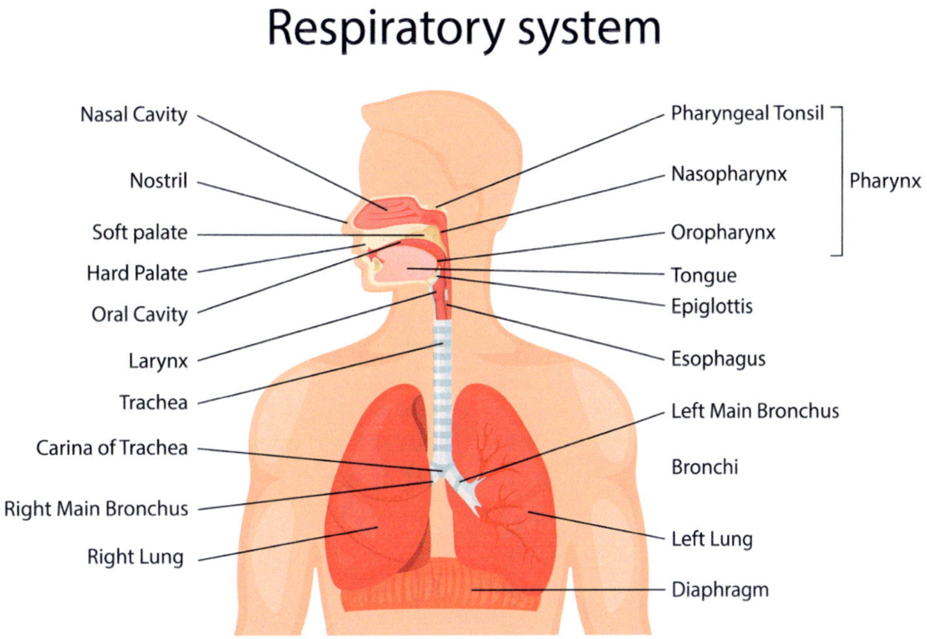

Figure 10.7. The intricate relationship between the throat and larynx and the respiratory system.

Source: https://img.livestrong.com/-/cme-data/getty/4c2353c0986b4d2c8381c8a624df96f5.jpg.

Test Your Knowledge

1. Explain the functions of the pharynx, including its roles in swallowing, respiration, and speech.
2. Describe the physiological mechanisms of swallowing and protection of the airway by the throat structures, including the soft palate and epiglottis.

10.4. Physiology of the Larynx

Learning Outcome

1. Sound Production and Modulation
2. Protective Functions During Swallowing
3. Role in Regulating Airflow

The larynx, also known as the voice box, is responsible for phonation or the generation of sound. The intricate structure is made up of a number of cartilages, muscles, and ligaments and rests at the top of the trachea, below the pharynx. The main cartilaginous framework consists of the thyroid, cricoid, and arytenoid cartilages. These structures are arranged strategically to facilitate movement while allowing the different movements needed to modulate pitch and volume during speech. The tension and positioning of the vocal folds are regulated by the coordination of intrinsic and extrinsic laryngeal muscles so that individuals may generate differentiated vocal tones. Besides this, the larynx also serves protective functions as a safeguard to keep food and foreign objects from entering the trachea when swallowing, a system crucial for not aspirating and keeping the respiratory process going. Apart from speech production, the larynx is also significant in the respiratory system. Its anatomical design permits the regulation of airflow during breathing. When air passes through the laryngeal passage, the vocal folds can adduct or abduct and thus control the passage of air during the process of vocalization. The mucous lining of the larynx contains sensory receptors that are sensitive to irritation or changes in airflow and trigger defense reflexes such as coughing or throat clearing. Furthermore, advances in medical science, particularly in otorhinolaryngology, have improved our understanding of laryngeal physiology, enabling more effective treatment of laryngeal diseases and conditions that interfere with voice quality and respiratory function (Américo et al., 2007). This combination of anatomical and physiological insights underscores the importance of the larynx beyond phonation. Its complex anatomy also allows it to fulfill its role in communication, not just in humans, but even in certain animal species. Its application in the source-filter theory of voice production proves that the larynx serves not just as a sound producer but also as a filter, modifying numerous acoustic properties based on physiological parameters and environmental conditions. For instance, the vocal behavior of domestic dogs demonstrates that barks can communicate specific information about emotional states and intentions, reflecting a deviation from their ancestral counterpart, the wolf (Adachi et al., 2014). That it occurs evidences the communicative function of voice structures, broadening the understanding of the role of the larynx beyond human phonation to an interspecies communication context. As research advances continue to intensify, there is no question that laryngeal anatomy and physiology have central roles in vocalization and social interaction among different species.

10.4.1. Sound Production and Modulation

The intricate processes of sound production and modulation in the larynx and pharynx are central to understanding human voice. Sound is primarily produced by the vibration of the vocal folds within the larynx as airflow from the lungs creates sound waves. The mechanism is governed by physiological factors, including the tension and length of the vocal folds, which can be manipulated to produce various pitch and intensity levels. Besides, the shape of the vocal tract, including the throat, mouth, and nasal chambers, is a resonating space that contributes significantly to the quality of voice. Hence, the structure of the larynx and its associated structures are significant in modulating sound to allow for subtle variation required in speech and other human vocal communication, compared to other animals that lack such complexity during sound production. The uniqueness of human vocalization is also emphasized by the absence of anatomical features in other primates, particularly lateral ventricular air sacs. These air sacs, retained in extant great apes, are involved in sound property modification, possibly adding resonance during production. On the contrary, the evolutionary loss of such sacks in human beings has been posited as a paramount aspect that triggered the development of advanced spoken language. Studies of great apes indicate that vocal production does not necessarily rely on these air sacs and may instead employ other physiological adaptations. The awareness of these variations improves our comprehension of sound modulation, suggesting that the evolution of the human larynx provided the foundation for complex communication, making human beings different from other creatures (Trenbeath, 2021). The modulation of sound does not only involve anatomy, but also encompasses learned behavior and environmental influences. For instance, human beings alter their speech based on social contexts, emotional cues, and even the presence of the audience. This ability to change pitch, tone, and volume based on varying stimuli has the effect of highlighting the cognitive aspect of vocalization. In addition, research with domestic dogs also demonstrates the way in which vocal outputs can convey some information, capturing physiological limitations and altering emotional states (Adachi et al.,

2014). Such communication, through such interaction, shows a high level of acoustic ability with animals, including human beings, to highlight the interplay between biology and behavior in generating sound. As studies on the production and modulation of sound continue to grow, they offer avenues of explanation not only for human speech but for vocalizations in other species and therefore add to knowledge of anatomy and physiology in a wider ecological background (Figure 10.8).

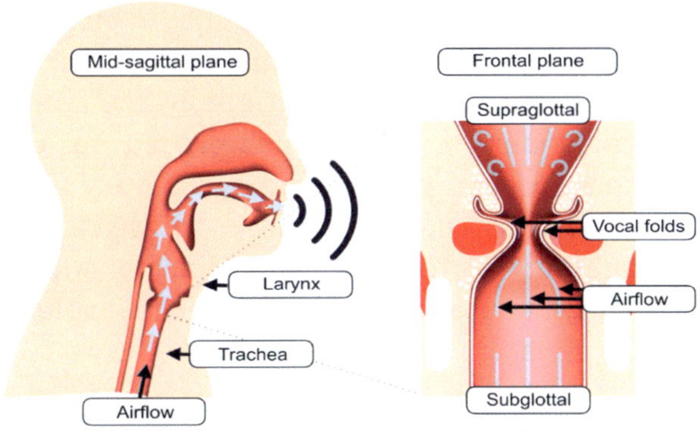

Figure 10.8. The intricate mechanisms of sound production and modulation in the throat and larynx.

Source: https://www.mdpi.com/applsci/applsci-09-01963/article_deploy/html/images/applsci-09-01963-g001.png.

10.4.2. Protective Functions During Swallowing

Swallowing is a highly developed physiological process that comprises numerous protective functions responsible for the prevention of aspiration and safe arrival of food in the stomach. The larynx and throat are central components of this process, managing muscular contractions and reflexes to safeguard the airway. The epiglottis, a cartilaginous flap found at the back of the tongue, is very important for swallowing; it folds down over the trachea and closes the passage, and in doing so, keeps the food or fluid from entering the lungs. This is particularly vital for the lungs, as any compromise here could lead to aspiration pneumonia, a serious complication because food particles can enter the trachea. As the swallowing reflex starts, oropharyngeal and laryngeal sensory input alerts the brainstem to trigger protective airway closure, exemplifying the highly developed interaction between structures and mechanisms. In pediatric swallowing, protective functions also include additional elements due to the unique challenges faced by young patients. Neonates exhibit reflexive patterns of swallowing, initially involuntary, which rely on the anatomy of the larynx and throat to pass through automatically during feeding. As development occurs in children, they gain voluntary control over the oral phases of swallowing but preserve involuntary response for the pharyngeal and esophageal phases. These protective mechanisms could be lost as a result of complications such as gastroesophageal reflux or congenital anomaly, which places children at high risk for aspiration. The significance of such protective processes is underscored in clinical evaluation, where procedures such as the Video Fluoroscopic Swallow Study (VFSS) enable clinicians to examine live swallowing behaviors and facilitate the identification of dysfunctions that can compromise these vital protective processes (Piazza D et al., 2019). Protective functions during swallowing extend beyond anatomical structures to include the implications of swallowing disorders. Protective mechanisms can be compromised severely by dysphagia and other disorders, leading to severe health implications like malnutrition and respiratory-related problems. The larynx and throat coordinate intricate reflexes during swallowing, thereby guarding the airway while allowing food and liquids to pass. With dysphagia, protective reflexes are compromised, and there is a greater chance of aspiration as well as complications. Therefore, the assessment and rehabilitation of swallowing functions are essential in clinical practice, particularly in high-risk populations such as children (Piazza D et al., 2019). This accounts for the significance of the interplay between anatomic integrity and physiological function in the upkeep of safe swallowing practices among various population groups.

10.4.3. Role in Regulating Airflow

The throat and larynx play a vital role in regulating airflow, an activity essential for numerous physiological processes, including respiration, phonation, and airway protection. The voice box or the larynx acts as a pathway for airflow from the trachea to the lungs. Its intricate structure, composed of various cartilages and muscles, allows it to open and close during breathing, thus allowing air to enter while preventing foreign material from penetrating the lower respiratory tract. Its selective control of airflow ensures oxygen is delivered to the lungs to the needed degree, and pharyngeal and laryngeal reflexes, such as coughing and swallowing, are properly coordinated in ensuring the airway is protected. This dynamic role underscores the significance of the larynx as not only a fundamental component of speech but also a critical component of respiratory health. The role of the throat in managing airflow is more than what occurs within laryngeal tissues. The pharynx is both an air passage and a food passageway that serves to direct airflow towards the larynx while simultaneously preventing food and fluids from entering. Its muscular walls can relax and close, permitting air to pass through it, and play an important role in phonation by modifying the shape and size of the airway. Additionally, as air passes through the pharynx, it plays an important role in modifying the quality of vocal resonance, and it is of paramount importance in singing and speaking. Equally important is the coordination of the throat and larynx. A normally functioning pharynx can optimize vocal quality and assist in efficient airflow regulation to enhance overall sound production ability in speech and singing—considerations further elaborated in Baum (2023). In the clinical setting, understanding how airflow regulation is utilized is central to most otolaryngological procedures. Laryngeal or pharyngeal surgery requires meticulous airway management to prevent compromising the airway patency and visibility during surgery. Anesthetic choice, that is, general or local, can potentially profoundly influence the patient's comfort level as well as the success of the surgery, as discussed in Cecot et al. (2024). For example, a local anesthetic can reduce operating time and hospital stays, which are particularly advantageous in cases involving narrow airway control. Additionally, the ability to manage airflow during such procedures can lead to improved postoperative recovery rates and patient satisfaction. Thus, the physiology and anatomy of the throat and larynx should be well understood, emphasizing their role in airflow control (Figure 10.9).

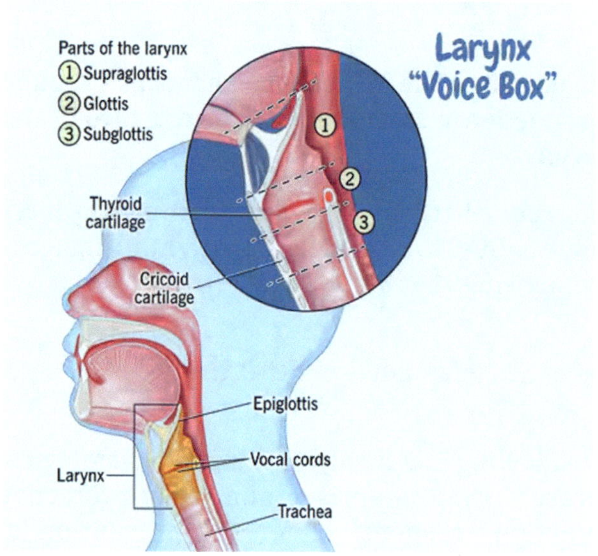

Figure 10.9. The throat and larynx play a pivotal role in regulating airflow.

Source: https://cache.careers360.mobi/media/articles/uploads/froala_editor/images/2024/8/21/1724249234579.png.

Test Your Knowledge

1. Explain the role of the larynx in phonation, including how the vocal cords produce sound and regulate pitch and volume.
2. Describe the functions of the larynx in respiration and airway protection, including mechanisms that prevent aspiration during swallowing.

10.5. Common Disorders of the Throat

Learning Outcome

1. Pharyngitis and Its Causes
2. Tonsillitis and Its Implications
3. Impact of Allergies on Throat Health

Throat disorders are also common disorders that encompass a wide variety of conditions capable of impeding vocal functioning as well as general health. Laryngitis, for example, is an inflammation and infection of the larynx caused by viral infections, voice overuse, or irritants, and which is characterized by hoarseness, sore throat, and difficulty in speaking. Chronic laryngitis occurs in individuals who regularly abuse their voice, such as professional speakers or singers. Recognition of the underlying relationship between anatomy and such disorders is essential for effective management and treatment. A precise understanding of laryngeal anatomy enhances vocal health and facilitates early diagnosis of conditions like laryngitis, thus decreasing long-term vocal handicap (Andrade et al., 2023). Teachers and healthcare professionals can better support individuals in voice-dependent vocations by raising awareness of common disorders and their physiological underpinnings. Another common throat condition is vocal cord nodules, also known as singers' nodules. This noncancerous growth occurs as a result of vocal strain or misuse and is characterized by the development of callous-like lesions on the vocal cords. Individuals with sustained or inappropriate vocal use, such as teachers and performers, are most vulnerable. The presence of nodules can lead to hoarseness, voice fatigue, and even voice pain during singing or speech. The relationship between vocal technique, laryngeal function, and nodule formation brings to the fore the importance of proper vocal hygiene habits (Vetter, 2016). Curricula in vocal pedagogy emphasize the study of vocal anatomy and throat hygiene, progressing from reactive methods to preventive measures that can minimize the risk of developing such disorders. Apart from laryngitis and vocal cord nodules, throat conditions such as gastroesophageal reflux disease (GERD) can affect the quality of the voice and throat health quite directly. GERD is when stomach acid frequently backs up into the esophagus, causing inflammation of the larynx and throat. The reflux creates symptoms such as chronic cough, throat clearing, and sensation of lump in the throat, also called globus sensation. Awareness of the physiologic mechanisms of GERD contributes to the recognition of its impact on vocal health. For vocal professionals, good vocal hygiene is critical, as poor habits exacerbate GERD. Educational interventions and awareness are necessary to ensure that singers and speakers adopt strategies to minimize reflux symptoms and protect voice health (Andrade et al., 2023).

10.5.1. Pharyngitis and Its Causes

Pharyngitis, an inflammation of the pharynx, is a prevalent disease seen among members of different age groups, often causing discomfort and various clinical manifestations. Mostly classified as acute or chronic, acute pharyngitis is typically caused by infectious agents, primarily viruses such as rhinoviruses, adenoviruses, and influenza viruses, although bacterial agents, such as Group A Streptococcus, may also significantly contribute to its pathogenesis. The inflammation leads to clinically apparent symptoms, like sore throat, dysphagia, and lymphadenopathy, which may profoundly affect the quality of life of affected individuals. This intricate interaction between infectious agents and the body's immune mechanisms complicates the clinical diagnosis and management of pharyngitis, underscoring the importance of the anatomy and physiology of the throat and larynx, as these organs are central to the disease's pathophysiology (Brancato et al., 2015). The pharyngeal anatomical configuration, including complex mucosal lining and positioning of lymphoid tissues, contributes to susceptibility and immune reaction against potential pathogens. Pharyngeal tonsils, located at the nasopharyngeal opening, function as a first line of defense by harboring invading microorganisms and initiating local immunity. This anatomical process is particularly evident in the context of infection, leading to inflammation and tonsillar hypertrophy in conditions such as pharyngitis. Moreover, the interrelationship between respiratory processes and immunity highlights the importance of understanding pharyngitis in the context of infections of the upper respiratory tract. Acute infections of the upper airways are prone to elicit a cascade of symptoms, making the presentation and treatment of pharyngitis both clinically challenging, and can also induce secondary processes such as sinusitis or otitis media, particularly in pediatric populations (Anubala, 2017). Chronic pharyngitis, as compared to the acute type, has a tendency to be associated with irritation over long periods or environmental exposures like smoking, allergens, or gastroesophageal reflux disease (GERD). These conditions can result in chronic irritation and inflammation, manifesting as a sensation of a lump in the throat, chronic cough, or hoarseness. Treatment for chronic pharyngitis needs a multidisciplinary approach, not just to relieve symptoms but also to treat the etiology. Lifestyle modifications like cessation of smoking, fluid intake, and dietary modifications can benefit patients to reduce reflux symptoms. Knowledge of the interrelationships between anatomical structures and the multifactorial pathogenesis of pharyngitis is critical to the development of effective treatment strategies, as it enables targeted interventions that improve symptoms and outcomes in patients with this condition (Brancato et al., 2015) (Figure 10.10).

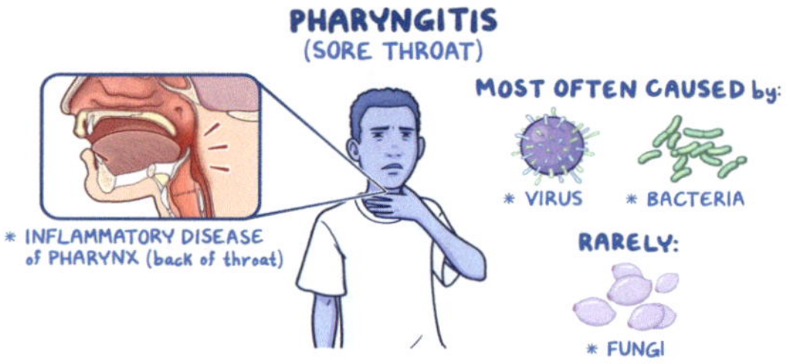

Figure 10.10. Pharyngitis, an inflammatory condition of the pharynx.

Source: https://d16qt3wv6xm098.cloudfront.net/4W8GpiltRN2F2UIjAdIcw5u5RcuA1Yvc/_.jpg.

10.5.2. Tonsillitis and Its Implications

Tonsillitis, characterized by the inflammation of the palatine tonsils, is a significant clinical condition that deals with the anatomy and physiology of the throat. Lymphoid tissue is a significant part of the body's immune defense against pathogens entering through the oral cavity and nasal pathway. When the tonsils become chronically inflamed, as in recurrent attacks of tonsillitis, they can cause a wide range of complications, including obstructive sleep apnea and swallowing dysfunction. Because of the anatomical position of the tonsils, in between the anterior and posterior oropharyngeal pillars, the tonsils are susceptible to infection, particularly by streptococcal and viral pathogens. Hence, understanding the underlying physiological mechanisms of tonsillitis is important for diagnosing and treating its myriad implications, particularly in children, who are most frequently affected. Aside from the initial physical discomfort, the implications of untreated or recurring tonsillitis can extend far and wide and affect quality of life and overall health. The chronically inflamed tonsils can potentially result in chronic mouth breathing, excessive snoring, and disruption of sleeping patterns, leading to neurocognitive and learning issues in pediatric patients. According to one study, chronic adenoiditis, most frequently associated with tonsillitis, may result in daytime somnolence and a deficiency in attention, hence supporting the need for acute symptom control and potential surgical treatment. Adenoidectomy, for instance, has been shown to be quite relieving, enhancing the quality of life in patients who have severe cases of *adenotonsillitis* (Jagan, 2017). The medical treatment not only addresses the immediate physical obstruction but also avoids the long-term health effects of undiagnosed tonsillar disease. In addition to physical health issues, the psychological aspects of tonsillitis need to be mentioned. Chronic throat infection may lead to heightened anxiety and tension, particularly for teenagers who face social ramifications, such as embarrassment or social isolation, due to their condition. Furthermore, there is greater awareness of the interconnection between chronic illness and mental well-being, closing the distance between physiological signs and psychological distress. Applying a holistic treatment strategy through combined medical and psychological interventions can enhance the overall recovery rate. This is an opinion that emphasizes seeing tonsillitis' multi-disciplinary effects, with collaboration between various disciplines such as otolaryngology, psychology, and education, whose aim is to achieve maximum patient outcomes (Sell, K., & Sell, K., 2003). Finally, extensive knowledge and management approaches are required to address the far-reaching effects that tonsillitis has on individuals, particularly those in vulnerable populations.

10.5.3. Impact of Allergies on Throat Health

Allergies greatly affect the throat's health and, in fact, induce inflammation and irritation in the throat or larynx. When people are exposed to allergens such as pollen, dust mites, or pet dander, they experience a line of physiological reactions, primarily the release of histamines. This reaction typically presents as throat swelling and soreness, making it difficult to speak or swallow. In severe cases, postnasal drip develops and can cause further irritation and an increased risk of laryngitis. Thus, individuals with allergy will tend to develop chronic throat conditions that may exacerbate underlying voice difficulties, particularly among professional voice users such as teachers and singers, who are already vulnerable to voice strain and vocal problems, as postulated in the associated literature (DOCKS N at University T of Carolina N at Greensboro et al., 2005). In addition, the relationship between throat health and allergy is further complicated by exposure to natural and environmental factors. For instance, living in highly allergenic or damp environments is likely to exacerbate the negative impact on the larynx and throat. In a study of teachers, the findings showed that awareness of the anatomy and physiology of the voice and vocal hygiene practices is essential in preventing voice disorders related to allergies (Vetter, 2016). Unmanaged allergies could lead to chronic throat irritation, thus complicating the process of vocal performance and training even more. This underscores the importance of integrating allergen management into voice teaching and encouraging the development of strategies to address the needs of individuals prone to throat-related health complications.

Preventive measures and effective management are necessary in cases of sufferers of allergies to ensure overall throat wellness. By educating individuals about their condition, including vocal hygiene and anatomical awareness, one can better adapt to the complications associated with allergies. Practices involving hydration maintenance, reduced exposure to known allergens, and the utilization of antihistamines can help alleviate the symptoms. Secondly, the voice teachers' and clinicians' discussion on the topic of allergy impacts can lead to opening the door for healthier vocal practices among professionals and students. A preventative approach to voice training, both in terms of anatomy and allergy control, has to be at the forefront of ensuring sustained long-term vocal well-being, ultimately enabling individuals to maintain a healthy and efficient vocal instrument (Vetter, 2016) (Figure 10.11).

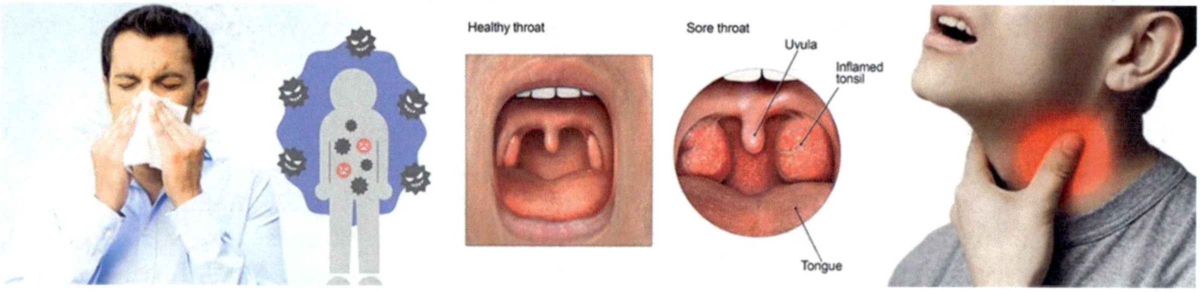

Figure 10.11. Allergies can significantly impact throat health.

Source: https://www.internationaldrugmart.com/wp-content/uploads/2024/02/1422024-Blog-Image-Can-allergies-cause-sore-throat-1024x236.webp.

Test Your Knowledge

1. How does the larynx contribute to voice production (phonation), and what roles do the vocal cords, respiratory airflow, and laryngeal muscles play in modulating sound?
2. Explain the protective functions of the larynx, including its role in preventing aspiration and regulating airflow during swallowing and respiration.

10.6. Common Disorders of the Larynx

Learning Outcome

1. Laryngitis and Its Symptoms
2. Vocal Cord Nodules and Their Effects
3. Cancer of the Larynx and Treatment Options

The larynx, the critical structure in the throat, is open to various common diseases that have a significant impact on voice production, breathing, and swallowing. Laryngitis is the most prevalent of these conditions, with redness of the laryngeal mucosa typically caused by viral infections, excessive vocal use, or irritants such as smoke. Acute laryngitis will typically have signs and symptoms of hoarseness, throat pain, and dry cough, while chronic laryngitis may result from prolonged exposure to irritants or gastroesophageal reflux disease (GERD). The cause and treatment of laryngitis must be known in order to prevent as well as treat further complications, for example, vocal cord nodules or polyps, in an extensive manner (Américo et al., 2007). Another common laryngeal condition is vocal cord nodules, benign growths that appear on the vocal folds due to chronic voice abuse or overuse, often in teachers and singers. Nodules produce distortion of normal voicing, leading to hoarseness, vocal fatigue, and reduction of vocal range. Vocal therapy is most often the initial treatment modality, with a focus on correcting vocal technique and relieving vocal strain. More severe cases where therapy fails may require surgery to remove the growths and restore normal functioning. Management of such disorders involves voice therapy, behavioral modification, and education on safe vocal use (Cook et al., 2019). Laryngeal cancer, although not as common as other disorders, is associated with great health risks and should be treated early. This malignancy also presents classically with the triad of hoarseness, dysphagia, and weight loss, typically in the background of lifestyle factors such as tobacco and alcohol abuse. Early detection by endoscopic examination and biopsy significantly improves prognosis, as treatment typically consists of multi-modality therapy with surgery, radiation, and chemotherapy. Knowledge of the risk factors and education regarding laryngeal health can contribute to early diagnosis and improvement of the patient's overall prognosis (Américo et al., 2007).

10.6.1. Laryngitis and Its Symptoms

Laryngitis refers to inflammation of the larynx, characterized by symptoms such as hoarseness, voice loss, and pain in the throat. The larynx, positioned at the apex of the respiratory tract, is an extremely significant structure for phonation and tracheal closure against food aspiration. Inflammation in the area will result in severe vocal strain and disrupt normal speech patterns. Most frequently caused by infection, overuse, or irritants such as smoke, laryngitis can become both acute and chronic. Its identification is also important, as acute presentations can often be readily managed with hydration and rest, whereas chronic laryngitis may indicate underlying conditions such as gastroesophageal reflux disease (GERD), which affects vocal quality and health.

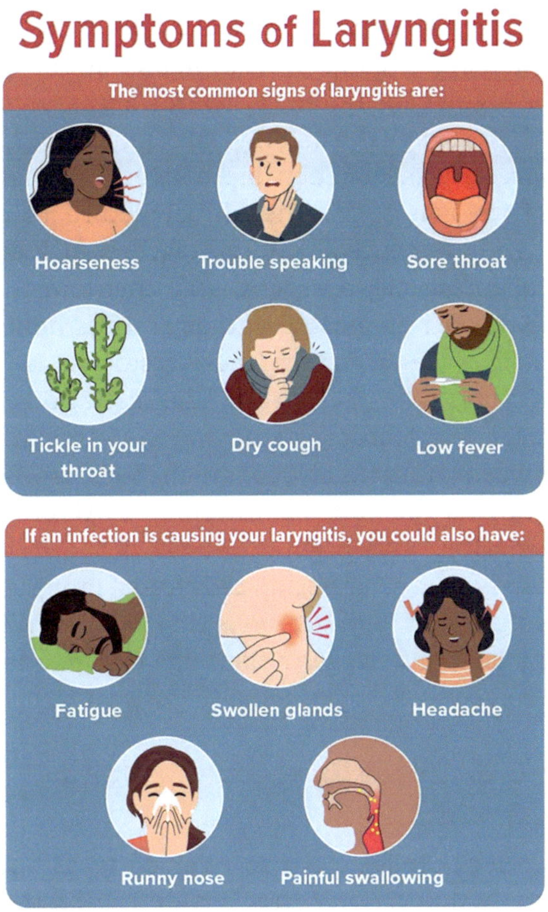

Figure 10.12. Laryngitis and its symptoms.

Source: https://img.lb.wbmdstatic.com/vim/live/webmd/consumer_assets/site_images/article_thumbnails/infographics/symptoms_of_laryngitis_infographic/650x1113_webmd_laryngitis_infographic.jpg.

Aside from hoarseness, laryngitis patients might also show symptoms such as a chronic cough, a parched throat, or a feeling of constriction. These result from swollen tissues and vocal folds, which impair airflow and sound output. For those engaged in vocally stressful jobs, such as teaching or singing, these symptoms can introduce serious work-related issues, creating a feedback cycle in which vocal stress worsens the condition. Furthermore, the tolerance of these symptoms can create anxiety and tension regarding performing with the voice, affecting personal as well as professional relationships. It is significant in the context of the laryngeal and pharyngeal anatomy and physiology to appreciate the relationship between laryngitis and its symptoms. The ultrastructure of the larynx is influenced by multiple factors, including viral infections, allergens, and environmental habits such as alcohol and cigarette smoking, which cause laryngitis. These factors must be appreciated for therapeutic administration and prevention. Moreover, studying the association between laryngitis and conditions such as GERD highlights the complex interplay between the respiratory and gastrointestinal systems. The inter-system relationship calls for an integrated resolution of laryngeal health as well as voice disorders and suggests thorough examinations in voice-related symptoms (Figure 10.12).

10.6.2. Vocal Cord Nodules and Their Effects

Singer's nodules are also referred to as vocal cord nodules. They are symmetric, bilateral nodules that develop on the vocal cords due to voice misuse or overuse. They are caused by prolonged vocal strain, which leads to an imbalance of the force of the vocal fold closure during phonation. This condition affects individuals in vocations that require extensive vocal use, such as teachers, singers, and public speakers. This ensuing inflammation could disrupt the regular vibratory activity of the vocal cords, thus affecting the voice quality. Vocal cord nodules can produce a number of different symptoms, such as hoarseness, vocal fatigue, and decreased ability to project, all in total their quality of life and communication. Physiologically, the implication of vocal cord nodules is significant because the lesions in themselves can change the aerodynamics of phonation. When nodules do appear, the altered mass and stiffness of the vocal fold cover create a maladaptive vibratory pattern, rendering the voice breathy or strained. This can create enhanced vocal effort and fatigue, as singers and speaker will attempt to compensate for voice change. Furthermore, prolonged exposure to vocal strain can further deteriorate the nodules, resulting in a vicious cycle of malfunction wherein the individual is no longer able to produce sound and consequently affects the vocal mechanics negatively. This understanding about the physiological outcome is necessary for developing an efficient treatment plan, such as vocal hygiene behaviors, to avoid risk and improve vocal wellness. Aside from the challenge posed by vocal cord nodules, other treatments, such as vocal hygiene training, have also been explored to facilitate recovery and improve voice quality. Research has shown that vocal hygiene training does not appear to cause large perceptual differences in voice quality rated by listeners, but it does offer important advantages to self-reporting patients who suffer from vocal complaints. In particular, directed vocal training methods, including relaxation techniques and altered phonation strategies, may be able to reduce tension and restore the vocal folds to optimal function. In cases when vocal strain cannot be avoided, for example, in the school or performance context, these methods can help people manage their vocal health themselves. As per related literature, one has to constantly enhance practices and knowledge concerning vocal health in order to help individuals affected by such disorders so that they may speak effectively and confidently (Wait, 1999).

10.6.3. Cancer of the Larynx and Treatment Options

Laryngeal carcinoma, a significant problem in the field of otorhinolaryngology, is predominantly expressed as squamous cell carcinoma, the cause of the majority of laryngeal cancers. Cancers can occur in the glottic, supraglottic, or subglottic regions, with variations in incidence rates mostly attributable to risk factors related to cigarette smoking and excessive alcohol consumption. A better understanding of laryngeal and throat anatomy and physiology has contributed significantly to the early diagnosis of this condition, which is crucial for effective therapy. Hoarseness, difficulty in swallowing, and a persistent sore throat are the characteristic symptoms that bring the patient to the doctor. Early diagnosis by laryngoscopy can identify lesions that guide further evaluation and treatment plans. Injustices typically arise where patients take a long time to undergo treatment due to a lack of appreciation for the importance of prompt early medical care, highlighting the imperative need for public education about this disease. The treatment of laryngeal cancer is based on the stage and location of the tumor and is a multidisciplinary process that could involve surgery, radiation therapy, and chemotherapy. Surgical therapy often includes laryngectomy, partial to complete laryngectomy, with the possibility of greatly affecting the patient's ability to produce sound. Adjuvant therapy after surgery, such as radiotherapy, can be employed to eliminate microscopically disseminated cancer cells and eliminate the possibility of recurrence. Chemotherapy also has an adjunctive function in advanced or recurrent disease, to shrink tumors before surgical resection or to manage metastatic disease. New methods, including endoscopic laser surgery, are being researched to provide less invasive therapies with promising outcomes. Progress in treatment modalities in laryngology underscores the importance of ongoing innovation in medical technology and intervention methods, thereby enhancing the quality of care for affected patients. Emerging research highlights the detrimental effects of smoking and electronic nicotine delivery systems. Studies suggest that ENDS users show a pattern of abnormalities in laryngeal appearance and function, indicating potential risks similar to traditional smoking, which has long been established as a leading cause of laryngeal cancer (Sample, 2019). This relationship underscores the necessity for comprehensive treatment plans that not only address the cancer itself but also the lifestyle factors contributing to its development. Public health initiatives encouraging cessation of tobacco use and education regarding the harm caused by smoking and vaping are crucial for reducing the occurrence of laryngeal cancer. With the expanding body of medical knowledge, including these preventive interventions along with existing state-of-the-art treatment protocols, will be essential for improving patient outcomes and reducing the social burden of laryngeal malignancies (Américo et al., 2007).

Test Your Knowledge

1. What are the common laryngeal disorders, such as laryngitis, vocal cord nodules, polyps, and laryngeal cancer, and what are their typical causes and clinical features?
2. Explain the diagnosis and management strategies for common laryngeal disorders, including medical treatment, voice therapy, and surgical intervention.

SUMMARY

It is apparent that these structures not only perform basic life processes but also perform complex functions, such as speech and swallowing. Their minute anatomical patterns reveal interactions among various systems, illustrating how body structures enable essential functions. The description of the interaction explains how coordination is essential in such functions. Additionally, the data provide a basis for exploring pathologies that may arise when any of these systems are affected, underscoring the need for more thorough research on individual elements and their influence on overall laryngeal and throat health. Advances in imaging technology have significantly expanded our understanding of the anatomy of these structures. Techniques such as contrast-enhanced computed tomography have enabled the visualization of the larynx and throat with remarkable accuracy, hence allowing for more informed medical practice. For instance, through the application of advanced imaging methods, scientists can analyze the intricate skeletal and soft-tissue anatomy that plays critical roles in assessing normal and disease states. These imaging modalities also have therapeutic implications, as evidenced by studies that use computational fluid dynamics (CFD) to analyze airflow patterns following surgery. These have significant clinical decision-making implications, illustrating how anatomical variations can affect the outcome of treatment (Dahl et al., 2017). Future research directions will most likely involve further integration of technological advances with traditional anatomical studies. Investigating the three-dimensional morphologies of the larynx and throat, combined with computer simulations, will provide further insight into biomechanics and functional capacities. As the scientists delve deeper into the highly tuned equilibrium of the throat and laryngeal apparatus, knowledge of how these anatomical structures interact with neighboring tissues will be essential. As demonstrated by model-organism research, including studies of the African clawed frog, increased understanding of these systems is possible; interspecific comparisons also improve our understanding of evolutionary adaptation (Ahn et al., 2017). The importance of these studies highlights the ongoing need for interdisciplinary collaboration in research as well as clinical settings.

Laryngeal and throat physiology and anatomy are central to understanding other medical conditions, particularly those involving vocalization and swallowing. The larynx serves as a significant passage for air as well as a major factor in sound production. Medical conditions such as dysphagia, or swallowing difficulty, result from abnormalities in this intricate system. As highlighted, the earlier identification of dysphagia is more important, especially due to its association with high morbidity and mortality. Furthermore, the inherent subtlety of silent dysphagia presents additional challenges, necessitating rigorous screening procedures. Allaying these issues is central to improved patient outcomes, especially due to the fact that many screening procedures are subjective self-estimation that fails to capture subtle physiological changes crucial for diagnosis (Henderson, 2018). Furthermore, advances in clinical devices for the evaluation of laryngeal function will be required to bridge existing gaps in screening for dysphagia. The prospect of developing portable, non-invasive technology brings optimism to enhance diagnostic sensitivity without subjecting patients to invasive procedures. Newer work has included the creation of easy-to-use instruments to monitor laryngeal motion, which has promise for the assessment of swallowing dynamics. These devices can significantly democratize access to effective screening, enabling clinicians to more consistently and earlier identify swallowing disorders. By employing non-invasive techniques, health care providers are able to gain valuable information about patients with varied physiological presentations, hence better able to tailor treatment interventions (Henderson, 2018). Therapeutic interventions like laryngeal manual therapy (LMT) have also proved useful in voice disorder recovery due to muscular tension. Research has indicated that the application of LMT can yield measurable improvements in vocal quality and reductions in vocal tract discomfort. The outcomes, evaluated using acoustic measurements and perception ratings, indicate that these therapies should be included in treatment protocols for voice disorders. As established in relevant studies, LMT significantly reduced perturbation in conversational speech following treatment, demonstrating improvement in vocal function. The optimistic findings highlight the importance of understanding the physiological processes of voice production, thereby necessitating the integration of anatomy, therapy, and patient management in the field of throat and laryngeal health.

KEY TERMS FROM THIS CHAPTER

- Pharynx
- Oropharynx
- Larynx
- Vocal Cords
- Glottis
- Arytenoid Cartilages
- Cricoid Cartilage
- Cuneiform Cartilages
- Cricothyroid Membrane
- Nasopharynx
- Laryngopharynx
- Epiglottis
- Vestibular Folds
- Subglottis
- Thyroid Cartilage
- Corniculate Cartilages
- Hyoid Bone
- Recurrent Laryngeal Nerve

CRITICAL THINKING QUESTIONS

1. **Inflammation of the tonsils is called:**
   a) Pharyngitis
   b) Tonsillitis
   c) Adenoiditis
   d) Laryngitis
2. **The most common causative organism of acute bacterial tonsillitis is:**
   a) Streptococcus pyogenes
   b) Staphylococcus aureus
   c) Haemophilus influenzae
   d) Pseudomonas aeruginosa
3. **Tonsillar exudate is most commonly seen in:**
   a) Viral pharyngitis
   b) Bacterial tonsillitis
   c) Allergic reaction
   d) Fungal infection
4. **Peritonsillar abscess is also known as:**
   a) Quinsy
   b) Ludwig's angina
   c) Retropharyngeal abscess
   d) Epiglottitis
5. **The most common complication of untreated bacterial tonsillitis is:**
   a) Rheumatic fever
   b) Sinusitis
   c) Otitis externa
   d) Labyrinthitis

Short Answer Questions

1. What are the common diseases of the tonsils and pharynx, such as tonsillitis, peritonsillar abscess, and pharyngitis, and what are their usual causes?
2. Describe the clinical features and symptoms of tonsillar and pharyngeal diseases, including sore throat, dysphagia, fever, and enlargement of tonsils.
3. Explain the diagnostic methods for tonsillar and pharyngeal disorders, including throat examination, throat swab culture, and imaging when indicated.
4. Discuss the treatment options for tonsillar and pharyngeal diseases, including antibiotic therapy, surgical interventions (e.g., tonsillectomy), and supportive care.
5. What are the possible complications of untreated or recurrent tonsillar and pharyngeal diseases, such as peritonsillar abscess, rheumatic fever, and obstructive sleep apnea?

Answers to Critical Thinking Questions

1. (b) 2. (a) 3. (b) 4. (a) 5. (a)

REFERENCES

1. Abdelal, A. (2013). *Voice as a Parameter of Emotional and Physical Health.* https://core.ac.uk/download/48830815.pdf (accessed on 7th August 2025).
2. Taylor, A. M., Ratcliffe, V. F., McComb, K., & Reby, D. (2014). Auditory communication in domestic dogs. In *Elsevier eBooks* (pp. 131–163). https://doi.org/10.1016/b978-0-12-407818-5.00005-xAhn, C., Burgess, S., Burggren, W., Cannatella, D., Cannatella, G., Clemente, C., Cline, M., et al. (2017). *Digital dissection of the model organism Xenopus laevis using contrast-enhanced computed tomography.* https://core.ac.uk/download/96600364.pdf (accessed on 7th August 2025).
3. Akbudak, İ. H., & Mete, A. (2018). *Functional Anatomy and Physiology of Airway.* https://core.ac.uk/download/322437486.pdf (accessed on 7th August 2025).
4. Américo, R. dos R., Barauna Filho, I. S., Hermann, D. R., Nogueira Júnior, E., et al. (2007). *A brief history of otorhinolaryngology: Otology, laryngology and rhinology.* https://core.ac.uk/download/37707315.pdf (accessed on 7th August 2025).
5. Andrade, P. A., Cornelius, P., Fereday, L., Hall, T., et al. (2023). *Seeing voices: A dynamic, interprofessional approach to teaching performing arts and speech-language pathology students about vocal anatomy and physiology.* https://core.ac.uk/download/587251825.pdf (accessed on 7th August 2025).
6. Anubala, B. (2017). *Clinical evaluation of Sirupulladi Ennai (a siddha drug) for the treatment of Neerkana Mantham (URI) in children.* https://core.ac.uk/download/235669211.pdf (accessed on 7th August 2025).
7. Baken, R. J., Epstein, R., Hirani, S. P., Mathieson, L., et al. (2009). *Laryngeal manual therapy: A preliminary study to examine its treatment effects in the management of muscle tension dysphonia.* https://core.ac.uk/download/20540189.pdf (accessed on 7th August 2025).
8. Brancato, A., Cannizzaro, C., Cannizzaro, E., Ferrara, M., et al. (2015). *Upper respiratory tract infections in children: From case history to management.* https://core.ac.uk/download/53300409.pdf (accessed on 7th August 2025).
9. Cecot, J., Grajnert, F., Głuszczyk, A., Holdun, M., et al. (2024). *Local anesthesia as an alternative to general anesthesia in ENT surgery – A review of selected procedures.* https://core.ac.uk/download/620863083.pdf (accessed on 7th August 2025).
10. Clemm, H., Halvorsen, T., Heimdal, J. H., Røksund, H., et al. (2016). *Exercise Inducible Laryngeal Obstruction: Diagnostics and Management.* https://core.ac.uk/download/pdf/81173666.pdf (accessed on 7th August 2025).
11. Cook, M. T., Hamdy, S., Liu, F., McAuley, M., et al. (2019). *The swallowing characteristics of thickeners, jellies and yoghurt observed using an in vitro model.* https://core.ac.uk/download/287582259.pdf (accessed on 7th August 2025).
12. Dahl, S. K., Johnsen, S. G., Jordal, M. R., Müller, B., et al. (2017). *Patient specific numerical simulation of flow in the human upper airways for assessing the effect of nasal surgery.* http://arxiv.org/abs/1706.02575 (accessed on 7th August 2025).
13. Di Piazza, A., Di Vittorio, M. L., Lo Re, G., Picone, D., et al. (2019). *Swallowing evaluation with videofluoroscopy in the pediatric population.* https://core.ac.uk/download/196288515.pdf (accessed on 7th August 2025).

14. Dobra Baum. (2023). *Singer's Voice Quality – Genetic or Environmental Influences?* https://core.ac.uk/download/616444343.pdf (accessed on 7th August 2025).

15. Dogaru, G., & Stanescu, I. (2014). *Swallowing disorders in clinical practice: Functional anatomy, assessment and rehabilitation strategies.* https://core.ac.uk/download/pdf/27195839.pdf (accessed on 7th August 2025).

16. Fondevila Gascón, J. F., Martorell Castellano, C. (Coordinador), Miotto, G., Polo López, L., et al. (2018). *Advertising and Evaluation of Voice Through Digital Media.* https://core.ac.uk/download/250239174.pdf (accessed on 7th August 2025).

17. Franczak, J. L. (2005). *An Investigation of Vocal Abuse in School Teachers.* https://core.ac.uk/download/542630068.pdf (accessed on 7th August 2025).

18. Greene, J. B. (1968). *Approaches to Breath Support and Control.* https://core.ac.uk/download/33363079.pdf (accessed on 7th August 2025).

19. Henderson, M. P. J. (2018). *Quantitative and portable instrumentation for the screening and assessment of pharyngeal dysphagia.* https://core.ac.uk/download/189723636.pdf (accessed on 7th August 2025).

20. Jagan, A. S. (2017). *Comparative study between conventional adenoid curettage and endoscopic assisted adenoid curettage.* https://core.ac.uk/download/288215689.pdf (accessed on 7th August 2025).

21. Kerkhoff, E. K. (2013). *Comparing the efficacy of voice restoration speaking options following laryngectomy.* https://core.ac.uk/download/60562057.pdf (accessed on 7th August 2025).

22. Lai, S. Y. S. (2007). *Laryngeal muscle activities during phonation and swallowing in non-dysphonic and dysphonic subjects.* https://core.ac.uk/download/37891825.pdf (accessed on 7th August 2025).

23. Maldhure, S. V. (2011). *Prevalence of gastroesophageal reflux disease in patient with voice disorders.* https://core.ac.uk/download/288215879.pdf (accessed on 7th August 2025).

24. Mohd Alip, R. (2011). *A study on outcome of intubation in Emergency Department, Hospital Universiti Sains Malaysia.* https://core.ac.uk/download/141499439.pdf (accessed on 7th August 2025).

25. Sample, H. G. (2019). *The Effect of Electronic Nicotine Delivery Systems on the Vocal Folds.* https://core.ac.uk/download/228304702.pdf (accessed on 7th August 2025).

26. Sell, K., & Sell, K. (2003). *The Disciplines of Vocal Pedagogy: Towards a Holistic Approach.* https://core.ac.uk/download/573857384.pdf (accessed on 7th August 2025).

27. Sonnenberg, L. L. (2005). *A therapeutic approach for improved vocal performance in individuals in teaching occupations.* NC DOCKS at The University of North Carolina at Greensboro. https://core.ac.uk/download/149229530.pdf (accessed on 7th August 2025).

28. Trenbeath, C. (2021). *Yakety Sacs: Laryngeal Air Sac Usage in Great Apes.* https://core.ac.uk/download/480449789.pdf (accessed on 7th August 2025).

29. Vetter, D. L. (2016). *Recommendations for vocal pedagogy curriculum based on a survey of singers' knowledge and research in vocal hygiene.* https://core.ac.uk/download/232574185.pdf (accessed on 7th August 2025).

TONSILLAR AND PHARYNGEAL DISEASES

11

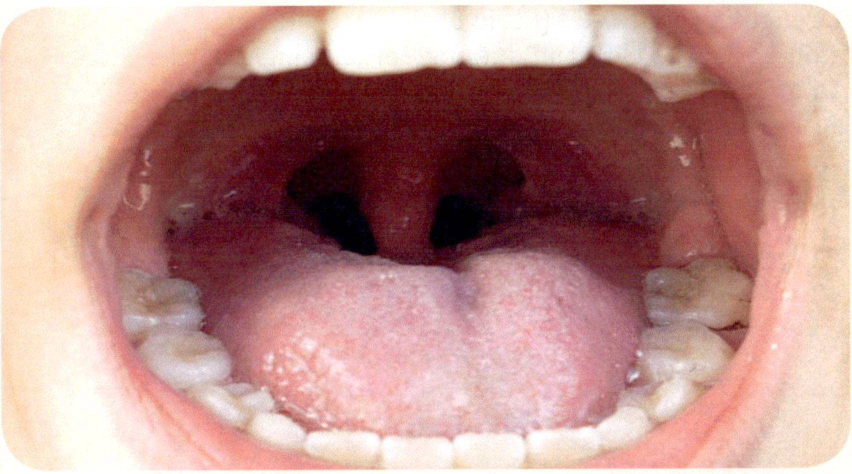

LEARNING OBJECTIVES

After studying this chapter, you will be able to:

1. Anatomy of the tonsils and pharynx.
2. Common tonsillar diseases.
3. Common pharyngeal diseases.
4. Diagnostic methods.
5. Treatment options.
6. Prevention strategies.

Introduction

The field of tonsillar and pharyngeal conditions encompasses a wide range of diseases involving the throat and its associated structures, notably the tonsils and the pharynx. The conditions may manifest in various ways, thereby making them challenging to diagnose and treat. Awareness of the anatomy and physiology of these structures is vital, as it provides knowledge of how they function and why they are susceptible to various pathologies. One of the most common examples is obstructive sleep apnea syndrome (OSAS), a widespread respiratory illness that is usually commented on in children. OSAS is caused by partial or complete obstruction of the upper airways during sleep and may have severe health implications if left untreated. Groups in pediatric populations are most vulnerable to sleep disorders, and thus the need for early detection and treatment programs is vital. In explaining the importance of tonsillar and pharyngeal disease, one must consider its multifaceted impact on overall health. In children, conditions such as large tonsils or recurrent tonsillitis can lead to strained breathing patterns, sleep disturbances, and associated auditory processing difficulties, as recent studies have shown. Likewise, presenting symptoms of tonsillar disease with other pathologies, including allergies and respiratory infections, also complicate diagnosis. This complexity underscores the need for an interdisciplinary approach that not only encompasses the observation of physical manifestations but also sensitivity to the potential systemic effects of these diseases, particularly on sleep and hearing functions. The interplay between breathing, sleep quality, and auditory processing has significant implications for a child's development and health. Administration of the tonsillar and pharyngeal conditions requires a multidisciplinary effort from various health providers, such as otolaryngologists, pediatricians, and most significantly, dental practitioners. The role of pediatric dentists and orthodontists has become more well-known, particularly in the discovery of early indicators of conditions like OSAS. The doctors serve as sentinels in the continuum of care, recognizing symptoms that require otolaryngology follow-up (Carlo et al., 2019). Research has also more recently investigated the association between OSAS and auditory processing disorder, with poorer performance on auditory tests in affected children described (Colella-Santos et al., 2006). This growing literature underscores the need for interprofessional care and active management of tonsillar and pharyngeal illnesses, with the long-term aim of optimizing outcomes in pediatric patients with these conditions (Figure 11.1).

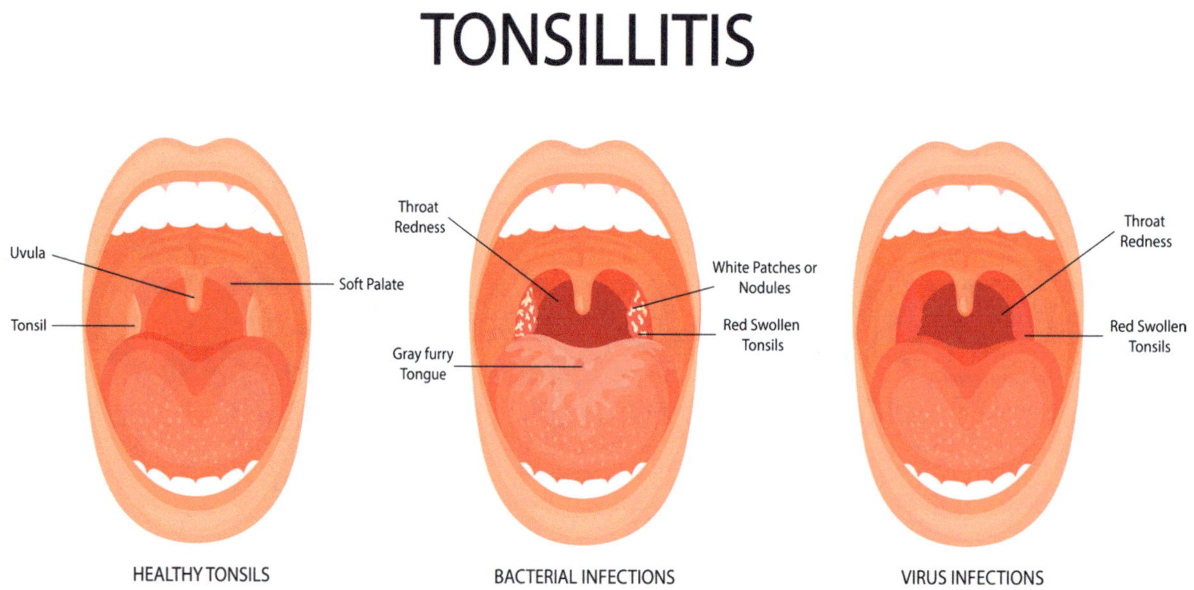

Figure 11.1. Tonsillar and pharyngeal diseases.

Source: https://external-content.duckduckgo.com/iu/?u=https%3A%2F%2Fstatic.vecteezy.com%2Fsystem%2Fresources%2Fpreviews%2F008%2F569%2F665%2Foriginal%2Fangina-pharyngitis-and-tonsillitis-tonsillitis-bacterial-and-viral-tonsil-infection-open-mouth-anatomy-vector.jpg&f=1&nofb=1&ipt=79d20ba6878e5c1a806cf0cfc3341fe0a66e8e32be37b1aa745b08c3f5c8b218.

Definition of Tonsillar and Pharyngeal Diseases

Tonsillar and pharyngeal disease embraces a wide variety of infections of the tonsils and the area of the pharynx, a critical part of the respiratory and gastrointestinal tract. The tonsils, part of the body's immune system, become infected or inflamed and lead to tonsillitis, characterized by sore throat, difficulty in swallowing, and fever. Pharyngeal diseases, or those that occur in the pharynx, can include infections such as pharyngitis, typically caused by viral or bacterial agents. An appropriate understanding of such diseases depends on separating between acute and chronic diseases since chronic diseases tend to bring about severe complications, impacting the well-being. The increase in cases of pharyngeal and tonsillar illnesses brings to the fore the importance of heightened awareness and early diagnosis to curtail the morbidity of these illnesses. There are a number of factors responsible for the cause and progression of pharyngeal and tonsillar illnesses. Infectious etiologies—ranging from viruses to bacteria and, in some cases, fungi—are prime culprits in the causation of these illnesses. For instance, streptococcal infection frequently results in tonsillitis, whereas pharyngitis is due to adenoviruses and respiratory syncytial virus. Being aware of the etiology of such disorders helps in targeted planning of treatment. Interestingly, underlying anatomic defects, that is, adenoids or hypertrophic tonsils, can predispose the patient to recurrent infection as well as obstructive sleep syndromes. Prevalence rates of such conditions can vary based on the population. Recent findings suggest a growing rate of head and neck cancers, particularly nasopharyngeal cancer, with significant implications for diagnosis and treatment of such cases, as explained in research on age and sex distribution among head and neck cancer patients (Hidanti, M. L., & Prasetyo, A., 2015). Furthermore, the adverse effects of untreated or chronic tonsillitis and pharyngitis can have significant health implications, including sleep disorders and airway obstructions. In children, for instance, obstructive sleep apnea syndrome (OSAS) is commonly linked to large adenoidal tissue, which may be a sign of concurrent tonsillar pathology (Bellini et al., 2019). In addition to affecting quality of life, these chronic diseases may have long-term effects on health, thereby necessitating holistic management plans. Clinical evaluation is commonly the first method of diagnosis, complemented by imaging or lab examination to differentiate between various pathologies. Early treatment is also crucial, either conservative or in the form of surgical interventions like tonsillectomy, to improve patient outcomes as well as compensate for the risks of these conditions. The definitions and meanings of tonsillar and pharyngeal diseases remain focal components in addressing the broader context of head and neck health.

Importance of Studying These Diseases

The relevance of studying tonsillar and pharyngeal disease transcends the realm of academia; it directly affects public health as well as one's own well-being. The disease, characterized by manifestations of sore throat, dysphagia, and sleep apnea, can significantly impair daily functioning and quality of life. Early treatment and proper management of such diseases are crucial, not only to relieve symptoms but also to prevent complications, such as reinfection or chronic disease. With knowledge of the epidemiology and pathophysiology of such diseases, healthcare providers can formulate targeted interventions, leading to more efficient and customized treatment approaches. As the prevalence of related diseases like obstructive sleep apnea syndrome (OSAS) is rising, it is important to emphasize research and information on these diseases for improved patient outcomes as well as to reduce healthcare burden (University, 2013). Moreover, tonsillar and pharyngeal disease research is significant in identifying and overcoming the involved risk factors that contribute to their development. These disorders are often linked with anatomical issues, such as hypertrophy of lymphoid tissue and craniofacial anomalies, as well as with functions such as neuromuscular disease (Balbani et al., 2005).

A thorough understanding of these etiologic conditions enables researchers and clinicians to detect populations that are more susceptible and to implement preventative measures. For instance, the realization of the relationship between adenotonsillar hypertrophy and sleep apnea in children has led to increased screening and earlier treatment. Raising families' and communities' awareness of these risks fosters a preventive approach to health, prioritizing prevention over reaction, thereby translating into healthier populations and reduced healthcare spending. Furthermore, exploring tonsillar and pharyngeal illnesses enables clinical practice and surgical innovation.

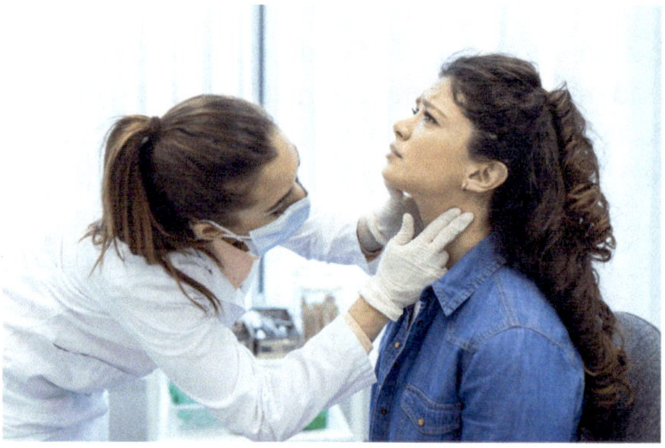

Figure 11.2. Studying tonsillar.

Source: https://external-content.duckduckgo.com/iu/?u=https%3A%2F%2Fmedtigo.com%2Fwp-content%2Fuploads%2F2024%2F06%2FUntitled-design-72.png&f=1&nofb=1&ipt=e1bdd0f86d080a87dcf0722a46f4af21cee385909010a19ab695465fc91f3c4b.

Through ongoing research, medical professionals are able to further enhance current treatment practices and create new methods of successfully managing such diseases. For example, the development of minimally invasive surgery has reduced recovery periods and complications, significantly enhancing the patient experience (Balbani et al., 2005). Furthermore, the addition of sophisticated diagnostic tools such as polysomnography and nocturnal pulse oximetry increases diagnostic precision to allow clinicians to offer tailored treatment plans based on individual patient needs. By investing in research time and effort to understand these diseases, we can look forward to increased clinical outcomes, as well as increased quality of overall patient care provided to patients with tonsillar and pharyngeal diseases, thereby making such research essential to the modern practice of medicine (University, 2013) (Figure 11.2).

11.1. Anatomy of the Tonsils and Pharynx

Learning Outcome

1. Description of the Tonsils and Their Functions
2. Overview of the Pharynx and Its Role in the Respiratory System
3. Relationship Between Tonsils and Pharyngeal Health

The pharynx and tonsils are involved in the immune system and respiratory-related life-threatening infections, providing a multiple-progression anatomical landscape. The tonsils, predominantly located at the oropharyngeal entrance, consist of the tubal, pharyngeal, lingual, and palatine tonsils, and each has special immunological roles.

Palatine tonsils are duplicated structures most commonly observed with tonsillitis, and the lingual tonsil lies posterior to the tongue and plays a role in immune response production. The pharyngeal tonsil, or adenoid, is located in the nasopharynx and is of greatest importance in the pediatric population, where it can hypertrophy and produce obstructive sleep apnea. Understanding their precise anatomical positions is important, as it enables the diagnosis and treatment of tonsillar and pharyngeal pathology, both of which remain vital to overall health. The comparative anatomy strategy reveals the variety of tonsillar organs across various animal species, with implications for veterinary and human medicine. Domestic animals possess six types of tonsillar tissue, variations of which influence immune responses and susceptibility to disease. As an example, sheep and goats possess all six forms of tonsils, which may make them respond more favorably to pathogens, while animals like the rat and pigeon possess no tonsils at all in certain instances (Breugelmans et al., 2011). Such differences in anatomy give relevance to learning about the functions of tonsils in different organisms and throw light on evolutionary responses. Comprehension of these differences not just aids veterinary practice, but also explains the intrinsic roles tonsils exhibit in man, where similar anatomical structures typically bear with them associated clinical conditions, for example, infection and cancer. Moreover, the relevance of pharyngeal patency may significantly affect disease incidence, particularly malignancy. The increasing incidence of oropharyngeal squamous cell carcinoma among traditionally lower-risk younger age groups attests to the significance of early intervention and detection (Eley et al., 2020). The anatomical overlap between the tonsil and critical structures such as the oropharynx has significant implications for understanding this region for therapeutic and diagnostic purposes. General dental professionals, through routine inspections, can be instrumental in detecting and thereby allowing early referral of possible lesions or abnormal growths. With increasing knowledge of tonsillar and pharyngeal anatomy, so too does our ability to deal with the diseases that develop, highlighting the imperative relationship between anatomical awareness and successful clinical practice in the fight against tonsillar and pharyngeal disease (Figure 11.3).

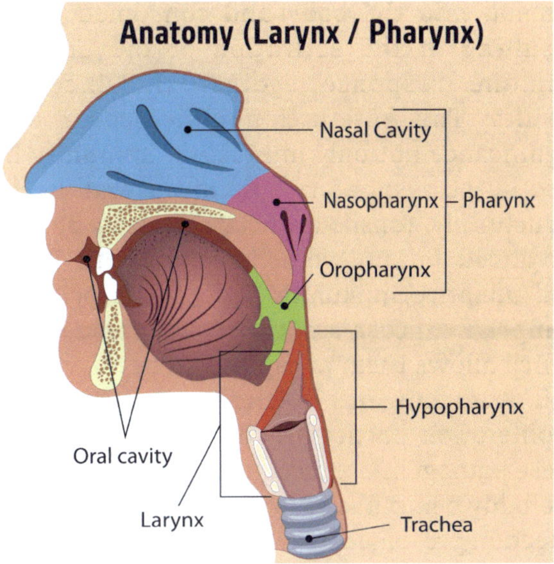

Figure 11.3. Anatomy of the tonsils and pharynx.

Source: https://external-content.duckduckgo.com/iu/?u=https%3A%2F%2Fatlantaheadandneck.com%2Fimages%2Fdefault-source%2Fpractices%2Fgettyimages-1204429898.jpg%3Fsfvrsn%3D5f1174c9_1&f=1&nofb=1&ipt= b45d6d18ba213af97b6ec4e98723 4fd938ce f47b0 015b398c02047bfc0686c9a.

11.1.1. Description of the Tonsils and Their Functions

The tonsils, being an integral part of the body's defense mechanism, are strategically located within the pharyngeal area and act as the body's first line of defense against pathogens entering from the oral and nasal cavities. There are primarily three pairs of tonsils: palatine tonsils on either side of the oropharynx; lingual tonsils on the posterior aspect of the tongue; and the pharyngeal tonsil, also called adenoid when enlarged. Each of these organs is composed of lymphoid tissue that produces and houses an extensive variety of immune cells. Their topological position enables them to effectively sample and respond to antigens inhaled into the body and consumed, hence resulting in the activation of the adaptive immune response against the incoming insults. This interaction underscores their significance not only in mucosal immunity but also in the respiratory system's overall health. Structurally, tonsils are characterized by their advanced immune mechanisms, both innate and adaptive immunity. The tonsils primarily comprise mucosa-associated lymphoid tissue, which allows them to capture bacteria, viruses, and other antigens. Tonsils trigger lymphocyte proliferation, particularly of B and T cells, when these pathogens are recognized, which organizes the body's immune response. Not only is acute infection prevented by this stimulation, but long-term immunity is also facilitated by memory cells that develop. This physiological role points to the importance of tonsillar health: disturbed tonsils lead to increased infection or chronic inflammation rates, for which medical treatment is required. Accordingly, understanding tonsillar functions is an understanding of the rationale behind procedures such as tonsillectomy and adenoidectomy, which are often indicated secondarily for recurrent infection and other disease processes. Recent studies have outlined several of the complexities surrounding tonsillar health, including viral infections and their interactions with local immunity. Research has identified tonsils to be the most frequent sites of virus infection in the respiratory system, with a high detection rate of up to 94% of samples from individuals having elective adeno-/tonsillectomy, which further indicates the role of tonsils in the operation of the immune system. Surprisingly, tonsillar tissues not only consist of immune cells but also possess a dynamic microbiome, which can be regulated by agents such as atopy, where differential microbial diversity has been observed between atopic and non-atopic individuals. Such findings indicate that the tonsils are more than mere passive bodies; they are actively involved in immune modulation and react to environmental stress, bearing testimony to their intrinsic role in pharyngeal health as part of the body's total immune architecture (Breugelmans et al., 2011; Ivaska, 2022) (Figure 11.4).

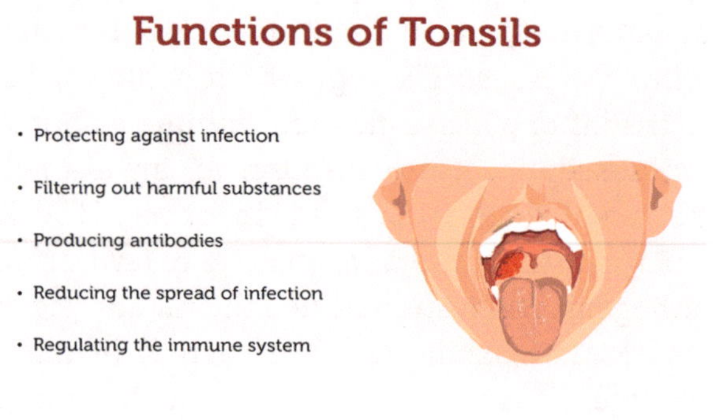

Figure 11.4. Description of the tonsils and their functions.

Source: https://assets.lybrate.com/imgs/tic/enadp/function-of-tonsils.jpg.

11.1.2. Overview of the Pharynx and Its Role in the Respiratory System

The pharynx is a vital anatomical structure of the digestive and respiratory systems, serving as a conduit for air and food. The muscular tube extends from the nasal passage to the esophagus and is divided into three sections: the nasopharynx, oropharynx, and laryngopharynx. The nasopharynx is almost totally responsible for breathing and contains the nasal passages and speech. Meanwhile, swallowing is aided by the oropharynx and laryngopharynx, and enables airflow. The pharynx plays a very critical role in achieving good respiration since any obstruction or illness within the segment will significantly impede airflow, leading to respiratory problems. Since it is involved in numerous physiological functions, a thorough understanding of the pharynx's anatomy and its related function in the respiratory system is vital in managing tonsillar and pharyngeal diseases. The tonsils, located within the pharyngeal cavity, are a part of the body's immune system as they house lymphoid tissue responsible for detecting and responding to infection. The adenoids and the palatine tonsils are also very active locations in which the immune response initiates. The presence of these tonsils and the pharynx signifies their role in respiratory health. For instance, hypertrophy of the tonsils or chronic tonsillitis may impair the airflow, leading to obstructive sleep apnea (OSA). OSA is characterized by the recurrent obstructions of the sleep airway, illustrating the direct effect tonsillar disease has on respiratory function (Dinesh et al., 2015). Hence, a straightforward examination of the pharynx informs the pathophysiology of tonsillar disease and how it has broader consequences for respiratory disease. Moreover, diseases that attack the pharynx, such as tonsillitis and adenoiditis, will often lead to systemic consequences. Such conditions are capable of inducing local and systemic inflammatory responses that impact global respiratory function as well as the incidence of comorbidities. Recent literature shows that recurrent tonsillar tissue infection is able to induce elevated airway resistance and impaired ventilation (Ivaska, 2022). This is particularly important in children because recurrent tonsillar and pharyngeal illness can disrupt normal development and result in long-term health consequences. Knowledge of the role of the pharynx in the respiratory system is significant in developing effective therapy for tonsillar and pharyngeal diseases with the final aim being to restore and preserve normal respiratory function.

11.1.3. Relationship Between Tonsils and Pharyngeal Health

The interaction between tonsils and pharyngeal health is multifaceted, including anatomical and immunological implications. Tonsils, lymphoid organs located at the back of the pharynx, play a crucial role in immune function, particularly during childhood, when the immune system is still developing. They function as first-line defense mechanisms against infection entering via the oral and nasal cavities. This function is significant because the tonsils are involved in antibody production, particularly in respiratory infections, thus relating their well-being to that of the overall pharyngeal condition. But when the tonsils hypertrophy or become repeatedly infected, they can cause pharyngeal dysfunctions like obstructive sleep apnea or persistent sore throats, showing the causal relationship between the well-being of the tonsils and the health of the pharyngeal environment. Chronic tonsillitis, or ordinary tonsillar disease, more accurately describes the relationship between the tonsils and pharyngeal health. It is a painful inflammatory process that not only affects the tonsils but can also have detrimental effects on adjacent pharyngeal tissue.

These studies have indicated that children with chronic tonsillitis are more likely to experience pharyngeal airway obstruction, which leads to respiratory disorders during sleep, such as obstructive sleep apnea syndrome (OSAS) (Colella-Santos et al., 2006). The condition of the tonsils is critical in maintaining optimal pharyngeal function and respiratory health. Moreover, the inflammatory responses of chronic tonsillitis tend to aggravate pharyngeal sensitivity, creating swallowing difficulties and a heightened susceptibility to recurrent infections, demonstrating the inseparability of such anatomical units. The histopathological study of tonsillar pathology further elucidates the condition's association with pharyngeal health. A review of tonsil biopsies reveals that the vast majority of patients referred for tonsillectomy present with benign lesions, such as reactive lymphoid hyperplasia, whereas a smaller proportion have malignancy (Essa, 2018). This finding suggests that recurrent infections and chronic irritation are able to cause significant changes in tonsillar tissue consistent with pharyngeal illness. Significantly, the incidence of tonsillar malignancies, although rare, underscores the need for caution in the evaluation of tonsillar disease, particularly among susceptible populations. This complex relationship between benign illness and potential malignancies bears witness to the crucial function that tonsils serve in maintaining pharyngeal health and marks the significance of precautionary medical treatment in preventing problems stemming from tonsillar dysfunction.

Test Your Knowledge

1. Describe the anatomical location, structure, and types of tonsils (palatine, pharyngeal, lingual, and tubal) and their role in the lymphatic system.
2. Explain the anatomical divisions of the pharynx (nasopharynx, oropharynx, laryngopharynx) and their relationships with surrounding structures.

11.2. Common Tonsillar Diseases

Learning Outcome

1. Acute Tonsillitis: Causes and Symptoms
2. Chronic Tonsillitis: Diagnosis and Treatment Options
3. Peritonsillar Abscess: Complications and Management

Among tonsillar infections, acute tonsillitis is among the most common illnesses, particularly among children and adolescents. Either the infection can be viral or bacterial in cause, and among the bacterial etiologies, Group A Streptococcus is a leading one. The presentation of the illness typically consists of sore throat, throat pain on swallowing, fever, and swollen lymph nodes. The clinical significance of acute tonsillitis lies in its potential to cause complications, such as peritonsillar abscess, that can obstruct the airway and require surgical intervention. Clinical assessment in most cases is reliant on diagnosis, supplemented by rapid tests for the detection of antigens to confirm streptococcal infection. Treatment is also generally supportive, though with analgesics or antibiotics if needed. Understanding the epidemiology and treatment of acute tonsillitis is relevant, since repeated attacks might prompt consideration of tonsillectomy in patients with chronic tonsillitis, thus highlighting controversy around management strategies in otolaryngology. Chronic tonsillitis, or chronic inflammation of the tonsils, is distinct from acute tonsillitis. It is typically manifested by recurring episodes of acute tonsillitis, leading to chronic symptoms such as halitosis, sore throat, and dysphagia without the severity of acute infections. Patients report a decline in quality of life due to persistent symptoms, which may impair daily activities and sleep. The role of tonsils in the modulation of immune responses comes into play because persistent infection can create a vicious cycle of inflammation and hypertrophy. Treatment decisions are diverse and may involve conservative treatment before contemplating surgery, such as tonsillectomy. More emergent is the requirement for surgery in cases in which chronic tonsillitis causes sleep apnea or significantly impacts quality of life, necessitating patient-specific therapy directed by symptom severity and clinical presentation. In addition to tonsillitis, peritonsillar abscess is a significant complication of tonsillitis. This infection is typically a local collection of pus adjacent to the tonsil, typically following an antecedent bout of acute tonsillitis. The complaints are typically a very tender throat, swelling, and "trilateral" symptoms such as ear pain and trismus. Clinical examination and imaging, when necessary, typically establish the diagnosis. Management requires prompt action, most commonly drainage of the abscess, typically needle aspiration or incision and drainage in serious cases. Fusobacterium nitrophorin has been reported in association with peritonsillar abscesses and is considered a pathogen of concern in such cases (Nygren, 2023). Understanding the pathophysiology and optimal management technique for peritonsillar abscess is important as early treatment will prevent more complex complications, emphasizing the necessity for continued research and clinical awareness in the management of tonsillar and pharyngeal disease (Figure 11.5).

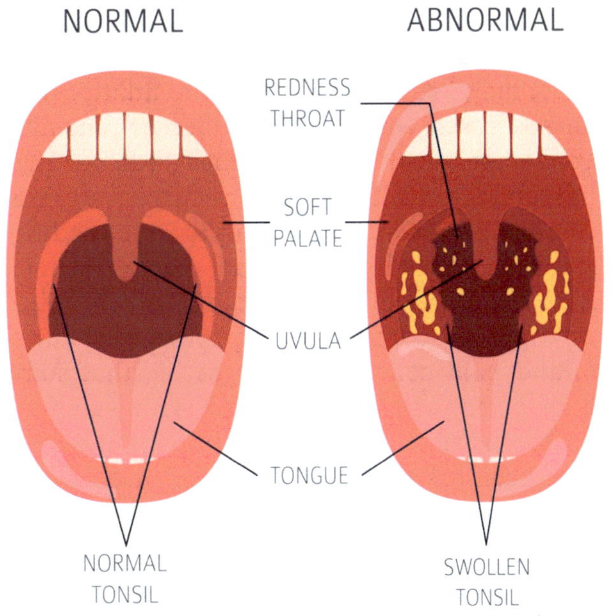

Figure 11.5. Common tonsillar diseases.

Source: https://smb.ibsrv.net/imageresizer/image/blog_images/1200x1200/51983/322727/009120100163138 7867.jpg.

11.2.1. Acute Tonsillitis: Causes and Symptoms

Acute tonsillitis is an infection of the tonsils by different pathogens, predominantly viral and bacterial infections. The most common viral etiology is adenovirus, influenza virus, and Epstein-Barr virus, while bacteria, particularly Group A Streptococcus, are the causative organisms of bacterial tonsillitis. The symptoms will typically develop rapidly, between one to two days after contact with the causative organism. The patients usually come with a sore throat, dysphagia, fever, and lymphadenopathy. On examination, the tonsils may reveal purulent exudate, suggesting a bacterial origin. The condition is most prevalent in children and adolescents but can occur at any age, thus requiring vigilance in children as well as adults to ensure effective intervention. A complete clinical assessment is required for acute tonsillitis diagnosis, beginning with a thorough medical history and physical examination. On physical examination, clinicians will note typical signs, such as red, swollen tonsils with whitish-yellow exudate, indicating a bacterial infection. Of note, less common pathogens also cause acute tonsillitis, such as *Neisseria gonorrhoeae*, although this is relatively rare. In one study examining oral gonococcal infection, tonsillitis as a result of gonorrhea is an unusual presentation, as few reported cases involved tonsillar infection (Balmelli, C., & Günthard, H., 2018). This highlights the importance of incorporating a broad differential diagnosis when an individual with tonsillitis is being evaluated, especially in sexually active individuals. Complications arise with acute tonsillitis, especially if left untreated, and hence require effective management. It may, in severe instances, lead to peritonsillar abscesses, which are surgically treated. Recurrent acute tonsillitis also results in chronic tonsillitis, and the affected person should have tonsillectomy. Besides the physical symptoms, the impact of acute tonsillitis can extend as far as the patient's quality of life in terms of days lost in school or work. Supportive measures such as hydration and pain control with analgesics are commonly given, and for bacterial tonsillitis, a course of antibiotics to decrease inflammation and avoid complications is also administered. Understanding both the etiology and complications of acute tonsillitis is critical in the effective management and prevention of the condition in the background of tonsillar and pharyngeal pathology.

11.2.2. Chronic Tonsillitis: Diagnosis and Treatment Options

Chronic tonsillitis is a challenging condition in the tonsillar and pharyngeal disease area, typically presenting as recurrent inflammatory episodes that adversely affect quality of life. Sore throat, dysphagia, and bad breath are frequent symptoms that can result in irreversible complications if untreated. The diagnosis of chronic tonsillitis usually consists of a thorough clinical evaluation, a comprehensive history of recurrent infection, and physical examination revealing enlarged tonsils with possible purulent exudate. Current clinical practice emphasizes the importance of distinguishing chronic tonsillitis from other similar conditions, as therapeutic methods may vary widely in effectiveness and patient outcomes. Clinicians usually make their diagnosis and management based on parameters such as symptom severity and frequency. Management of chronic tonsillitis is complex, with predominantly conservative and surgical approaches. A conservative treatment approach may initially include the administration of antibiotics for bacterial infections, along with analgesics to manage pain and inflammation. Tonsillectomy, however, becomes a common recommendation when patients have repeated episodes of tonsillitis despite these measures. Studies indicate that tonsillectomy decreases the recurrence of throat infections and related healthcare spending significantly in the long term. Recent studies on the microbiological etiology of chronic tonsillitis have identified Staphylococcus aureus as a common pathogen, suggesting that some cases are unlikely to be cured with standard antibiotics because the bacterium can evade host defense mechanisms (Zautner et al., 2010).

Thus, surgery is often regarded as an absolute cure for those with persistent conditions. More recent treatment modalities must also be considered, particularly regarding more recent modalities such as Ayurveda, which offers herbal formulations to manage symptoms of chronic tonsillitis. For instance, the drug Tonsenorm has been evaluated in relation to its promise in the management of Tundikeri, a related disorder of chronic tonsillitis, indicating potential for herbal therapy as a safe and cost-effective intervention for the patient (Pushkar et al., 2023). With progressive studies, it becomes all the more important to integrate these adjunct therapies into formal treatment modalities to deliver holistic care to patients. Finally, the management of chronic tonsillitis requires an individualized approach based on the patient's history, symptomatology, and preferences to improve outcomes and enhance patient satisfaction (Figure 11.6).

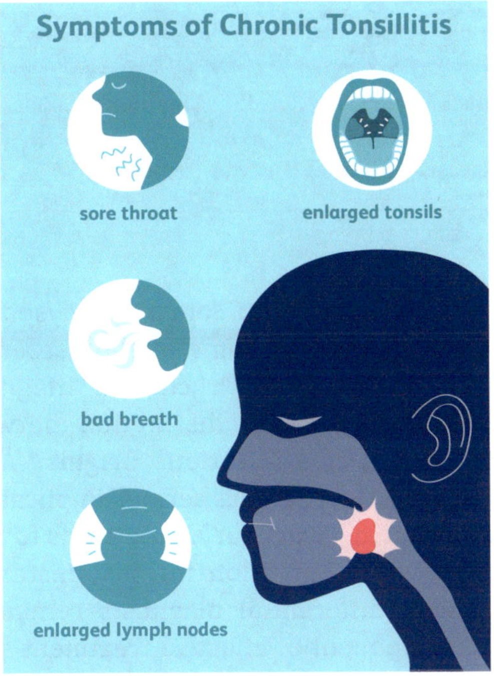

Figure 11.6. Chronic tonsillitis: diagnosis and treatment options.

Source: https://www.verywellhealth.com/thmb/mD1TRUa7Ua2CPQigLddlC1SFp98=/1500x0/filters:no_upscale():max_bytes(150000):strip_icc()/1191984-chronic-and-recurrent-tonsillitis-5afded720e23d9003715ffb9.png.

11.2.3. Peritonsillar Abscess: Complications and Management

The peritonsillar abscess is a familiar complication of acute tonsillitis and most often the sequel of chronic infection of the palatine tonsils. It is characterized by the accumulation of pus in the peritonsillar tissues and typically presents as an acute sore throat, dysphagia, and trismus. As the abscess enlarges, it may result in serious airway obstruction and require urgent treatment. With *Fusobacterium necrophorum* being an important pathogen in some cases, the condition emphasizes the need for thorough microbiological investigations. For its role in future systemic infections, such as *Lemierres* syndrome, awareness of the etiology and early treatment of peritonsillar abscess is crucial in the prevention of fatal complications (Nygren, 2023). Its treatment is mainly surgical, either by drainage by incision or puncture with a needle. The effectiveness of these interventions cannot be overstated, as early drainage not only alleviates symptoms but also avoids complications like aspiration pneumonia or sepsis. Antibiotic therapy is supplementary to surgery, and regimens typically consist of polymicrobial-active agents with beta-lactam and anaerobic coverage. Despite declining antibiotic use for non-streptococcal infections, the rising incidence of peritonsillar abscesses underscores the need for clinicians to remain vigilant regarding appropriate treatment protocols. Optimal management requires a multimodal strategy that pairs surgical treatment with appropriate pharmacotherapy to optimize patient outcomes in potentially serious complications (Jackson, 2009). Finally, one should be cognizant of the possible long-term consequences of untreated peritonsillar abscesses. Patients can experience repeated infections and other morbidity concerning the upper airway and swallowing functions. Also, historical review indicates increasing trends in *F. necrophorum* infections, which highlights the necessity for ongoing research and surveillance in this area. Awareness of the geographic and demographic variability in pathogen prevalence can inform targeted prevention, particularly for high-risk groups. Finally, active management of peritonsillar abscesses, including early drainage, appropriate antibiotic therapy, and patient education, is imperative to prevent complications and improve patient care quality for tonsillar and pharyngeal disease (Nygren, 2023).

Test Your Knowledge

1. What are the common diseases of the tonsils, such as acute tonsillitis, chronic tonsillitis, and peritonsillar abscess, and what are their causes and clinical features?
2. Explain the diagnosis and management of common tonsillar diseases, including medical treatment, indications for tonsillectomy, and postoperative care.

11.3. Common Pharyngeal Diseases

Learning Outcome

1. Pharyngitis: Viral vs. Bacterial Causes
2. Allergic Pharyngitis: Triggers and Symptoms
3. Pharyngeal Cancer: Risk Factors and Early Signs

The pharynx, a central component of the upper respiratory tract, is frequently affected by diseases that have significant consequences for respiratory and auditory health. Obstructive sleep apnea syndrome (OSAS) is a prevalent disease that is particularly troublesome in children. Since the repetitive blocking of the airway during sleep, OSAS has several complications like intellectual disability and behavioral defects. Early detection and intervention are essential as uncomplicated OSAS may progress to a more advanced presentation. Pediatricians and orthodontists have significant roles to play as point-of-entry; they are able to identify early presentations of upper airway obstruction during clinical assessment and refer patients at an early stage to specialists for further evaluation and treatment (Carlo et al., 2019).

Aside from OSAS, other pharyngeal disorders have the propensity to present with a constellation of symptoms that make clinical management difficult. A good example is acute pharyngitis, one of the most common reasons for patients to seek the services of the health care system, primarily due to its association with bacterial or viral infection. Sore throat, dysphagia, and fever are usually some of the presenting features. Difficulty with clinical diagnosis largely hinges on the distinction between infectious and non-infectious origins. While streptococcal infection has serious implications if left untreated, viral pharyngitis tends to have a less severe progression in most instances. Either way, differential diagnosis remains a critical component of effective treatment since targeted treatments can alleviate symptoms and prevent complications from occurring as a result of a lack of treatment (Colella-Santos et al., 2006). Further, hypertrophy of adenoids and tonsils can lead to recurrent pharyngeal obstruction, introducing a complicating factor to the usual clinical presentation of pharyngeal disease. This typically manifests in children and may be attributable to sleep disturbance, facial growth changes, and auditory processing disorder. Evidence indicates a correlation between hypertrophic tonsils and adenoids and impaired auditory function, warranting a comprehensive otolaryngologic evaluation in these children. Management ranges from conservative observation to surgery, for example, tonsillectomy and adenoidectomy, particularly where obstruction causes serious health issues. The challenge of tonsillar and pharyngeal diseases, therefore, requires an interprofessional collaboration among medical practitioners to optimize patient outcomes and avoid long-term complications (Colella-Santos et al., 2006) (Figure 11.7).

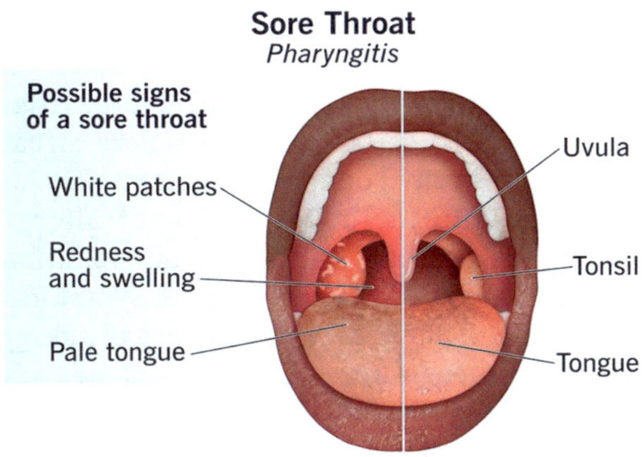

Figure 11.7. Common pharyngeal diseases.

Source: https://my.clevelandclinic.org/-/scassets/images/org/health/articles/8274-sore-throat-pharyngitis-signs.

11.3.1. Pharyngitis: Viral vs. Bacterial Causes

Among tonsillar and pharyngeal diseases, pharyngitis or inflammation of the pharynx is a frequent condition that will most often present patients with a reason to consult a healthcare facility. The primary distinction between viral and bacterial pharyngitis lies with their etiologic agents. Viral pharyngitis is most commonly caused by infections with adenoviruses, rhinoviruses, and influenza viruses, which tend to have classically milder illnesses with associated upper respiratory tract illness such as *rhinorrhoea* and cough. Bacterial pharyngitis is predominantly caused by group A Streptococcus (GAS), which can produce more severe presentations, for example, fever and exudative tonsillitis. The clinical presentation and causality of these pathogens strongly influence treatment protocols, making accurate diagnosis essential in the management of this prevalent disease (Ahmed et al., 2013). The epidemiology of pharyngitis shows a high rate of bacterial infection among certain groups, particularly children. There is firm evidence from a large body of research that the carriage rates of group A streptococcus can be considerably high, with estimates ranging from 10 to 50% in children from low-income groups (Okello et al., 2017). The carriage of the organism is generally asymptomatic, serving as a reservoir of infection that can be transmitted to others, particularly in groups of close contact such as schools. An understanding of the environmental and sociological determinants of bacterial pharyngitis is valuable, as it allows for the identification of risk populations and the implementation of directed public health measures.

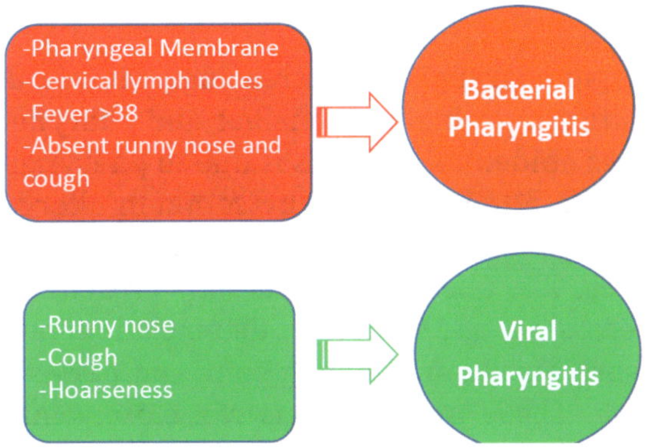

Figure 11.8. Pharyngitis: viral vs. bacterial causes.

Source: https://www.researchgate.net/publication/330873916/figure/fig3/AS:722868702818311@1549356737572/Bacterial-Vs-Viral-Pharyngitis.ppm

Consequently, the prevalence of bacterial pharyngitis poses unique challenges for clinicians diagnosing and managing pharyngitis in high-risk groups. In the clinical setting, making the distinction between viral and bacterial pharyngitis is critical, in that it dictates management strategies. Viral infections are typically self-limiting and can be treated with symptomatic relief, that is, painkillers and throat lozenges, while bacterial pharyngitis calls for antibiotics to clear the infection and prevent rheumatic fever complications. The causative agent determination is based on a combination of clinical examinations and, if needed, laboratory diagnostic procedures. Additional sophisticated techniques, such as throat culture and rapid antigen detection tests, play a critical role in making the diagnoses. Based on an informed understanding of pharyngitis' viral and bacterial origins, clinicians have the knowledge they need to optimize care and avoid potential complications arising from the ubiquitous sore throat (Ahmed et al., 2013) (Figure 11.8).

11.3.2. Allergic Pharyngitis: Triggers and Symptoms

Allergic pharyngitis is increasingly viewed as a significant problem in tonsillar and pharyngeal illness epidemiology. This is due to pharyngitis, which is often triggered by common allergens such as pollen, dust mites, pet dander, and mold spores. The allergic patients may present with several signs and symptoms that include scratchy or sore throat, swallowing pain, and persistent cough. These presentations can closely mimic viral or bacterial infections and thus complicate clinical diagnosis. Allergic pharyngitis is often associated with other allergic diseases, such as allergic rhinitis and asthma, suggesting a broader immunological background that clinicians should consider when assessing throat illnesses (Ahmed et al., 2013). The pathogenesis of allergic pharyngitis is multifaceted and is an interplay between allergens and the immune system. When exposed to allergens, the IgE antibodies trigger the release of histamines and other mediators of inflammation from mast cells, resulting in the characteristic symptoms of patients. Healthcare practitioners must differentiate allergic pharyngitis from other etiologies of pharyngitis, for instance, infection, since treatment procedures are significantly different. Although environmental control and antihistamines are generally employed in the treatment of allergic pharyngitis, infectious causes can be treated with antibiotics or other therapeutic measures (Ivaska, 2022). The rationale for this distinction emphasizes the importance of meticulous clinical evaluation to identify the cause of pharyngeal sore throat. Furthermore, environmental factors play an important role in the causation of allergic pharyngitis. Seasonal variations, air pollution, and passive smoking can worsen the symptoms, particularly in patients with a history of allergy. Control of these environmental variables can be of great significance in the prevention and treatment of allergic pharyngitis. Treatment modalities are most effective if they are not just pharmacological but also entail lifestyle modifications, such as a decrease in exposure to the allergens, as well as the utilization of home air cleaning devices. It is significant that clinicians dealing with pharyngeal and tonsillar disease understand thoroughly these symptoms as well as the triggers, since it enables them to provide tailored care that minimizes pain while attending to the cause of the disease (Ahmed et al., 2013).

11.3.3. Pharyngeal Cancer: Risk Factors and Early Signs

Pharyngeal cancer is a significant health concern with numerous risk factors predisposing to this condition. Notable among these are cigarette smoking and heavy alcohol consumption, which have been identified as the major etiologic agents of pharyngeal cancer. Cigarette smoking subjects pharyngeal epithelial cells to numerous carcinogens that can cause dysplasia and neoplastic transformation in the long run. Also, alcohol and tobacco interaction has been found to have enhanced carcinogenic effects synergistically, thus contributing to an elevated risk of pharyngeal cancer. Human papillomavirus (HPV) infection has also been known to be a major risk factor, predominantly among the young generation. The virus is a sexually transmitted disease that leads to cellular transformation of the oropharynx, thereby necessitating vaccination among adolescents (Blaxhult et al., 2009). Therefore, understanding these complex risk factors is vital to prevention and early detection efforts aimed at reducing the incidence of pharyngeal cancers. Pharyngeal cancer symptoms may be subtle and therefore difficult to diagnose at an early stage. Persistent sore throat, dysphagia, and weight loss are common presentations. They can also experience voice changes, earaches, or the feeling of a lump in the neck due to lymphadenopathy. They are often misdiagnosed as other mild conditions and thus delayed appropriate medical evaluation. Awareness by the patients and medical practitioners is important for earlier detection and improved patient outcomes. Additionally, patients with high-risk behaviors, such as those exhibited by men who have sex with men (MSM), should remain vigilant to these warning signs (Nygren., 2023). Patient education and regular follow-ups can lead to early symptomatic case detection, which will eventually enhance the prognosis of pharynx cancer. Clinical advancements in imaging diagnostics and screening methods are improving pharyngeal cancer detection in earlier stages. Endoscopy and imaging procedures, such as CT and MRI scans, provide clearer visualization of the pharyngeal region and enable the identification of malignant lesions. Also, the inclusion of HPV testing among risk groups has been promising in the detection of those at risk of pharyngeal cancer, effectively doubling the rationale for preventing the disease. By increasing awareness of risk factors and precancerous symptoms, and improving diagnostic capabilities, healthcare systems can better combat pharyngeal cancer. Continued research on the pathogenesis and epidemiology of the disease will be significant in the formulation of appropriate intervention approaches against pharyngeal cancer outbreaks and occurrences (Blaxhult et al., 2009) (Figure 11.9).

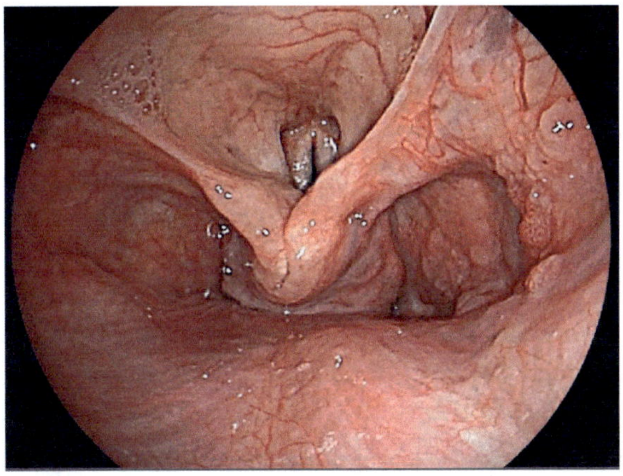

Figure 11.9. Pharyngeal cancer.

Source: https://www.researchgate.net/publication/273164396/figure/fig1/AS:651176773156865@1532264049723/The-endoscopic-view-of-the-primary-pharyngeal-cancer-There-was-no-another-cancer-under.png.

Test Your Knowledge

1. What are the common diseases of the pharynx, such as acute pharyngitis, chronic pharyngitis, and peritonsillar abscess, and what are their typical causes and clinical features?
2. Explain the diagnostic approach and management strategies for pharyngeal diseases, including medical treatment, surgical interventions when necessary, and supportive care.

11.4. Diagnostic Methods

Learning Outcome

1. Physical Examination Techniques
2. Laboratory Tests and Imaging Studies
3. Differential Diagnosis of Tonsillar and Pharyngeal Diseases

Diagnosing tonsillitis and pharyngitis requires a robust diagnostic framework to ensure accurate diagnosis and guide therapeutic intervention. Physical examination, combined with evaluation of the patient's history, is among the most vital diagnostic measures. Detailed questioning and examination of complaint-persevering throat soreness, swallowing pain, or recurring infections provide pertinent information regarding the course of disease and its potential causes. Moreover, clinicians can use imaging techniques such as ultrasound or computed tomography (CT) scans to obtain images of the anatomical structures within the throat and surrounding tissues. The imaging modalities enhance detection of abnormal findings, for example, hypertrophy of palatine tonsils or pharyngeal obstruction, which are usually observed with obstructive sleep apnea syndrome (OSAS) and associated disorders, as noted by Carlo et al. (2019). These comprehensive diagnostic evaluations play a crucial role in formulating an optimal treatment plan tailored to the patient's needs. In children, understanding the impact of tonsillar and pharyngeal illness extends beyond coarse physical symptoms; it also involves attention to their effects on domains of developmental functioning, such as auditory processing. One should evaluate children with sleep-disordered breathing using polysomnography (PSG) to identify the severity and occurrence of OSAS. PSG provides measurable indices of sleep disturbances and respiratory events, thereby enabling a thorough analysis of sleep airway obstruction. As the research conducted by Colella-Santos et al. (2006) establishes, children with abnormal PSG typically have widespread hypertrophy of palatine tonsils and nasal turbinates, which is the cause of their symptoms. Such interaction underscores the necessity of comprehensive diagnostic approaches that consider, in addition to clinical data, the influence of sleep disorders on children's health and development. Furthermore, enhanced diagnostic methods, such as flexible fiberoptic endoscopy, have revolutionized tonsillar and pharyngeal illness examination. This technique provides direct visualization of the oropharynx and larynx, enabling accurate diagnosis of structural abnormalities or infection. Endoscopic testing may identify underlying pathologies contributing to sleep-disordered breathing or other adverse effects. Additionally, integrating audiometric and auditory processing tests may provide definitive evidence of the correlation between tonsillar hypertrophy and impaired auditory processing in children, as demonstrated by research (Colella-Santos et al., 2006). These multidimensional diagnostic methods not only validate clinical decisions but also maximize patient outcomes by implementing targeted interventions based on comprehensive assessments, emphasizing the vital interdependencies among sleep, hearing, and overall health in the context of tonsillar and pharyngeal disease.

11.4.1. Physical Examination Techniques

Effective physical examination techniques are necessary in correct diagnosis and management of tonsillar and pharyngeal disorders. Because the oral cavity is an entrance to the respiratory and gastrointestinal tracts, a thorough examination begins with a visual inspection that assesses the health of the tonsils and their surrounding structures. This assessment can incorporate the lookout for evidence such as redness, swelling, or exudate, which may indicate infection or pathology. In addition to visual inspection, a thorough history is required to put findings in context. The patient's symptoms, that is, throat soreness, difficulty in swallowing, and so forth, can guide the clinician to appropriate investigation and interventions and hence enhance diagnostic yield. Thus, visual inspection and patient history form a good foundation for the subsequent stages of examination and treatment in the care of tonsillar and pharyngeal disease. Having carried out the visual inspection, physicians are then obliged to apply palpation techniques to uncover further diagnostic information regarding tonsillar and pharyngeal conditions. On deliberate palpation of the neck, lymphadenopathy can be identified, a common sign of systemic infection or regional disease. By using gentle pressure to palpate submandibular and cervical lymph nodes, clinicians can assess swelling and tenderness, which are relevant clinical findings that may reveal the extent of disease. In addition, examination of the temporomandibular joint and mastication muscles can be helpful in assessing referred pain or function issues related to pharyngeal disease. Such a broad understanding of these physical examination techniques, as highlighted in literature relevant to this subject, plays a crucial role in arriving at accurate diagnoses, consequently resulting in appropriate treatment modalities for diseases affecting the tonsils and pharynx (Bellini et al., 2019; Burgess et al., 2017). Finally, the role of some physical examination techniques in arriving at a diagnosis of tonsillar and pharyngeal disease cannot be downplayed, particularly cranial nerve examination. Testing of the cranial nerves is to determine the neurosensory and neuromuscular function that is compromised with severe disease. Testing, such as the assessment of the gag reflex, which utilizes both glossopharyngeal and vagus nerves, is quite crucial in finding abnormalities that can occur as a result of infectious or inflammatory processes. An investigation should also include evaluation of the patients' capacity to make sounds, which can reflect involvement of the nerves in speech and swallowing. Implementation of these extended examination procedures not only boosts the accuracy of diagnosis but also provides critical details on tonsillar and pharyngeal disease functional implications that enhance proper intervention measures provision (Burgess et al., 2017; Bellini et al., 2019) (Figure 11.10).

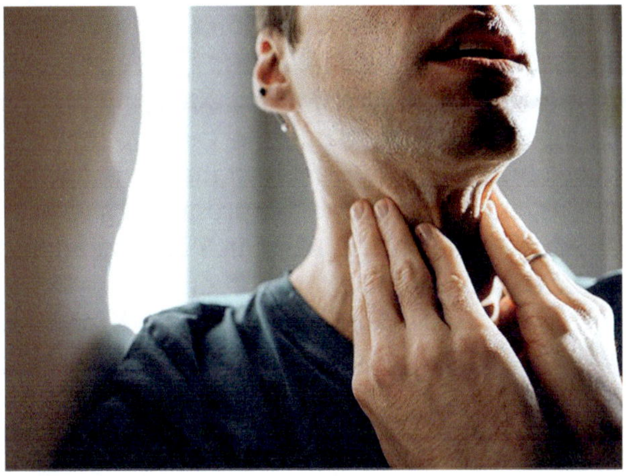

Figure 11.10. Physical examination techniques Pharyngeal cancer.

Source: https://media.post.rvohealth.io/wp-content/uploads/2023/03/close-up-man-touching-his-throat-neck-732x549-thumbnail.jpg.

11.4.2. Laboratory Tests and Imaging Studies

Laboratory tests and imaging procedures play a very crucial role in tonsillar and pharyngeal disease diagnosis and treatment. Laboratory tests can be the initial step in the evaluation, with throat cultures and complete blood counts used to identify infectious causes. They can help in differentiating between viral and bacterial tonsillitis etiology, thus guiding appropriate treatment decisions. Furthermore, the use of rapid antigen testing can provide early results for streptococcal infections, thereby avoiding unnecessary antibiotics. Identification of the underlying etiology is essential since it not only determines the treatment but also the potential complications of untreated infections. Besides laboratory examinations, imaging tests also have a vital role in the diagnosis of tonsillar and pharyngeal illnesses. Imaging modalities such as ultrasound, CT, and MRI can provide excellent resolution of pharyngeal anatomy and pathology. For example, imaging can be instrumental in cases of suspected abscess or deep neck space infections, where early diagnosis is important in the prevention of complications. (Abramo et al., 2012) highlights the significance of imaging in the diagnosis of severe infections, especially among susceptible groups, such as immunocompromised patients, who may present atypically. Such studies enable demarcation of the scope of disease spread, which serves to guide operative and medical interventions efficiently. In addition, combining laboratory investigations and imaging studies improves the overall clinical management of tonsillar and pharyngeal illnesses by a more personal approach. This integration makes it possible for healthcare providers to assess the efficacy of therapy and disease resolution or worsening. For instance, imaging follow-up is needed to exclude a residual abscess, whereas serial laboratory examinations can track inflammatory markers in a disease of chronic duration. In pediatric patients, in whom conditions like obstructive sleep apnea can be secondary to tonsillar hypertrophy, a critical understanding of clinical presentation in relation to laboratory and imaging findings is most critical for optimal management. (Bellini et al., 2019) emphasizes the manner in which the occurrence of such conditions highlights the necessity for exhaustive diagnostic workup to direct appropriate therapeutic interventions.

11.4.3. Differential Diagnosis of Tonsillar and Pharyngeal Diseases

Pharyngeal and tonsillar illness differential diagnosis involves a strong understanding of several clinical presentations that can have overlapping signs and symptoms. Acute tonsillitis, which is commonly viral in etiology, can present in a manner similar to bacterial disease, such as streptococcal pharyngitis. The clinical presentation is the most significant differentiator, where bacterial infections are typically found to have worse presentations in the form of high fever, sore throat, and exudate on the tonsils. Contact history with the pathogenic agents can be utilized to enhance the diagnostic sensitivity. The utilization of rapid antigen detection tests or throat cultures is included in the diagnosis of streptococcal infections. Recognition of viral versus bacterial differences is necessary, as inappropriate use of antibiotics in virus-induced disease encourages evolving patterns of resistance and complicates treatment (Blaxhult et al., 2009). Other more severe illnesses, such as infectious mononucleosis, should also be considered in the differential.

This Epstein-Barr virus (EBV)-associated disease can have a presentation that mimics bacterial tonsillitis, leading to significant confusion in clinicians. Interestingly, infectious mononucleosis most often presents with generalized lymphadenopathy, prostration, and splenomegaly, characteristics less commonly associated with typical bacterial infections. Heterophile antibody tests and other diagnostic processes are useful in identification. Discrimination of the two diseases is important as improper treatment would have serious implications for the patient's recovery. Besides, other viral diseases, allergies, and even leukemia may present with tonsillar hypertrophy or pharyngeal symptomatology, underscoring the broad differential to be comfortably familiar with in clinical practice (Aluas et al., 2019). Merging patient history, physical exam findings, and adequate diagnostic studies forms the foundation of a successful differential diagnosis of tonsillar and pharyngeal illness. For example, throat ulcers or lesions, as well as difficulty in swallowing, may point towards more dangerous conditions like oropharyngeal malignancy or systemic infection. Careful evaluation for other systemic symptoms, such as weight loss, night sweats, or persistent hoarseness, can suggest malignancy. Hence, professionals should be very suspicious and adopt a multidisciplinary strategy in the management of patients with recurrent or chronic tonsillar and pharyngeal conditions. This strategy provides comprehensive patient care and optimal outcomes through timely interventions and tailored treatments that account for the full spectrum of potential etiologies (Blaxhult et al., 2009; Aluas et al., 2019).

Test Your Knowledge

1. What conditions should be considered in the differential diagnosis of tonsillar and pharyngeal diseases, and how can clinicians distinguish between bacterial tonsillitis, viral pharyngitis, peritonsillar abscess, and other oropharyngeal lesions?
2. Describe the clinical features, investigations, and key distinguishing signs that help differentiate tonsillar and pharyngeal diseases from systemic infections or neoplastic conditions.

11.5. Treatment Options

Learning Outcome

1. Pharmacological Treatments: Antibiotics and Analgesics
2. Surgical Interventions: Tonsillectomy and Adenoidectomy
3. Home Remedies and Lifestyle Modifications

Treatment of tonsillar and pharyngeal disease varies with the severity and nature of the underlying disease. Symptomatic treatment with analgesics and antibiotics in the case of presumed bacterial etiology is the generally conservative approach for acute tonsillitis in patients. Recurrent or chronic tonsillitis, however, is more often treated with tonsillectomy when frequency and severity disrupt patients' quality of life. This procedure not only removes chronic inflammation but also reduces the danger of potential complications such as peritonsillar abscess. Thus, the treatment option needs to be tailored to the patient's presentation, and therefore, careful assessment is important in maximizing outcomes. In obstructive sleep apnea (OSA) patients secondary to tonsillar hypertrophy or related pharyngeal tissues, more aggressive treatment modalities are necessary. Uvulopalatopharyngoplasty (UPPP) with tonsillectomy is an effective surgical procedure to correct the condition. Research indicates that it can provide significant symptomatic relief from severe obstructive sleep apnea syndrome, particularly in individuals with a normal body mass index. In a retrospective study, a remarkable 78% of the patients reported a total response to the therapy, emphasizing the efficacy of the procedure as a therapy in serious cases (Ballacchino et al., 2009). Surgical treatments such as UPPP thus improve significantly with significant benefits, and thus individualized treatment according to the patient's own particular presentation of disease becomes justified. In addition to surgery, non-surgical approaches are essential in the management of tonsillar and pharyngeal disease. The most common use of Continuous Positive Airway Pressure (CPAP) is in patients with obstructive sleep apnea, particularly when surgery is not indicated or when it is used as an adjunct to surgery. CPAP is employed to keep the airway patent during sleep and thus prevent the occurrence of attacks of apnea. Besides, lifestyle measures like weight loss and posture correction can be combined with surgical and medical treatments, especially in obese patients, where fatty deposition around the neck aggravates airway obstruction (Calero et al., 2012). In conclusion, a multidisciplinary strategy that combines surgical and non-surgical treatments is effective for treating a variety of tonsillar and pharyngeal diseases (Figure 11.11).

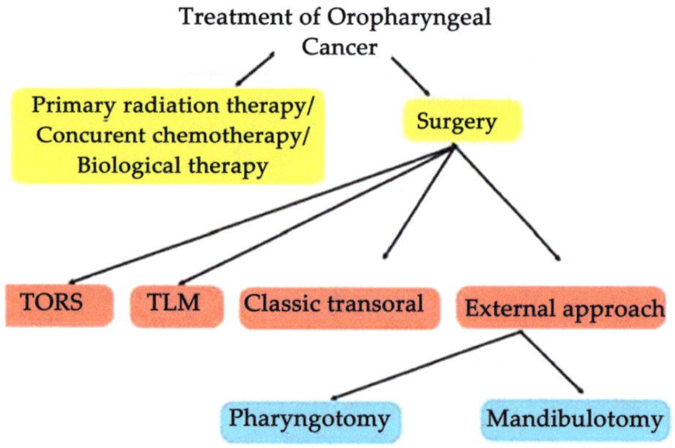

Figure 11.11. Treatment options for tonsillar and pharyngeal diseases.

Source: https://www.frontiersin.org/files/Articles/430151/fonc-09-00388-HTML/image_m/fonc-09-00388-g001.jpg.

11.5.1. Pharmacological Treatments: Antibiotics and Analgesics

In pharmacological treatment of tonsillar and pharyngeal infections, antibiotics play a central role, particularly in cases caused by bacterial infection such as streptococcal pharyngitis. These infections are highly likely to lead to complications for patients if left without treatment, and thus urgent antibiotic therapy is recommended. Administration of drugs like penicillin and amoxicillin has proved to be effective in eradicating the pathogenic bacteria of such infections, reducing the duration and severity of the symptoms. Furthermore, early therapy not only alleviates the pain associated with sore throats but also reduces the risk of sequelae, such as rheumatic fever and peritonsillar abscesses. Understanding how to effectively use antibiotics is also essential because its misuse can lead to resistance, making future treatment impossible and opposing public health measures against common bacterial pathogens of tonsillar diseases. In addition to antibiotics, analgesics constitute a significant portion of the pharmacological management of tonsillitis and pharyngitis. These medications, including over-the-counter agents like ibuprofen and acetaminophen, provide symptomatic relief from pain and inflammation and enable patients to remain hydrated and consume proper nutrition as healing progresses. Analgesics may be antipyretic in their action and assist in the management of fever that often occurs with infections. Even though they do not treat the true bacterial etiology itself, administration of the same does serve a major role in improving the overall quality of life in the patient with acute pharyngitis or tonsillitis. It is crucial that the healthcare providers educate the patients on the appropriate dosages and duration of administering analgesics to avoid potential side effects or misinterpretation of their condition, whereby a harmonious form of treatment is achieved. Antibiotics and painkillers need to be utilized judiciously in order to deliver maximum outcomes in patients with tonsillar and pharyngeal disease. The combination of selective antibiotic therapy with supportive painkillers is a double-barreled strategy towards curing the pathogen as well as the symptomatic pain that the patient is currently experiencing. Research has established that those patients who received combined antibiotics and effective analgesics have greater symptom remission and quality of life compared to patients receiving symptomatic treatment alone. As an illustration, a study highlighted the substantial reduction of recovery time among patients who were administered osteopathic manipulation alongside pharmacological treatment for tonsillitis, which can further enhance the efficacy of the standard treatments (Luceño-Mardones et al., 2021). Moreover, patient-related factors, including age, comorbidities, and potential drug interactions, must also be considered in order to tailor pharmacological regimens suitably for the purposes of safety and efficacy in tonsillar and pharyngeal diseases (Fehrm, 2020).

11.5.2. Surgical Interventions: Tonsillectomy and Adenoidectomy

Surgical interventions of tonsillectomy and adenoidectomy are important components of treating tonsillar and pharyngeal diseases, particularly in the case of pediatric patients with obstructive sleep apnea (OSA). OSA, characterized by repeated episodes of airway obstruction during sleep, has significant health morbidities, including neurobehavioral and cardiovascular morbidities. Adenotonsillectomy (T&A) remains the first line of treatment as it entails direct removal of hypertrophied tonsils and adenoids responsible for airway obstruction. By eliminating these obstructions, T&A not only enhances the child's quality of sleep but also plays a preventative role in minimizing the development of adult OSA. Early intervention via surgery is therefore necessary in young patients to promote optimum craniofacial growth as well as prevent further complications due to recurrent airway obstruction, as noted in recent literature (Ameli et al., 2010). The methods employed in tonsillectomy have evolved with advances in medical technology, particularly with the advent of colposcopy, which offers inherent advantages over dissective methods. Collation tonsillectomy consists of the removal of tonsil tissue with low-temperature radiofrequency energy, which results in much less intraoperative bleeding compared to traditional methods. A recent study demonstrated that patients who underwent collation had intraoperative blood loss of approximately 18.74 ml, compared with 43.44 ml with the traditional procedure (Sathish, 2014). Moreover, patients suffered less postoperative pain with the application of collation, which means an improved recovery process. While operation times may initially be increased, the benefits of reduced pain and bleeding highlight the paradigm shift in procedures for the surgical management of tonsillar disease. Postoperative care and follow-up are equally as significant components of such surgical treatments as tonsillectomy and adenoidectomy. Close follow-up of residual disease and complications is critical in securing successful outcomes, particularly with the rising prevalence of such ailments as OSA among children, which has a tendency to coincide with obesity rates. In the recovery stage, lifestyle factors, including control of weight, need to be treated to ensure optimal overall success in surgical interventions as well as possible recurrence. In this context, coordinated multidisciplinary care among otolaryngologists, pediatricians, and nutritionists can create an environment for comprehensive care. Not only does it facilitate the management of acute postoperative complications, but it also leads to long-term health benefits for children with tonsillar and pharyngeal conditions.

11.5.3. Home Remedies and Lifestyle Modifications

In the management of pharyngitis and tonsillitis, home treatments and lifestyle modifications are extremely crucial in prevention and in symptom reduction. Simple practices, such as ensuring hydration with adequate fluid intake, can significantly relieve a sore throat. Herbal teas flavored with honey, ginger, and lemon are extremely well known for being soothing therapeutic agents, providing moisture and nutrients with healing properties to irritated throat tissues. Furthermore, saltwater gargles are an ancient remedy that helps to reduce inflammation as well as clean the throat of harmful pathogens. These measures may not replace medical measures but can deliver palliative relief, addressing the overall health of patients with such conditions. Lifestyle adjustments also have a huge contribution to making tonsillar and pharyngeal disease manageable. For instance, an equilibrated diet that is rich in vitamins and minerals will provide nutrition to the immune system, thereby minimizing susceptibility to infections. Incorporation of food sources rich in vitamins C and D and zinc should be accomplished to fortify immune functions. Moreover, avoidance of smoking and restriction of alcohol intake are essential lifestyle changes that can minimize the risk of chronic throat illness. Both smoking and alcoholism are proven irritants that kill throat health, giving rise to conditions such as chronic pharyngitis and increasing the occurrence of tonsillitis. Effectuation of these alterations not only prevents sickness but also facilitates recovery. In addition to dietary alteration and modification of behavior, rest and stress relief are also an integral part of a unified system for tonsillar and pharyngeal health. Studies indicate that sleep disorders have the potential to complicate throat-related ailments and underscore the importance of quality sleep for immune system functioning and overall wellness. On the same note, stress management through mindfulness practice, such as meditation and yoga, has a significant influence on physical well-being through its ability to counteract inflammation and relax the body. The symbiotic nature of endocrine functionality and sleep quality helps underscore the importance of a holistic lifestyle treatment regimen for regulating such conditions. By adopting these home remedies and dietary changes, individuals can build immunity against tonsillar and pharyngeal infections and aid in the recovery from existing conditions (Vimmerová-Lattová, 2013; Berg, 2022).

Test Your Knowledge

1. What are the indications for using antibiotics and analgesics in the management of tonsillar and pharyngeal diseases, and how is the choice of antibiotic determined?
2. Explain the principles of antibiotic therapy and pain management, including dosage, duration, and potential side effects in treating ENT infections.

11.6. Prevention Strategies

Learning Outcome

1. Vaccination and Its Role in Prevention
2. Hygiene Practices to Reduce Infection Risk
3. Dietary Considerations for Maintaining Throat Health

Tonsillar and pharyngeal disease prevention requires a multidisciplinary approach, with priority on reducing infectious agent transmission rates. As an example, knowledge of the epidemiology of STIs is important since the trend of increasing syphilis and hepatitis infection among MSM reflects serious health concerns. Appropriate education about risks and pathways of transmission is necessary since the oral cavity can be a reservoir of asymptomatic infection without any evident symptoms. Routine STI testing when patients present with symptoms or during routine health checks will help reduce the incidence of such infections. Health care professionals should raise awareness of the urgency of testing for asymptomatic STIs, especially among risk groups, thereby reinforcing the demand for early diagnosis and treatment to reduce complications from tonsillar and pharyngeal infections (Blaxhult et al., 2009).

Vaccination is a vital method of prevention against reducing the incidence of viral and bacterial pathogens involved in tonsillar and pharyngeal diseases. The availability of highly effective vaccines against hepatitis B and A, as well as the potential for boys to be included in human papillomavirus (HPV) vaccination programs, is a valuable public health intervention. Not only do vaccines protect individuals, but they also play a significant role in providing herd immunity needed to hinder the transmission of viruses within communities. Besides this, healthcare practitioners should make public awareness programs more robust to highlight the importance of vaccination against infectious conditions such as these. This preventive activity can be particularly useful when combined with educational interventions that inform populations about the risks of STIs and also about the preventive value of vaccines. In this manner, vaccination becomes a central part of a broader set of preventive measures against tonsillar and pharyngeal disease (Cano-Pumarega et al., 2019).

In addition to vaccination and education, lifestyle modification is part of the prevention of tonsillar and pharyngeal diseases. Initiatives such as promoting safe sex practice, that is, regular condom barrier method use, are needed in an effort to reduce the risk of STIs that have adverse effects on the throat and tonsils. Moreover, individuals should be motivated to achieve comprehensive health through regular exercise, a well-balanced diet, and adequate hydration, as these practices support a robust immune system. Smoking and alcohol also decrease, aiding in lowering the number of chronic throat illnesses. Combining these lifestyle changes with periodic medical visits promotes an integrative preventive process, in which individuals are proactive in maintaining their health, thereby minimizing the prevalence of tonsillar and pharyngeal diseases in the population. Lastly, these strategy implementations renew the significance of a holistic approach in disease prevention (Cano-Pumarega et al., 2019) (Figure 11.12).

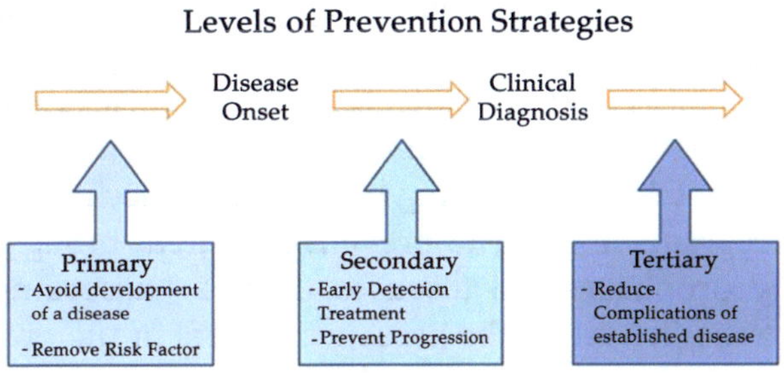

Figure 11.12. Prevention strategies for tonsillar and pharyngeal diseases.

Source: https://external-content.duckduckgo.com/iu/?u=https%3A%2F%2Fi.pinimg.com%2F736x%2F7f%2F3c%2F24%2F7f3c2426d9bd7e7e4b8291db282a8a17.jpg&f=1&nofb=1&ipt=79c2f741910235dad8e35157d50dafcb5bd61264165eb60fcd4ad2df1f3ffd17.

11.6.1. Vaccination and Its Role in Prevention

Vaccination is a key part in the prevention of infections of the tonsils and the pharynx, particularly in the case of the immune processes facilitated by Walleye's ring lymphoid tissue. This area, which includes the palatine and adenoid tonsils, serves as the first line of defense against pathogens entering via inhalation and ingestion. Vaccines, by their capacity to elicit mucosal immunity, can augment earlier detection of such antigens, thus providing for an effective adaptive immune response. For instance, vaccination against such a pathogen as *Streptococcus pneumoniae* has been critical in preventing the occurrence of acute pharyngitis and tonsillitis, thereby easing the burden of these infections on public health. Enhanced immunization interventions can reduce the incidence of infections that cause complications such as abscesses and chronic tonsillitis, ultimately improving the health outcomes of vulnerable groups. Vaccinations and their association with STIs are key issues in the understanding of the broader effects of immunization. HPV and hepatitis vaccines, which have both been shown to affect the oropharyngeal region, provide the best illustration of how immunization indirectly influences tonsillar disease. The evidence that has been discovered through research indicates a high correlation between HPV and tonsillar cancer that reveals the need for vaccinating boys in HPV vaccination programs in order to prevent the threat brought by oropharyngeal diseases. Besides, according to the literature, the presence of STIs in the oral cavity can predispose subsequent infections to easier development, adding to the complexity of the clinical presentation of tonsillar disease. With the resolution of these interconnected ailments via mass vaccination, it is then possible to decline the incidence of both STIs and their resultant complications, further strengthening the value of preventive health programs. In the promotion of prevention, the incorporation of vaccination into public health policies for tonsillar and pharyngeal diseases is essential. Novel vaccine strategies, in conjunction with innovative techniques such as single-cell genomic technologies, enhance understanding of the immune response in Walleye rings. These technologies allow researchers to characterize the heterogeneous immune cell populations and their roles in combating upper aerodigestive tract infections, leading to improved vaccine constructs. Furthermore, as the association between immunization and reduced infections becomes clearer, public health campaigns will need to pay special attention to education on the benefits of vaccination with respect to both common and rare pathogens. By encouraging a culture of vaccination, public health institutions can ensure the integrity of mucosal immunity in the populace, ultimately lowering the occurrence and severity of tonsillar and pharyngeal illness and enhancing the well-being of the community in general (Blaxhult et al., 2009; Chahal et al., 2024).

11.6.2. Hygiene Practices to Reduce Infection Risk

Good hygiene habits help reduce the risk of infection associated with tonsillar and pharyngeal disorders. Handwashing is one of the most essential but effective preventive measures. By washing hands properly with soap and water, it is possible to lower the level of transmission of germs that can cause infections in the tonsils and throat. Dental hygienists are particularly critical as health care providers in informing patients about the importance of hygiene processes in preventing oral and pharyngeal diseases. A survey reported that a large percentage of dental hygienists perform intraoral examinations as a routine measure, yet many do not discuss key topics such as the risk for oral cancers by viruses like HPV. Hence, establishing a culture in which hygienists feel that they have the expertise to teach patients is essential to establish community awareness and reduce infection hazards related to tonsillar and pharyngeal diseases (Anesi, 2013). Other than hand hygiene, the use of personal protective equipment (PPE) in clinical settings is essential to reduce infection risk. When feasible, using face shields, gloves, and masks protects health workers and their patients from contamination, particularly during oropharyngeal procedures. The practice not only protects health workers but also minimizes the spread of pathogens that may cause tonsillar or pharyngeal disease to worsen. In primary care visits, particularly to dental care professionals, infection control standards should be maintained to avoid injury to the patient and provider. One study emphasized the need for greater knowledge and comfort levels among dental hygienists to inform patients about risks of infection, including oral HPV risks. By strengthening education on such treatments, clinicians can enhance patient awareness and compliance, thereby reducing the risk of infection (N/A). Vaccination and its application in preventing infection is another fundamental hygiene habit that can significantly reduce risks of tonsillar and pharyngeal diseases. Vaccines such as the meningococcal conjugate vaccine are essential for preventing infections that may result from throat infection and thus protect individuals at greater risk. Comprehensive vaccination education can encourage individuals, particularly adolescents, to take proactive steps to protect their health. This is in agreement with evidence for low meningococcal carriage rates among high school students, which are largely attributed to vaccination campaigns. Therefore, educational programs must be designed for both providers and patients to increase awareness and dispel misconceptions about vaccinations. By facilitating vaccine-informed dialogue and associated hygiene practices, the medical fraternity can work towards decreasing risks of infection spread for tonsillar and pharyngeal disease (Anesi, 2013) (N/A).

11.6.3. Dietary Considerations for Maintaining Throat Health

Nutritional factors play a critical part in maintaining throat health, particularly in individuals prone to tonsillar and pharyngeal illness. A healthy diet containing appropriate nutrients supports the proper functioning of the immune system, which plays a crucial role in warding off infections that lead to tonsillitis or pharyngitis. These nutrients, such as vitamins C and D, zinc, and antioxidants, ensure an antioxidant function and improve the mucosal immunity of the throat. Moreover, adequate hydration cannot be overstressed; sufficient fluid keeps the throat moist, facilitating the prevention of inflammation and irritation. In patients who already have conditions, such as dysphagia or tonsillitis, understanding the impact of diet on throat health can result in improved outcomes and quality of life. Stroke or neurologic patients with dysphagia, a common condition in populations from a wide range of groups, must make food choices that guarantee safe swallowing. As seen in existing literature, stroke or neurologic patients are particularly at risk for dysphagia with serious implications in obtaining adequate nutrition and hydration (Kohler, E., & Love, K. M., 1990). Foods and more concentrated fluids are often ordered to reduce the risk of aspiration, which can lead to infection, such as aspiration pneumonia. Therapeutic dietary changes incorporating pureed vegetables, fruits, and soft protein preserve nutrients while compensating for the mechanical difficulties in swallowing. Individualized dietary interventions of this type are critical in the management of throat health with continued medical evaluation and treatment. In children's groups, certain dietary behaviors may also be significant for throat health, as children are particularly susceptible to infection. Sources indicate that nutritional advancement may improve general health outcomes, including those regarding the diseases of the throat (Bernasconi et al., 2019). Dietary interventions with probiotics and prebiotics can enhance gut health, hence indirectly contribute to the immune system's ability to respond against pharynx and tonsil infections. The addition of foods with anti-inflammatory capacity, that is, omega-3 fatty acids in fatty fish, can reduce the incidence and severity of throat infections. Parents must be informed about the role of these dietary components in promoting preventive health behaviors to prevent tonsillar and pharyngeal infections in children.

Test Your Knowledge

1. What personal hygiene practices can help reduce the risk of ENT infections, including hand hygiene, nasal care, and oral hygiene?
2. Explain the role of environmental and lifestyle measures, such as avoiding exposure to smoke, allergens, and crowded places, in preventing infections of the tonsils, pharynx, and nasopharynx.

SUMMARY

The anatomy of tonsillar and pharyngeal disease illustrates a complex interrelationship among anatomical considerations, clinical symptomatology, and therapeutic approach. As emphasized throughout this chapter , tonsillar hypertrophy and its attendant diseases, such as obstructive sleep apnea syndrome (OSAS), have a profound impact on the overall health and welfare of pediatric patients. Most intriguing is the association between enlarged tonsils and difficulty with auditory processing, and we discuss the necessity of comprehensive ear, nose, and throat studies in children presenting with such findings. Practitioners must be aware of the far-reaching consequences of tonsillar diseases and their often underrecognized effects on auditory function and overall quality of life. Besides, acknowledgement of the prevalence of these disorders in children, approximately 2% for OSAS in the ages of 2 through 8, emphasizes the importance of early identification and intervention. The contribution of anatomical causes, in particular the effect of adenoid tissue size, is an important etiologic factor in the condition of sleep-disordered breathing in children. The existing controversies surrounding their management necessitate a multidimensional approach that integrates surgical and nonsurgical modalities to facilitate personalized therapies tailored to patient needs. This is necessary for optimal outcomes and the minimization of long-term consequences of untreated tonsillar diseases. Ultimately, the importance of this thorough review of tonsillar and pharyngeal diseases extends far beyond simply current clinical matters. The implications of untreated OSAS, for instance, can be far-reaching in terms of neurocognitive dysfunction and behavioral disturbances and can represent increased risks of cardiovascular disease among children and adults. As further evidence emerges elucidating the intricacies of these syndromes, future research should focus on integrative management models that optimize medical and surgical treatments through synergy. Lastly, the goal is not merely to alleviate symptoms but also to enhance the general quality of life for affected patients, reaffirming the importance of treating these often under-diagnosed diseases in clinical care and public health interventions.

The multifaceted interaction between tonsillar and pharyngeal disease and their etiologic microorganisms has continued to be the focus in recent studies. Notably, *Fusobacterium necrophorum*, heretofore considered nonpathogenic, has emerged as a pathogen of interest that is implicated in terminal infections like Lemierre's syndrome. The organism, often present in asymptomatic carriers, can lead to lethal complications during an otherwise mild initial oropharyngeal infection. Studies have established that *F. necrophorums* prevalence is not geographically uniform, with the carriage rate among Swedish adolescents being considerably higher than that of Zambian adolescents. This geographic variation indicates the need for heightened vigilance and additional research into the epidemiology of this pathogen and its role in the progression of pharyngeal disease, particularly among young adults, the most affected group (Nygren, 2023). In addition to the microbiological parameters, the treatment and management of tonsillar and pharyngeal diseases require an astute observation of evolving surgical techniques and therapeutic management. Oral and maxillofacial surgery plays a crucial role in the management of head and neck pathologies, including those arising from pharyngeal and tonsillar infections. Due to the potential for very lethal complications arising from these diseases, surgical intervention cannot be overstressed. The specialty encourages surgeons to be aware of current surgical trends and practices in order to ensure thorough treatment of patients with such diseases. The specialty not only ensures successful treatment but also better patient outcomes, confirming the perfection of the intersection between surgical knowledge and oral and maxillofacial disease management (N/A, 2021). Appreciation of the relationship between microbial pathogens and the clinical manifestation of tonsillar and pharyngeal illness also sheds light on the broader public health implications. In recent years, invasive infections with *F. necrophorum* have increased, raising concern about a potential change in the clinical presentation of these infections. Additionally, the recognition that antibiotic treatment of non-streptococcal pharyngotonsillitis has decreased as complications increased establishes the importance of re-assessing current treatment protocols. The evidence of thrombogenic pathways for *Lemierres* syndrome patients continues to endanger management and underscores the importance of ongoing investigation into the pathogenesis of such diseases. This combined treatment approach, incorporating epidemiologic data, clinical experience, and modern surgical practices, will need to advance the diagnosis, management, and prevention of tonsillar and pharyngeal disease over the next several years (N/A, 2021; Nygren, 2023).

KEY TERMS FROM THIS CHAPTER

Tonsillitis
Chronic Tonsilliti
Quinsy
Acute Pharyngitis
Follicular Tonsillitis
Diphtheritic Pharyngitis
Streptococcal Pharyngitis
Adenotonsillitis
Parapharyngeal Abscess
Acute Tonsillitis
Peritonsillar Abscess
Pharyngitis
Chronic Pharyngiti
Membranous Tonsillitis
Viral Pharyngitis
Tonsillar Hypertrophy
Retropharyngeal Abscess
Ludwig's Angina

CRITICAL THINKING QUESTIONS

1. **The first-line treatment for bacterial tonsillitis is:**
   a) Antivirals
   b) Antibiotics
   c) Antifungals
   d) Surgery
2.. **Chronic tonsillitis is defined as:**
   a) Recurrent episodes of acute tonsillitis
   b) Tonsillitis lasting >3 months
   c) Any bacterial infection of tonsils
   d) Viral infection of tonsils
3. **The most common age group affected by tonsillitis is:**
   a) Infants
   b) Children 5–15 years
   c) Adults 30–40 years
   d) Elderly
4. **A white membrane over the tonsils suggests:**
   a) Viral infection
   b) Diphtheritic tonsillitis
   c) Allergic tonsillitis
   d) Chronic tonsillitis
5. **The surgical removal of the tonsils is called:**
   a) Adenoidectomy
   b) Tonsillectomy
   c) Laryngectomy
   d) Myringotomy

Short Answer Questions

1. What are the common tonsillar and pharyngeal diseases, such as acute tonsillitis, chronic tonsillitis, pharyngitis, and peritonsillar abscess, and what are their usual causes?
2. Describe the clinical features and symptoms of tonsillar and pharyngeal diseases, including sore throat, fever, dysphagia, and enlargement of tonsils.
3. Explain the diagnostic approaches for tonsillar and pharyngeal disorders, including throat examination, throat swab culture, and imaging when indicated.
4. Discuss the treatment options, including medical management (antibiotics, analgesics), surgical intervention (tonsillectomy, drainage of abscess), and supportive care.
5. What are the potential complications of untreated or recurrent tonsillar and pharyngeal diseases, such as peritonsillar abscess, rheumatic fever, or airway obstruction, and how can they be prevented?

Answers to Critical Thinking Questions

1. (b) 2. (b) 3. (b) 4. (b) 5. (b)

REFERENCES

1. Abogunrin, S., Di Tanna, G. L., Keeping, S., Carroll, S., & Iheanacho, I. (2014). Prevalence of human papillomavirus in head and neck cancers in European populations: a meta-analysis. *BMC Cancer, 14*(1), 968. https://doi.org/10.1186/1471-2407-14-968Abramo, A., Ferri, E., Spinato, G., Tirelli, G., et al. (2012). *Necrotizing fasciitis of the posterior cervical compartment: An atypical case due to Streptococcus agalactiae.* https://core.ac.uk/download/pdf/9634056.pdf (accessed on 7th August 2025).
2. Ahmed, K., Akram, M., Asif, H. M., Khan, M., et al. (2013). *Pharyngitis and Sore Throat: A Review.* https://core.ac.uk/download/478326442.pdf (accessed on 7th August 2025).
3. Aluas, M., Bordea, R. I., Budin, C. E., Ciumarnean, L., et al. (2019). *Therapeutic Alternatives with CPAP in Obstructive Sleep Apnea.* https://core.ac.uk/download/232440313.pdf (accessed on 7th August 2025).
4. Ameli, F., Bhattacharjee, R., Brietzke, S. E., Brigance, J., Brouillette, R. T., Capdevila, O. S., Cho, J. H., et al. (2010). *Treatment of Obstructive Sleep Apnea in Children.* https://core.ac.uk/download/pdf/8500828.pdf (accessed on 7th August 2025).
5. Anesi, L. (2013). *Dental hygienists' role in education of oropharyngeal cancers caused by human papillomaviruses: A thesis.* https://core.ac.uk/download/230644779.pdf (accessed on 7th August 2025).
6. Azagra Calero, E., Barrera Mora, J. M., Espinar Escalona, E., Llamas Carreras, J. M., et al. (2012). *Obstructive sleep apnea syndrome (OSAS): Review of the literature.* https://core.ac.uk/download/71024828.pdf (accessed on 7th August 2025).
7. Balasubramanian, T. (2025). *Endoscopic Orbital Decompression.* https://core.ac.uk/download/pdf/10673379.pdf (accessed on 7th August 2025).
8. Balbani, A. P. S., Montovani, J. C., & Weber, S. A. T. (2005). *Update in Obstructive Sleep Apnea Syndrome in Children.* https://core.ac.uk/download/pdf/82010675.pdf (accessed on 7th August 2025).
9. Ballacchino, A., Dispenza, F., Gallina, S., Kulamarva, M., et al. (2009). *Uvulopalatopharyngoplasty with tonsillectomy in the treatment of severe OSAS.* https://core.ac.uk/download/53269545.pdf (accessed on 7th August 2025).
10. Balmelli, C., & Günthard, H. (2018). *Gonococcal Tonsillar Infection—A Case Report and Literature Review.* https://core.ac.uk/download/159144812.pdf (accessed on 7th August 2025).
11. Bellini, C., Cammaroto, G., Colizza, A., & de Vincentiis, M., et al. (2019). *Risk factors for obstructive sleep apnea syndrome in children: State of the art.* https://core.ac.uk/download/231747914.pdf (accessed on 7th August 2025).
12. Berg, L. M. (2022). *Treatment success with continuous positive airway pressure or mandibular advancement splints in non-severe obstructive sleep apnea: A randomized controlled clinical trial on sleep quality, health-related quality of life and clinical predictors of treatment success.* https://core.ac.uk/download/523298069.pdf (accessed on 7th August 2025).
13. Bernasconi, S., Borrelli, M., Caffarelli, C., Corsello, G., Di Pinto, R., Gaeta, V., Iovane, B., et al. (2019). *Report on advances for pediatricians in 2018: Allergy, cardiology, critical care, endocrinology, hereditary metabolic diseases, gastroenterology, infectious diseases, neonatology,*

nutrition, respiratory tract disorders and surgery. https://core.ac.uk/download/286528671.pdf (accessed on 7th August 2025).

14. Blaxhult, A., Bratt, G. A., Cullberg, M., Edlund, M., et al. (2009). *Sexually transmitted infections (STI) in men who have sex with men (MSM).* https://core.ac.uk/download/76980648.pdf (accessed on 7th August 2025).
15. Breugelmans, S., Casteleyn, C., Simoens, P., Van den Broeck, W., et al. (2011). *The tonsils revisited: Review of the anatomical localization and histological characteristics of the tonsils of domestic and laboratory animals.* https://core.ac.uk/download/pdf/8608468.pdf (accessed on 7th August 2025).
16. Burgess, J., Eisen, D., Lynch, D. P., Nordlund, J. J., et al. (2017). *Oral Examination.* https://core.ac.uk/download/213072873.pdf (accessed on 7th August 2025).
17. Cano-Pumarega, I., Castillo-García, M., García-Río, F., Martínez-Sánchez, J. M., et al. (2019). *Obstructive sleep apnea: Emerging treatments targeting the genioglossus muscle.* https://core.ac.uk/download/323287760.pdf (accessed on 7th August 2025).
18. Chahal, M., Clatworthy, M. R., Coates, M., Haniffa, M., Mather, M. W., & Talks, B. J. (2024). *Mapping Human Immunity and the Education of Waldeyer's Ring.* https://core.ac.uk/download/617062088.pdf (accessed on 7th August 2025).
19. Colella-Santos, M. F., Fujita, R. R., Monteiro, V. G., Moreira, R. R., et al. (2006). *Auditory processing assessment in children with obstructive sleep apnea syndrome.* https://core.ac.uk/download/37706494.pdf (accessed on 7th August 2025).
20. Di Carlo, G., Ierardo, G., Luzzi, V., Polimeni, A., et al. (2019). *Obstructive sleep apnea syndrome in the pediatric age: The role of the dentist.* https://core.ac.uk/download/196295362.pdf (accessed on 7th August 2025).
21. Dinesh, S. P. S., Ramamurthy, J., Srinivas, A., Viswanath, D., et al. (2015). *Obstructive Sleep Apnea: Awakening the Hidden Truth.* https://core.ac.uk/download/478302321.pdf (accessed on 7th August 2025).
22. Eley, K. A., Hopper, C., Hussain, F., McMillan, K., et al. (2020). *What the general dental practitioner needs to know about HPV-related oropharyngeal malignancy.* https://core.ac.uk/download/323054211.pdf (accessed on 7th August 2025).
23. Essa, R. (2018). *A review of adult tonsil histopathology and the effect of concomitant human immunodeficiency viruses infection.* https://core.ac.uk/download/188772584.pdf (accessed on 7th August 2025).
24. Fehrm, J. (2020). *Surgical treatment of obstructive sleep apnea: Randomized controlled studies in children and adults.* https://core.ac.uk/download/334508182.pdf (accessed on 7th August 2025).
25. Hidanti, M. L., & Prasetyo, A. (2015). *Head and neck cancer trends in Semarang: An analysis of ASR and ASCR.* https://core.ac.uk/download/76929358.pdf (accessed on 7th August 2025).
26. Ivaska, L. (2022). *Tonsils as an in Vivo Model: Virus Infections, Microbiome, and Immune Responses.* https://core.ac.uk/download/535017364.pdf (accessed on 7th August 2025).
27. Jackson, J. C. (2009). *Peritonsillar Abscess.* https://core.ac.uk/download/62772203.pdf (accessed on 7th August 2025).

28. Kohler, E., & Love, K. M. (1990). *Management of swallowing disorders: A program for professionals working in rural areas.* https://core.ac.uk/download/267583226.pdf (accessed on 7th August 2025).

29. Luceño-Mardones, A., Luceño-Rodríguez, I., Oliva-Pascual-Vaca, J., Oliva-Pascual-Vaca, M., et al. (2021). *Effects of osteopathic T9–T10 vertebral manipulation in tonsillitis: A randomized clinical trial.* https://core.ac.uk/download/459221665.pdf (accessed on 7th August 2025).

30. N/A. (2021). *Oral and Maxillofacial Surgery.* https://core.ac.uk/download/478137874.pdf (accessed on 7th August 2025).

31. N/A. (2025). *J Infect Dis.* https://core.ac.uk/download/153362519.pdf (accessed on 7th August 2025).

32. Nygren, D. (2023). *Fusobacterium necrophorum – From tonsillar carriage to Lemierre's syndrome.* https://core.ac.uk/download/587248190.pdf (accessed on 7th August 2025).

33. Okello, E., Ndeezi, G., Nayiga, I., & Lwabi, P. (2017). *Prevalence of group A streptococcus pharyngeal carriage and clinical manifestations in school children aged 5–15 yrs in Wakiso District, Uganda.* https://core.ac.uk/download/pdf/81606752.pdf (accessed on 7th August 2025).

34. Pushkar, A. K., Vardhan, P., Rajkumar, R. K. N., Pushkar, S., Kumawat, S., & Rani, S. (2023). *Efficacy of Tonsenorm Compound in the management of Tundikeri with special reference to chronic tonsillitis in children.* https://core.ac.uk/download/617189655.pdf (accessed on 7th August 2025).

35. Sathish, R. (2014). *Prospective Comparative Study of Coblation Versus Conventional Tonsillectomy.* https://core.ac.uk/download/235654569.pdf (accessed on 7th August 2025).

36. The Rockefeller University. (2013). BenchMarks 2013, July 26. https://core.ac.uk/download/519866528.pdf (accessed on 7th August 2025).

37. Vimmerová-Lattová, Z. (2013). *Endokrinní a metabolické aspekty vybraných spánkových poruch.* https://core.ac.uk/download/401794403.pdf (accessed on 7th August 2025).

38. Zautner, A. E., Podbielski, A., Kreikemeyer, B., Maletzki, C., Stropahl, G., Frickmann, H., Pau, H. W., et al. (2010). *Intracellular persisting Staphylococcus aureus is the major pathogen in recurrent tonsillitis.* https://core.ac.uk/download/pdf/8383843.pdf (accessed on 7th August 2025).

TRAUMA RECONSTRUCTION IN FACIAL COSMETIC

12

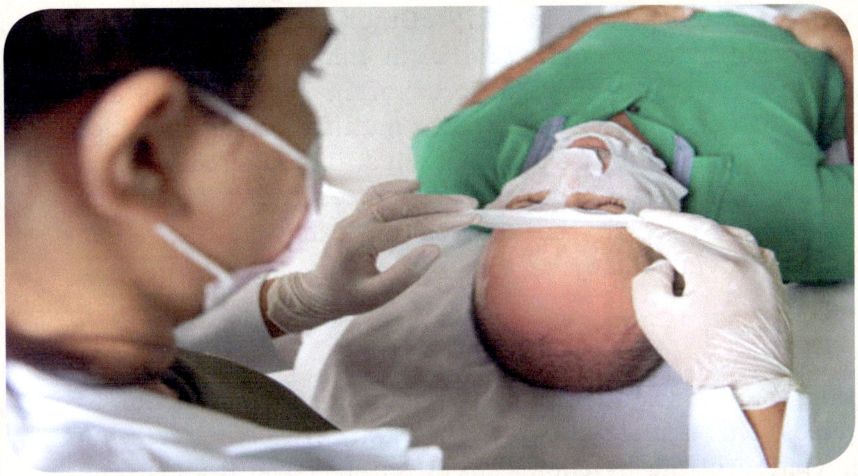

Introduction

The discipline of trauma reconstruction in the field of facial cosmetic surgery has gained significant interest owing to the increasing number of cases of facial trauma, either from accidents or violence or surgery. Facial structures are very important in both aesthetic and functional demands; efforts to reconstruct such structures to their pre-trauma state are prioritized. The face's reconstruction complexities are not just physical reconstruction of bone and tissue, but also the psychological effects of trauma. The most optimal reconstructive outcomes are capable of improving patients' self-esteem and quality of life, thereby highlighting the need for developments and innovations in surgical techniques and materials during the process of trauma management. Autologous grafting has been the gold standard in these situations for many years, providing good cosmetic outcomes at low risk of rejection from foreign substances (Abbott et al., 2003). The more demand there is for improved reconstructive techniques, the greater the quest for alternative techniques and materials. Though autologous bone

LEARNING OBJECTIVES

After studying this chapter, you will be able to:

1. Discuss facial trauma types;
2. Describe the psychological impact of facial trauma;
3. Highlight surgical methods of facial reconstruction;
4. Describe the cosmetic procedure contribution to reconstruction;
5. Understand a multidisciplinary treatment approach;
6. Know ethical issues in facial reconstruction.

grafting possesses numerous benefits, such as optimal biocompatibility and mechanical durability, its potential drawbacks, such as donor-site morbidity and protracted operation time, led to the development of alloplastic materials. These attempts to prevent the attendant complications of acquiring bone from the donor site while offering sufficient structural support and ultimately leading to increased patient recovery times. Clinical studies have yielded promising results regarding the use of synthetic bone substitutes and their ability to complement or even replace autologous grafts in certain instances (Neovius, 2016). Therefore, understanding the risks and benefits of traditional and new reconstruction techniques is paramount to achieving optimal surgical outcomes and lowering the rate of complications. Also, the integration of surgical and technical developments into trauma reconstruction processes is proof of the evolving nature of the field. The incorporation of minimally invasive surgical processes along with high-tech image-making technologies has allowed the surgery process to make more precise and effective restorations. Other seminal research in bioactive materials includes the bone morphogenetic proteins (BMPs) in enhancing bone repair and regeneration, but caution should be exercised in the variable reported success rates and complications with the use of such therapy. Further, comprehension of the multifaceted complexities of facial trauma involves an individualized consideration of each patient's unique circumstance, taking into account the type of injury, psychological issues, and long-term expectation for function. This multidisciplinary approach emphasizes the necessity of research and extensive training in trauma reconstruction (Abbott et al., 2003; Neovius, 2016).

Definition of Trauma Reconstruction

Trauma reconstruction is a multidisciplinary approach attempting to restore form and function to the facial form following traumatic injuries. This subject of study is not only critical for treating physical deformity but also for the alleviation of the psychological effects of facial trauma. The reconstructive process entails careful examination of the condition of the patient, as well as an appreciation of the cause of injury, for instance, vehicular accident, falling, or assault. Effective trauma reconstruction entails interdisciplinary cooperation between surgeons, orthodontists, and other healthcare workers as they strive to achieve the best aesthetic outcome while ensuring the underlying structural integrity of the facial bony skeleton. The nature of such cases often demands a combination of surgical techniques, like bone graft and soft tissue repositioning, to address both short-term and long-term needs at the same time. One of the most important features of trauma reconstruction is implementing advanced surgical techniques to restore facial aesthetics and function. Among those techniques, the facial artery perforator (FAP) flap has been attracting attention due to its unique advantages. Based on reports, this new technique has the potential to transform a normally two-stage procedure into a more efficient one-stage operation, therefore reducing the time and risks associated with surgery. FAP flaps are favored since they can provide better aesthetic results, especially for those patients seeking trauma reconstruction. Extensive use is, however, constrained by the need for extensive knowledge of the requisite anatomical features, which form the basis of successful application. Through cadaveric dissections, vast data regarding the facial artery, its perforating branches, and their diameter have been gathered, with better consistency of FAP flaps in reconstructive surgery on various parts of the face (Fogg et al., 2010). The psychological aspects of facial trauma cannot be ruled out, as they also hold equal value to the physical aspect. Trauma reconstruction not only aims at reversing the form of a patient but also restoring self-worth and rehabilitating them to re-integrate them into society. Patients typically experience shame or embarrassment resulting from external deformities that lead to social isolation or emotional distress. The multi-disciplinary aspect of trauma reconstruction emphasizes the coordination of care that includes emotional and psychological care in addition to surgical control. Comprehensive treatment regimens must also consider the application of adjunctive treatments, such as counseling or support groups, which are also able to supplement the healing process. Prioritizing both physical and psychological recovery is what makes trauma reconstruction such a crucial stepping stone towards achieving the quality of life in patients who have endured facial injuries (Bosio et al., 2008) (Figure 12.1).

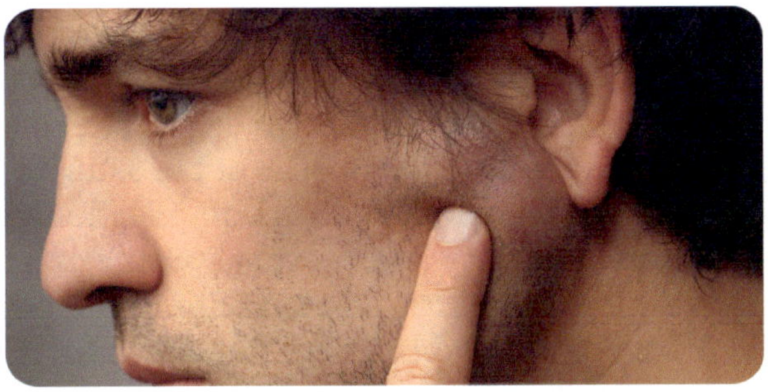

Figure 12.1. Trauma reconstruction.

Source: https://external-content.duckduckgo.com/iu/?u=https%3A%2F%2Fswosa.com%2Fwp-content%2Fuploads%2F2024%2F06%2FSWOSA_Procedures_Facial-Trauma-1024x512.png&f=1&nofb=1&ipt=e2abe8f4acbd96208c2452e8cc5e1722a10508118bdc347e84953073e717fa61.

Facial Aesthetics In Psychological Rehabilitation

The function of facial aesthetics in psychological rehabilitation cannot be overstated, especially in trauma reconstruction. In patients who have experienced disfiguring conditions or injuries, rebuilding of facial appearance generally leads to increased levels of self-esteem and self-confidence. It has been researched that an aesthetically pleasing face significantly contributes to how people see us, and thus affects interpersonal relationships as well as social interactions. In addition to cosmetic changes, a successful outcome in terms of facial aesthetics following trauma can also be a driver of emotional recovery. Patients are often said to feel psychologically more well when they perceive a return to a more familiar self, connecting physical presentation with mental health recovery on a direct level. This connection between beauty and emotional hardiness emphasizes the need for holistic methods that maximize facial aesthetics as fundamental aspects of psychological recovery. In craniofacial reconstruction, advancements in surgical techniques and technology have greatly improved the outcomes of aesthetic repair. The use of new devices, such as ultrasound-guided osteotomes, has enabled surgeons to perform fine procedures in the craniofacial region more accurately. For all this, studies have evidenced that such advanced devices lead to more quality micromorphological outcomes in bone healing, i.e., a smoother healing process for patients who are reconstructing (Anesi et al., 2014). These advancements are necessary since they improve not only the cosmetic results but also the psychological status of individuals. By reducing recovery time and complications, such strategies allow for an early return to regular life, thereby eliminating worry and providing confidence to patients who undergo traumatic facial injury. In addition, the exploration of tissue engineering and stem cell therapy also provides promising pathways for facial aesthetic enhancement and psychological healing. Recent studies indicate that stem cell therapy can regenerate damaged craniofacial tissue more effectively than existing methods (Hughes & Song, 2016). New technology aligns therapeutic goals and esthetic goals with a common emphasis on the structure and function of the face throughout the healing process. The integration of scientific findings with craniofacial surgery not only optimizes physical rehabilitation but also addresses the psychological implications of trauma. With patients finding new hope and identity from such cutting-edge treatments, psychological resilience is also increased. The convergence of cosmetic enhancement with medical technology ultimately underscores the reality that creation of facial aesthetics constitutes a key component in the overall rehabilitation of traumatized patients (Figure 12.2).

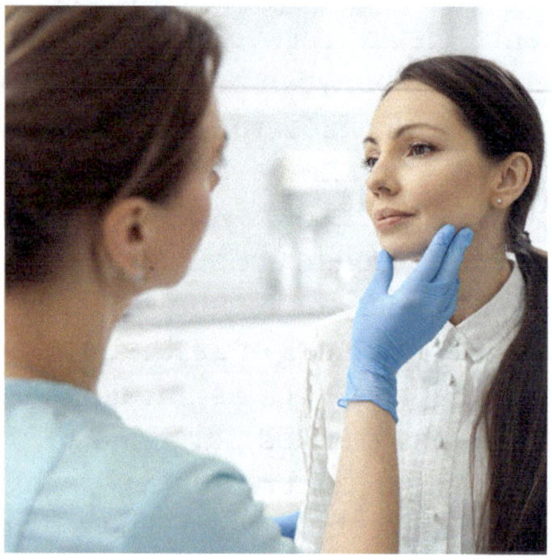

Figure 12.2. Importance of facial aesthetics in psychological recovery.

Source: https://external-content.duckduckgo.com/iu/?u=https%3A%2F%2Fthedentalsurgeries.co.uk%2Fwp-content%2Fuploads%2F2023%2F08%2Ffacial-aesthetics-consultation-1024x1024.jpeg&f=1&nofb=1&ipt=a9c2630f6869873a72c1b477add4378aeb0778b5db7bf51331462480354f0960.

12.1. Types of Facial Trauma

Learning Outcome

1. Common Causes of Facial Injuries
2. Classification of Facial Trauma
3. Impact of Trauma on Facial Structure

Facial trauma is a very critical area of investigation in the domain of trauma reconstruction due to its involvement with various types of trauma that have different implications on function and aesthetics. Facial trauma can occur in a variety of common forms, namely, soft tissue trauma, fracture, and laceration, each of which presents unique challenges during reconstruction. Soft tissue injury most commonly creates defects that compromise both protective and aesthetic roles of facial structures, necessitating advanced reconstruction techniques for optimal recovery. One such example is when trauma results in extensive lacerations that not only disrupt the skin but also involve underlying muscle and vascular components, which affect both cosmetic and functional outcomes, e.g., speech and swallowing. Understanding of the individual mechanisms and implications of such trauma is significant in the development of effective reconstructive methods, particularly in the restoration of facial integrity and patient confidence. Fractures are also a broad category of facial trauma involving bones of the skull and mandible, which would lead to complications if not attended to early and effectively. Some of the most commonly fractured facial bones include the nasal bones, zygomatic arch, and maxilla. All types of fractures require proper realignment and stabilization, which is typically done via surgery. Methods of reconstruction employed can make use of plates, screws, or grafts to restore harmony in the architecture and maintain functionality intact. Delayed intervention can exacerbate complications such as malocclusion or asymmetry, thus making later reconstruction more difficult. This timing value is also stressed by research that shows delayed intervention is expressed in greater aesthetic failures and increased patient morbidity, which necessitates that surgical procedures for facial fractures be timely and effective. When it comes to facial reconstructive modalities, the significance of newer surgical modalities cannot be overstated, particularly when facial injuries are very severe (Bodiwala et al., 2025). Newer surgical techniques, such as the pedicled forehead flap, have become indispensable tools in the quest for form and function restoration, particularly in challenging cases where standard methods are not effective. For example, the pedicled forehead flap has pertinent advantages regarding vascular assistance to enable the reconstruction of large traumatic soft tissue deficits. It has been shown to provide not just cosmetic rehabilitation but also functional recovery, as evidenced by the gain in improved oral competence and facial symmetry post-surgery. These methods emphasize how crucial it is for surgeons to have a clear knowledge of the nature of facial trauma, as clearly explicated in recent studies, revealing that personalized approaches concerning the nature of injury exhibit the best outcomes in trauma reconstruction in facial cosmetic conditions (Yu et al., 2022) (Figure 12.3).

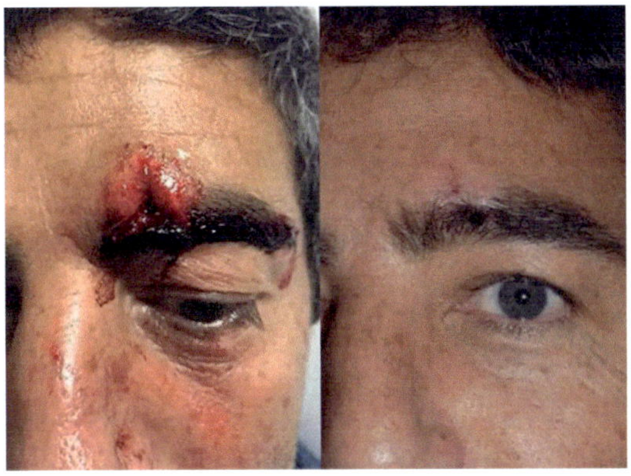

Figure 12.3. Facial trauma.

Source: https://www.darrensmithmd.com/wp-content/uploads/2023/08/facial-trauma-ba-2.webp.

12.1.1. Common Causes of Facial Injuries

Facial trauma is more common, and it most frequently results from different accidents and traumatic injuries. Car accidents are among the most common causes, whereby crashes result in high impact forces leading to fractures of the facial bones or damage to the soft tissues. Facial trauma from car crashes constitutes a high percentage of emergency department presentations and typically mandates complex surgical treatment, as witnessed in a review of trauma data. The degree of the injury can be highly variable, ranging from lacerations of soft tissue to fractures involving the mandible or maxilla. In treating these injuries, it is critical to understand the mechanisms of injury as they directly affect the reconstruction techniques used in trauma surgery. Understanding these allows surgeons to plan successful reconstruction in order to restore function and aesthetic appearance in patients with such traumas. Interpersonal violence, such as physical assaults and cases of domestic violence, is also a significant cause of facial injuries. Statistics indicate that facial trauma due to brawls or domestic disputes is very high, particularly among certain populations. Injuries of this nature are most commonly reported as midface fractures, zygomatic bone fractures, and lacerations. Management of such injuries often entails unique challenges as patients not only require physical therapy but also psychological counseling due to the nature of their trauma. Furthermore, facial nerve and vascular exposure during surgeries requires cautious attention to avoid long-term consequences of aesthetic and functional deficits. Therefore, classification of various etiologies of facial trauma introduces the topics of prevention and management with emphasis on particular strategies in reconstructive trauma. Injuries secondary to sports are a frequent cause of facial trauma seen in patients of all ages. Contact sports such as football, hockey, and boxing have a high incidence of facial injuries, mainly due to direct blows, falls, or impact against another participant. They most commonly present as fractures of the nasal and zygomatic bones and soft tissue damage in the patterns of contusions and lacerations. Protective equipment, such as helmets and face masks, plays an important role in reducing the number and degree of injuries. Rates are still high with precautions, emphasizing the need for continued research and development in preventive techniques and surgery. As trauma reconstruction emerges, advanced imaging modalities and minimally invasive surgical approaches must be included to enhance recovery outcomes in athletes with facial injuries due to sporting activities (Figure 12.4).

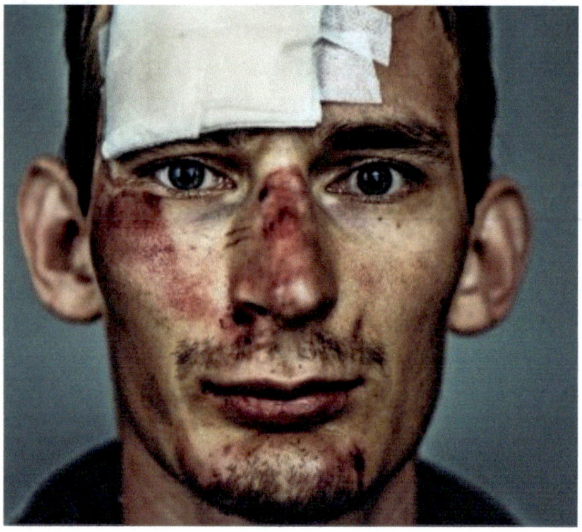

Figure 12.4. Facial injuries.

Source: https://external-content.duckduckgo.com/iu/?u=https%3A%2F%2Fhpasolicitors.com%2Fwp-content%2Fuploads%2Felementor%2Fthumbs%2FFace-Injury-Claims-r0agjx97hbzl4y5mzi3yr0z6s29s2emlymrirc940s.jpg&f=1&nofb=1&ipt=d1525ea2115a227695fcb5f8623e492020b521257da5146f4cb6fa09b0853bda.

12.1.2. Classification of Facial Trauma

Facial trauma must be classified in order to guide treatment plans in trauma reconstruction. Facial trauma can in general be classified into soft tissue and hard tissue trauma, both with varying implications for reconstruction surgery. Soft tissue damage typically involves laceration, abrasion, and contusion that represents a continuum of injury to the skin, muscles, and underlying structures. It is classically divided into depth and distribution, with special emphasis on preserving function and aesthetic outcome. Conversely, hard tissue injuries entail fractures of facial bones such as the maxilla, mandible, and zygomatic arch that can potentially significantly impact function and aesthetics. Proper classification helps in determining the most appropriate reconstructive approach depending on the severity and extent of the injuries, thus ensuring better patient outcomes for reconstructive procedures. In the area of facial trauma, a broad-based classification system attempts to address the variability of numerous injury patterns found in the clinical environment. Tuli et al.'s suggested broad-based system distinguishes facial fractures as either high-energy or low-energy forms and offers insights regarding mechanisms of trauma based on impact forces. This differentiation is crucial for reconstructive surgeons when scheduling operations, as high-energy trauma causes more extensive damage that may require advanced techniques and materials for reconstruction (Desai et al., 2020). Second, understanding the location and pattern of mandibular and maxillary fractures, which are most common in facial trauma, allows for a more tailored treatment strategy whereby not only structural reconstruction but also aesthetic restoration of the patient's face can be addressed by surgeons. Such subtle classification allows surgeons to optimize surgical procedures effectively. The growing application of technological advancements, such as three-dimensional (3D) printing, is reshaping facial trauma classification and reconstruction. While traditional classifications are significantly reliant on clinical examination and imaging, 3D models from Digital Imaging and Communications in Medicine (DICOM) data are ultimately more accurate in preoperative planning and education. Through the production of three-dimensional models of intricate fractures, reconstructive surgeons can comprehend facial anatomy and spatial relationships more clearly in a trauma environment. Not only does this new modality improve the precision of surgical procedures, but it is also beneficial for patient counseling and visualization of anticipated results. As proposed in recent literature, there is some expectation that use of 3D-printed models will grow in reconstructive procedures, particularly cementing further the association between innovative technologies and maximized classification in the management of facial trauma (Mitsouras et al., 2015).

12.1.3. Impact of Trauma on Facial Structure

Trauma radically transforms facial structures, both in terms of appearance as well as functional integrity. Facial trauma can be brought about by a variety of reasons like road accidents, falls, and violent confrontations. The traumatic injury is prone to cause fractures, cuts, and displacements of the bone as well as soft tissue. These alterations can provide overt deformities as well as impaired functions, such as chewing, speech, and breathing. Also, the psychological impact of facial trauma is prominent, with patients showing reduced self-esteem and withdrawal from society. Hence, learning about the different methods by which trauma affects facial contours is necessary to incorporate clinical interventions and psychological therapy as part of the reconstruction process. Reconstruction of facial trauma encompasses numerous surgical techniques and cutting-edge technology to recapture both the contour and function. One of the notable advancements in this field is the use of piezosurgery, which offers a more precise method for osteotomies compared to traditional instruments. Studies have established that techniques like Piezosurgery Medical® result in more precise incisions without injuring surrounding tissues such as the dura mater and nervous tissue. The reduced trauma to the surrounding tissues promotes better healing and reossification of the injured bone surfaces, addressing not just the short-term cosmetic problems but also long-term sustainability of the bone and associated tissues (Anesi et al., 2014). The improvements point to the necessity of selecting proper surgical methods that are crafted based on the unique character of the trauma, as well as the desired outcomes of the reconstruction. Secondly, the integration of 3D body-surface scanning technology has revolutionized the planning and assessment stages. Advanced imaging modalities such as these facilitate the accurate visualization and measurement of a patient's facial anatomy, which remains critical for the creation of individualized treatment plans. The accurate information provided by 3D scanning aids surgeons' predictions and designs prosthetics or grafts required for effective reconstruction (Figure 12.5).

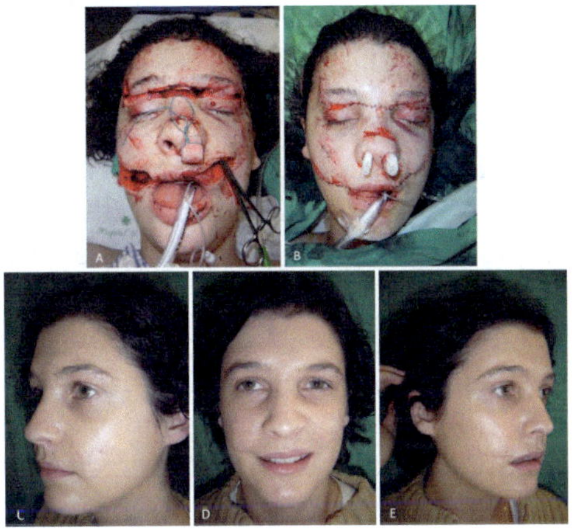

Figure 12.5. Trauma on the facial structure.

Source: https://media.springernature.com/lw685/springer-static/image/chp%3A10.1007%2F978-3-642-38482-0_133-2/MediaObjects/272888_0_En_133-2_Fig2_HTML.jpg.

Test Your Knowledge

1. How do different types of facial trauma, such as soft tissue injuries, fractures, and burns, differ in terms of severity, treatment, and recovery outcomes?
2. What are the most common causes of facial trauma, and how do they influence the pattern and classification of facial injuries?

12.2. Psychological Effects of Facial Trauma

Learning Outcome

1. Emotional and Mental Health Implications
2. Social Stigma and Its Effects on Recovery
3. Role of Self-image in Psychological Healing

The psychological consequences of facial trauma are profound and intricate, typically leading to extreme emotional pain that impacts individuals' quality of life. Facial traumas, when they occur, not only jeopardize physical appearances but also challenge personal identity and social relationships. Patients may experience a range of psychological reactions, including anxiety, depression, and post-traumatic stress disorder (PTSD), as they cope with altered self-concept and social perceptions. Research indicates that the seriousness of facial injury correlates with the seriousness of psychological symptomatology observed, illustrating an intricate relationship between physical and psychological well-being. The unique form of each individual's experience calls for a personalized approach to trauma reconstruction, where the overriding priority lies in psychological support as well as physical rehabilitation. The psychological trauma has to be treated in the patient with facial trauma so that complete recovery can be facilitated. Cosmetic reconstructive surgery can play a pivotal role in facilitating this process, both restoring the physical damage and healing emotionally as well. As discussed, utilization of autologous bone grafting in facial reconstruction has distinctive advantages, including improved aesthetic outcomes that are able to significantly boost a patient's self-esteem and psychological rehabilitation (Abbott et al., 2003). Successful surgery can lead to enhanced social contact and reduced social isolation, thus allowing individuals to restore their sense of identity. However, the psychological recovery cannot be left out because the patients can still go on struggling to get used to the new appearance and cope with social interactions after the surgery. Additionally, advances in surgical techniques, for example, utilization of Piezosurgery® for surgical osteotomies, have been shown to have potential positive outcomes for both physical and psychological recovery (Anesi et al., 2014). Maintenance of the surrounding tissues during surgery with meticulousness minimizes complications and improves cosmetic results, which can minimize recovery-related anxiety. By improving not just the structural support for facial structures but also the psychosocial aspect of healing, such technologies can result in better overall outcomes for patients. Ultimately, there is a need for an effective global approach that addresses both physical and psychological consequences of facial trauma in trauma reconstruction, giving the person assistance in their healing process and reintegration into society (Figure 12.6).

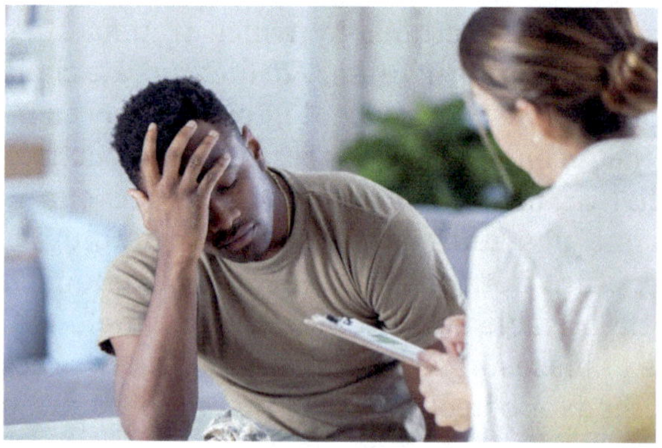

Figure 12.6. Psychological effects of facial trauma.

Source: https://www.sanantoniobehavioral.com/wp-content/uploads/2021/12/psychological-trauma.jpg.

12.2.1. Emotional and Mental Health Implications

Facial cosmetic surgery, particularly in trauma reconstruction, has emotional and mental health implications which are myriad and extensive.

Patients undergoing such procedures often wish for changes that not only aim to restore the physical but also to heal the psychological. Research has established that patients who undergo reconstructive surgeries such as rhinoplasty are likely to experience extensive alterations in mental health status, particularly with regard to depression. In a trial of 200 rhinoplasty patients, there was a great decline in depression scores at six months after the operation ($p=0.032$) (Bazgir et al., 2023). The finding illustrates how cosmetic surgery can enhance emotional well-being by addressing feelings of inadequacy or social embarrassment that could be caused by facial disfigurements or injuries. But it is also critical to look at the psychological factors why and how these procedures are done so that maladaptive body views do not result from them. In addition, all emotional outcomes are not positive. The interplay between early life and body image can be a deciding factor in whether cosmetic procedures work for an individual's mental health. Surgery patients with a history of childhood trauma and neglect may have deep-seated body shame-related issues, which thus manifest as body dysmorphic disorder after surgery. Body dysmorphic disorder is characterized by obsessive concerns regarding perceived flaws and persistent dissatisfaction regardless of surgery (Constantian, 2022). If the patients carry unresolved psychological trauma related to their concept of self, then the expectation that cosmetic surgery will be an overall increase in mental health may remain unfulfilled. Thus, resolution of the psychological concerns on which a patient's motivation for surgery lies is of special significance for trauma reconstruction in the field of facial cosmetic surgery. In general, the emotional and psychological impacts of facial cosmetic surgery trauma reconstruction must be tackled with complex insight. Although evidence has shown that these procedures can lead to improvement in mental well-being, it is also important to note that the psychological factors and individual histories play significant roles in such cases. A careful assessment concerning patients' pre-surgery mental health may potentially identify at-risk individuals for ill effects, for instance, anxiety or body dysmorphic disorder. By including psychological counseling and guidance in the cosmetic surgical intervention, clinicians are better able to make certain that the benefits of trauma reconstruction transition from physical changes to facilitate long-term emotional recovery (Figure 12.7).

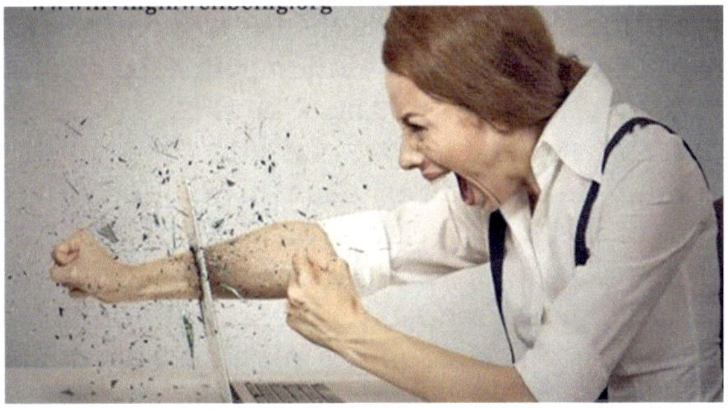

Figure 12.7. Emotional and mental health implications of facial cosmetic procedures.

Source: https://www.livinginwellbeing.org/wp-content/uploads/2019/05/Emotional-Mental-Health-Problems-1200x675.jpg.

12.2.2. Social Stigma and Its Effects on Recovery

The process of healing from facial trauma is normally tainted by the pervasive social stigma that accompanies altered appearances. Victims of extreme facial injuries are often confronted with current social attitudes that characterize them as different or unfortunate. Stigma does this to cut one off and make them feel inferior, and over time, this impedes emotional healing. Research demonstrates that the psychosocial effects of facial disfigurements have a tendency to surpass the bodily injuries, extending to affect self-esteem and interpersonal relations. The stigma is also bolstered by the cultural emphasis on aesthetics and beauty, which tends to enhance the psychological disturbance in recovering patients. Identification of these dynamics is important, given the fact that the social world has a profound impact on one's ability to metabolize trauma and react positively to rehabilitative efforts. The effects of social stigma are multifaceted and function differently across different demographic populations. Individuals recuperating from facial trauma, be it due to accidents or medical procedures, may be subjected to gendered nuances in the practice and perception of stigma. For example, women may experience more judgment over their looks and the beauty standards of society. Men may experience stigmas related to challenging their sense of masculinity and being strong. Both populations have to navigate complex social environments that can either reinforce healing or disrupt healing. Because of this, supportive networks are needed that take into consideration the individual needs of each population. These types of networks can promote dialogue and sharing of experience, thereby reducing the stigmatizing segregation of recovery paths. In cosmetic reconstruction, addressing social stigma is not only demanded for cosmetic improvement but also for general recuperation. The innovation of prosthetic design and production, for instance, custom-made artificial eyes, is a demonstration of collaboration of technological advancement and social acceptance in recuperation. Despite these advances, studies indicate that there is still limited knowledge of the psychosocial impacts of wearing appearance-transforming devices, such as artificial eyes, which can perpetuate stigma (Chinnery et al., 2016). At the same time, what cisgender and transgender patients go through in the performance of cosmetic surgeries is found to be parallel as far as motivation and postoperative satisfaction are concerned, but accentuates differential access to support systems along gender status (Windsor, 2011). This means a demand for certain therapeutic techniques with stigmatization of altered aesthetics in mind for purposes of encouraging broader understanding and acceptance within society.

12.2.3. Role of Self-image in Psychological Healing

The relationship between self-image and psychological healing is of profound significance, specifically in facial cosmetic surgery of trauma reconstruction. Self-concept, one's own definition of one's own physical appearance and one's overall worth, is a deciding factor in the direction of mental health outcomes. In cosmetic facial patients, the desire to improve is typically linked with a past history of traumatic incidents in which their self-concept has been negatively impacted. This interaction suggests that individuals who perceive a disparity between the inner being and outward appearances may suffer from low self-esteem as well as social anxiety. Thus, treating these elements through surgery is not only able to alter an individual's outer appearance but also invoke powerful psychological healing. The psychological effects of bodily deformity or perceived ugliness can manifest in the form of social anxiety, depression, and a severe effect on inter-relations. The majority of individuals who experience trauma, particularly where the facial aesthetics are altered or disfigured, do have self-view concerns that affect their mental health. Recovery towards redefinition of one's self-perception involves a sensitive therapy process where people can modify their pre- and postoperative selves. To reiterate, incorporating psychological care into the cosmetic surgical process cannot be overstressed. These treatments benefit patients not only through the physical changes but also through the emotional effects that accompany them, so that a very holistic approach to reconstruction of trauma in facial cosmetic surgery is possible. Furthermore, self-image extends beyond the individual and into interpersonal relationships and social interaction. Following reconstructive surgery, patients may have higher self-esteem, which translates into more positive social interactions and relief from feelings of disconnection and isolation that the surgery client may have experienced before surgery. Research indicates that a positive change in self-image can lead to tangible benefits in a person's overall quality of life, such as healthier relationships and an increased social support network. Furthermore, successful outcomes from reconstructive surgery can confirm a patient's identity and agency, restoring their resilience to previous traumas. It is where the role of self-image not just facilitates psychological healing but develops a new sense of self, enabling individuals to regain control over their lives following trauma (Anesi et al., 2014; Cheung et al., 2014) (Figure 12.8).

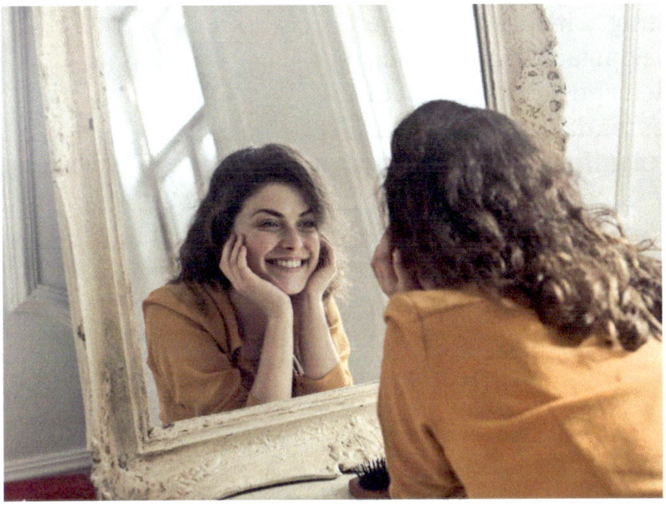

Figure 12.8. Role of self-image in psychological healing.

Source: https://cdn2.psychologytoday.com/assets/styles/manual_crop_4_3_1200x900/public/teaser_image/blog_entry/2024-11/pexels-olly-774866.jpg?itok=jiIeR7Fe.

Test Your Knowledge

1. How does facial trauma affect a patient's self-esteem, body image, and social interactions?
2. What psychological support strategies are most effective in helping patients cope with emotional distress following facial trauma?

12.3. Surgical Techniques in Facial Reconstruction

Learning Outcome

1. Overview of Surgical Options Available
2. Innovations in Surgical Technology
3. Importance of Personalized Treatment Plans

Accuracy of surgical technique is the essence of facial cosmetic surgery for the restoration of form and function, as well as aesthetic form, in the process of trauma reconstruction. The multidisciplinary nature of facial plastic surgery, which involves composite techniques from otolaryngology, oral maxillofacial surgery, dermatology, ophthalmology, and plastic surgery, provides a complete approach to the management of traumatic injury. Reconstructive surgery often entails the use of new flap techniques, which aim to restore the integrity of the cutaneous and promote healing with minimal scarring. These techniques are continually evolving since they are governed by advances in surgical skills and adjunctive technologies, necessitating surgeons to remain updated on existing practice of facial reconstruction to enhance patient results (Chuang et al., 2016). Among the many surgical techniques, the bicoronal flap technique has emerged as a so-called catch-all procedure when dealing with troublesome facial and skull fractures. Popularized by Tessier, the technique offers wide exposure to the field while preserving all the essential neurovascular structures intact, thus significantly reducing postoperative morbidity. Bicoronal incision is where the incision is made within the area of hair-bearing skin, which not only gives the necessary exposure to the site of surgery but also optimizes the cosmetic outcome upon recovery.

Each case of the application of this technique has underscored its versatility, in that it may be tailored to suit different pathological conditions within the frontal region (Balachandar et al., 2012). The benefits of this flap operation extend beyond enhancing aesthetic looks; it provides potential for functional reconstruction that is critical in reconstructive trauma. Beyond traditional flap techniques, the integration of minimally invasive procedures is transforming the component of facial reconstruction surgery. Techniques such as injectables and lasers have gained popularity to the extent that they provide surgeons with the ability to enhance facial aesthetics with fewer traumatic maneuvers. These methods can correct texture defects, soft tissue deficiency, and aging alterations that can occur after trauma. The incorporation of these non-surgical adjuncts into practice complements surgery, allowing for a more extensive solution to facial reconstruction. Surgeons are thus encouraged to integrate highly innovative surgical techniques with innovative cosmetic procedures in order to attain optimal recovery and patient satisfaction when patients need trauma reconstruction in facial cosmetics (Chuang et al., 2016) (Figure 12.9).

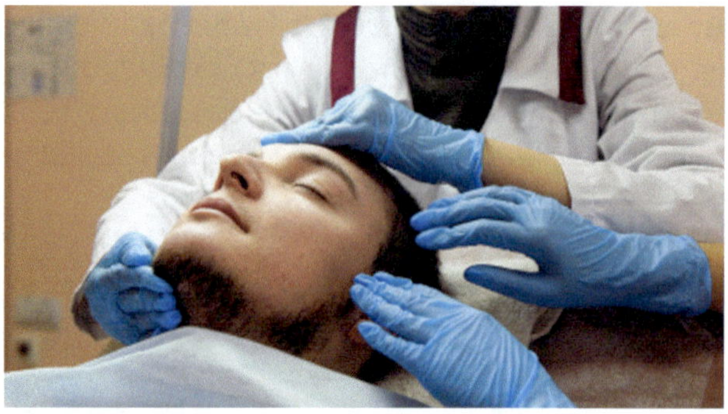

Figure 12.9. Surgical techniques in facial reconstruction.

Source: https://www.medstarhealth.org/-/media/project/mho/medstar/services/h1_doctor-examining-paitents-face.jpg?h=410&iar=0&w=730&hash=7108613E91018EEFFD7F7F490816C63D.

12.3.1. Overview of Surgical Options Available

For trauma reconstruction within facial cosmetic purposes, surgical options vary significantly based on the severity and nature of injuries incurred. One of the more significant techniques employs autologous bone grafts, which are harvested from the patient's own body to facilitate the reconstruction of facial shape and function. This technique is particularly suited to the repair of craniomaxillofacial fractures, as it ensures biological compatibility and low risk of rejection. However, there are consequences, as harvesting these grafts runs the risk of additional surgical sites and complications. With the aim to enhance the results of surgery, the application of emerging technologies such as 3D printing has emerged as a viable option, allowing for the fabrication of personalized implants and surgical guides to fit the unique anatomical features of the patient's face, resulting in improved function and aesthetics. Along with 3D printing and bone grafting, other surgical techniques have also been established to address the different needs of patients undergoing facial reconstruction. As an example, soft tissue grafting is used to restore volume and shape, especially in the area of trauma. This can involve the transfer of skin, muscle, or fat from the rest of the body, tailored to fit the defect resulting from injury. The success of the procedure relies largely on the meticulous planning of the surgical site and the source of donor tissues. Besides, technology in microsurgical techniques has also enhanced the precision of soft tissue reconstruction to the extent that the complex anastomosis of veins and arteries, and also nerves, can be achieved with good perfusion and function of the transplanted tissue.

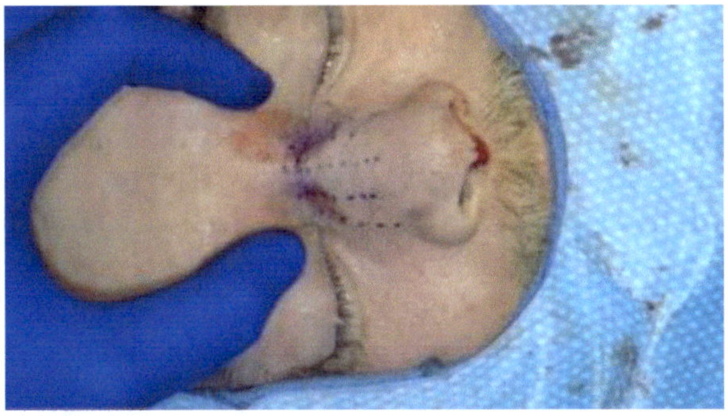

Figure 12.10. Surgical options for trauma reconstruction.

Source: https://cfvod.kaltura.com/p/1315631/sp/131563100/thumbnail/entry_id/1_x80jwhen/version/100011/height/197/width/350.

The evolving techniques make it possible for a better quality of life for patients through the enhancement of both form and function. The application of technology and emerging techniques in trauma reconstruction recognizes the need for a multidisciplinary approach between surgical teams. Craniofacial, plastic, and reconstructive surgeons also often work with specialists from other fields to offer comprehensive care of facial trauma. Teamwork is crucial, especially when treating complex trauma that can involve bones, soft tissue, and ocular tissues. For instance, in cases like anterior staphyloma, where complicated ocular deformities resulting from trauma develop, surgery and prosthetic rehabilitation afterward have been successful, as shown in comparative studies (Yadav et al., 2025). Besides, the use of 3D-printed devices has been effective in producing patient-specific results, which contribute to facial symmetry and functional capacity restoration (Oley et al., 2024). These novel techniques reflect the ongoing evolution of surgical methods observed in trauma reconstruction of facial cosmetic surgery, ending in enhanced patient outcomes and experience (Figure 12.10).

12.3.2. Innovations in Surgical Technology

The recent technological advancements in surgical technology have significantly changed the dynamics of trauma reconstruction in facial cosmetics. Developments such as minimally invasive surgery, computer-assisted surgical planning, and newer imaging technologies have vastly improved surgical outcomes and recovery of the patient. One of them is the development of ultrasonic osteotomes that have replaced traditional cutting technologies in craniofacial surgeries. These devices make precise cuts with minimal trauma to the encompassing tissue, promoting better healing and less intraoperative complications. As a result, the application of such technologies not only ensures optimal aesthetic results but also enhances functional restoration of facial morphology. This convergence of innovation serves to put the central role of technology into focus to revolutionize the standard practice of reconstructive surgery to offer new hope for patients with facial trauma and deformities (Chuang et al., 2016). Developments in 3D printing technology have also changed preoperative planning and intraoperative control for facial cosmetic reconstruction. Surgeons can now create patient-specific facial anatomy models to allow precise surgical plans individualized to specific needs. These models are capable of being used to develop custom-designed implants, reducing the risk of biocompatibility complications and allowing for greater ease of integration with the surrounding tissues. Coupled with virtual reality environments for simulating operations, accuracy in trauma reconstruction has never been greater. These customized methods not only enhance the surgeon's capability for predicting complications but also improve the patient's experience through enhanced translucence of the surgical process. To this end, these innovations introduce a paradigm shift in solving facial cosmetic procedures, leading to improved patient outcomes and satisfaction (Anesi et al., 2014).

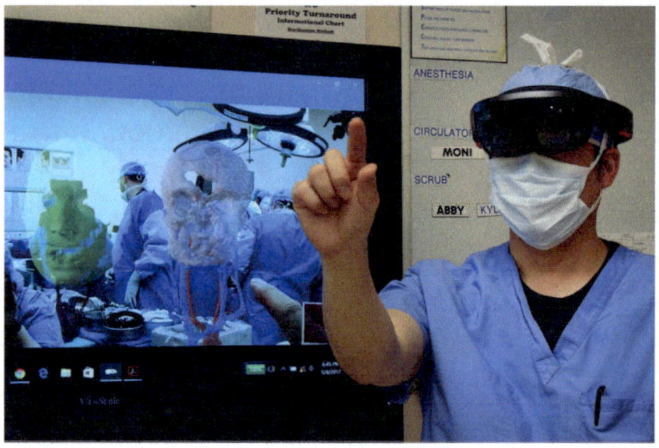

Figure 12.11. Innovations in surgical technology.

Source: https://medical-technology.nridigital.com/medical-technology/medical_technology_yb20/how_is_technology_transforming_facial_reconstruction_surgery/788339/Researcher_using_Halo_Lens.960_0_1.jpg.

Aside from the surgical devices themselves, the use of artificial intelligence and digital technology in patient management and postoperative care also contributed to advancements in the field. Predictive analytics using patient data analysis can ensure better selection of surgical procedures and interventions after surgery, resulting in a more tailored approach to recovery. The use of augmented reality is on the agenda to assist surgeons in actual surgery, providing immediate feedback and visualizations of critical anatomical structures. The application of digital technology in the surgical workflow is not a plus but is becoming pivotal to the achievement of trauma reconstruction excellence. Constant research into the newest technological advances is an allegiance to refine surgical methods, ultimately resulting in decreased complications, faster recovery times, and better overall patient results in facial cosmetic surgery (Chuang et al., 2016) (Figure 12.11).

12.3.3. Importance of Personalized Treatment Plans

Personalized treatment planning and its execution are of the highest priority in the practice of trauma reconstruction in cosmetic facial surgery. Every patient possesses a one-of-a-kind set of anatomical features, medical background, and aesthetic aspirations that must be carefully planned for in order to achieve optimal results. Personalized approaches allow for customized intervention that not only addresses the physical component of the trauma but also the psychological needs of the patient. This personalized care improves patient satisfaction and creates the illusion of control, thereby facilitating a better healing process. It has been established through research that the psychological status of patients who are about to undergo reconstructive procedures can also have a tangible effect on their recovery, and therefore, the treatment plan should not only be physically responsive to the patients' needs but also psychologically. Technological advancements, such as the application of precision surgical equipment and the use of artificial intelligence, have further emphasized the need for such customized plans. As an example, technologies such as ultrasonic osteotomes have shown benefits over traditional osteotomes when used to prevent damage to surrounding tissues and enhance bone healing results. These advancements allow surgeons to choose methods most appropriate to the specific requirements of the trauma being treated, ensuring high levels of precision and efficiency in reconstructive surgery. The ability to individualize operative procedures both to the anatomy of the patients as well as the nature of the trauma puts personalized treatment protocols in the very center of modern facial cosmetic surgery. The inclusion of technology such as AI can automate this process further, ultimately leading to better surgical planning and treatment of patients (Aguayo et al., 2024). Moreover, the incorporation of data-driven insights within individual treatment plans can significantly increase the predictability of surgery outcomes. Advanced imaging techniques and analysis help create deep profiles of patients, leading to improved decision-making. They can also outline realistic cosmetic expectations in harmony with the patient's lifestyle and wants, which can directly impact postoperative satisfaction. Personalization even extends to the postoperative recovery, where customized rehabilitation programs can enable functional recovery and emotional well-being. Therefore, not only is it helpful, it is a critical practice of reconstructive facial cosmetic surgery for trauma that acknowledges the diverse realities and fantasies of patients, ultimately leading to improved care and outcomes (Anesi et al., 2014) (Figure 12.12).

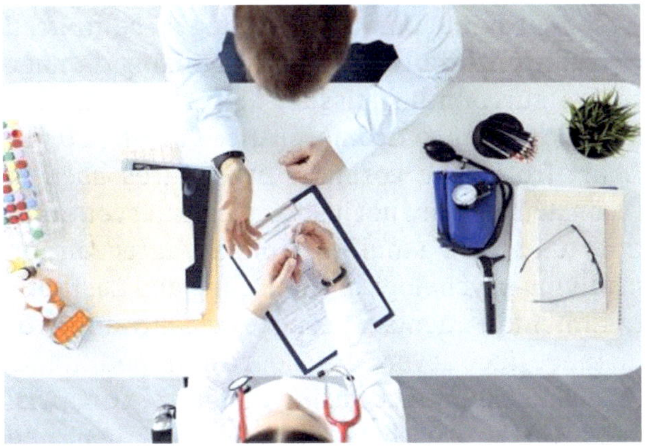

Figure 12.12. Importance of personalized treatment plans.

Source: https://www.indiapharmaoutlook.com/uploaded_images/newstransfer/r6e2Captureujiklo.JPG.

Test Your Knowledge

1. What are the different surgical methods used in facial reconstruction, and how do surgeons decide which technique is most appropriate for a specific facial injury?
2. How do procedures such as skin grafts, local flaps, and free tissue transfer help restore both function and appearance in facial reconstruction patients?

12.4. Role of Cosmetic Procedures in Reconstruction

Learning Outcome

1. Integration of Cosmetic Techniques in Trauma Recovery
2. Non-Surgical Options for Facial Enhancement
3. Patient Satisfaction and Quality of Life Improvements

The use of cosmetic surgery in reconstruction is a crucial element in enhancing the welfare of patients suffering from facial trauma. Psychological and emotional effects of the trauma are extremely debilitating, leading to significant psychosocial disabilities. For instance, facial deformities caused by trauma can significantly alter one's image and interpersonal functioning, and thus reconstruction is not merely a physical restoration issue but also a mental health emergency. By applying new cosmetic surgery techniques, surgeons attempt to reestablish not only the structure but also the aesthetic appearance of the face. These procedures typically utilize new technology and techniques, where the accuracy and success of surgical operations are further enhanced. This is best observed through the implementation of ultrasonic osteotomes, which provide unique advantages compared to traditional tools through minimizing damage to the surrounding tissue, thereby promoting better healing outcomes (Anesi et al., 2014). Apart from that, cosmetic procedures used in reconstruction are not just surgical interventions; they tend to be a multidisciplinary intervention involving psychological counseling and aesthetic treatments. Patients exposed to ocular trauma, for instance, face severe psychosocial impediments that can be minimized using customized artificial eyes. Such prosthetic devices are designed to rehabilitate not just the visual aspect but also the emotional and social aspects of the wearer's existence (Chinnery et al., 2016). The present report and technological advances in the design and construction of these artificial prosthetics signify the heightened acceptance of the psychosocial aspects that accompany facial trauma. As such, the integration of cosmetic aspects in reconstructive surgery has a considerable role to play in ensuring patient satisfaction and quality of life by meeting both the functional and aesthetic needs of the patient. Finally, the role of cosmetic surgery in reconstruction points to the importance of considering the needs and wishes of individual patients during recovery. Individualization of the reconstructive processes ensures physical restoration is compatible with the psychological as well as social desires of the patient. Physicians are becoming more patient-focused, engaging individuals in discussions about their expectations and goals. This cooperative process enhances patients' feelings of agency and empowerment, which contribute to improved psychological outcomes after surgery. With the progress of cosmetic surgeries, not only do they have the potential to enhance physical looks, but they also allow emotional recovery, thereby changing the trajectory of recovery from trauma. Thus, the combination of cosmetic procedures with reconstructive surgery clearly evinces a sense of the subtle interaction between physical rehabilitation and psychosocial restoration (Figure 12.13).

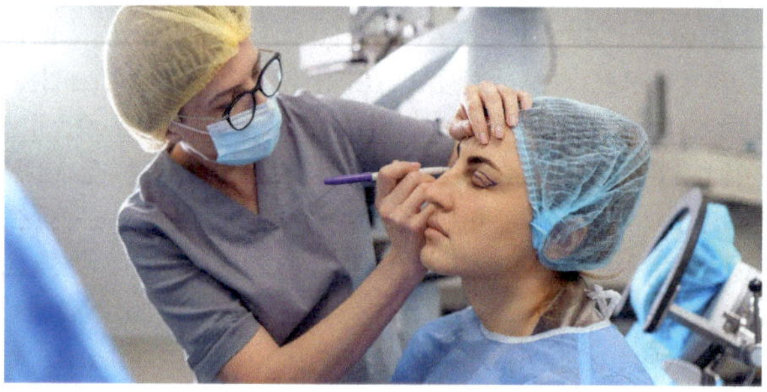

Figure 12.13. Cosmetic procedures.

Source: https://cachevalleyent.com/storage/2023/10/Reconstructive-Surgery-by-Cache-Valley-ENT-in-Logan-UT-scaled-2560x1280.jpeg.

12.4.1. Integration of Cosmetic Techniques in Trauma Recovery

Combining cosmetic methods with trauma recovery has emerged as an essential component in facial reconstruction, with important benefits on both aesthetic results and functional performance. As patients recover from traumatic facial injuries, focus shifts more and more to restoring physical appearance and psychological well-being. This dual strategy is important because the external consequences of trauma are capable of seriously degrading self-esteem and social interactions. Through the application of cosmetic techniques that prioritize careful tissue handling and aesthetic enhancement, caregivers can reduce scarring and maximize overall facial symmetry. These treatments are usually supplemented by technological advances that enable proper surgical techniques, thereby optimizing recovery avenues for patients with facial trauma, finally bridging the gap between medical necessity and esthetic demand, evident in today's research on craniofacial surgery (Neovius, 2016). The application of advanced surgical techniques, including ultrasonic osteotomes, has totally revolutionized the practice in the treatment of facial trauma. In contrast with traditional methods that can injure surrounding tissues, the innovative devices not only enhance bone cut precision but also preserve essential soft tissue morphology. Research indicates that piezosurgical procedures not only achieve improved micromorphology of osteotomized surfaces but also facilitate better healing and reossification (Anesi et al., 2014). This is particularly advantageous in trauma healing, where aesthetics and integrity of bone are simultaneous objectives. These developments highlight the importance of integrating cosmetic principles during trauma surgery, equipping surgeons with the tools to achieve optimal functional and aesthetic results, ultimately enhancing patients' quality of life following injury and rebuilding their bodies and also their resilience. Moreover, a full system of trauma rehabilitation entails multidisciplinary teamwork between surgeons, psychologists, and rehabilitation professionals. Such an association not only assures to focus on the physical aspects of recovery through advanced cosmetic treatments but also underscores the necessity of mental health treatment for trauma victims. Because facial trauma can profoundly affect self-concept, psychological ramifications need to be addressed for complete recovery. By integrating cosmetic with psychosocial treatments, treatment planning can be tailored to individual patient needs to create an environment conducive to healing and personal growth. Lastly, the synthesis of cosmetic surgery with trauma recovery is an innovative paradigm shift in facial reconstruction, demonstrating how aesthetic artistry in cosmetic surgery can smoothly complement medical treatments to provide greater degrees of patient satisfaction and improved general outcomes in trauma treatment (Anesi et al., 2014; Neovius, 2016).

12.4.2. Non-Surgical Options for Facial Enhancement

In contemporary facial cosmetic surgery, enhancement without surgery is a dominant trend, particularly with trauma reconstruction. The procedures allow patients to achieve their desired appearance without exposing themselves to the risks and recovery times associated with invasive interventions. One of the most popular non-surgical procedures is dermal fillers, which can easily restore the cheeks and lips, among other features, to make the face appear young. Besides, neuromodulators like Botox are often employed to minimize the appearance of wrinkles by paralyzing specific facial muscles for a temporary period of time. The rapid result and relative simplicity of these procedures render them attractive for individuals desiring quick changes after facial injury, allowing for more prompt return to social functioning and regular activity, as well as to aesthetic considerations. Another fundamental feature of non-surgical facial enhancement involves the role of advanced skin treatments. Chemical peels and laser resurfacing, along with other treatments, have the potential to dramatically improve skin texture, tone, and overall appearance. These procedures induce collagen production and are employed to manage many of the sequelae of trauma, such as scarring or dyspigmentation. In cases of facial trauma, these treatments offer a non-invasive alternative to restoring skin integrity and thereby maximizing facial form. Furthermore, their tailoring to the individual requirements and skin types proves their adaptability and renders them a consideration in trauma reconstruction cases worth exploring. Non-surgical treatment can be tailored, raising its effectiveness and providing a more holistic means of facial recreation. While celebrating all these triumphs, though, it should be remembered that there are limitations and complications to non-surgical facial augmentation techniques. Though normally safe, procedures such as fillers and Botox can produce side effects such as swelling, bruising, or allergic reactions. Moreover, since favorable outcomes usually depend on the practitioner's skill set and level of experience, extensive consultations and examinations prior to treatment are required. As highlighted in more current studies, incorporating new technologies into planning and conducting non-surgical procedures can diminish some of these risks as well as improve outcomes (Xu et al., 2022). This is particularly important in reconstructive cases where precision is of utmost importance. With growth in the field, ongoing study and development will undoubtedly shape the new face of non-surgical facial enhancement (Figure 12.14).

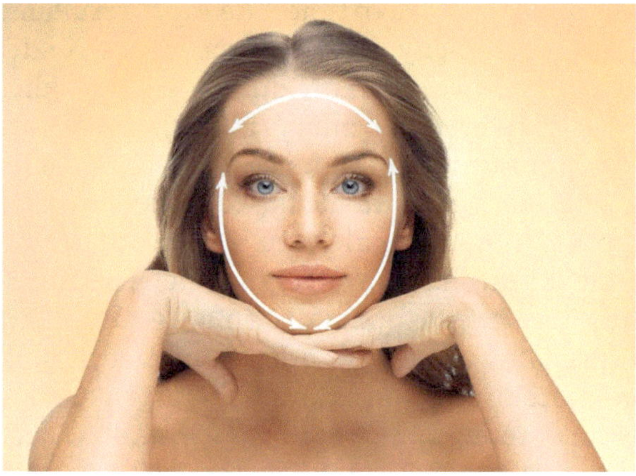

Figure 12.14. Non-surgical options for facial enhancement.

Source: https://drkaranshetty.com/wp-content/uploads/2024/04/non-surgical-facelift-glasgow-e1712837681310-1024x752.jpg.

12.4.3. Patient Satisfaction and Quality of Life Improvements

The complementarity of patient satisfaction and quality of life improvement for cosmetic facial surgery in the reconstruction of trauma is increasingly valued in reconstructive surgery. Correction of aesthetic as well as functional defects is required for enhanced overall patient care, with successful outcomes significantly affecting psychological function and social rehabilitation. Various surgical techniques, such as utilizing cutting-edge ultrasonic osteotomes, have been developed to enhance surgical precision and minimize postoperative complications. These advancements not only optimize the structural stability of the reconstructed facial framework but also facilitate a better healing process, ultimately leading to enhanced patient satisfaction. Studies that examine the micro-morphologies and roughness values of osteotomized surfaces, as published in Anesi et al. (2014), are just one of the ways technological advancement in operating tools is tantamount to improved patient outcomes, lending credence to the fact that innovation in surgery improves quality of life. Furthermore, understanding patient experience is important when evaluating the effectiveness of trauma reconstruction treatments. The focus shifted from merely achieving surgical success to incorporating patient-reported outcomes. For instance, autologous fat grafting studies in the eyelid have focused on the improvement rate overall among recipients of such procedures, and this has revealed that most of the patients indicate significant improvement not just in terms of looks but also in emotional and social areas of life. The systematic review outlined in Bannani et al. (2016) elaborates on the relationship between reconstructive surgeries and enhanced patient satisfaction, underscored by the crucial role of subjective experience in determining the success of surgery. Improved patient experience, testified to in the form of minimal complication rates and satisfactory aesthetic results, necessarily extends to enhanced quality of life, thus patient satisfaction being a fundamental aspect of reconstructive surgery. The repercussions of these findings extend beyond the patient to shape the overall healthcare practice. As patient satisfaction increasingly becomes a metric for successful outcomes with trauma reconstruction, healthcare providers are increasingly tasked with tailoring interventions to the individual. This patient-centered approach facilitates communication between the patient and the surgeon that fosters trust and goal-driven treatment. The insights obtained from recent advances, for example, as reported in Anesi et al. (2014) and Bannani et al. (2016), not only shape clinical practice but also further enhance surgical procedure and protocol improvement. Lastly, as these technologies are applied to work in the context of improved patient experiences, the face of medicine will experience an enormous paradigm shift towards prioritizing patient satisfaction as a driving force of quality-of-life improvements in facial cosmetic trauma reconstruction (Figure 12.15).

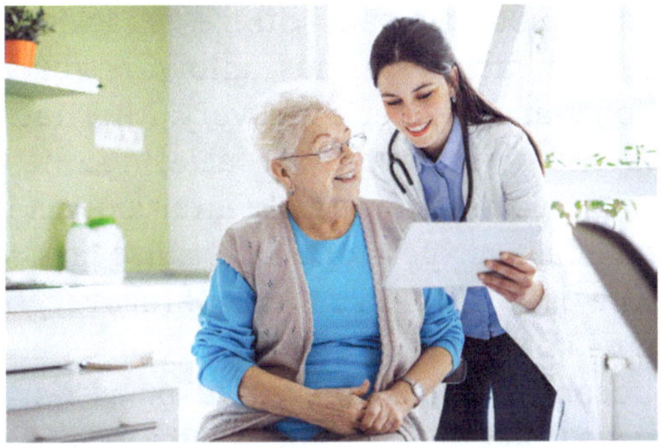

Figure 12.15. Patient satisfaction and quality.

Source: https://external-content.duckduckgo.com/iu/?u=https%3A%2F%2Fwww.performancehealthus.com%2Fhubfs%2Fimproving%2520patient%2520satisfaction.png&f=1&nofb=1&ipt=d7323a349af5ab66debc1ae5dbfb239ded792fd4fce622ba6867a732b08e5d96.

Test Your Knowledge

1. How do cosmetic procedures such as skin grafting, scar revision, and rhinoplasty contribute to restoring facial appearance after trauma?
2. What is the role of modern cosmetic techniques in improving both functional and aesthetic outcomes in facial reconstruction?

12.5. Multidisciplinary Approach to Treatment

Learning Outcome

1. Collaboration Between Surgeons, Psychologists, and Therapists
2. Importance of a Holistic Treatment Plan
3. Case Studies Demonstrating Successful Multidisciplinary Outcomes

The complexity involved in trauma reconstruction for facial cosmetics necessitates a multidisciplinary approach to treatment through the application of respective specialists' expertise. Facial trauma patients require orthodontists, prosthodontists, and oral and maxillofacial surgeons to collaborate closely to produce optimal outcomes. Initial stages often involve surgical reconstruction, during which maxillofacial and oral surgeons manage fractures and soft tissue injury. Orthodontic therapy may be required after surgery to correct misalignments, both through trauma and surgical methods. This cooperation guarantees that function and esthetic outcomes are optimized together, treating both the jaw's structural stability and the patient's appearance. This broad-based care ultimately enhances patient satisfaction and emotional health, reflecting the importance of a team-based approach in efficiently addressing the complex aspects of facial trauma. In addition, the incorporation of other medical professionals, including physical therapists and psychologists, adds to the overall treatment. While the surgeons focus on reconstructing the face, physical therapists can aid in rehabilitation, dispelling any functional limitation that can hinder the patient's recovery.

The therapists typically utilize exercises that strengthen facial muscles, allowing for both functional and cosmetic recovery. Alternatively, the psychological impact of facial trauma may be enormous, which requires intervention from mental health professionals. It is also critical to treat the psychological aspects of recovery, such as body image and self-esteem, because patients may become anxious, depressed, or withdrawn. The development of a cohesive treatment plan incorporating these various disciplines not only improves physical well-being but also assists in the emotional recovery process, critical to successful recovery. In the specific instance of facial trauma, management of complications such as open gingival embrasures also demonstrates the necessity of a multidisciplinary approach. The fact that such cosmetic complications, typically the aftermath of periodontal disease or surgical intervention, will arise only serves to highlight the importance of involving the services of orthodontists and periodontists in treatment. Management of the aesthetic ramifications of such conditions can significantly enhance patient results and satisfaction. As noted by research, there are multiple means of treating open gingival embrasures, but it is the cooperation of the interdisciplinary team that usually yields the most successful results (Bosio et al., 2008). Thus, incorporating multiple specialties ensures that not just the surgical defects, but also the esthetic components are carefully addressed, fulfilling the holistic demands of trauma reconstruction patients.

12.5.1. Collaboration Between Surgeons, Psychologists, and Therapists

The very intricate task of reconstructing trauma in facial cosmetic surgery necessitates a multidisciplinary approach, emphasizing the importance of cooperative work among surgeons, psychologists, and therapists. Surgeons provide the technical expertise necessary to perform the physical reconstruction of facial structures affected by trauma. However, the psychological impact of facial disfigurement tends to be profound, more than just physical appearance, affecting individuals' self-esteem, interpersonal relationships, and mental health. This beautiful dance of physical and emotional recovery calls for the integration of psychologists who can assess and treat the psychological well-being of patients. With an integration of surgical techniques and psychological treatment, teams can offer patients complete care, leading to improved outcomes and building resilience to adversity. The alliance extends beyond the operating theatre and into rehabilitation and psychological preparation. Psychologists are engaged in prepping patients for reality surgery and potential results, reducing anxiety and emotional barriers to recovery. Speech and occupational therapy-trained therapists intervene further by addressing the functional and rehabilitative aspects of recovery. Patients' physiological and psychological demands are, in this manner, coordinated, making it possible to treat trauma reconstruction as an overall phenomenon. Such multidisciplinary interaction is paramount in minimizing the risk of post-operative complications as patients are mentally prepared to cope with the changes that surgery creates. The work of these professionals ultimately leads to improved patients' quality of life during recovery. The newer trend towards trauma reconstruction highlights the importance of building strong networks between facial transplantation and reconstruction professionals, as reported in the face allotransplantation literature (Coiante et al., 2022). A network of surgeons, psychologists, and therapists enables the sharing of information, strategies, and best practices that work to enhance patient care and outcomes. By creating a synergy of professionals, cross-disciplinary education has the potential to bring forth novel approaches and therapies to match each patient's needs. Also, ethical considerations that stem from such sophisticated procedures demand integrated debates among these experts. Patient choice, rejection management, and long-term follow-up are best managed by honest communication and collaboration to maintain the ethical standards of treatment while advancing the specialty of facial cosmetic surgery trauma reconstruction (Cimasi et al., 2011). By such an approach of collaboration, the procedure is legitimized, and a support system is made stronger on a holistic level for the patient during their recovery processes.

12.5.2. Importance of a Holistic Treatment Plan

In reconstructive trauma in facial cosmetic surgery, the role of a holistic treatment plan becomes even more evident. A holistic approach not only deals with the physical aspects of the procedure but also deals with the emotional and psychological well-being of the patient. With the disfiguring impact facial injury and reconstruction can have on a patient's self-esteem, a comprehensive approach must be employed to effectively recover. This involves a detailed work-up that incorporates medical history, psychological evaluations, and the patient's wants, facilitating more individualized surgical planning that addresses particular concerns. Such a holistic approach is most frequently linked with enhanced patient satisfaction and improved results, which underscore the requirement that surgeons anticipate more than mere technical skill when redefining facial structures. Moreover, through an overall treatment plan, the medical team can design a facilitating environment that answers the multifaceted challenges inherent in trauma reconstruction for patients. The coordination between surgeons, mental health specialists, and rehabilitation specialists is crucial in the process of ensuring that all recovery facets of a patient are properly addressed. The multidisciplinary care not only ensures optimum surgical results but also provides emotional healing and coping skills to tackle psychological effects. Evidence has shown that when patients feel supported emotionally during recovery, they will be more likely to take additional rehabilitative measures and adhere to post-operative instructions, thus working towards even better long-term results in facial appearance and self-esteem (Anesi et al., 2014). It is also important to observe the strange interplay of medical care and emotional support within the overall treatment plan, particularly in cases such as the O'Donnabhain case, which shows how competing ideas of medical necessity can affect patient treatment (Pratt, 2016). In patients who are reconstructing facial trauma, cosmetic benefit is usually entangled with psychological well-being. The experts should be aware of the psychological impact of surgical outcomes and social stigmatization. Thus, by the incorporation of elements such as counseling, peer counseling, and patient education into treatment protocols, surgeons can enhance the healing process so that people can recover not only their physical appearances but also self-confidence. Consequently, physical and psychological care as well constitute a vital component of an integrated treatment plan for trauma reconstruction.

12.5.3. Case Studies Demonstrating Successful Multidisciplinary Outcomes

Integration of various medical specialties has been found crucial in providing effective outcomes for trauma reconstruction, particularly in cosmetic surgery of the face. Recent case studies depict how a multidisciplinary approach enhances recovery and patient satisfaction. For instance, collaborative works between oral and maxillofacial surgeons, plastic surgeons, and rehabilitation specialists assure functional and esthetic reconstruction of facial trauma. Not only do these collaborative works make surgery more effective, but they also maximize postoperative care to an optimum extent, resulting in a reduction of complication rates and improved overall patient satisfaction. The effectiveness of such an approach is evidenced by a report indicating the necessity of integrating multiple expertise to achieve the best surgical outcomes in complicated facial reconstructions. Finally, a synergistic team setting encourages innovative solutions, as evidenced by perfect multidisciplinary outcomes in trauma reconstruction. Extraprimordial attention to innovative surgical approaches, such as Piezosurgery® use for osteotomies, underscores the innovation achieved by working in multidisciplinary teams. Comparative research on the micromorphologies and roughness values of bone surfaces after osteotomies has shown that ultrasound-assisted osteotomes have definite advantages over conventional practice. The use of Piezosurgery® allows selective cutting of mineralized tissue with preservation of the surrounding soft tissues, a key to maximizing healing and minimizing complications in craniofacial surgery. This technological application is an example of how surgical innovation and collaboration can bring superior outcomes in structural and functional rehabilitation. These findings point to the continuous evolution of techniques mixed with interdisciplinarity controversy to enable surgeons to further establish practices on empirical evidence. Therefore, the application of such modern techniques reflects the viability of successful multidisciplinary practice in facial trauma reconstruction. The inquiry into bone substitutes in craniofacial reconstruction further substantiates the benefit of multidisciplinary management. Conventional methods often involve the use of autologous bone to avoid donor-site morbidity, but studies indicate growing interest in artificial bone substitutes as a means of addressing this problem (Neovius, 2016). For instance, current studies on the comparison of the healing potential of next-generation materials, such as BMP-2 in hydrogel, reveal promising results that are equivalent to conventional autograft results. These analyses highlight the central role of coordination between material scientists and surgeons to streamline treatment modality. Such evolving practices not only aim to eliminate donor site complications but also enhance the efficacy of bone healing. The cross-fertilization of knowledge among disciplines is thus a vision-oriented effort towards achieving fruitful results in the realm of trauma reconstruction, heading towards optimum patient care and surgery success.

Test Your Knowledge

1. Why is a multidisciplinary team important in the management and rehabilitation of patients with facial trauma?
2. How do different healthcare professionals collaborate to ensure comprehensive recovery for facial trauma patients?

12.6. Ethical Considerations in Facial Reconstruction

Learning Outcome

1. Informed Consent and Patient Autonomy
2. Balancing Aesthetic Desires with Medical Needs
3. Addressing Disparities in Access to Care

The ethical issues of facial reconstruction, particularly after trauma, serve to underscore the nuance of patient autonomy and consent. Because reconstructive surgery of the face tends to be extensive in terms of altering the patient's appearance, it is very important that practitioners engage patients in lengthy preoperative discussions. These discussions must not only address the medical aspect of the procedure but also the emotional and psychological consequences that may arise due to cosmetic change. Ethical practice demands that patients are properly informed and that they provide consent freely, without coercion, so that they know about the probable outcome and risks of the procedure. Moreover, respecting a patient's wish where trauma has already resulted in emotional distress is paramount to establishing trust and feelings of control in the reconstructive process. Another basic ethical issue is the allocation of resources and access to facial reconstruction services. Notably, the disparities of access to healthcare can significantly decide who benefits from ideal advanced reconstructive treatments. Ethical issues necessitate that professionals critically examine the socio-economic determinants of quality of care received and patient care. The professionals must engage in the struggle to provide equal access to these life-critical reconstructive services, particularly among patients who are less affluent and therefore would be least able to pay for these services. The approach is consistent with the general healthcare equity framework that each patient, irrespective of socio-economic standing, ought to be provided with sufficient care. Thus, efforts to narrow these disparities can significantly improve aggregate patient outcomes and adherence to ethical standards in the medical profession. Finally, integrating leading-edge technologies into facial reconstruction comes with ethical concerns about the ramifications of such technologies. Although techniques like free tissue transfer and advanced imaging significantly enhance surgical precision and patient results, they also pose challenges. Informed consent questions arise when patients have to make decisions about new technology that has not been widely tried. The ethical burden on surgeons is to be up to date on the most current studies and to freely discuss the potential benefits and limitations of new procedures. Additionally, the evolving nature of reconstructive surgery requires ongoing debate in medicine in terms of best practices, ethics, and the patient-centered care mandate, which underlies the argument for sustaining clinical excellence while ensuring patients undergoing trauma reconstruction come first (Turner et al., 2021; Morales et al., 2023).

12.6.1. Informed Consent and Patient Autonomy

In trauma reconstruction for cosmetic facial surgery, informed consent is a paramount principle in maintaining patient autonomy. This ethical principle enables patients to make decisions about their medical care, so they are better informed about the risks, benefits, and options of their treatment regimen. The complexities of facial reconstructive surgery mandate extensive consultations between the surgeon and the patient, establishing an environment in which the patients are able to express their fears and expectations. The nuances of informed consent involve not just a detailed understanding of the procedures themselves, but also an understanding of the psychological impact of trauma and body changes. This ensures that patients are engaged in shared decision-making, which is essential in maintaining their autonomy and enhancing their satisfaction after surgery. Furthermore, the cosmetic surgery environment is also influenced by varied legal settings that decide how paramount informed consent is. The growing evaluated nature of cosmetic treatments has provoked debate on the medical professional's ethical role to prioritize patient understanding. Regulations and legislation are quite diverse throughout jurisdictions, which mirrors the evolving understanding of consent throughout the surgical fields. Comparative research highlights that it is crucial for medical professionals to be well educated about local and international practices, as Levon & Valančienė (2021) stress. This is a sign that there is a need to create a standard model of informed consent that responds to best practices and in the long term, allows patients to take charge of their health decisions while safeguarding their rights.

The history of surgical practices also provides an impetus for upholding the importance of informed consent and patient autonomy, especially where treatments before were not disclosed. For instance, routine recommendation of sex reassignment surgery for intersex infants is ethically questionable in terms of consent because the majority of parents were persuaded to enroll for radical procedures without being fully aware of everything they stood to risk. This cautionary tale, quoted in Beh et al. (2000), necessitates a paradigm shift from the response to patient autonomy employed in modern medicine, particularly in trauma reconstruction. By putting informed consent first, healthcare professionals can establish trust and a culture of respect for patient autonomy, opening the way for ethical practice in healthcare in line with evolving conceptions of autonomy in medical advancement.

12.6.2. Balancing Aesthetic Desires with Medical Needs

There is a special challenge in the field of trauma reconstruction in facial cosmetic surgery in balancing aesthetic desires and medical needs. Reconstructive patients typically possess intense emotional and psychological motivations behind their interest in appearance, resulting from trauma. A desire for beauty can at times conceal underlying medical factors, and there can be conflict where the medical need is overshadowed by a desire to attain standards of beauty. The ramifications of this conflict are far-reaching; not only do they complicate surgical planning and patient consultation, but they also raise ethical concerns regarding the prioritization of aesthetic want over authentic medical need. By closely examining these dynamics, practitioners are able to determine a framework that respects patients' aesthetic wants while keeping clinical imperatives as the priority for treatment planning. The globalized beauty of cosmetic surgery is a cultural trend whereby aesthetic interventions are becoming normalized, imposing societal pressures to maintain the need for cosmetic upgrades. In such an environment, the reasons for elective surgeries, even in the context of trauma, can be shaped by wider social constructs such as economic means and cultural ideals of beauty. As highlighted by studies, historical and sociopolitical backgrounds hold significant relevance for patient expectations, notably in developing nations where Western beauty perception is likely to affect personal aspiration (Riggs et al., 2012). The combined presence of the aforementioned factors makes the healthcare decision-making process challenging for healthcare providers, as they must balance patients' sociocultural demands with their medical needs. Reconstructive surgeons are thus confronted with ethical dilemmas, with a clear understanding of the social constructs that define what desires in a patient are, to provide holistic, ethical treatment. The problem of differentiating between medical and cosmetic motivations for surgical use also implies that there must be an apprehensive process of patient assessment and surgical planning. Research indicates that the majority of patients request treatments with both dental and cosmetic problems in mind, often driven by psychosocial reasons not always easily identifiable to practitioners (Broers, 2025). This highlights the importance of strict screening processes with mental health in view, and post-surgery long-term satisfaction in mind. Surgeons must establish an environment that fosters open communication about expectations, in which patients are fully informed of risks associated with any surgery. By highlighting ethical principles such as nonmaleficence and patient autonomy, clinicians can establish a work environment for teamwork whereby aesthetic desires are openly discussed without compromising medical integrity. Therefore, achieving an optimal equilibrium between cosmetic desires and medical needs is based on an integrated understanding of patients' motivations, hence enhancing outcomes and patient satisfaction.

12.6.3. Addressing Disparities in Access to Care

The accessibility of healthcare, particularly trauma reconstruction for facial cosmetic surgery, is highly disproportionate. Socioeconomic standing, geographical location, and systematic inequalities are significant determinants of an individual's access to necessary surgery. Patients from disadvantaged groups often face obstacles that not only hinder their access to timely treatment but also influence the quality of treatment they attain. As an example, those in rural communities might have limited specialized services available, which would require a lot of travel to access, thus discouraging patients from seeking proper treatment. Besides, inequalities also often stem from weak insurance coverage, which can significantly affect patients' decisions regarding whether or not to access reconstructive surgeries, thus limiting their potential for successful treatment of trauma. This dynamic of interdependence perfectly illustrates the actual need to reform policies to eliminate these inequalities and ensure equal access for everybody. Another aspect of complexity in achieving access imbalances is identity intersectionality, i.e., gender, race, and socioeconomic status, which overlaps with the existing healthcare disparities. Transgender individuals, for instance, have specificity of experiencing difficulties in accessing reconstructive services that might not be clearly understood by the health professionals. Evidence shows that the majority of practitioners are given minimal extensive training on the specific requirements of transgender patients, thus leading to misperceptions and suboptimal treatment choices. In addition, gender-affirming operations, normally inseparable from reconstructive and cosmetic procedures, are less likely to be taken care of by insurance programs, creating additional barriers in terms of access. Patient reluctance to seek healthcare for fear of discrimination or stigmatization denies them the opportunity to address trauma on time. Addressing the disparities requires a multi-disciplinary approach that is sensitive and responsive to differences in patient identity and experiences within the healthcare system. To reduce inequalities in access to trauma reconstruction care, advanced measures need to be taken that prioritize patient-centered strategies. Policymakers and healthcare professionals need to make committed efforts toward broad educational endeavors that heighten awareness of the singular needs of various populations, including gender-diverse populations. This is imperative in creating an environment that is helpful in delivering quality care and healing. In addition, leveraging technology to offer remote consultation services can potentially transcend spatial differences in access. Having community-based programs that offer financial assistance or sliding scales for the underinsured can enhance equity of healthcare access as well. Further, longitudinal studies are essential to an understanding of how these differences impact patient outcomes over the longer term and emphasize the importance of targeted interventions. Such attempts not only presage greater direct access to care but also promote a more sensitive healthcare system to the diverse needs of patients navigating through trauma reconstruction in facial cosmetic surgery.

Test Your Knowledge

1. What ethical considerations must surgeons address when performing facial reconstruction procedures?
2. How does informed consent play a critical role in ensuring ethical decision-making in facial reconstruction?

SUMMARY

The complexities of trauma reconstruction in facial cosmetics attest to a rich interaction between cutting-edge surgical technology and patient-centered outcomes. With the advent of new tools such as ultrasound-guided osteotomes, the potential for improving surgical precision and restricting trauma to surrounding tissues has increased. Literature has revealed considerable differences in osteotomized bone surfaces using outdated versus newer techniques, suggesting that technologies such as Piezosurgery might aid in promoting more favorable patterns of postoperative healing and reducing donor-site morbidity. The development of such surgical tools plays an important role in the greater objective of attaining not only aesthetic improvement but functional reconstruction as well, thus validating the motivation for continued research and innovation in facial trauma surgeries (Anesi et al., 2014). In addition, growing interest in artificial bone substitutes is a turning point in the art of facial reconstruction. Historically, the autologous bone grafting has been considered the gold standard, but donor-site morbidity limitations and complications make it essential to search for alternative solutions. Results from research emphasize the necessity of assessing risks and complications following craniofacial surgeries, thereby simplifying surgical protocols for enhancing patient safety. The relative comparison between grafting techniques, e.g., the effectiveness of BMP-2 in hydrogel systems, illustrates the complex interplay between innovation and resilience in bone healing progress. These results bring the field closer to the implementation of safer and more efficient biomaterials for reconstructive surgery (Neovius, 2016). Finally, the future of trauma reconstruction in facial cosmetic surgery lies at a crossroads, with emerging evidence still defining best practices and surgical methodologies. With continuing evolution, the focus must be put on minimizing sequelae like diplopia and sensory impairment, which have a profound impact on patients' quality of life after trauma. Advanced surgical techniques and minimal-access modalities promise to minimize complications while still achieving aesthetic and functional outcomes. However, keeping the synergism of sound clinical studies and patient participation active is critical to advancing treatment protocols to a level of comprehensiveness. Ultimately, it is by holding to a vision of innovation and patient-centricity that the topic of study in facial trauma reconstruction is actually able to advance, making outcomes effective as well as enduring over the long term (Neovius, 2016).

A balanced overview of trauma reconstruction in aesthetic facial surgery illustrates several important aspects of surgical methods and their implications for patient outcomes. Among the primary issues has been technology in surgical instruments, specifically the advent of ultrasonically activated devices, such as Piezosurgery®, that revolutionized the practice of osteotomy. Studies highlight the disparity in micromorphology and roughness of bone surfaces attainable by standard methods compared to modern ultrasonic osteotomes. The latest technology facilitates the selective removal of mineralized tissues with the maintenance of the integrity of surrounding soft tissues, which is especially important for optimal recovery and healing in facial reconstruction. The evaluation of such tools reflects high potential to improve cranio-facial surgery outcomes, as is the demand for cosmetic reconstruction and functional rehabilitation of facial beauty from trauma patients (Anesi et al., 2014). Rhinoplasty remains at the core of trauma reconstruction as it addresses aesthetic and functional grievances that have their origin in facial trauma. The book Contemporary Rhinoplasty provides a clear insight into the complexities of orbital reconstruction surgery, discussing various points such as nasal beauty, and how to plan for the operation. This source highlights the importance of identifying the interaction between the surgery techniques and patient-specific anatomical differences, particularly in cases where skeletal abnormalities caused by trauma are a factor. In particular, correcting deformities like saddle nose deformity requires not only technical competence but also an intuitive understanding of morbidities underlying them, which can be sleep breathing disorders or cleft diseases. Adequate consideration of these factors during the surgical process guarantees enhanced results and patient satisfaction in trauma reconstruction (Kalaskar et al., 2016). With evolving experience in cosmetic reconstruction of the face, the incorporation of new methods and a deeper understanding of anatomical issues is critical. There is an obligation for surgeons to remain current with the latest happenings in surgical technology and technique, such as the efficacy of various osteotomes and the value of individualized rhinoplasty. Ongoing research into the impact of different surgical techniques on healing processes even more underscores the necessity for critical review and adaptation within the practice of surgery. This commitment to continued education ultimately ensures enhanced patient outcomes, validates the relevance of trauma reconstruction, and determines its role within the restoration of both form and function in facial trauma patients. With these technologies, clinicians can make a significant difference in the trajectory of healing from trauma by incorporating goals of cosmetic repair with the required aspects of patient rehabilitation and care.

KEY TERMS FROM THIS CHAPTER

- Facial Fractures
- Zygomaticomaxillary Complex (ZMC)
- Maxillofacial Trauma
- Avulsion Injuries
- Open Reduction and Internal Fixation (ORIF)
- Titanium Plates and Screws
- Soft Tissue Reconstruction
- Facial Symmetry Restoration
- Functional Rehabilitation
- Orbital Floor Repair
- Mandibular Fracture Fixation
- Soft Tissue Laceration Repair
- Contusion Management
- Rigid Fixation
- Bone Grafting
- Nerve Injury Assessment
- Scar Revision
- Ocular Protection

CRITICAL THINKING QUESTIONS

1. **The main goal of facial trauma reconstruction is to:**
   a. Reduce wrinkles
   b. Restore anatomy, function, and aesthetics
   c. Improve facial pigmentation
   d. Increase skin thickness
2. **The first priority in managing facial trauma is:**
   a. Aesthetic evaluation
   b. Airway assessment and stabilization
   c. Scar revision
   d. Bone grafting
3. **The "golden period" for primary closure of facial lacerations is usually within:**
   a. 6–8 hours
   b. 24 hours
   c. 48 hours
   d. 72 hours
4. **Which bone is most commonly fractured in facial trauma?**
   a. Nasal bone
   b. Frontal bone
   c. Zygoma
   d. Mandible
5. **Blowout fractures typically involve which structure?**
   a. Nasal septum
   b. Orbital floor
   c. Zygomatic arch
   d. Mandibular symphysis

Short Answer Questions

1. What are the primary goals of facial trauma reconstruction?
2. How does the concept of "functional and aesthetic subunits" influence facial reconstruction planning?
3. What imaging modality is most commonly used to evaluate facial fractures and why?
4. What is the role of rigid fixation in facial fracture reconstruction?
5. How does soft tissue swelling affect surgical timing in trauma reconstruction?

Answers to Critical Thinking Questions

1. (b) 2. (b) 3. (a) 4. (a) 5. (b)

REFERENCES

1. Abbott, Amstutz, Arden, Arnaud, Arnaud, Asano, Axhausen, et al. (2003). *Bone autografting of the calvaria and craniofacial skeleton: Historical background, surgical results in a series of 15 patients, and review of the literature.* https://core.ac.uk/download/pdf/53848962.pdf (accessed on 14th July 2025).

2. Aguayo, S., García-Huidobro, R., Villena, F., Véliz, et al. (2024). *Generative artificial intelligence in dentistry: Current approaches and future challenges.* http://arxiv.org/abs/2407.17532 (accessed on 14th July 2025).

3. PRELIMINARY FINDINGS OF A POTENZIATED PIEZOSURGERGICAL DEVICE AT THE RABBIT SKULL / Anesi, A;Palumbo, C; Ferretti, M; Salvatori, R; Cavani F, .; Chiarini, L. - (2014). ((Intervento presentato al convegno 22° Congressof European Association for Cranio-Maxillofacial Surgery (EACMFS) tenutosi a Praga (Repubblica Ceca) nel 23-26September 2014(accessed on 14th July 2025).

4. Anger, J. T., Case, L. K., Baranowski, A., Berger, A., Craft, R. M., Damitz, L. A., Gabriel, R. A., et al. (2024). Pain mechanisms in the transgender individual: A review. *Frontiers in Pain Research, 5.* https://doi.org/10.3389/fpain.2024.1241015 (accessed on 14th July 2025).

5. Balachandar, L., & Thiagarajan, B. (2012). *Versatility of bicoronal flap approach in head and neck surgeries.* https://core.ac.uk/download/pdf/9634063.pdf (accessed on 14th July 2025).

6. Bannani, S., Bertheuil, N., Boureaux, E., Carloni, et al. (2016). *Eyelid fat grafting: Indications, operative technique and complications; a systematic review.*

7. Chuang, J., Barnes, C., & Wong, B. J. F. (2016). Overview of Facial Plastic Surgery and Current Developments. *Surgery journal (New York, N.Y.), 2*(1), e17–e28. https://doi.org/10.1055/s-0036-1572360 (accessed on 14th July 2025).

8. Bazgir, N., Fazli, M., Gachkar, L., Ghazizadeh Hashemi, et al. (2023). *Comparison of depression and anxiety levels before and after rhinoplasty: A longitudinal study.* https://core.ac.uk/download/643598101.pdf (accessed on 14th July 2025).

9. Beh, H. G., & Diamond, M. (2000). *An emerging ethical and medical dilemma: Should physicians perform sex assignment surgery on infants with ambiguous genitalia?* https://core.ac.uk/download/32299494.pdf (accessed on 14th July 2025).

10. Beneti, I. M., Rezende, L. S., & Sena Sobrinho, M. A. de. (2023). *Access to the upper third of the face: A literary review of indications, techniques, and intercurrences.* https://core.ac.uk/download/622811946.pdf (accessed on 14th July 2025).

11. Bodiwala, N., Bhola, N. D., Gupta, C. S., & Anukula, H. S. (2025). Single-staged islanded forehead flap for cheek defect in recurrent buccal mucosa cancer: A case report. *Journal of Clinical and Diagnostic Research.* https://www.semanticscholar.org/paper/f7a004a2d47c79169392b6345cfe58ed1b40559b (accessed on 14th July 2025).

12. Bosio, J. A., Furquim, B. D'Aurea, Maruo, H., Pascotto, et al. (2008). *The dilemma of the open gingival embrasure between maxillary central incisors.* https://core.ac.uk/download/213084039.pdf (accessed on 14th July 2025).

13. Broers, D. L. M. (2025). *Is the customer king?: Ethical and psychological considerations regarding tooth removal.* https://core.ac.uk/download/655140725.pdf (accessed on 14th July 2025).

14. Cheung, L. K., Ho, M. Y. S., Luk, W. K., McGrath, et al. (2014). *Psychosocial and quality of life outcomes of prosthetic auricular rehabilitation with CAD/CAM technology*. https://core.ac.uk/download/38046618.pdf (accessed on 14th July 2025).

15. Chinnery, H., Dyer, B., Noroozi, S., Thompson, et al. (2016). *Scoping review of the development of artificial eyes throughout the years*. https://core.ac.uk/download/163076643.pdf (accessed on 14th July 2025).

16. Cimasi, R. J. (2011). *Adviser's Guide to Health Care: Volume 2, Professional Practices*. https://core.ac.uk/download/335347929.pdf (accessed on 14th July 2025).

17. Coiante, E., D'Andrea, F., Hersant, B., La Padula, S., Longo, B., Meningaud, J. P., Pensato, R., et al. (2022). *Face transplant: Indications, outcomes, and ethical issues—Where do we stand?* https://core.ac.uk/download/636949002.pdf (accessed on 14th July 2025).

18. Constantian, M. B. (2022). *Childhood Abuse, Body Shame, and Addictive Plastic Surgery*. https://core.ac.uk/download/520261637.pdf (accessed on 14th July 2025).

19. Dean, J. H., Hoch, C. C., Wollenberg, B., Navidzadeh, J., Maheta, B., Mandava, A., Knoedler, S., et al. (2025). Advancements in bioengineered and autologous skin grafting techniques for skin reconstruction: A comprehensive review. *Frontiers in Bioengineering and Biotechnology, 12*. https://doi.org/10.3389/fbioe.2024.1461328 (accessed on 14th July 2025).

20. Desai, S. C., & Seth, R. (2020). Shifting paradigms in head and neck reconstructive surgery during the COVID-19 crisis. *Facial Plastic Surgery & Aesthetic Medicine, 22*, 152–154. https://doi.org/10.1089/fpsam.2020.0186 (accessed on 14th July 2025).

21. Fogg, Q., Ng, Z. Y., & Shoaib, T. (2010). *Where to Find Facial Artery Perforators: A Reference Point*. https://core.ac.uk/download/10521.pdf (accessed on 14th July 2025).

22. Hughes, D., & Song, B. (2016). Dental and Nondental Stem Cell Based Regeneration of the Craniofacial Region: A Tissue Based Approach. *Stem cells international, 2016*, 8307195. https://doi.org/10.1155/2016/8307195 (accessed on 14th July 2025).

23. Kothandaraman, S., Nair, V. B., & Narasiman, S. (2013). *'Old Foley's in a new bottle' – Use of Foley's catheter in anterior maxillary wall fractures*. https://core.ac.uk/download/pdf/9634091.pdf (accessed on 14th July 2025).

24. Levon, J., & Valančienė, D. (2021). *Ar pasaulinės kosmetinės chirurgijos teisinės problemos aplenkia Lietuvą?* https://core.ac.uk/download/479942901.pdf (accessed on 14th July 2025).

25. Mitsouras, D., Liacouras, P., Imanzadeh, A., Giannopoulos, A. A., Cai, T., Kumamaru, K. K., George, E., et al. (2015). Medical 3D printing for the radiologist. *Radiographics, 35*, 1965–1988. https://doi.org/10.1148/rg.2015140320 (accessed on 14th July 2025).

26. Deepak M. Kalaskar, Peter E. Butler, Shadi Ghali. (2016). *Textbook of Plastic and Reconstructive Surgery*. ISBN: 978-1-910634-37-0 (Hbk.) https://core.ac.uk/download/79526588.pdf

27. (accessed on 14th July 2025).

28. Neovius, E. (2016). *Development of Surgical Techniques in Craniofacial Reconstruction*. https://core.ac.uk/download/70344167.pdf (accessed on 14th July 2025).

29. Oley, M. H., Oley, M., Sukarno, V., & Faruk, M. (2024). Advances in three-dimensional printing for craniomaxillofacial trauma reconstruction: A systematic review. *The Journal of Craniofacial Surgery, 35*, 1926–1933. https://www.semanticscholar.org/paper/21a3e3ce98ec2c77b146be237e9136f3c4ae035a (accessed on 14th July 2025).

30. Pratt, K. (2016). *The tax definition of medical care: A critique of the startling IRS arguments in O'Donnabhain v. Commissioner.* https://core.ac.uk/download/232700370.pdf (accessed on 14th July 2025).

31. Riggs, L. E. (2012). *The Globalization of Cosmetic Surgery: Examining BRIC and Beyond.* https://core.ac.uk/download/216977885.pdf (accessed on 14th July 2025).

32. Turner, B., Collin, J., & Fernandes, R. (2021). Soft tissue reconstruction of the maxillofacial region. *Oral and Maxillofacial Surgery for the Clinician.* https://www.semanticscholar.org/paper/7fa97a061fae0906be70c91e2a8c23ee0518c768 (accessed on 14th July 2025).

33. Vega Morales, A. Q., Lara Pérez, M. A., & Ruiz Reyes, D. P. (2023). Advancements in plastic surgery and facial reconstruction: A comprehensive review of surgical techniques and outcomes. *International Journal of Medical Science and Clinical Research Studies.* https://www.semanticscholar.org/paper/971665dbda7c1828e2089ce662d4c434d4fb8f13 (accessed on 14th July 2025).

34. Windsor, E. J. (2011). *Regulating healthy gender: Surgical body modification among transgender and cisgender consumers.* https://core.ac.uk/download/71423075.pdf (accessed on 14th July 2025).

35. Xu, Y., Zhang, F., Zhai, W., Cheng, S., Li, J., & Wang, Y. (2022). *Unraveling of advances in 3D-printed polymer-based bone scaffolds. Polymers, 14,* 566–566. https://doi.org/10.3390/polym14030566 (accessed on 14th July 2025).

36. Yadav, N. K., Singhal, S., Sadaphale, S. V., & Srivastava, A. K. (2025). Cosmetic reconstruction of post-traumatic anterior staphyloma by customized ocular prosthesis. *International Journal of Research and Scientific Innovation.* https://www.semanticscholar.org/paper/078ba885b3e5eada4add5f573b1d7bb73cf7d8c4 (accessed on 14th July 2025).

37. Yu, A., Ference, E., Ge, M., Su, P., Smith, S., Moayer, R., Levin, K. M., et al. (2022). Facial plastic and reconstructive surgery poster presentations. Otolaryngology–*Head and Neck Surgery, 167,* P182–P192. https://www.semanticscholar.org/paper/e467d5d0d3f13c11f7cf2c4402802ca47316c419 (accessed on 14th July 2025).

38. Zhou, G., Jiang, H., Yin, Z., Liu, Y., Zhang, Q., Zhang, C., Pan, B., et al. (2018). In vitro regeneration of patient-specific ear-shaped cartilage and its first clinical application for auricular reconstruction. *EBioMedicine, 28,* 287–302. https://doi.org/10.1016/j.ebiom.2018.01.011 (accessed on 14th July 2025).

CONGENITAL AND DEVELOPMENTAL DEFORMITIES IN FACIAL COSMETIC

13

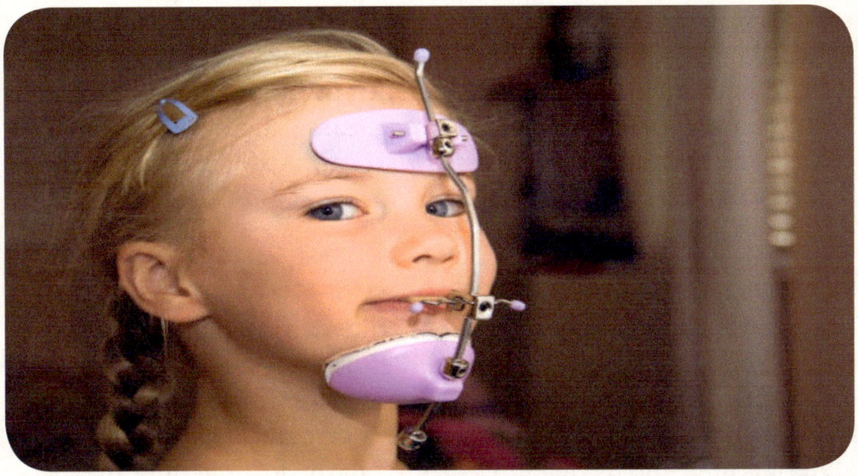

Introduction

The facial aesthetics are an interdisciplinary combination of biological, aesthetic, and psychological problems, particularly when we talk about congenital and developmental deformities. These are likely to occur during childhood and can potentially have a significant impact on a person's quality of life. Such studies address not just the morphological aspect of facial shape but also the social and emotional impact of such conditions on patients. Advances in surgical techniques, including orthognathic surgery, have led to improved patient outcomes, modifying the concept of aesthetic beauty and function. A complete understanding of these deformities calls for an examination of the genetic histories, fetal influences, and neonatal developments responsible for their occurrence, ultimately informing treatment methodologies as well as prevention in craniofacial deformities, thus breaking up the normal development (Zammit et al., 2023). Wherever facial deformities intersect with neurodevelopmental processes, it is a critical field of research to explore. Evidence suggests

LEARNING OBJECTIVES

After studying this chapter, you will be able to:

1. Discuss the type of congenital deformities;
2. Describe the type of developmental deformities;
3. Assess causes of the congenital deformities;
4. Understand the psychological impact of facial deformities;
5. Highlight treatment of facial deformities;
6. Know advancements in facial aesthetic procedures.

that stomatognathic abnormalities are either a cause or a consequence of neurological illnesses. Because facial growth is intricately interwoven with neural inputs, it is important to know how such correlates with facial growth, especially in diagnosing and managing congenital defects. The presence of the "brain-oral axis" highlights the intricate intertwining of neurological and facial beauty, necessitating multidisciplinary management of such conditions. An understanding of the crosstalk between the nervous system and facial deformities can reveal the processes of congenital anomaly formation, thus shaping therapy intervention and enhancing the quality of care (Wu et al., 2023). Lastly, evaluation of congenital and developmental deformities of facial aesthetics is a multi-faceted task of careful assessment of physical as well as psychological conditions. Practitioners must seek out comprehensive treatment protocols that address not only structural abnormalities but also the psychosocial ramifications that these impose on patients. The growing number of studies warrants intervention measures that are supplementary to surgical procedures, psychological treatment, and patient education at an initial stage. As technology improves and multidisciplinary approaches evolve, the aim is to encourage better patient outcomes for patients suffering from such complex deformities. Achieving harmony in both form and function remains an inherent goal in the domain of facial aesthetics, and this ensures that afflicted patients can lead productive lives irrespective of their status (Zammit et al., 2023).

Definition of Congenital and Developmental Deformities

Congenital and developmental deformities represent a significant area of study within medical and aesthetic disciplines, particularly regarding facial aesthetics. Congenital deformities are structural growth developmental anomalies that arise during fetal development and growth, which are usually caused by genetic defects, environmental exposure, or both. The deformities can manifest in many forms, such as but not limited to cleft palate, cleft lip, and auricular deformity in the form of microtia. On the other hand, developmental deformities are often brought about by an interruption in typical postnatal patterns of growth due to nutrition, disease, or trauma. The differentiation between the two categories is significant to health professionals, as this influences intervention choices and strategies in surgical reconstruction, rehabilitation, and psychological counseling of individuals who possess such conditions. In studying the specific form of facial deformities, scholars observed that certain conditions, including microtia, significantly alter functional and aesthetic attributes of the face. Microtia, or the deformation of the outer ear, is a congenital malformation that can threaten hearing abilities and affect an individual's self-esteem and social interactions. As illustrated through existing research, the complexity of auricular deformities transcends outward physical appearance; they also impact psychological well-being as well as social growth in children. This multifaceted impact is a persuasive argument in favor of an interdisciplinary approach to considering the etiology and implications of such deformities. Understanding how the developmental origin and formation of such deformities take place is valuable in designing effective clinical methods specifically tailored to restore form and function in patients presenting with such conditions (Lin et al., 2024). The advancement of medical technology has also enhanced our ability to diagnose and assess congenital and developmental deformities better. For instance, novel imaging technologies and automated measuring algorithms, the focus of recent research, provide for a precise evaluation of facial structures that allows for customized treatment plans to be devised. These new technologies are significant in standardizing methods of assessment, hence improving clinical outcomes for auricular malformation patients. Moreover, the use of objective measuring devices provides for uniform tracking of treatment performance over time, thereby culminating in improved patient confidence and satisfaction. With heightened awareness of congenital and developmental deformities, medical practitioners are better positioned to advocate for the needs of the affected individuals, putting restoration of function and aesthetic enhancement at the top throughout the treatment continuum (Lin et al., 2024) (Figure 13.1).

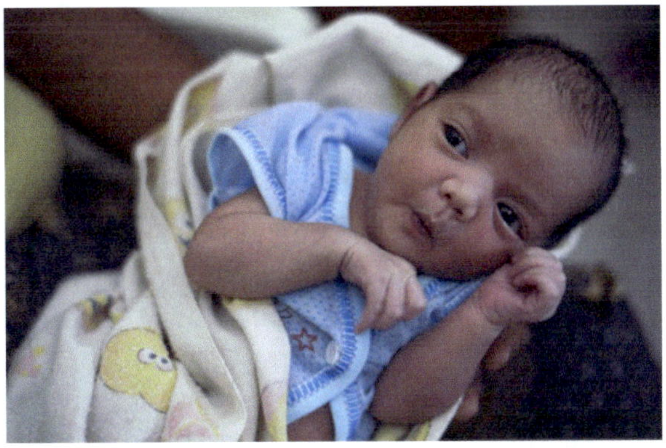

Figure 13.1. Congenital and developmental deformities.

Source: https://cdn.who.int/media/images/default-source/mca/maternal-nb/un0304684.tmb-479v.jpg?sfvrsn=d91cee2_3%20479w.

Importance of Facial Aesthetics in Social Interactions

Facial beauty is of utmost significance in social encounters, as facial beauty determines the way people see one another and are treated. The human face is a principal vehicle of emotion and attachment expression; therefore, positive facial beauty has the ability to shape social experiences greatly. Individuals who have congenital and developmental disfigurements, such as hemifacial microsomia (HFM), tend to struggle with peer relationships because their typical facial appearance is disrupted. Research confirms that HFM children tend to struggle to form social relationships and are extremely susceptible to peer rejection, which will have adverse effects on their self-esteem and mental health. These issues underscore the paramount importance of not only the medical management of facial deformities' physical conditions but also their psychosocial effects, as espoused in research connecting the face's appearance and social acceptability and developmental traits (Pniak et al., 2024). Moreover, facial aesthetics' impacts continue into peer relations during adolescence and adulthood. Teenagers with congenital facial abnormalities are likely to be more socially isolated and may face challenges in establishing romantic relationships, as they are perceived to be lacking aesthetically. Social challenges in such instances are most likely accompanied by internalized stigma that causes individuals to avoid social engagements altogether. The impact of such isolation is extremely profound; it might hamper emotional and cognitive development, resulting in widespread educational and career inequalities in later life. As observed in follow-up studies on psychosocial adaptation among individuals with facial deformities, the interventions that optimize physical appearance and confidence can be decisive in cushioning against such adverse effects and overall quality of life (Lone et al., 2023). The pressure for facial beauty during interactions is also increased by cultural and societal expectations that strongly favor symmetry and beauty. In the majority of social interactions, individuals with conventionally attractive facial structures are assessed as more competent, honest, and likable. This halo effect leads to unfair treatment in all aspects of life, including employment opportunities and social standing. Thus, individuals carrying facial congenital malformations can resist preconceptions and stereotypes that reduce their social standing. Understanding these dynamics is central to developing comprehensive support programs aimed at fostering acceptance and accommodation for individuals with abnormal facial aesthetics. Awareness, education, and empathy-driven programs can be central in shifting attitudes in society and supporting social interactions for individuals affected by congenital and developmental facial abnormalities, ultimately leading to a more accommodating society (Lone et al., 2023) (Figure 13.2).

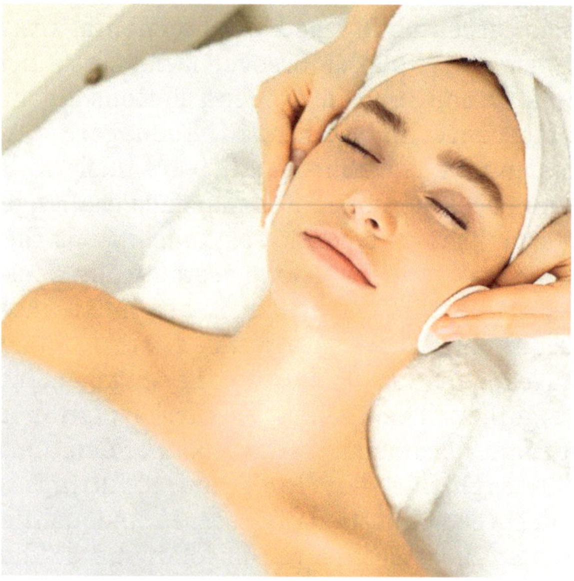

Figure 13.2. Facial aesthetics in social interactions.

Source: https://www.bellissimaclinic.com/wp-content/uploads/2023/05/facial-aesthetics-blog.jpg.

13.1. Types of Congenital Deformities

Learning Outcome

1. Cleft Lip and Palate
2. Craniosynostosis
3. Hemifacial Microsomia (HFM)

Congenital deformities occur in varied forms and have a strong impact on facial appearance, presenting individualistic difficulties in diagnosis, treatment, and psychosocial acceptance. The most common types are craniofacial microsomia and cleft lip and palate. Craniofacial microsomia occurs as a result of underdevelopment of the mandible and ear, resulting in asymmetry as well as functional disability, especially speech and mastication. By comparison, cleft lip and palate are due to a failure of facial structures to fuse early in development, usually resulting in conspicuous aesthetic discrepancies and feeding and speech problems. A perspective on these specific deformities is necessary to establish effective intervention protocols that maximize both functional and aesthetic results in affected patients. A second crucial category of congenital deformities involves the more complex syndromic presentations, like Treacher Collins syndrome and Pierre Robin sequence. Treacher Collins syndrome can be associated with a combination of facial dysmorphisms, e.g., underdeveloped jaw and cheekbones, that lead to impaired facial symmetry and hearing deficit. Conversely, the Pierre Robin sequence is primarily defined by a triad of anomalies: a decreased jaw size, cleft palate, and tongue displacement, which will occlude the airway. Both conditions have significant influences on the developmental trajectory and social experience of the affected, as facial appearance is a central ingredient in both social interaction and self-concept. These syndromic congenital anomalies need a multi-disciplinary treatment plan to optimize treatment protocols based on both the external and functional aspects of facial appearance (Rutger ter Horst et al., 2021). Congenital anomalies also happen on the basis of genetic and environmental factors, like hemifacial microsomia, where the face is underdeveloped on one side, affecting overall symmetry and aesthetic balance. The presentation and severity of the condition can widely differ from one individual to the next, emphasizing the importance of individualized treatment approaches. Treatment approaches tend to involve surgical corrections to restore symmetry to the face and enhance functional abilities, as well as psychological counseling to manage the emotional impact of having a visible difference. Hence, a comprehensive treatment plan is required, keeping in view not only the physical rectification but also the psychosocial well-being of patients, thereby facilitating a holistic approach to care in the domain of congenital and developmental deformities of facial aesthetics (Rutger ter Horst et al., 2021) (Figure 13.3).

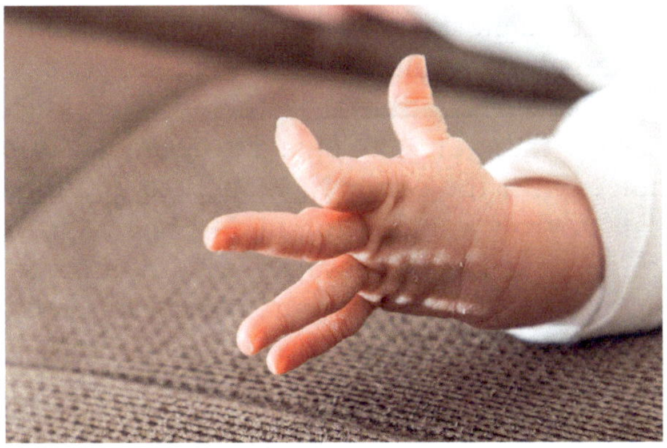

Figure 13.3. Congenital deformities manifest.

Source: https://www.spirehand.com.sg/wp-content/uploads/2024/04/spire-blog-congenital-hand-scaled.jpeg.

13.1.1. Cleft Lip and Palate

The impact of cleft lip and palate extends much further than mere physical characteristics, affecting numerous aspects of a child's life and health. The birth defects happen in fetal formation during early pregnancy when tissues employed to form the lip and palate fail to fuse together. Prevalence of cleft lip and palate also varies geographically, from 1 in 500 to 1 in 2,500 live births, reflecting a significant health concern that necessitates all-embracing intervention strategies. The nuances of these deformities tend to give rise to a complex set of functional deficits, such as feeding disorders and speech pathology, and psychological and social implications, yet further complicate the life of the affected person. This heterogeneity of cleft lip and palate highlights the need for multidisciplinary treatment and care, which introduces the significance of addressing the physical and psychological needs of patients. Multidisciplinary care coordination is the key to the care of cleft lip and palate since it maximizes treatment outcomes and facilitates overall rehabilitation. These children are typically cared for by an interdisciplinary team of professionals, including surgeons, orthodontists, speech therapists, and psychologists, to address the broad variety of issues presented by the deformity. Available literature suggests that integrated management with a tiered system is extremely useful, allowing for increased functional potential and restorative esthetics. For instance, Eshiev et al. (2025) emphasize the necessity of interdisciplinary collaboration on an everyday basis, one that is not only necessary in surgical operations but also in constant observation and treatment throughout childhood.

This active interprofessional collaboration guarantees the development of a practice arena in which healthcare professionals can work collaboratively toward solving the physical and psychosocial problems involved in treating children for cleft lip and palate. Apart from the direct issue resulted by cleft lip and palate, patients also bear a higher risk for dental abnormalities, such as Molar-Incisor Hypomineralization (MIH), complicating orthodontic treatment and oral health overall (Pérez Sánchez et al., 2022). Such dental anomalies bring about high burdens, affecting the psychosocial outcomes of children in dealing with their own circumstances. Effective and prompt dental care becomes inevitable, not just for the reason that untreated dental conditions exacerbate underlying functional deficits but also because they are likely to induce compromised social acceptance and self-confidence. It is thus necessary that the healthcare practitioners apply methods with the priority of employing holistic treatment approaches involving dental rehabilitation with other modalities to optimize facial aesthetics, function, and quality of life in these patients. By adopting a comprehensive approach to treatment and rehabilitation, the medical community can improve the life course of the victims of cleft lip and palate (Figure 13.4).

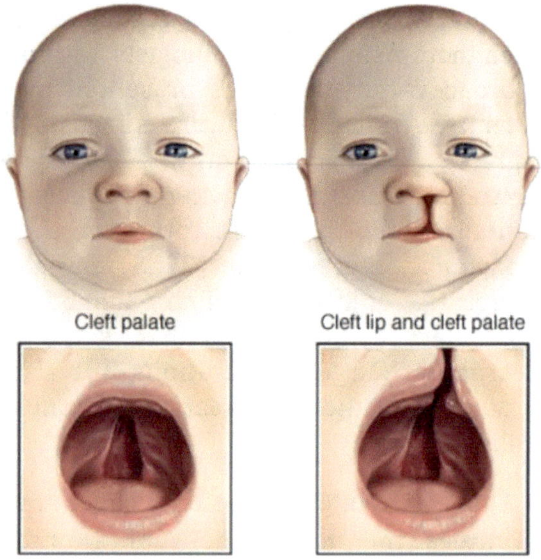

Figure 13.4. Cleft lip and palate.

Source: https://www.mayoclinic.org/-/media/kcms/gbs/patient-consumer/images/2013/08/26/10/45/ds00738_ds00998_im02607_fl7_cleft_palatethu_jpg.png.

13.1.2. Craniosynostosis

Craniosynostosis is a severe congenital abnormality resulting from the premature closure of an individual or more cranial sutures. This abnormal fusion restricts skull expansion and can lead to elevated intracranial pressure and potential developmental delays, ultimately influencing overall facial appearance. The illness most frequently occurs in multiple forms, the most common of which is single-suture craniosynostosis. For instance, sagittal synostosis results in a short, narrow head form, while coronal synostosis results in asymmetrical skull features. These deformities not only may jeopardize the cosmetic shape of the skull but also facial architecture, with significant social implications for the manner in which an individual is perceived. As such, craniosynostosis necessitates careful evaluation and multi-modal therapy to prevent aesthetic as well as functional morbidity. Craniosynostosis is typically diagnosed in infancy with the aid of imaging modalities such as X-rays or CT scans for assessment of suture involvement. Prompt diagnosis is crucial, as it will dictate the treatment plan aimed at the remodeling of skull shape and alleviation of intracranial pressure. Surgical intervention remains the modality of choice, with the surgery planned to allow the skull to grow and develop in a normal fashion. Prompt treatment is associated with improved neurological function and cosmetic results. Additionally, thorough care will sometimes go beyond surgery, including continued observation and possible orthodontic work as the child matures. As indicated in companion research, treatment for such cranial deformities can radically improve quality of life and psychosocial adjustment, especially among children as they continue to cope with social interactions.

The psychosocial nature of craniosynostosis is important and too often underemphasized in clinical reports. Kids with typical cranial morphologies may be stigmatized or bullied, in turn influencing their social relationships and self-perception. These issues must be approached from a multidisciplinary point of view, not only from medical and surgical treatment but also from psychological intervention. Family counseling and education play an important role in developing patients' and families' resilience. For instance, the importance of psychosocial intervention coupled with physical therapy has been highlighted in order to achieve the best possible developmental results. Research shows that by integrating these factors into care, clinicians can significantly improve the quality of life in affected individuals, ultimately leading to increased overall function and form, combining both therapeutic and aesthetic results (Figure 13.5).

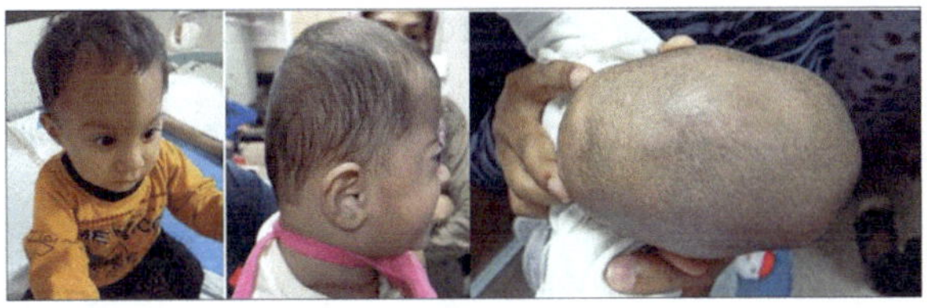

Figure 13.5. Craniosynostosis.

Source: https://www.researchgate.net/publication/363687463/figure/fig1/AS:11431281085248531@1663688286727/Abnormally-shaped-head-as-a-presentation-of-craniosynostosis-in-a-child-of.ppm.

13.1.3. Hemifacial Microsomia (HFM)

HFM is a significant congenital craniofacial deformity, with clinical presentations that can dramatically impact an individual's aesthetic and functional features. Second only to cleft lip and palate as the most frequent congenital facial deformity, HFM is characterized by a vast spectrum of facial asymmetry, typically including the mandible, maxilla, and associated soft tissue. The heterogeneity of presentation creates complex challenges like underdevelopment of the jaw, malformations of the ear, and potential hearing impairment. In addition to the physical status, the psychosocial impact of having HFM can significantly contribute to the patient's self-concept, communication, and interpersonal relationships. Facilitating early intervention and appropriate management strategies reduces such problems, which proves that there is a need for a multidisciplinary team in the delivery of care, including operative interventions as well as psychosocial intervention. The impact of HFM extends even into the area of neurodevelopment and education, particularly for the affected children. Studies indicate that HFM patients are at a higher risk of verbal, non-verbal, and educational problems, particularly if accompanied by other anomalies such as microtia and mandibular hypoplasia. These challenges can hinder skills that are crucial to social interaction and mental development, and cause feelings of isolation or peer rejection to persist. Although some children get by in the beginning, research states that as they progress with their education, they experience declining outcomes later. This also emphasizes the need for early assessment and targeted interventions that enhance social and language skills, eventually improving the quality of life of patients with HFM (Pniak et al., 2024). Recent advances in surgical techniques have promising potential in the treatment of HFM, and more importantly, the use of virtual surgical planning (VSP) and 3D-printed surgical assistants, which have been used to great benefit in reconstructive procedures.

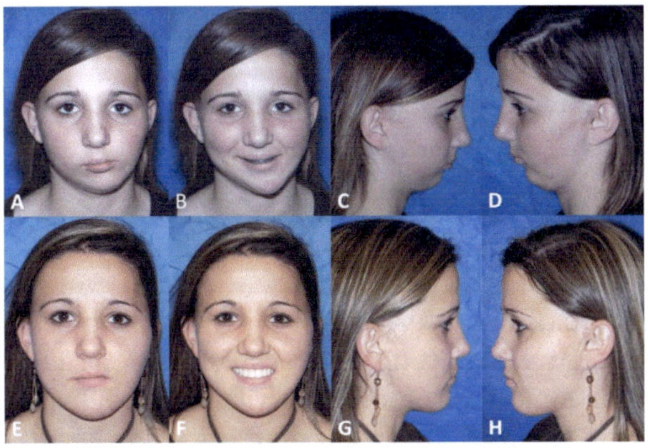

Figure 13.6. Hemifacial microsomia (HFM).

Source: https://drlarrywolford.com/wp-content/uploads/2015/01/Screenshot-2015-02-14-12.14.48.png.

Through the application of modern technology, surgeons are able to accurately plan and execute surgical procedures that rectify deformity, in addition to obtaining the most optimal aesthetic outcomes. Combined application of 3D-printed titanium mesh and iliac cancellous bone grafts, for instance, has been found to significantly improve facial function and symmetry. The precision that these tools provide not only enhances the efficacy of surgery but also decreases the rate of complications and postoperative bone resorption. As additional research continues to illuminate the benefits of such new techniques, the possibility for improved surgical results in patients with HFM grows, ultimately leading to a more favorable prognostic profile in congenital facial anomalies (Zhao et al., 2023) (Figure 13.6).

Test Your Knowledge

1. What are the most common types of congenital facial deformities, and how do they affect facial structure and function?
2. How do congenital deformities such as cleft lip and cleft palate differ in their presentation and clinical management?

13.2. Types of Developmental Deformities

Learning Outcome

1. Facial Asymmetry
2. Acquired Deformities Due to Trauma
3. Deformities Resulting from Medical Conditions

Developmental facial deformities are grouped in facial aesthetics as a broad range of conditions that may be caused by genetic, environmental, or multifactorial etiologies. Of these, craniosynostosis, or deformity through premature closure of one or more of the cranial sutures, has profound effects on the development of the face. Irregular head shapes often ensue from this deformity, and facial structure position and symmetry can be compromised. In some cases, surgery is required to prevent elevated intracranial pressure and permit normal craniofacial growth. The significance of treatment and diagnosis at an early stage is rendered evident by the possibility of more favorable aesthetic and functional outcomes, illustrating the relationship of developmental processes and beauty of the face within the broader framework of congenital deformity. Another extremely prevalent category of developmental anomalies is cleft lip and palate, which results from an incomplete closure of the lip and/or palate during embryogenesis. Incidence of this syndrome varies across the globe but is among the primary indications for surgical repair in children. Along with the main cosmetic defect, cleft lip and palate will have major impacts on the acquisition of speech, oral health of the dentition, and psychosocial adaptation. Medical specialists have a penchant for adopting an interdisciplinary strategy, combining surgical correction with orthodontic treatment and speech therapy in order to address the numerous challenges posed by these deformities. This integrated mindset is dedicated to the intricate relationship between congenital conditions and the resulting effect on facial morphology, and the importance of patient-specific interventions to achieve functional and esthetic goals. More complex developmental deformities, such as those requiring advanced surgical techniques, have been enhanced by recent advances in technology. One prime example of a useful improvement to craniofacial surgery is the introduction of ultrasound-guided osteotomes, such as Piezosurgery®. Comparing research on traditional osteotomes with the new devices has shown advantages in terms of micromorphological precision and preservation of surrounding tissues, which can enhance healing outcomes (Anesi et al., 2014). Additionally, new treatments utilizing stem cells hold promising directions for regenerating specific craniofacial structures, providing solutions for what may not best heal with conventional surgical intervention (Hughes & Song, 2016). With the continued advancement of scientific research in the field, it is clear that the nature of developmental facial appearance deformities is complex, thus necessitating continued study of new remedies and methods for improving patient outcomes (Figure 13.7).

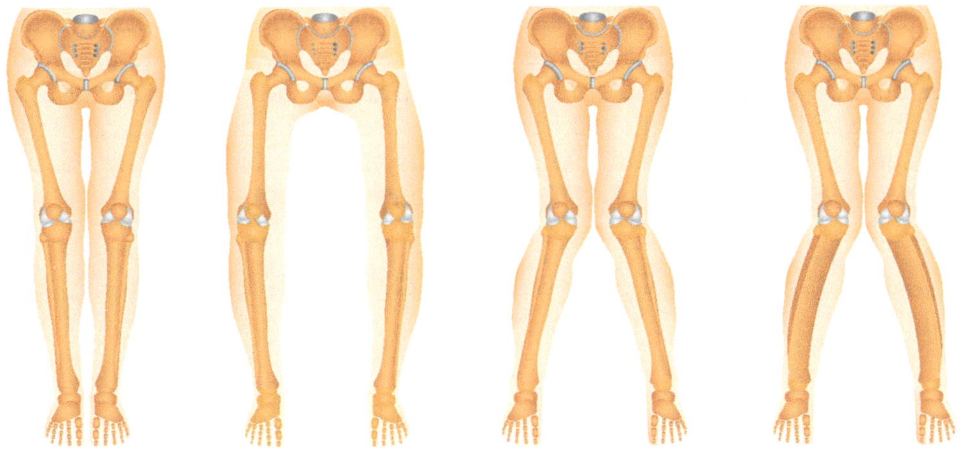

Figure 13.7. Types of developmental deformities.

Source: https://external-content.duckduckgo.com/iu/?u=https%3A%2F%2F1.bp.blogspot.com%2F-L97YYXcp5qA%2FXcCK1_EYsGI%2FAAAAAAABtz8%2F-a3whpQ_oV8EGT8bClZILJ60fL1SuqWSQCLcBGAsYHQ%2Fs1600%2FDevelopment%252Bof%252BAngular%252BDeformities.jpg&f=1&nofb=1&ipt=57e9a35a2d56658834412bb8fb783e71468808cff84e9b844a07f0e77d636de6.

13.2.1. Facial Asymmetry

Facial asymmetry is very prevalent in facial aesthetics, particularly as it relates to how congenital and developmental deformities look on individuals. As described as a non-symmetrical appearance between the two sides of the face, asymmetry can be brought about by some different factors, including genetic influences and environmental pressures on developmental critical periods. In the case of patients with congenital deformities such as microtia, facial asymmetry may bear severe consequences not only on their outward appearance but also on their psychological condition, typically presenting as self-esteem and social integration issues. Uncovering the etiology of facial asymmetry is essential in formulating specific therapeutic interventions, either through surgery or other means of enhancing facial symmetry and beauty. In the examination of specific conditions that lead to facial asymmetry, auricular deformities like microtia come to mind. Microtia is characterized by the underdevelopment of the outer ear and typically also by asymmetry of both the auricle and the facial complex closely related to it. Current research highlights the necessity for a precise measurement technique in the assessment of such deformities, as conventional techniques may not detect minor asymmetries, which potentially can affect the outcome of treatment. New technologies, such as a newly developed computerized 3D surface-based measurement of the auricle, offer higher accuracy in auricular feature and bilateral asymmetry measurement. This new technology is likely to be able to better optimize facial deformity patient diagnostic and treatment algorithms, such as those responsible for high levels of asymmetry, with the ultimate aim of improved aesthetic results and higher psychological benefit (Lin et al., 2024). Apart from surgical repairs, the psychological impacts of facial asymmetry should not be taken lightly. Individuals who have visible asymmetries, either congenital or acquired, are subject to societal bias, which can cause tremendous influences on their mental health as well as their general well-being. It has been shown through research that beauty is highly correlated with facial symmetry, thus placing more burdens on individuals with asymmetrical facial anatomy. Awareness of these psychological effects encourages a more sympathetic and integrated treatment approach that confronts not only the physical realignment of asymmetries but also the social and emotional ramifications of living with these conditions. By integrating psychological support with aesthetic procedures, medical experts can prescribe a more complete treatment program to patients with facial asymmetry, encouraging better body image and acceptance among patients (Lin et al., 2024) (Figure 13.8).

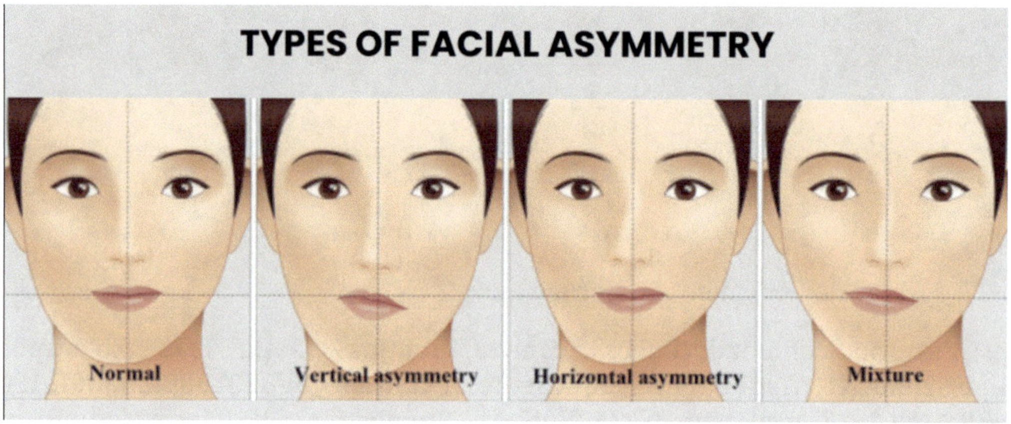

Figure 13.8. Facial asymmetry.

Source: https://external-content.duckduckgo.com/iu/?u=https%3A%2F%2Fgotobeauty.com%2Fwp-content%2Fuploads%2F2024%2F01%2FTYPES-OF-FACIAL-ASYMMETRY-1024x576.png&f=1&nofb=1&ipt=62b957f72b3f1d3b3d184b415ca0c9fd192030d0c09876f08b459a5db959fff4.

13.2.2. Acquired Deformities Due to Trauma

Trauma-caused deformities are a key issue of the field of facial aesthetics, distinguishing them from developmental or congenital deformities. These resulting conditions are a result of a variety of injuries, including accidents, athletic accidents, or brutal attacks, that can alter facial bone and soft tissue structural integrity. Trauma tends to have profound effects, as not only do they alter one's looks but also the psychological health of the patient. Patients can suffer chronic emotional distress resulting from disfigurement, which decreases quality of life. It is essential to understand the consequences of such deformities in the development of therapeutic interventions aimed at correcting both function and esthetics. It is frequent that the treatment of acquired facial deformities is carried out by a multidisciplinary team. Maxillofacial reconstruction surgeries are crucial in the correction of the underlying bony structure and esthetic contour of the face. Evolutionary facial jaw surgery techniques, which seek to repair structural deformities caused by trauma, have been introduced to achieve maximum patient benefit (Ugli, 2024). These treatments can involve the use of advanced imaging technologies and biocompatible materials to achieve maximum benefit. Rehabilitation operations following treatment are critical in ensuring normalcy in recovery, as well as to facilitate patients to restore their physical form, as well as self-belief when interacting with people. With such comprehensive care, the aftermath of trauma-related deformities can be effectively addressed. Furthermore, rehabilitation in patients with facial acquired deformities is a complex process that is generally not possible surgically. Prosthetic is also widely used to address aesthetic and functional deficits, particularly in children and adolescents who are victims of such injury at formative stages (Wojtyńska et al., 2024). Such prosthetics are not only used to cover the deformities but also to enable the normal facial movement during social interaction. With the treating clinicians interacting with these patients, it becomes necessary to assess their individualized needs and formulate a personalized care regimen involving both surgical and prosthetic components. This move emphasizes the importance of integral treatment models that take into account the multidimensional impact of acquired deformities on individuals who are in pursuit of aesthetic balance in facial appearance.

13.2.3. Deformities Resulting from Medical Conditions

The intersection of congenital disease and facial aesthetics is a complicated issue, particularly as it involves the treatment of deformities due to medical conditions. Congenital conditions such as cleft lip and palate are significant concerns due to their pervasive impact on both aesthetics and functionality. These disfigurements may disrupt essential activities such as feeding and speech and need intricate, multidisciplinary treatment. The psychosocial impact of the visibility of disfigurements may disrupt social interaction and self-esteem, further making the experience of affected individuals more complicated. As with studies among patient populations with heterogeneity, benefits from cooperative work among surgeons, orthodontists, and speech pathologists underscore the necessity for an integrated rehabilitation care strategy beyond the correction of aesthetics (Eshiev et al., 2025). In addition to birth conditions, acquired facial deformities due to illnesses such as trauma or surgery also significantly impact facial appearances. For instance, the results of injuries that manifest as craniofacial trauma can result in extreme asymmetry and malformation. The conditions reflected in such instances normally demand advanced reconstructive processes specifically designed to correct both the function and the aesthetics. Moreover, facial asymmetry, resulting from an array of medical conditions—such as developmental disorders—should be thoroughly analyzed in order to determine the etiology of the conditions. Understanding of the underlying causes can facilitate proper surgical planning and management, ultimately improving aesthetic outcomes. As research emphasizes, convergence of novel imaging technologies in diagnosis as well as surgical planning is crucial to providing optimal facial balance and patients' quality of life (Boymuradov et al., 2025). The role of interdisciplinary integration cannot be overemphasized in the treatment of deformities resulting from medical conditions. Effective management of conditions like cleft palate and lip involves a lifelong effort from an interdisciplinary team of skilled health professionals, bringing together both physical and psychological components of treatment. Corrective surgery is usually staged, and ongoing reevaluation and intervention are required as the patient grows. Furthermore, participation of mental health professionals may help address the psychological burden of having visible defects and enhance the general therapeutic process. A treatment plan that is methodical in scope and incorporates not only operative correction, but also psychological guidance and rehabilitative therapy, realizes massive benefits both aesthetically and in terms of patients' overall well-being. Such a holistic model is crucial to instill resilience and foster an optimistic self-image among patients with congenital and developmental deformities (Eshiev et al., 2025).

Test Your Knowledge

1. What are developmental facial deformities, and how do they differ from congenital deformities?
2. How can abnormal growth of facial bones lead to developmental deformities such as jaw misalignment or asymmetry?

13.3. Causes of Congenital Deformities

Learning Outcome

1. Genetic Factors
2. Environmental Influences
3. Maternal Health During Pregnancy

Congenital deformity pathogenesis is multifactorial and includes genetic, environmental, and epigenetic factors contributing to the adverse impact on fetal development. The majority of cases are caused by genetic defects in the forms of chromosomal and single-gene disorders. For instance, trisomy 21 disorders like Down syndrome are characterized by several physical deformities and predominantly facial structures. In addition, environmental influences, such as teratogenic agents, ranging from drugs to infectious diseases, have major roles to play in fetal morphology during periods that are critical for gestation. Maternal alcohol or drug exposure has been found to be a causative agent of facial deformities and therefore contributes importantly to the induction of disorders such as fetal alcohol syndrome. Therefore, an understanding of both environmental stimuli and genetic susceptibility is paramount in the development of the multifaceted processes of congenital deformities. In addition to environmental and hereditary causes, maternal health or nutrition also play a key role in the prevention of congenital disabilities. Deficiencies in some critical nutrients early in pregnancy have been found to increase vulnerability to neural tube defects and other birth defects. Pregnancy-associated maternal conditions like obesity and diabetes are additional threats, not only causing potentially fatal pregnancy-related complications but also increasing the chances of congenital facial abnormalities in offspring. As more research pours in, what becomes apparent is that the integration of a multidisciplinary strategy of maternal care can assist in reducing risk for congenital malformation. By promoting maximum prenatal health and filling in defects, doctors can improve outcomes and eventually reduce the prevalence of congenital deformities. Advances in medical technology and genetic counseling have opened up new avenues for education about and possibly avoiding the dangers of congenital deformities. For example, the application of orthognathic surgery has evolved significantly, so that treatment of facial deformities resulting from congenital conditions is more successful. Midface and mandible osteotomies are routinely done now, and the aesthetic and functional outcome is improved. Additionally, as craniofacial deformities (CFDs) as a science are continually changing, corrective procedures based on regenerative medicine and tissue engineering are of immense potential to correct severe deformities. However, congenital deformities still remain a challenge in the form of complex anatomical structures and individualized management. Consequently, ongoing research is an integral part of fine-tuning treatment modalities and enhancing patient outcomes within facial aesthetics, ultimately improving quality of life among congenital patients (Tahmasebi et al., 2023; Zammit et al., 2023) (Figure 13.9).

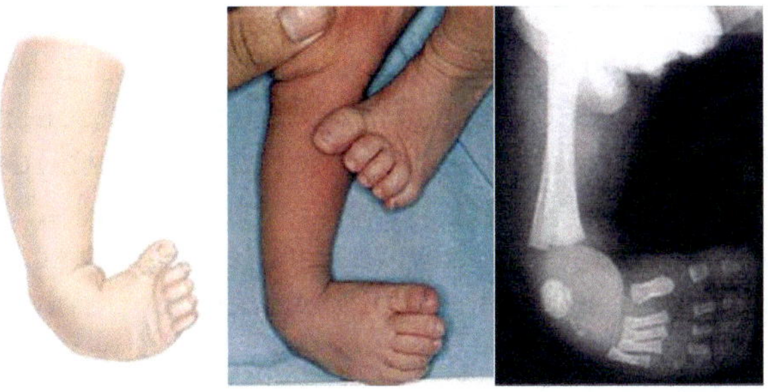

Figure 13.9. Causes of congenital deformities.

Source: https://external-content.duckduckgo.com/iu/?u=https%3A%2F%2Farchive.cdc.gov%2Fwww_cdc_gov%2Fncbddd%2Fbirthdefects%2Fsurveillancemanual%2Fphoto-atlas%2Fmuscu_html_files%2FCongenital-deformities-of-feet.jpg&f=1&nofb=1&ipt=963b6b0fbdcba7b2d99e63f1f664504c98c205a57ae886d08dac6b9a1986f979.

13.3.1. Genetic Factors

Genetic contributions towards the cause of congenital and developmental facial deformities are extensive and multifaceted. Genetic predispositions can lead to various craniofacial anomalies, which manifest through complex interactions among a number of genes. Studies have indicated that certain genetic diseases are directly related to abnormal facial patterns, i.e., cleft lip and palate, caused not only due to environmental reasons but also by the hereditary contributions of the genes. With continuous progress in genomic studies, determining the specific genetic markers and their role in craniofacial morphogenesis becomes increasingly important. With the identification of these genetic factors, clinicians are better able to assess risks, provide early interventions, and plan personalized treatment for patients who are facing such congenital challenges, thus optimizing clinical as well as aesthetic results in facial reconstruction. Exceeding isolated congenital deformities, the influence of genetic factors is present across a vast spectrum of facial aesthetic conditions that manifest themselves during the course of an individual's lifetime. For example, facial structures can be asymmetrical because they have both genetic and environmental influences. Facial directional asymmetry (DA) research indicates that genetic predispositions toward certain face shapes will work with the influence of aging to create unique developmental trajectories between populations. Three-dimensional measurements of DA over different ages are used in research to demonstrate how genes are involved in morphological change over time. In reviewing these findings, it is apparent that ongoing studies of genetic influences may shed light on the maintenance of facial beauty and the repair of a hereditary etiology of deformity, and ultimately the overall quality of life in such cases. Finally, neurodevelopmental genetics plays a part in the expression of facial beauty as the very interactive relation between nervous and stomatognathic systems. Genetic abnormalities may interfere with the highly complex processes of craniofacial development, causing congenital disorders that require in-depth clinical treatment. Recent research has highlighted the significance of the "brain-oral axis" in elucidating these connections, with a view to underlining that deviations from normal neural development can have downstream effects on facial features and overall aesthetic result. Diseases such as periodontitis were discovered in conjunction with neurodegenerative diseases, shedding light on the bidirectional interaction of the nervous and facial systems. As progress is made in science, it becomes increasingly important to combine genetic and neurological knowledge, fostering an interdisciplinary approach to treating congenital facial abnormalities and improving patient care in aesthetic and reconstructive surgery (Harnádková et al., 2023; Wu et al., 2023).

13.3.2. Environmental Influences

Environmental conditions are of utmost significance in the development and congenital deformities, particularly facial appearance. Various environmental factors, including maternal health, teratogenic effects, and nutrient deficiencies, have been shown to influence fetal development in a significant way. Malnutrition in pregnant women, for instance, has been shown to affect the craniofacial structures, leading to asymmetry and other types of deformities. The environmental role ranges from chemical exposure to psychosocial stressors known to influence fetal health. Therefore, it is paramount to comprehend these influences so that populations at risk can be identified and preventive interventions can be instated that can counteract adverse developmental impacts. Advances in imaging techniques have facilitated better comprehension and diagnosis of facial asymmetry and environmental deformities. As emphasized by recent research, discrimination between true and false facial asymmetries is important in formulating effective treatment plans. Diagnostic methods such as 3D CBCT scanning, cephalometry, and facial photometry enhance the clinician's ability to identify structural defects resulting from environmental causes (Boymuradov et al., 2025). Further, these assessments facilitate the correct preoperative evaluation so that the intervention provided is done in accordance with the precise needs of the patient, taking into consideration both aesthetic and functional deformities. The multifactorial nature of congenital and developmental deformities makes treatment a process that demands a holistic approach where genetic predispositions are balanced against environmental factors. Even though genetics might initiate the tendency towards the formation of facial deformities, environmental conditions are more likely to be the provocateurs of expression. For instance, environmental exposure in utero to pollutants or behavioral factors like smoking may worsen genetic susceptibilities to conditions such as facial asymmetry or cleft lip and palate (Boymuradov et al., 2025). Understanding these intersections is important for designing successful intervention strategies that treat both the genetic and environmental aspects, which in turn contributes to better treatment outcomes and enhancing the general quality of life of patients. With continued research continuing to reveal more and more of these factors, it highlights the importance of integrated healthcare policies which incorporate genetic counseling as well as environmental health literacy.

13.3.3. Maternal Health During Pregnancy

Pregnancy maternal health is a significant determinant of fetal as well as maternal outcomes, particularly regarding congenital and developmental defects. The intricate interrelationship among maternal diet, mental health, and environmental exposures plays a significant role in determining the trajectory of fetal health. Maternal nutrition plays a critical role in fetal development because dietary deficiency can make infants susceptible to congenital malformations, including orofacial clefts. For example, research has established that supplementation with folic acid can reduce the occurrence of neural tube defects, which highlights the importance of maternal food factors. The psychological well-being of the mother also cannot be overlooked since high levels of stress and anxiety during pregnancy have been proven to produce negative outcomes for the fetus, making pregnancy even more complicated during this period of maternal development. The challenges to neonate mothers with congenital abnormalities, such as cleft lip and palate, extend beyond the body's health. Such aberrations in anatomy are often complicated by a need for a multimodal care continuum, ranging from surgical intervention to a sophisticated feeding regimen. In cleft lip and palate, for instance, the issues of breastfeeding are compounded by the infant's characteristic anatomical deficits. Their management requires a multidisciplinary approach with surgical reconstruction and psychological treatment of mothers. Mothers must cope with the psychological aftermath of caring for a child with a congenital deformity. Stress and emotional status in mothers are two significant variables that not only affect lactation success but also the overall developmental outcome for the child. Therefore, emotional support and resources specific to these mothers can have a valuable impact on their capacity to care for their infants effectively. Furthermore, the prevalence of cleft lip and palate differs amongst populations, posing individual challenges based on genetic and environmental components. Insight into the epidemiology of these congenital anomalies can inform public health efforts towards enhancing maternal health practices and outcomes. For example, evidence shows that in Asian communities, clefting is more common than in African communities, which highlights the relevance of culturally sensitive healthcare provisions. The multifactorial etiology of these deformities implies that genetic vulnerabilities as well as maternal health behaviors during pregnancy, including smoking and alcohol consumption, play a major role in their occurrence. Controlling these risk factors by strengthening maternal health education and steering interventions can introduce more effective prevention strategies in congenital anomalies, thus guaranteeing optimum facial aesthetics as well as overall wellness of the affected person (Figure 13.10).

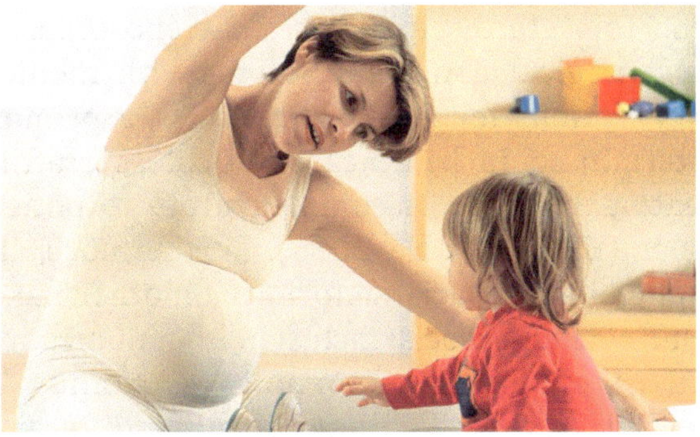

Figure 13.10. Maternal health during pregnancy influences a child's autism.

Source: https://external-content.duckduckgo.com/iu/?u=https%3A%2F%2Fsurvivethenews.com%2Fwp-content%2Fuploads%2F2025%2F03%2FHow-maternal-health-during-pregnancy-influences-a-childs-autism-risk.jpg&f=1&nofb=1&ipt=08feedd083146c2228509090a7ea26a8c19ce82abe3e4b1775af54dcf68268f5.

Test Your Knowledge

1. What genetic and environmental factors contribute to the development of congenital facial deformities?
2. How do maternal health, nutrition, and exposure to harmful substances during pregnancy influence congenital deformities?

13.4. Psychological Impact of Facial Deformities

Learning Outcome

1. Self-esteem and Body Image Issues
2. Social Stigma and Discrimination
3. Mental Health Implications

The psychological impact of facial deformities is quite wide-reaching beyond considerations of aesthetics alone, affecting the individual's self-esteem and relationships with others considerably. Congenital and developmental facial deformity patients usually express high levels of social distress and distress relating to their appearance. Research has demonstrated that individuals with craniofacial deformities experience higher levels of psychological distress than the general population, pointing to the fact that exterior stimuli of their look can lead to interior tension with their self-concept and identity. Negatively affecting mental health are depression, social withdrawal, and anxiety, which can significantly reduce quality of life. Emergence of addressing these psychological considerations underscores the need for interdisciplinarity that encompasses psychological counseling along with medical interventions for facial deformities, a primary determinant in healthcare providers crafting treatment protocols commensurate to patient needs (Bessell et al., 2015). Furthermore, the implications of facial deformity on other facets of life, including social inclusion, communication, and employment opportunities, cannot be ignored. As individuals with visible difference will struggle with negative stereotypes or prejudice, they are likely to face barriers that constrain full inclusion in many social contexts. Studies establish that such barriers lead to loneliness and a diminished sense of community, which further complicates mental illness. For instance, difficulties with chewing and speaking can generate feelings of inadequacy and anxiety, amplifying the impact their facial look has on social interactions. Incredibly, rehabilitative intervention, although beneficial, may still not restore people's self-esteem and quality of life to a position where they can be equated with nondisfigured counterparts. Along this line, it is crucial to pursue rehabilitation with a holistic perspective of the psychological dimension of facial beauty (Palmeiro et al., 2013). Last but not least, the issue of support systems is a significant one in mitigating psychological distress caused by facial deformity. Supportive comments from parents, peers, and health professionals can foster individuals' sense of self-concept and resilience in coping with adversity in society. Counseling and support groups may serve as a useful means of promoting acceptance and coping strategies, enabling one to cope with the intricacies associated with appearance in an improved manner. By building accepting environments that are centered on acceptance and understanding, the stigmatization of facial deformities can be reduced. Consequently, alongside the treatment of the physical aspect, the provision for the emotional and psychological aspects of the individual can significantly aid their general well-being and social incorporation, an essential process towards empathetic practice in facial aesthetics (Bessell et al., 2015) (Figure 13.11).

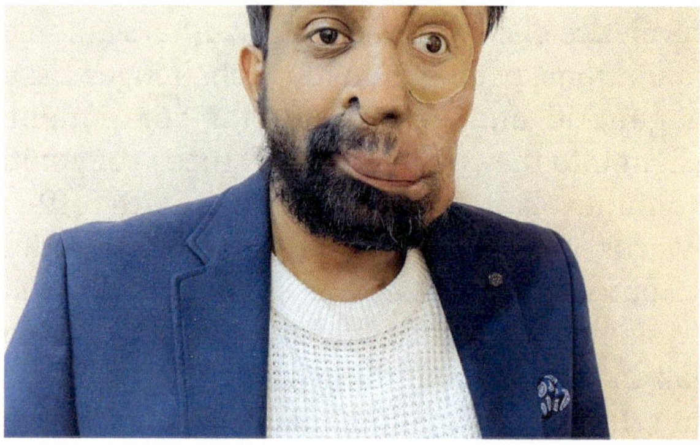

Figure 13.11. Psychological impact of facial deformities.

Source: https://www.camraredisease.org/wp-content/uploads/2023/08/image_50368513-1080x675.jpg.

13.4.1. Self-esteem and Body Image Issues

Facial aesthetic deformities, whether developmental or congenital, have a significant impact on body image issues and low self-esteem. The overwhelming majority of individuals with conditions such as hemifacial microsomia experience the adverse views of their appearance and subsequently suffer from low self-esteem. Facial deformity has the greatest psychological impact at adolescence—a tender time marked by enhanced sensitivity to social acceptance and body image. As the research shows, hemifacial microsomia children have social integration problems and the risk of rejection by their peers, which aggravates their self-esteem issues. These issues are strongly entangled with their facial features, where perceived cosmetic abnormalities influence their interpersonal relationships and mental health results, which makes it critical to provide them with psychological help at the earliest stage in order to improve their general quality of life (Michał Pniak et al., 2024). In addition, the relationship between appearance and self-esteem may be seen in the higher rates of anxiety and depression in patients with congenital facial deformity. Abnormal facial appearance most often leads to feelings of inadequacy and isolation, which impede social relationships and reinforce negative self-concepts. In adolescents and young adults, these consequent impacts cause social avoidance or unwillingness to engage in relationships, perpetuating the cycle of low self-esteem. Moreover, individuals internalize cultural ideals of beauty, become unhappy with their own looks and distressed about their state. Resolution of such psychological and emotional problems is pivotal in developing self-acceptance and resilience in targeted groups, emphasizing the need for integrated treatment responses that involve psychological well-being (Pniak et al., 2024). As part of effective interventions, recognition of the part played by healthcare professionals in managing issues related to self-esteem and body image is important. Clinicians are also required to have attention not only to the physical treatments but also to the psychosocial consequences that accompany facial congenital deformities. The therapy may include working on open conversations about one's image, providing access to counseling interventions, and applying education as a strategy of achieving de-stigmatization by society. Studies have shown that patients suffering from conditions such as hemifacial microsomia, when provided with proper psychosocial support, show improved emotional functioning and an increased sense of belongingness among peers. Moreover, active intervention in the form of programs such as community awareness and outreach aids in creating a positive attitude towards diversity in facial aesthetics, in the end aiding affected individuals to enhance their body image and self-esteem in the long run (Pniak et al., 2024) (Figure 13.12).

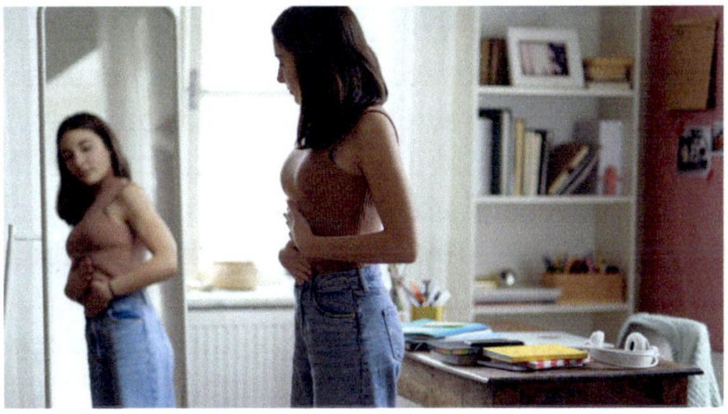

Figure 13.12. Self-esteem and body image issues.

Source: https://www.servicesforeducation.co.uk/wp-content/uploads/2024/07/Body-Image-and-Self-Esteem-1400x775.png.

13.4.2. Social Stigma and Discrimination

The social stigma that accompanies congenital and developmental deformities, particularly those affecting the beauty of the face, has drastic effects on the person's psychological and social well-being. Victims of deformity endure discrimination that gets to define their lifestyle and relationships. Social exclusion exists in the form of offensive statements, social rejection, and overall negative generalization. All these external forces tend to create the overwhelming emotional pain with resulting low self-esteem and mental illness. Drawing from research on oral reconstructive surgery, bullying and social experiences of loneliness persist to influence people before undergoing surgery, further underlining the urgent need for addressing these social perceptions of physical appearance (Sablada & Amparado, 2020). Not only do such stigmatizations undermine a person's feeling of belonging, but these stigmatizations also form a vicious cycle of discrimination that can deter individuals from accessing necessary medical or psychological care. Physical appearance discrimination is widespread in multi-ethnic social settings, including schools, the workplace, and healthcare facilities. Where those with facial disfigurements are discriminated against, their opportunities for social mobility, professional development, and access to basic services are compromised. A review of literature on cleft lip and/or palate individuals reveals that while the overall impact of these disorders on psychological adaptation was found to be low, the multigene nature of social experiences indicates significant barriers in terms of acceptance and satisfaction with appearance (Stock & Feragen, 2016).

This dissonance between self and societal expectations generally increases feelings of isolation. Eradicating these inequalities requires an understanding of the stigma that exists and deliberate steps to bring inclusivity, thereby providing a space where individuals are valued for what they are able to do rather than being attacked based on their physical appearance. Steps towards avoiding social stigma and discrimination against individuals with congenital and developmental deformities require a holistic approach that includes education, advocacy, and community action. By raising awareness of the psychological impacts of experiencing such, society can demolish prevalent stereotypes surrounding physical appearance. Inclusivity and empathy programs can significantly improve the lives of people with facial deformities. Support groups and peer workshops, for instance, can allow individuals to voice their experiences, develop resilience, and overcome loneliness. In addition, medical personnel and teachers need to be educated on identifying and confronting biases in their settings, developing a more supportive environment for patients and students. Encouraging empathy and understanding can play a critical role in shifting societal attitudes and ensuring that individuals with congenital and developmental deformities are given the respect and support they need (Figure 13.13).

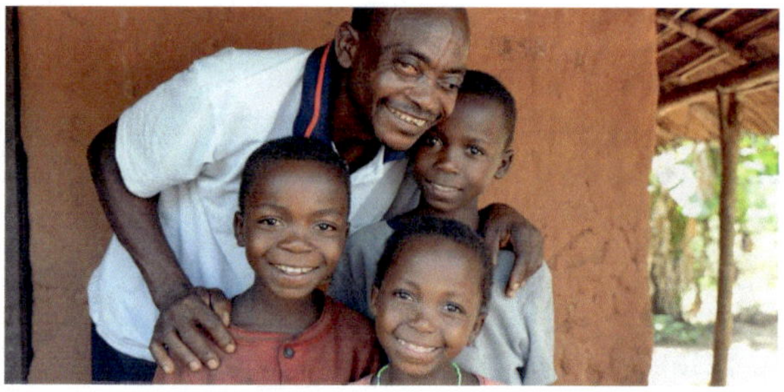

Figure 13.13. Social stigma and discrimination.

Source: https://www.infontd.org/sites/default/files/styles/crop_freeform/public/2020-05/CBM-Onchocerciasis-0011.JPG?h=34e69bba&itok=jOS2gSx1.

13.4.3. Mental Health Implications

The psychological effect on congenitally or developmentally deformed individuals who have facial aesthetic deformities is profound and intricate. Research shows that patients with craniofacial anomalies have heightened issues concerning their appearance, leading to high social anxiety and a diminished quality of life. For instance, such patients have been found to register higher negative psychological impacts in terms of their appearance compared to patients presenting without deformities. Specifically, interventions using the Psychological Impact of Dental Aesthetic Questionnaire (PIDAQ) and the Derriford Appearance Scale (DAS) identify that patients with craniofacial abnormalities experience much more distress over their looks, which may prompt avoidance of social interaction and fear of others' reactions (Bessell et al., 2015). Hence, the psychological impact from it does not just manifest at the subjective level of well-being but also in the general capacity to engage in normal social rituals. Also adding to the intricacies of handling mental health among this population is the long-term nature of the issues they have. Individuals with congenital deformities also tend to have issues with chewing, speech, and social integration, all impacting their quality of life (QoL) vitally. The oral presentation of such deformities tends to be so complicated that it requires extensive rehabilitation to restore function and aesthetics. However, studies have shown that even with interventions like oral rehabilitation, patients with conditions like cleft lip and palate (CLP) continue to have impaired masticatory function and lower QoL scores than healthy controls. Therefore, the inability of rehabilitation efforts to completely achieve both functional and psychosocial needs underscores the importance of interdisciplinary-based care; integrating psychological support with physical treatments (Palmeiro et al., 2013). Generally, the psychological aspects of congenital and developmental deformities must be addressed with a comprehensive approach that values and addresses the emotional needs of the afflicted. Effective interventions should aim not just to correct physical appearance, but also to promote emotional ease through counseling and outreach. By self-acceptance and the strengthening of coping mechanisms, mental health treatment can improve social integration and quality of life among such people. It is critical to have such an integrated approach, for it realizes that the journey towards accepting one's appearance is as significant as the medical or surgical intervention that has already been done. The psychological climate for the cases of facial deformity, therefore, can be favorably altered, initiating enhanced overall results.

Test Your Knowledge

1. How do facial deformities affect an individual's self-confidence, emotional well-being, and social life?
2. What role does psychological counseling play in helping patients cope with facial deformities?

13.5. Treatment Options for Facial Deformities

Learning Outcome

1. Surgical Interventions
2. Orthodontic Treatments
3. Psychological Support and Counseling

Treatment of facial deformities is case-specific and multidisciplinary in nature. Certain of the surgical options, such as orthognathic surgery, have also emerged as vital instruments in orthodontic correction of mismatched jaws and overall facial aesthetics. This type of surgery allows for the accurate realignment of facial bones to both restore functional deficits and address aesthetic concerns. Advances in technology, including computer planning and patient-specific fixation, have significantly enhanced the outcome of these operations. Surgeons are now better able to plan complex osteotomies with better predictability of outcome. Apart from this, the operations are also able to cure obstructive sleep apnea in a manner that makes the treatment doubly beneficial for patients who have both cosmetic and functional problems with their facial structures (Zammit et al., 2023). Apart from surgery, orthodontic treatments form part and parcel of facial deformity treatment, particularly in malocclusion. Malocclusion can interfere with one's oral function and also the aesthetic appearance, and identification and treatment of malocclusion have become extremely important in contemporary dentistry. Malocclusions were acknowledged by the World Health Organization as a main oral disorder that occurs with a high prevalence rate among the community. Interference at an early stage during the primary dentition period is capable of preventing the development of severe malocclusion into adulthood. The various malocclusion classifications, particularly the Angles classification system, enable understanding of unique dental alignment deviation forms to help orthodontists select the best treatment modalities based on specific cases (Lone et al., 2023). Lastly, non-surgical methods such as facial fillers and orthodontic appliances are becoming increasingly used to minimize or correct minor facial deformities and improve aesthetic results without surgery. For those patients who are not surgical candidates or wish less intrusive options, aligners and braces provide excellent improvement in facial form and function. Facial fillers are also an extremely viable option for volume and contour restoration of birth-defected areas. These treatments can enhance facial looks by providing rapid results with minimal downtime, which is appealing to those who appreciate rapid and effective treatments. With the development of facial aesthetics, possessing a general understanding of the variety of treatment modalities provides patients with the capacity to make informed choices regarding their treatment (Zammit et al., 2023) (Figure 13.14).

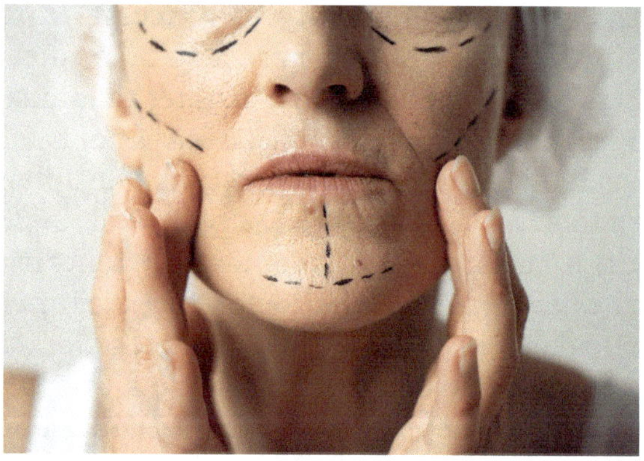

Figure 13.14. Treatment options for facial deformities.

Source: https://reconfaceindia.in/wp-content/uploads/elementor/thumbs/Post-trauma-facial-deformities-qf6ws1lmuvx33nip0n7m7qjv3gpywk5af1b92wtw5c.png.

13.5.1. Surgical Interventions

Surgical procedures play a pivotal role in the treatment of congenital and developmental facial aesthetic deformities, particularly for cases such as hemifacial microsomia (HFM). This is an asymmetric underdevelopment of first and second branchial arch components and is characterized by a variety of craniofacial anomalies that include mandibular hypoplasia, ear deformities, and other related structures. Surgical intervention generally requires a multidisciplinary approach to ensure holistic management and optimal aesthetic results. Several methods are utilized, including rib or fibular bone grafting, distraction osteogenesis, and orthognathic surgery, all of which collectively attempt to address functional and aesthetic deformities. The efficient synergism of such surgical techniques has far-reaching implications for improving not only the facial structural dimensions but also the psychosocial quality of life of the patients at a young age (Behnia et al., 2023). In addition to traditional surgical modalities, technological advancements have created sophisticated surgical instruments that further enhance the accuracy and efficacy of these interventions. Ultrasonic osteotomes, such as Piezosurgery, offer obvious advantages over conventional rotary or sawing devices. Studies have demonstrated that these ultrasonic devices yield smoother bone surfaces, which may enhance tissue healing and reduce injury to surrounding soft tissues during osteotomies. Such accuracy is crucial in the correction of complex craniofacial malformations, wherein collateral injury has to be avoided to preserve important anatomical structures. The comparative outcomes between ultrasonic and traditional osteotomes reveal a dramatic contrast in micromorphological features, again confirming the application of newer technology in operations to correct facial deformity (Anesi et al., 2014). The long-term benefits of surgical intervention in correcting congenital and developmental facial deformity extend beyond aesthetic purposes. Successful surgical outcomes can significantly enhance the psychosocial aspect of patients' lives, particularly at the time of adolescence, when perceptions of the peer group have an increasingly powerful influence. Procedures to correct jaw straightening or facial asymmetry have been found to enhance self-esteem and social function, producing a more positive self-concept. The integration of functional orthodontics along with surgical treatment, as validated by the findings of longitudinal follow-up in the instances of HFM, underscores the importance of a strictly planned treatment regimen that attempts to offer optimal facial esthetics and restoration of function. This multi-disciplinary strategy supports the imperative for ongoing research and communication among specialists to continue improving surgical techniques and overall patient care within the field of craniofacial surgery (Behnia et al., 2023) (Figure 13.15).

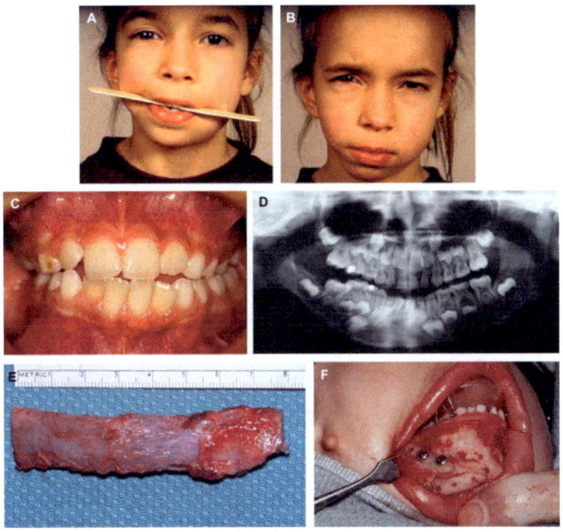

Figure 13.15. Surgical interventions play a pivotal role in addressing congenital and developmental deformities in facial aesthetics.

Source: https://ars.els-cdn.com/content/image/1-s2.0-S1042369907000386-gr7af.jpg.

13.5.2. Orthodontic Treatments

Orthodontics is a key component in the management of congenital and developmental facial aesthetic deformities. Orthodontic treatment has a tendency of aligning teeth, correcting issues with bites, and improving overall dental function, which can significantly improve a patient's facial appearance. With patients who have diseases such as Apert syndrome, which includes facial and dental abnormalities, orthodontics plays a crucial role. Early treatment using braces or other orthodontic devices can help in the proper alignment of the teeth and jaws, which in turn results in a more balanced facial esthetic profile. Since most of the congenital conditions can produce secondary functional impairment, orthodontic treatment not only has a purely aesthetic function but also corrects the underlying functional impairment and hence supports a better quality of life for the patients. With the progress in orthodontic treatments, integration of surgical treatments has become the standard, particularly if skeletal discrepancies exist. Orthognathic surgery is typically used in conjunction with orthodontic treatments to achieve optimum benefits. Improvements in surgical techniques in today's time, such as computer-aided planning and patient-specific fixation, have tailored the process in the correction of severe deformities (Zammit et al., 2023). This partnership between orthodontists and oral surgeons allows the face and oral structures to be treated more accurately and effectively, not only for their appearance, but also for the functional dynamics of the bite. Such comprehensive care is the focal point in multidisciplinary treatment plans for those with congenital deformities and strives to enhance aesthetic outcomes as well as oral health. Moreover, the psychosocial impact of orthodontic treatment cannot be overlooked, especially on individuals with obvious congenital or developmental deformities. Orthodontic therapy of dental and facial deformities exercises a significant influence on self-perception and social acceptance. Patients become less embarrassed and more confident following the treatment, which is evidence of the psychological significance of facial beauty (Kumari et al., 2023). By improving the symmetry and alignment of their smile, orthodontic treatments contribute to a satisfactory self-image, thereby maximizing the quality of life as a whole. To this end, healthcare providers are required to plan for treatment holistically, taking into consideration the emotional and psychological health of the patients along with the technical know-how of care in aesthetic dentistry (Figure 13.16).

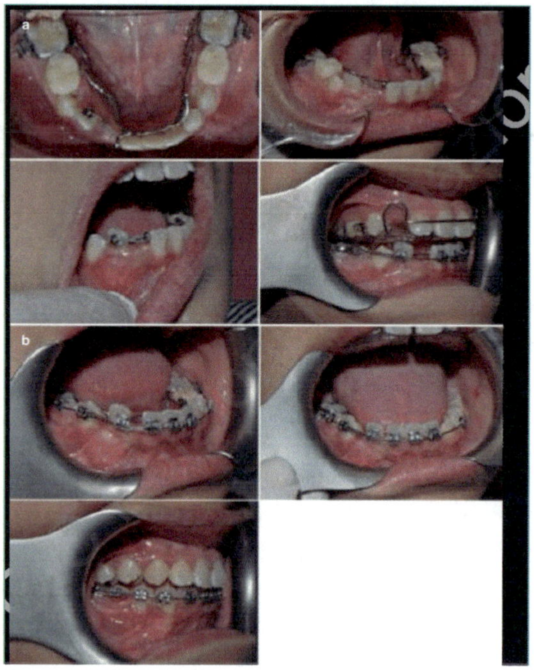

Figure 13.16. Orthodontic treatments.

Source: https://www.researchgate.net/profile/Biagio-Rapone/publication/320432128/figure/fig2/AS:580206029176833@1515343305438/a-Pictures-of-the-different-phases-of-the-orthodontic-treatment-b-Orthodontic.png.

13.5.3. Psychological Support and Counseling

Psychological guidance and support are of critical significance in the rehabilitation of congenital and developmental facial deformities in aesthetics, with direct impacts on emotional state as well as social integration. These individuals are often more anxious, self-conscious, and disabled in daily social contact, and hence they have a poorer quality of life. It entails the development of a therapeutic relationship between the patient and the mental health professional, in which the latter creates a comfortable environment where the patient can express their concerns and emotions. This kind of support is not only important in coping with the immediate emotional disturbance caused by their condition but also in preparing individuals to prepare for potential treatments or procedures that can alter the appearance of individuals, as the psychological impact can be as profound as the physical alterations inherent within these medical interventions. Counseling interventions specific to those with facial deformity should also take into account the special needs of this group. Cognitive-behavioral therapy (CBT) and other forms of therapy can successfully correct negative self-perception and distorted thinking about appearance. These therapeutic interventions assist patients in changing their perceptions and improving self-acceptance, thus building resilience against social stigma. In addition, support groups can prove to be priceless because they allow people to bond with their peers who are going through the same issues, fostering mutual healing. Sharing such group experiences not only offers emotional encouragement but also leads to the sharing of coping mechanisms and personal experiences, which ultimately strengthen people to deal with and overcome their fears concerning their facial looks, bolstering their mental strength. Further, the need for interprofessional teamwork among treatment professionals cannot be overemphasized when it comes to psychological care of patients with congenital and developmental deformities. Interprofessional collaboration ensures an integrated approach, involving plastic surgeons, mental health professionals, and genetic counselors to design an integrated plan of care. Interprofessional collaboration allows providers to address not only physical but also psychological issues, thus enhancing overall outcomes of treatment. As has been demonstrated in current literature, holistic management practices can lead to better patient outcomes and experiences, with the importance of shared decision-making in treatment highlighted. This inter-disciplinary strategy mirrors evidence regarding the complexity of most congenital conditions, highlighting the promise that integrated care networks hold to improve dramatically the quality of life for such individuals, allowing them to better navigate the complexity of their conditions with a lot more support and understanding, as in the management of neurofibromatosis type 1 (Bergqvist et al., 2020) and congenital heart disease (Pierpont et al., 2018).

Test Your Knowledge

1. What are the main surgical and non-surgical treatment options available for correcting facial deformities?
2. How does early diagnosis and treatment improve the functional and aesthetic outcomes of facial deformities?

13.6. Advances in Facial Aesthetic Procedures

Learning Outcome

1. Innovations in Surgical Techniques
2. Role of 3D Imaging and Modeling
3. Non-Surgical Aesthetic Enhancements

The field of facial aesthetics has experienced great advances that have widened the treatment options for patients with developmental and congenital deformities. Traditional practices, which were primarily surgical, have been revolutionized with the introduction of minimal access procedures that enhance safety and recovery. Emerging three-dimensional imaging and computer simulations have also become valuable in pre-surgical planning and patient education. These innovations provide professionals with a greater understanding of craniofacial anatomy, enabling them to provide customized treatment options better suited to individual patient needs. With fewer invasive and more precise surgeries, patients can expect improved functional and aesthetic results. More patient-centered treatment modalities for facial aesthetics place increased focus on improvements that assist in diminishing the psychological effect of congenital deformity, promoting overall quality of life for individuals so involved. Further, the development of non-surgical approaches to aesthetic enhancement has had a profound impact on the facial reconstruction and enhancement arena. Technologies such as fillers, neurotoxins, and other biocompatible agents in soft tissue augmentation provide some alternatives that can reduce the necessity for more invasive surgeries. For patients with congenital deformities, these technologies can correct the anomalies immediately, enhancing facial contours and symmetry without the extensive downtime associated with surgery. Also, the growing availability of Piezosurgery®, among other ultrasound-assisted osteotomes, adds the benefits of precision in osteotomies that provide smoother bone surfaces to heal and produce more acceptable aesthetics following surgical interventions (Anesi et al., 2014). With growing technological developments, the use of these non-surgical techniques not only transforms patterns of treatment but also opens a new frontier for the return of confidence in patients with congenital and developmental facial disorders. Cosmetic procedures' clinical practices have expanded due to a better understanding of the physiological and psychological details of congenital deformities. More advanced prosthetic therapies, including individually customized orthodontic appliances, address both functional and cosmetic problems maximally. These devices have a vital role in treatment regimens for patients with conditions such as cleft lip and palate, where rehabilitation is multifaceted and requires close consideration in terms of the optimal balance between form and function. Novel non-surgical treatment options, including novel orthodontic techniques, can now offer patients more comfortable and functional solutions for coping with extreme deformity and optimizing oral function (McNeil, 1951). As research ever more illuminates the correlation between aesthetic perfection and emotional well-being, it is increasingly evident that innovation in facial aesthetic surgery is paramount for transforming not just the physical topographies but also the psychosocial existence of individuals with congenital and developmental facial disfigurements (Figure 13.17).

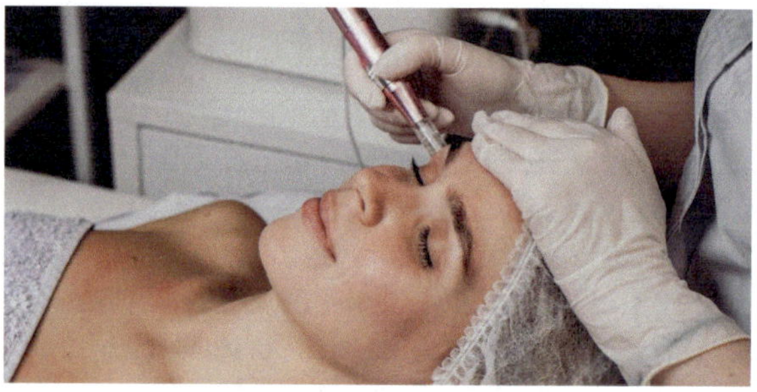

Figure 13.17. Facial aesthetics.

Source: https://iicad.org/wp-content/uploads/2024/01/IICAD-7.png.

13.6.1. Innovations in Surgical Techniques

Craniofacial surgery has witnessed significant new development as far as surgical techniques addressing congenital and developmental facial aesthetics deformities are concerned. Among the most promising of these is the use of stem cell therapy with tissue engineering. As highlighted in recent literature, this technique has immense potential for regrowing some craniofacial tissues but remains at its nascent stage of advancement in its clinical applications. The unique type of various stem cell sources makes personalized treatments for complicated facial deformity patients, hence promising improved surgical outcomes. While researchers seek to study the most appropriate cell sources, challenges that are unique to these new types of treatment need to be addressed to increase their efficacy and availability in clinics (Hughes & Song, 2016). The second essential innovation of surgical techniques is the application of ultrasonic osteotomes to enhance precision for osteotomies in craniofacial surgery. The traditional method of using turning or sawing tools will cause damage to the surrounding soft tissue, thus causing postoperative complications. However, studies have established that Piezosurgery, a technique assisted by ultrasound, not only preserves the integrity of adjacent tissues but also enhances bone healing and reossification. Micromorphological surface features of osteotomized surfaces mirror increased roughness values, which are crucial for effective healing and incorporation of graft materials. The minimally invasive surgery has monumental advantages, eventually leading to improved aesthetic and functional outcomes for individuals with craniofacial deformities (Anesi et al., 2014). With improving surgical techniques, integration of advanced imaging modalities and computer-aided design (CAD) has transformed preoperative planning as well as intraoperative navigation. Technological advances in 3D imaging make it possible to have personalized surgical strategies, and through this, surgeons are able to design patient-specific models that closely approximate the anatomical complexities of individual patients. Such precision guarantees that surgical procedures are customized to correct the specific deformities involved, as well as to maximize aesthetic outcome and functional abilities of reconstructions. Supported by intraoperative navigation devices, these developments facilitate accurate execution of surgical plans to the minimum possible extent, ensuring reduced opportunities for errors and overall patient safety. With growing popularity, these advances are likely to transform the quality of care for the correction of congenital and developmental facial anomalies (Anesi et al., 2014; Hughes & Song, 2016).

13.6.2. Role of 3D Imaging and Modeling

The intersection of three-dimensional (3D) imaging and modeling technology has revolutionized the field of reconstructive surgery for developmental and congenital facial aesthetic deformities. Advances in 3D imaging provide advanced visualization of craniofacial anatomy, which allow clinicians to examine deformities with unmatched precision. Such technological advances enable virtual surgical planning (VSP), which transforms cumbersome anatomical data into efficacious surgical plans. For instance, in the management of conditions such as hemifacial microsomia, 3D modeling enables planning of osteotomy lines and cutting guides that are tailored to the individual anatomical features of the patients. The technique enhances intraoperative precision and minimizes intraoperative complications, hence dramatically improving patient outcomes. This innovation serves to underscore the basic significance of 3D imaging in transforming traditional surgical practices into more precise, streamlined procedures, ultimately resulting in enhanced success rates for reconstruction surgeries. In terms of orthognathic surgery, 3D imaging has facilitated unprecedented advances in the planning and execution of treatment. Surgeons can now execute precise osteotomies of the midface and mandible, aligning their surgical goals with an individually designed treatment plan. The precise combination of patient-specific fixation systems and advancing imaging technologies provides a rational approach to treating both functional and cosmetic issues in facial aesthetics. In the past two decades, this paradigm has seen enhancements in the fidelity of computer-assisted planning, making it simpler for surgeons to predict and avoid potential complications during surgery. These improvements have enabled improved integration of orthodontic treatments with surgical procedures, generating synergistic methods for treating congenital and acquired facial deformities (Zammit et al., 2023). This development strongly suggests growing prevalence and reliance on 3D imaging among the surgical community. As craniofacial surgery continues to advance, the significance of 3D imaging and modeling technology is bound to increase even more. The utility of such technologies is not just restricted to successful surgeries; they also enhance postoperative assessment and long-term follow-up of facial shape and function. In successful reconstructions, for instance, with 3D-printed surgical implants in hemifacial microsomia treatments, systematic evaluations show promising decreases in asymmetry parameters (Zhao et al., 2023). The use of digital software not only impacts the short-term results of surgeries but also contributes to ongoing learning and improvement in surgical procedures. As more use of 3D imaging techniques is seen, novel progress in the future may simplify surgical procedures, improve reconstructive procedures, and increase the standard of patient care in facial aesthetic surgery. Overall, the use of 3D imaging and modeling remains at the core of defining the future of craniofacial reconstructive surgery, particularly for complex congenital malformations.

13.6.3. Non-Surgical Aesthetic Enhancements

Non-surgical aesthetic enhancement has emerged as a flagship procedure in the facial aesthetic industry, particularly for individuals with congenital and developmental anomalies. Such enhancements, such as dermal fillers and neurotoxin injections, provide versatile solutions that can subtly remodel facial features without the dangers of surgical procedures.

For those who have congenital asymmetries or facial development abnormalities, non-surgical interventions can be utilized to establish balance and aesthetic appeal. Procedures are favored because they are minimally invasive, recovery time is brief, and treatments can be individually designed to focus on particular facial issues. This adaptability not only empowers the patients but also promotes a more personalized modus operandi of aesthetic treatment in the scenario of congenital facial deformities. The increasing popularity of non-surgical augmentation of beauty evokes serious ethical concerns, particularly in children or congenital deformity cases. Although these interventions are effective in restoring self-esteem and enhancing quality of life, careful assessment must be conducted in order to determine the appropriateness of treatment and reality of treatment expectations. The practitioners must engage the patients in lengthy discussions of potential outcomes, risks, and limitations. Also, the fleeting nature of the majority of non-surgical enhancements necessitates repeated sessions, and this results in a continuous commitment, which could complicate the decision-making process by individuals with developmental disabilities. Healthcare providers then must walk the thin line between supporting self-betterment and making interventions match the psychosocial needs and maturity levels of the patients. Despite the efficacy of non-surgical measures, they should not be regarded as a substitute for complete surgical treatment for severe congenital and acquired facial deformities. For instance, conditions requiring extensive structural realignment, e.g., those being managed by orthognathic surgery, cannot rely on cosmetic enhancement alone to yield curative benefits. The overlap of non-surgical and surgical procedures indicates a growing pattern towards an amalgamation of the two in aesthetic medicine, both helping to complement each other. Both developments hold the potential for inter-disciplinary interaction, enhancing patient results and quality of life for sufferers of congenital conditions. As ongoing research and technological advancements continue, facial aesthetics will likely continue evolving, and non-surgical treatment will become a component of treatment modalities in harmony with the patient's individual profile and needs (Zammit et al., 2023; Ugli, 2024).

Test Your Knowledge

1. How have modern technologies improved the safety and effectiveness of facial aesthetic procedures?
2. What is the role of minimally invasive procedures in enhancing facial appearance and reducing recovery time?

SUMMARY

One can see in summarizing the complexity of congenital and developmental deformities in facial aesthetics that there must be a multi-dimensional approach to the successful treatment and rehabilitation. These deformities, such as cleft lip and palate, critically disrupt not only the facial beauty but also the functional aspect of speaking, breathing, and swallowing. By analyzing various case studies, the importance of interdisciplinary collaboration among the specialists, i.e., surgeons, orthodontists, speech therapists, and psychologists, is emphasized. Thus, successful treatment methods should be holistic to facilitate recovery of function and aesthetics equivalent to those of healthy children, thereby enhancing the quality of life in children so affected. Results from 1,415 children indicate that an integrated approach has a profound impact on outcomes of recovery, which is an indication that orderly methodological endeavor plays a pivotal role in addressing such multifaceted challenges (Eshiev et al., 2025). Also, facial symmetry issues are paramount to the art of maxillofacial surgery, most notably in the surgical correction of congenital deformities. Specifically, facial asymmetry requires careful diagnostic methodologies to formulate effective preoperative strategies. For 87 patients that were analyzed for skeletal malocclusions, of which 28 were asymmetries, advanced diagnostic tools such as 3D CBCT analysis and cephalometry were exceedingly useful. Such procedures not only allow for complete information regarding the deformities but also contribute to the precision of surgical restoration for restoring facial symmetry. Differentiation of authentic versus non-authentic asymmetries is crucial for the optimization of treatment planning. Addition of advanced imaging modalities, thus, has a direct impact on surgical procedures, affirming the need for individualized examination before intervention (Boymuradov et al., 2025). In essence, the landscape of treating congenital and developmental deformities in facial aesthetics is dynamically evolving, and this illustrates the necessity for consistent research and integration of varied disciplines. The profound impact of these deformities on an individual's functional and emotional well-being necessitates a concerted effort at treatment and rehabilitation. The future plans need to incorporate evolving technologies and methods in order to facilitate holistic care. These issues will not merely be alleviated with improved aesthetic and functional outcomes but also provide an environment where affected individuals can fulfill their full potential in social and personal domains. The integrated conclusions of studies from multiple fields corroborate the argument for systemic integration of treatment, yielding a path to enhance not just aesthetic appearance but also general quality of life for individuals afflicted by these complex disorders.

The study of congenital and developmental deformities in facial attractiveness reveals essential implications for physical and psychological well-being. Deformities can result from genetic, environmental, or combined causes and can lead to an array of disorders impacting craniofacial morphology. It is important to recognize the multifaceted character of such deformities, as they have the capacity not only to influence the facial structural qualities but also the functional capabilities such as speech and mastication. Visible deformities can be accompanied by stigma, leading to severe psychological torment, hence the importance of early diagnosis and treatment in children. A holistic strategy involving interdisciplinary collaboration by geneticists, psychologists, and maxillofacial surgeons is needed in an effort to address the intricate requirements of patients with such conditions both aesthetically and psychologically. Other types of maxillofacial injuries, which are often the outcomes of violence or accidents, are significant in explaining how facial deformity develops. There is a high correlation between social behaviors and the prevalence of such injuries, as evident from the pattern of incidence during events like the COVID-19 pandemic, when social distancing led to physically observable declines in such injuries (Canzi et al., 2023). Study of these injuries provides insight into the mechanical factors that shape facial morphology, in addition to the way surgical treatments may be used to restore form and function. Trauma-related deformity patients need advanced surgical techniques, continuous research, and new forms of therapy to achieve the best results and quality of life. Moreover, interdependency between neurological and developmental disorders complicates the facial aesthetic domain even further. The coordination between the stomatognathic system and the nervous system stresses gaining knowledge about congenital anomalies through the neural approach (Wu et al., 2023). Abnormalities in this complex interaction can result in severe craniofacial malformations, which can further exacerbate or cause neurological disorders. It illustrates the two-way effect of the two systems on health as well as form, suggesting that treatment approaches to the former should be made keeping these interdependencies in mind. Finally, the progression of clinical practice and research in the neurological complications of facial deformity will be very crucial in setting comprehensive care pathways for impacted patients, which consequently will yield improved aesthetic outcomes and psychological resilience.

KEY TERMS FROM THIS CHAPTER

- Cleft Lip
- Craniofacial Anomalies
- Micrognathia
- Craniosynostosis
- Midface Hypoplasia
- Multidisciplinary Management
- Cleft Palate
- Hemifacial Microsomia
- Macrognathia
- Syndromic Deformities
- Functional Impairment

CRITICAL THINKING QUESTIONS

1. **The most common congenital facial deformity requiring surgical correction is:**
   a. Craniosynostosis
   b. Cleft lip and palate
   c. Hemifacial microsomia
   d. Microtia
2. **The optimal age for primary cleft lip repair is usually:**
   a. At birth
   b. 2–3 months
   c. 1 year
   d. 5 years
3. **The "rule of 10s" for cleft lip repair includes all EXCEPT:**
   a. 10 weeks old
   b. 10 lbs weight
   c. Hemoglobin of 10 g/dL
   d. Oxygen saturation of 100%
4. **Hemifacial microsomia primarily affects which structure?**
   a. Orbit
   b. Maxilla
   c. Mandible
   d. Zygoma
5. **Goldenhar syndrome is a variant of:**
   a. Treacher Collins syndrome
   b. Hemifacial microsomia
   c. Cleft palate
   d. Pierre Robin sequence

Short Answer Questions

1. What are the common congenital deformities of the face that require cosmetic or reconstructive correction?
2. How does the concept of facial growth influence the timing of surgical intervention in congenital deformities?
3. What is the role of multidisciplinary care in managing congenital facial deformities?
4. What are the key principles for correcting craniofacial asymmetry?
5. How does hemifacial microsomia typically present clinically?
6. What types of grafts or implants are commonly used to correct congenital midface deficiencies?

Answers to Critical Thinking Questions

1. (b) 2. (b) 3. (d) 4. (c) 5. (b)

REFERENCES

1. Anesi, A., Cavani, F., Chiarini, L., Ferretti, et al. (2014). *Preliminary findings of a potenziated piezosurgical device at the rabbit skull.* https://core.ac.uk/download/80171725.pdf (accessed on 14th July 2025).
2. Behnia, H., Dehghani Soltani, A., Tehranchi, A., Zahedipour, et al. (2023). *Hemifacial Microsomia: A Mini-Review and Case Report.* https://core.ac.uk/download/588468504.pdf (accessed on 14th July 2025).
3. Bergqvist, C., Servy, A., Valeyrie-Allanore, L., Ferkal, S., Combemale, P., & Wolkenstein, P. (2020). Neurofibromatosis 1 French national guidelines based on an extensive literature review since 1966. *Orphanet Journal of Rare Diseases, 15.* https://doi.org/10.1186/s13023-020-1310-3 (accessed on 14th July 2025).
4. Bessell, A., Itthagarun, A., Marcusson, A., Thompson, A., Silva Da, A. P., McWilliams, B. J., Lorenzzaoni, D., et al. (2015). *Psychological impact of visible differences in patients with congenital craniofacial anomalies.* https://core.ac.uk/download/323891118.pdf (accessed on 14th July 2025).
5. Boymuradov, S. A., Yusupov, S. S., Rakhmanov, S. A., & Madraimova, K. (2025). The role of accurate diagnosis of the aesthetic parameters of the face in preoperative planning and successful surgical treatment for patients with asymmetric jaw deformities. *Frontline Medical Sciences and Pharmaceutical Journal.* https://www.semanticscholar.org/paper/cae33d20836eceafdb28638fab942820a03bfc73 (accessed on 14th July 2025).
6. Boymuradov, S. A., Yusupov, S. S., Rakhmanov, S. A., & Madraimova, K. (2025). The role of accurate diagnosis of the aesthetic parameters of the face in preoperative planning and successful surgical treatment for patients with asymmetric jaw deformities. *Frontline Medical Sciences and Pharmaceutical Journal, 5,* 11–17. https://doi.org/10.37547/medical-fmspj-05-05-03 (accessed on 14th July 2025).
7. Boymuradov, S. A., Yusupov, S. S., Rakhmanov, S. A., & Madraimova, K. (2025). The role of accurate diagnosis of the aesthetic parameters of the face in preoperative planning and successful surgical treatment for patients with asymmetric jaw deformities. *International Journal of Medical Sciences and Clinical Research, 5,* 29–36. https://doi.org/10.37547/ijmscr/volume05issue05-07 (accessed on 14th July 2025).
8. Canzi, G., Novelli, G., Mirabella, S., & Sozzi, D. (2023). The Comprehensive Facial Injury (CFI): A modern communication tool on maxillo-facial traumas characteristics. *Hellenic Archives of Oral and Maxillofacial Surgery, 24.* https://doi.org/10.54936/haoms242p74 (accessed on 14th July 2025).
9. Harnádková, K., Kočandrlová, K., Kožejová Jaklová, L., Dupej, J., & Velemínská, J. (2023). The effect of sex and age on facial shape directional asymmetry in adults: A 3D landmarks-based method study. *PLoS ONE, 18,* e0288702–e0288702. https://doi.org/10.1371/journal.pone.0288702 (accessed on 14th July 2025).
10. Hendrijantini, N., Dahlan, A., Husniya, J., Farha, M., Aziza, H., Rasheed, N., Joseph, S., et al. (2022). *Indonesian Journal of Prosthodontic, 3.* https://doi.org/10.46934/ijp.v3i2 (accessed on 14th July 2025).
11. Hughes, D., & Song, B. (2016). Dental and Nondental Stem Cell Based Regeneration of the

Craniofacial Region: A Tissue Based Approach. *Stem cells international, 2016*, 8307195. https://doi.org/10.1155/2016/8307195(accessed on 14th July 2025).

12. Jar, A. A., Alotaibi, A. S., Alqahtani, H. A., Alshaqaqeq, G. A., Alandanoosi, H. I., Alsulami, S. R., Alosaimi, L. A., et al. (2023). Breastfeeding in children with cleft lip and palate and its effect on surgical outcomes. *International Journal of Community Medicine and Public Health, 10*, 4957–4961. https://doi.org/10.18203/2394-6040.ijcmph20233522 (accessed on 14th July 2025).
13. Katanaki, N., Makrygiannakis, M. A., & Kaklamanos, E. G. (2024). The prevalence of congenitally missing permanent teeth in a sample of orthodontic and non-orthodontic Caucasian patients. *Healthcare, 12*, 541–541. https://doi.org/10.3390/healthcare12050541 (accessed on 14th July 2025).
14. Kumari, K., Saleh, I., Taslim, S., Ahmad, S., Hussain, I., Munir, Z., Javed, T., et al. (2023). Unraveling the complexity of Apert syndrome: Genetics, clinical insights, and future frontiers. *Cureus*. https://doi.org/10.7759/cureus.47281 (accessed on 14th July 2025).
15. Lin, Y. (2024). *Objective analysis of anthropometric parameters of the auricle in health and disease*. https://core.ac.uk/download/631131682.pdf (accessed on 14th July 2025).
16. Lone, I. M., Zohud, O., Midlej, K., Awadi, O., Masarwa, S., Krohn, S., Kirschneck, C., et al. (2023). Narrating the genetic landscape of human class I occlusion: A perspective-infused review. *Journal of Personalized Medicine, 13*, 1465–1465. https://doi.org/10.3390/jpm13101465 (accessed on 14th July 2025).
17. McNeil, C. K. (1951). *Congenital malformation and acquired deformity of the oral and facial structure*. https://core.ac.uk/download/286712032.pdf (accessed on 14th July 2025).
18. Palmeiro, M. R. L. (2013). *Quality of life and masticatory ability of selected foods in cleft lip and palate subjects and maxillary denture wearers*. https://core.ac.uk/download/48139729.pdf (accessed on 14th July 2025).
19. Pérez Sánchez, C. F., Sierra Perilla, N., Inostroza, F., & Palomares, M. (2022). LATICFA abstracts. *The Journal of Craniofacial Surgery, 33*, 2276–2320. https://www.semanticscholar.org/paper/f0267c5d8c075cda6abe9b85fd5da8940b95efd7 (accessed on 14th July 2025).
20. Pierpont, M. E., Brueckner, M., Chung, W. K., Garg, V., Lacro, R. V., McGuire, A. L., Mital, S., et al. (2018). Genetic basis for congenital heart disease: Revisited: A scientific statement from the American Heart Association. *Circulation, 138*. https://doi.org/10.1161/cir.0000000000000606 (accessed on 14th July 2025).
21. Pniak, M., Miklis, P., Mawlichanów, M., Ciesielska, A., Sieradzka, A., Szerej, K., Czaplińska-Paszek, Z., et al. (2024). Understanding the educational and social difficulties in children with hemifacial microsomia – A literature review. *Quality in Sport, 36*, 56644–56644. https://doi.org/10.12775/qs.2024.36.56644 (accessed on 14th July 2025).
22. Renkema, R. W. (2020). European guideline craniofacial microsomia. *Journal of Craniofacial Surgery, 31*, 2385–2484. https://doi.org/10.1097/scs.0000000000006691 (accessed on 14th July 2025).
23. Sablada, J. R. P., & Amparado, M. A. P. (2020). *Living changed lives: Experiences of individuals after oral reconstructive surgery*. https://doi.org/10.31219/osf.io/xep6a (accessed on 14th July 2025).

24. Stock, N. M., & Feragen, K. B. (2016). Psychological adjustment to cleft lip and/or palate: A narrative review of the literature. *Psychology and Health, 31*, 777–813. https://doi.org/10.1080/08870446.2016.1143944 (accessed on 14th July 2025).

25. Tahmasebi, E., Mohammadi, M., Alam, M., Abbasi, K., Gharibian Bajestani, S., Khanmohammad, R., Haseli, M., et al. (2023). The current regenerative medicine approaches of craniofacial diseases: A narrative review. *Frontiers in Cell and Developmental Biology, 11*. https://doi.org/10.3389/fcell.2023.1112378 (accessed on 14th July 2025).

26. Ter Horst, R., van Weert, H., Loonen, T., Bergé, S., Vinayahalingam, S., Baan, F., Maal, T., et al. (2021). Three-dimensional virtual planning in mandibular advancement surgery: Soft tissue prediction based on deep learning. *Journal of Cranio-Maxillofacial Surgery, 49*, 775–782. https://doi.org/10.1016/j.jcms.2021.04.001 (accessed on 14th July 2025).

27. Ugli, Y. B. D. (2024). Advancements in facial jaw surgery: Exploring surgical interventions and management of facial jaw diseases. *International Journal of Medical Sciences and Clinical Research, 4*, 74–81. https://doi.org/10.37547/ijmscr/volume04issue02-11 (accessed on 14th July 2025).

28. Wojtyńska, E., Bączkowski, B., Cierech, M., & Mierzwińska-Nastalska, E. (2024). Assessment of children and "young" adult patients' quality of life after prosthetic treatment of disorders of the craniofacial region—A retrospective study. *Journal of Clinical Medicine, 13*, 339–339. https://doi.org/10.3390/jcm13020339 (accessed on 14th July 2025).

29. Wu, Y., Lan, Y., Mao, J., Shen, J., Kang, T., & Xie, Z. (2023). The interaction between the nervous system and the stomatognathic system: From development to diseases. *International Journal of Oral Science, 15*. https://doi.org/10.1038/s41368-023-00241-4 (accessed on 14th July 2025).

30. Zammit, D., Ettinger, R. E., Sanati-Mehrizy, P., & Susarla, S. M. (2023). Current trends in orthognathic surgery. *Medicina, 59*, 2100–2100. https://doi.org/10.3390/medicina59122100 (accessed on 14th July 2025).

31. Zhao, Z., Bao, J., Shen, G., Cai, M., & Yu, H. (2023). Integrating virtual surgical planning and 3D-printed tools with iliac bone grafts for orbital and zygomatic reconstruction in hemifacial microsomia patients. *Journal of Clinical Medicine, 12*, 7538–7538. https://doi.org/10.3390/jcm12247538 (accessed on 14th July 2025).

32. Zumba. C. N. E., Macas Caamaño, L. J., Cueva Flores, R. A., Sarmiento Ávila, S. A., Franco, P. F., Ayala, A., Lombeida Arias, J. J., et al. (2023). Cleft lip and palate, scoping review. *EPRA International Journal of Multidisciplinary Research (IJMR)*. https://doi.org/10.36713/epra14264 (accessed on 14th July 2025).

33. Eshiev, M., Khalmurzaev, D., Eshiev, N., Azimbaev, N., Taalaibekov, N., & Myrzasheva, N. (2025). A comprehensive approach to the treatment of patients with congenital defects and deformities of the maxillofacial area. *Bulletin of Science and Practice*. https://www.semanticscholar.org/paper/a7289489049c5bc9fb2f32a8327f2c2462834b7e (accessed on 14th July 2025).

ONCOLOGIC AND POST-TUMOR RECONSTRUCTION IN FACIAL COSMETIC

14

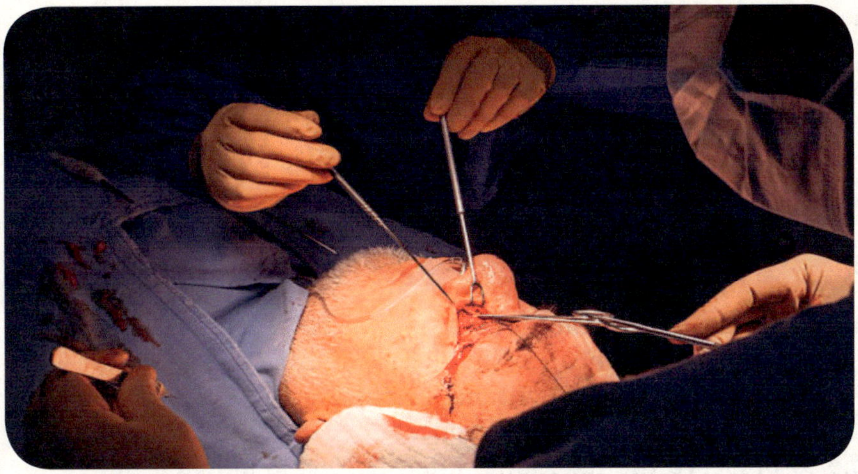

LEARNING OBJECTIVES

After studying this chapter, you will be able to:

1. Understand oncologic surgery;
2. Discuss reconstruction's role in facial cosmetic surgery;
3. Identify preoperative considerations;
4. Describe surgical techniques in reconstruction;
5. Identify postoperative care and recovery;
6. Understand ethical considerations in oncologic and reconstructive surgery.

Introduction

The intricate interplay between oncologic surgery and subsequent cosmetic reconstruction has been a matter of considerable interest in the medical literature. In association with the evolution of facial cosmetic surgery, it increasingly recognizes the value of not only removing malignant tumors but also rehabilitating form and function post-surgery. Oncologic treatments have a great impact in changing facial structure and function, and therefore there has to be a holistic approach that transcends the primary operation. Therefore, measures of reconstruction must be pursued to reverse the physical and psychological impacts of such treatments. This dual focus on excision of cancer and cosmetic reconstruction underscores the importance of innovative surgical techniques that can optimize patient quality of life in the setting of oncologic surgery. To this end, there should be a clear understanding of the spectrum of reconstructive modalities. One of the watershed moments in post-tumor and oncologic reconstruction is the management of facial defects due to tumor excision, especially when defects compromise critical zones affecting function as much as aesthetics. The reconstructive surgeon must very carefully weigh the specific nuances of the tissue loss, the extent of resection, the facial site, and patient-specific anatomical subtleties. This comprehensive analysis of interest, since inadequate reconstruction can lead to psychosocial sequelae and compromised function. Techniques such as the use of pedicled perforator flaps have come under the spotlight based on their capacity to restore both volume and cutaneous integrity. Most importantly, an algorithm for partial breast reconstruction with these flaps demonstrated successful outcomes, serving as a model that can be used in facial reconstruction following tumor excision (Cillino et al., 2010). In addition, functioning impairment treatment, such as paralysis of the face resulting from oncologic therapy, is still within the realm of post-tumor cosmetic surgery. Facial nerve paralysis can significantly impair a patient's quality of life by interfering with their emotional expression, as well as with simple activities such as eating and speaking. Restorations that will restore facial movement need to incorporate a thorough assessment of nerve integrity and muscular function. Various types of surgeries, including nerve grafts and dynamic muscle transfers, can be employed to yield good results (Anderson et al., 2012). But the complexity of facial anatomy and nerve courses is a huge hindrance to achieving maximum functional recovery. Thus, it is necessary that there should be more research and surgical development in oncologic and post-tumor reconstruction to help patients by improving outcomes and enhancing their quality of life.

Definition of Oncologic Surgery

Oncologic surgery is a significant branch of surgical oncology that focuses on the resection of tumor, especially malignant tumors, which are harmful to health. The most critical aim of oncologic surgery is to ensure the removal of the cancer completely without sacrificing the surrounding healthy tissue to the extent possible. Not only is maintaining this delicate balance crucial for the success of the treatment, but it is done to preserve the functional integrity of the afflicted body part. The character of such an operation requires an operative multidisciplinary team in which radiologists, oncologists, and surgeons all work together to establish a correct surgical plan for each individual patient's condition. This teamwork is essential in determining the optimal timing and the extent of the surgical procedure, ultimately guiding prognosis, enabling postoperative recovery, and enhancing the overall results. Following tumor excision by surgery, post-tumor reconstruction is also a critical factor in the restoration of the shape and function of the involved anatomical structures. In facial aesthetic surgery, this is regarding the correction of oncologic surgical defects and attempting to permit the patient to regain their preoperative appearance or to obtain an improved aesthetic result. Free tissue transfer, local flaps, and fat grafting are a few of the refined techniques that are utilized in order to overcome these reconstructive challenges. Use of pedicled perforator flaps, such as in the reconstruction of breasts, also indicates advancement in the surgical technique of regaining volume and form after oncologic surgery (Cillino et al., 2010). These methods not only aim at eliminating the physical deformities in surgery but also help to reduce the psychological impact of cancer therapy-induced disfigurement. Further, the inclusion of new techniques such as fat grafting also introduces more potential for successful reconstruction in oncologic surgery. By means of transferring autologous adipose tissue to sites of deficiency, the surgeons can improve the contour deformities with the additional benefit of using the patient's tissue, thereby eradicating the foreign body complications (Vyas et al., 2016). This twofold benefit outlines the manner in which contemporary oncologic and reconstructive therapies are evolving with regard to both cosmetic and functional needs of patients. However, use of adipose-derived stem cells (ASCs) within fat grafting also raises oncological concerns regarding cancer microenvironments and possible tumorigenesis, and will continue to require more investigation to offer protection for patients and efficacy for reconstructive outcomes. Thus, the oncologic surgery definition goes beyond simple cancer removal, embracing restoration and rehabilitation as well, ultimately targeting the enhancement of the quality of life for post-treatment patients (Figure 14.1).

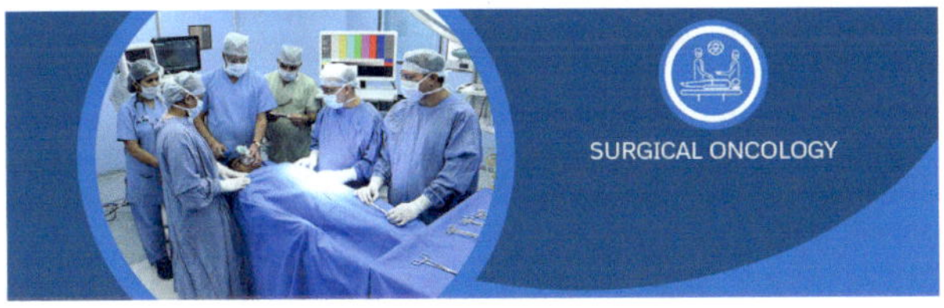

Figure 14.1. Oncologic surgery.

Source: https://external-content.duckduckgo.com/iu/?u=https%3A%2F%2Fwww.venkateshwarhospitals.com%2Fblog%2Fwp-content%2Fuploads%2F2019%2F04%2Fsurgical-oncology.jpg&f=1&nofb=1&ipt=0c7f13233510321641ccb59ff65dc731528d600152aa40d37b354d80017caa4e.

Role of Facial Cosmetic Surgery

Facial cosmetic surgery plays a -affected facial structures. Post-surgical procedures, for example, maxillectomy, may lead to severe issues in the form of altered facial beauty and functional impairment in patients. Disfigurement has a psychological impact, leading to decreased self-esteem and withdrawal from society. To overcome such problems, effective post-tumor reconstruction is necessary, which facilitates not only physical construction but also psychological healing. Evidence indicates that through intensive cooperation among reconstructive surgeons and oncologists, results are likely to significantly improve both the cosmetic results and functional capacities of patients. Such collaboration fosters personalized prosthetic treatments to restore normalcy to speech, mastication, and social interaction, thus supporting the role of facial cosmetic surgery as an integrated component of worldwide cancer care (Fattah et al., 2012). Use of modern cosmetic surgical techniques also facilitates the other general aim of enhancing the life quality of cancer survivors. Reconstruction of tumors, particularly on the face, necessitates sophisticated techniques that provide natural appearances and appropriate restoration of function. Certain procedures by pedicled perforator flaps, for instance, have been used to recreate breast forms but have striking contrasts when translated to facial reconstruction (Cillino et al., 2010). Like breast tissue, facial structures need to be handled with great care so that both volume and shape are harmonized with surrounding tissue. With the use of these techniques, compromised structural form can be restored, enabling patients to re-enter their social milieu and feel normal. The psychological effects of successful restorative appearance cannot be underestimated, as patients report heightened confidence and improved mental well-being following such reconstructive therapy. Moreover, facial cosmetic surgery has more than just cosmetic consequences, penetrating into social and working life. In the majority of cases, appearance-based social biases may have negative effects on career opportunities as well as social relationships. Because cosmetic surgery enables individuals to represent themselves in a more conventionally approved manner, it can prevent discrimination or prejudice against individuals who are different physically. Recognition of this intersection between aesthetics and social dynamics highlights facial cosmetic surgery as a priority for individuals who are recovering from oncologic disease. Indeed, it provides them with the ability to more effectively manage social expectations, ultimately leading to reintegration and improved life satisfaction. Therefore, the role of facial cosmetic surgery is not one-dimensional but instead multi-dimensional and involves restoration of beauty, enhancement of function, and reintegration into society for oncologic and post-tumor reconstruction (Fattah et al., 2012) (Figure 14.2).

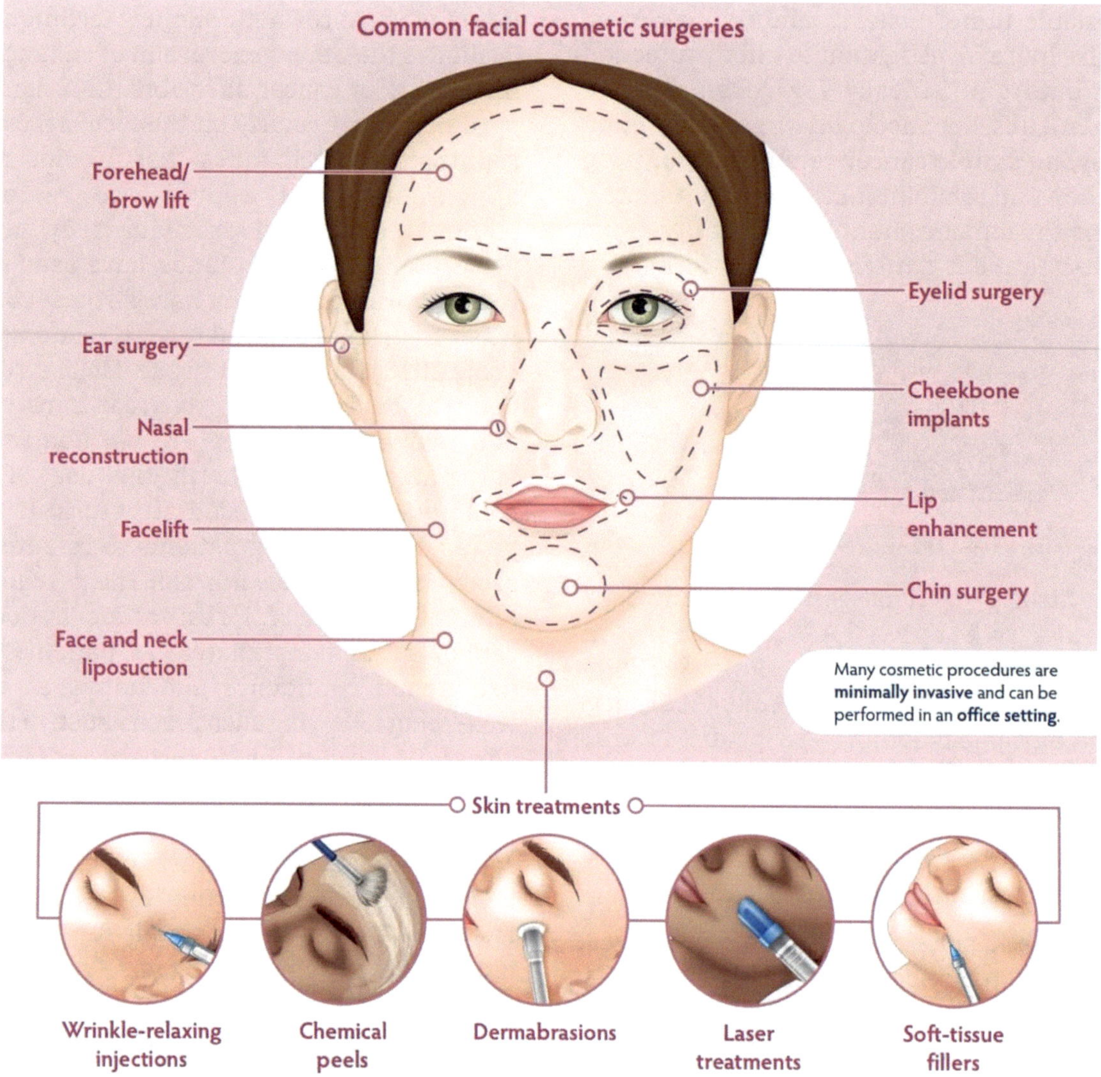

Figure 14.2. Facial cosmetic surgery.

Source: https://ekbybzt92zq.exactdn.com/wp-content/uploads/2021/12/facial_cosmetic_surgery-662x1024-1.jpg?strip=all&lossy=1&ssl=1.

Overview of the Relationship Between Oncology and Reconstruction

That the evolving nature of facial cosmetic surgery, particularly tumor post-reconstruction, is highlighted by the intricate relationship between reconstruction and oncology is noteworthy. The oncologic procedures have a propensity to result in huge loss of tissue, particularly in cases of head and neck cancers, and thus necessitate innovative reconstructive techniques to enable both function and aesthetics. These procedures not only make the patients look more beautiful but also have a significant role to play in their psychological rehabilitation. Through the integration of reconstructive techniques with oncologic treatment, surgeons are able to offer a more complete approach to patients, emphasizing the necessity for multidisciplinary patterns of care for cancer survivors. The collaboration between these fields ensures that the functional and psychological outcomes of tumor resection are adequately accounted for, thereby improving the overall quality of life for treated individuals. Among the new areas of interest in oncologic and reconstructive surgery is the use of advanced technologies, such as ultrasonic osteotomes and lipotransfer techniques. Comparison of different instruments, including Piezosurgery®, reveals potential advantages in reducing tissue trauma during procedures. For example, micromorphology and roughness values comparisons between osteotomized bone surfaces indicate that ultrasound-assisted procedures can assist in maintaining significant structures intact while facilitating successful healing. These innovations not only facilitate better surgical outcomes but also improve understanding of bone regeneration and soft tissue integration in reconstructive surgery. The more researchers explore these new methods, the more their oncologic considerations deepen, enriching the armamentarium of surgery after tumor reconstruction. As with lipotransfer, concerns arise regarding the effects of interactions between lipoaspirates and tumor beds. While lipofilling has improved certain aspects of plastic surgery, foremost breast reconstruction, its cancer recurrence implications remain obscure. Research has shown that while the adipose-derived regenerative tissues have been found to promote healing and tissue repair, they may interact with latent cancer cells, raising an issue about the long-term safety of the procedure. Thus, extensive clinical studies are urgently required to clarify such interactions and secure the safety of lipotransfer in oncologic patients. It is only by an exhaustive amount of research that the oncology-reconstruction interface can be better described, with surgery advancements complementing the principles of cancer treatment and maximizing patient safety and efficacy of treatment results (Goldhirsch et al., 2011; Anesi et al., 2014).

14.1. Understanding Oncologic Surgery

Learning Outcome

1. Types of Cancers Affecting the Facial Region
2. Surgical Techniques Used in Oncologic Procedures
3. Goals of Oncologic Surgery in Facial Aesthetics

Oncologic surgery forms a critical intersection between reconstructive surgery and cancer treatment. The final intent of oncologic surgery is to excise tumors with minimal sacrifice of surrounding normal tissue, a norm especially important in facial structure surgery. The intricacy of oncologic surgery is amplified by the intricate anatomy of the face, where small error can result in aesthetic and functional compromise of significant magnitude. Surgeons also have to plan for the excision of the tumor with careful planning for the subsequent reconstructive procedure to avoid disfigurement. With advancing technology and technique, procedures such as ultrasonic osteotomes are now available, with the promise to minimize damage to the surrounding tissues while effectively facilitating the removal of cancerous cells (Anesi et al., 2014). The goal is to achieve maximum healing and functional preservation, which serves as the foundation for further aesthetic restoration with cosmetic techniques. In facial cosmetic surgery after oncologic surgery, the two pillars of reconstructive surgery are involved in the restoration of appearance and function. With oncologic lesion extirpation, most patients have physical difficulties and profound psychological sequelae resulting from changes in appearance. This necessitates a tailored method of reconstruction, such as through the application of advanced techniques, such as pedicled perforator flaps, which have been proven to effectively improve volume and revise skin envelope deformities after tumor excision. It has been proven that the flaps are capable of reconstructing breast volume and shape with minimal noticeability at the donor site (Cillino et al., 2010). This philosophy is then carried over to facial regions, where symmetry and the maintenance of natural contours take precedence; aesthetic issues are therefore harmoniously incorporated into the reconstructive design. Lastly, the importance of multidisciplinary team effort in cancer and reconstructive surgery cannot be stressed enough. Oncologists, surgeons, and cosmetic professionals must all work together to devise integrated treatment regimens involving the removal of the cancer as well as reconstruction afterward. This common model facilitates better-informed decision-making regarding when and how to integrate cosmetic procedures into oncologic surgery and therefore, enhance patient outcomes.

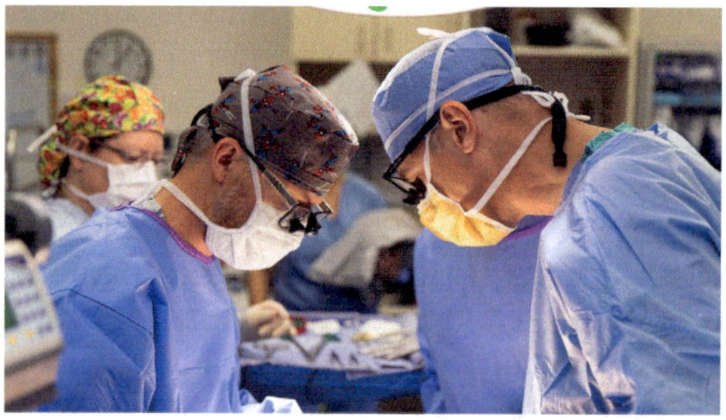

Figure 14.3. Oncologic surgery represents a critical intersection between cancer management and reconstructive techniques.

Source: https://www.childrenscolorado.org/globalassets/departments/surgical-oncology/2023-04-12-surgical-oncology_cost_roach_61_cropped.jpg?v=49ba92&width=1440&height=810&rxy=0.5,0.49.

Patient education and psychological counseling are also an integral part of care, as they address the emotional aftermath of cancer therapy. With the integration of a holistic model addressing both the technical and emotional aspects of surgery, the field of oncologic and post-tumor reconstruction itself expands, with the added emphasis on not only the extirpation of disease but also the reconstruction of patients' dignity and quality of life through successful cosmetic reconstruction (Figure 14.3).

14.1.1. Types of Cancers Affecting the Facial Region

Facial cancers are a diverse group of malignancies that mostly affect the skin, mucous membranes, and facial adnexal structures. Two of the most frequent types are basal cell carcinoma (BCC) and squamous cell carcinoma (SCC), often the consequence of prolonged exposure to ultraviolet (UV) radiation. BCC, while typically slow-growing and rarely metastasizing, can lead to extensive local tissue destruction if left untreated. On the other hand, SCC is at a higher risk of metastasis, particularly if it is on the lip or ear. In addition, melanoma, the more malignant skin cancer, develops from melanocytes in the epidermis and is notorious for the manner in which it rapidly spreads through the body. Awareness of these cancers is important in developing an effective oncologic treatment plan and later reconstructive plan in cosmetic facial surgery. Aside from skin cancers, oral cavity and salivary gland cancers also have a significant effect on the facial region. Oral squamous cell carcinoma (OSCC) arises from the mucosal lining of the oral cavity and is due to many risk factors, some of which include tobacco use and human papillomavirus (HPV) infection. OSCC commonly exhibits an aggressive nature and therefore most of the time needs wide resection surgically, which significantly damages the aesthetic as well as functional functions of the face. Salivary gland tumors, while uncommon, are also clinically formidable since their behavior is unpredictable and their histological subtypes may be extremely variable. These tumors may prove very difficult to operate on from a standpoint of intricate surgical techniques, and so the introduction of sophisticated postoperative reconstruction procedures must be utilized to optimize patient quality of life. Conquering these difficulties is an important step towards improving clinical outcomes in facial cosmetic surgery. Further, the intersection of oncologic treatment and post-tumor reconstruction testifies to the effectiveness of cooperative surgical approaches. Facially cancer therapy often requires an interdisciplinary group of oncologists, maxillofacial surgeons, and prosthodontists. More specifically, pre-prosthetic surgical conditioning in primary resections, i.e., maxillectomy, plays a pivotal role in the subsequent prosthetic rehabilitation process. Effective rehabilitative outcomes are much dependent on strategic planning and execution of reconstructive surgeries, rebuilding facial contours and function. With evidence provided by Fattah et al. (2012), incorporation of pre-prosthetic surgery with oncologic therapy optimizes patient rehabilitation, not only allowing for aesthetic recovery but also improving social interactions and quality of life. Therefore, optimal care encompassing both oncologic and reconstructive components is essential in addressing the implications of facial cancers (Figure 14.4).

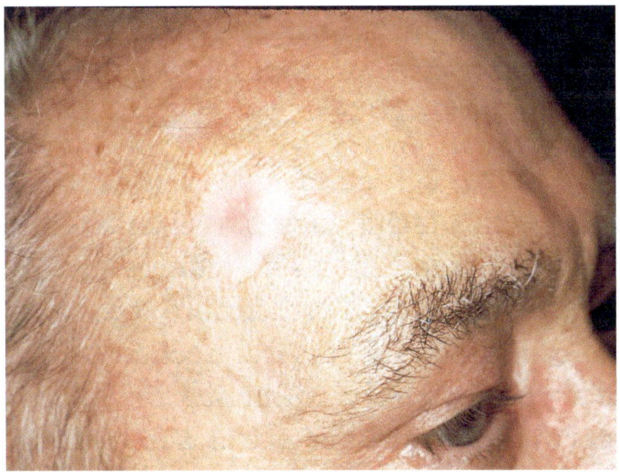

Figure 14.4. Cancers affecting the facial region.

Source: https://www.verywellhealth.com/thmb/z2UTB9_KBcE47gPA3R8Oe2PXzc0=/998x759/filters:no_upscale():max_bytes(150000):strip_icc()/basal-cell-carcinoma-4-scar-5304337d6b3e4b3b8c601fde7a0880f8.jpg.

14.1.2. Surgical Techniques Used in Oncologic Procedures

The trend in surgical oncologic procedures mainly utilizes advancements with the focus of efficiently removing the tumors while preserving functionality and aesthetics within the involved region. Techniques such as Mohs micrographic surgery are focal, especially in skin cancer treatment, and ensure complete removal of the tumor without causing excessive damage to the surrounding tumor tissue. This technique allows for real-time histological evaluation, eliminating the risk of recurrence to a large degree and allowing for more cosmetically pleasing results. Mohs surgery's precision specifically demands comprehensive knowledge of facial anatomy and demands reconstruction proficiency following excision.

These principles further align with oncologic and post-tumoral reconstruction practices in stressing the preservation of the facial tissues' fine details as a way of achieving oncologic clearance. Another key area of concern for surgical techniques in oncologic treatments is the management of complications, in this case, in relation to facial nerve integrity. Surgical intervention for head and neck cancer can inadvertently cause facial paralysis of the nerves, providing unique challenges in post-operative rehabilitation and restoration of function. Such complications need to be addressed with individualized interventions, ranging from neurotization to facial reanimation procedures, to restore function as well as aesthetics. The complex anatomy of the facial nerve makes reconstruction difficult, but new and innovative methods keep appearing, allowing improved quality of life for patients post-treatment. As stated, extensive study and patient-specific treatment are most significant in developing effective management regimens in patients with nerve deficits following tumor removal (Anderson et al., 2012). Reconstructive interventions following oncologic surgeries are significant in modifying patient outcomes and enhancing psychological well-being. Pedicled perforator flaps are one of the effective methods employed in breast cancer surgery that enable the maintenance of breast volume following quadrantectomy. Thoraco-dorsal and intercostal perforator-based flaps were found to be effective in restoring the natural breast contour with fewer complications at the donor site. These not only reconstruct the physical contours of the breast, but also correct the emotional impact cancer patients must endure. As shown, all flap procedures in a study had total survival, giving proper restoration in size, shape, and volume without requiring extra corrective surgery of the opposite breast (Cillino et al., 2010). This shows the profound intersection between patient care and surgical progress in oncologic treatment (Figure 14.5).

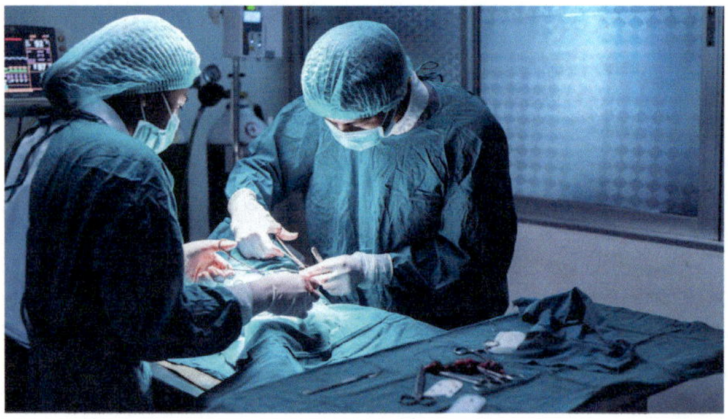

Figure 14.5. Surgical techniques used in oncologic procedures.

Source: https://www.krupamayihospitals.in/wp-content/uploads/2023/06/Onco-Surgery.jpg.

14.1.3. Goals of Oncologic Surgery in Facial Aesthetics

In oncologic surgery, particularly in facial beauty, one of the most critical aims is the complete eradication of malignant tumors without compromising the facial structure. Surgeons' target is not only successfully removing the malignant tissues but also preserving the functional and aesthetic components of the face. This dual focus is important as the face is at the core of individual identity and social interaction. Patients often suggest that alterations in facial attractiveness carry considerable psychological implications, affecting self-esteem and eliciting emotional distress. Thus, a successful integration of oncologic and aesthetic concerns is paramount to achieving not only physical but also psychological well-being in patients who are treated for facial oncologic reconstruction. Aside from the removal of the tumor, another critical goal of oncologic surgery with facial esthetic consideration is the meticulous reconstruction of the surgical defect. Reconstruction plays a crucial role in restoring the functional capacity of the deficient area, such as speech, swallowing, and breathing. Techniques like locoregional flaps are frequently used in order to do so, as these allow surgeons to work with surrounding tissues in order to correct defects without excessive extraneous scarring and with optimal aesthetic results. Research suggests that certain types of flaps, such as infrahyoid and nasolabial types, provide good results for both medium-sized and smaller defects, which supports the concept that well-planned reconstruction has the power to greatly improve postoperative appearances (Accorona et al., 2024).

By wise selection and application of reconstructive techniques, surgeons attempt to usher patients toward a symphonic equilibrium of healing and beauty. Furthermore, technological advancements and surgical techniques have had a revolutionary influence on oncologic surgery philosophy for facial aesthetics. The use of new practices such as preoperative planning of surgeries with Mixed Reality (MR) and navigation has been shown to enhance the success of procedures. MR technology provides improved visualization of anatomy, which may help surgeons to deliver more precise results, and also enhance patient communication on the outcome of their procedures (Kalaskar et al., 2016). Besides making surgery more accurate, these technological advances can also help in enhancing the aesthetic outcome. Thus, the goals of oncologic surgery increasingly are a combined policy that supports both cancer removal and, where feasible, restoration of facial form, with the ultimate aim to improve patients' quality of life after tumor excisions (Figure 14.6).

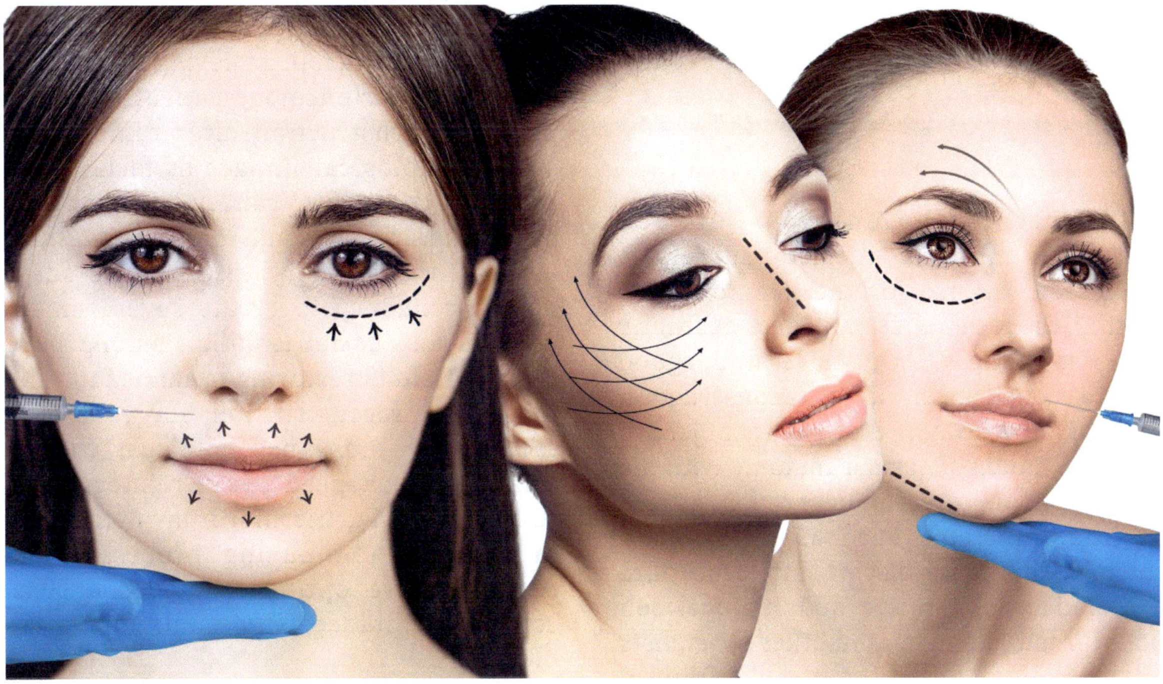

Figure 14.6. Goals of oncologic surgery in facial aesthetics.

Source: https://external-content.duckduckgo.com/iu/?u=https%3A%2F%2Fwww.boutiquedental23.com%2Fwp-content%2Fuploads%2F2022%2F10%2Fwhat-is-facial-aesthetics-1.jpg&f=1&nofb=1&ipt=3d30e27f00610de9a5f4e621d21adf8ddc11ce383a58a381fb2b20b0986969a3.

Test Your Knowledge

1. What is oncologic surgery, and how does it help in the treatment of facial cancers?
2. How does the removal of cancerous tissue during oncologic surgery affect facial structure and function?

14.2. The Role of Reconstruction in Facial Cosmetic Surgery

Learning Outcome

1. Definition and Purpose of Reconstructive Surgery
2. Techniques Used in Facial Reconstruction
3. Psychological Impact of Facial Reconstruction on Patients

The intricate relationship between reconstruction and facial cosmetic surgery is of utmost significance for the promotion of restoration of both functional and aesthetic outcomes in patients who have undergone oncologic surgery. In the facial reconstruction following tumor resection, the primary objective is the establishment of normal anatomy with the encouragement of preservation or enhancement of essential functions such as speech and swallowing. This multi-disciplinary procedure often includes cooperative activity between surgeons, prosthodontists, and other specialists to create individualized solutions tailored to unique needs. For instance, in maxillary defect reconstruction following maxillectomy, careful pre-prosthetic surgery planning plays a crucial role in the success of prosthetic rehabilitation. As pointed out by the study of Fattah et al. (2012), such preps would be able to enhance facial profile and overall aesthetic results, offering a foundation for successful rehabilitation and increased quality of life among patients suffering from cancer. Moreover, advancements in surgical tools and techniques likewise confirm the importance of innovation in facial reconstruction. Introduction of new technology, such as ultrasonic osteotomes, has revolutionized the field of bone manipulation for reconstructive surgery. Comparative studies on traditional rotating instruments and ultrasound-based systems illustrate natural differences in micromorphology and surface roughness of osteotomized bones and thus impact healing and functional restoration. Such technologies not only preserve soft tissue covering but also enhance osseointegration and health of the tissue and consequently deliver dramatically better outcomes for surgery. As highlighted in the work by Anesi et al. (2014), the application of such advanced devices in cranio-facial surgery is essential in achieving optimal results, particularly for oncology patients who require precise reconstruction after tumor excision. The psychological impact of facial cosmetic reconstruction after cancer treatment cannot be overstated. Facial disfigurements and alterations secondary to oncologic surgeries have a tendency to create severe emotional distress and social isolation among patients. By successfully restoring facial beauty through meticulous reconstruction, surgeons are able to mitigate these psychological challenges, facilitating enhanced social reintegration and self-concept. Furthermore, involving patients in the decision-making process for their reconstructive options provides a sense of control, facilitating wholesome mental health outcomes.

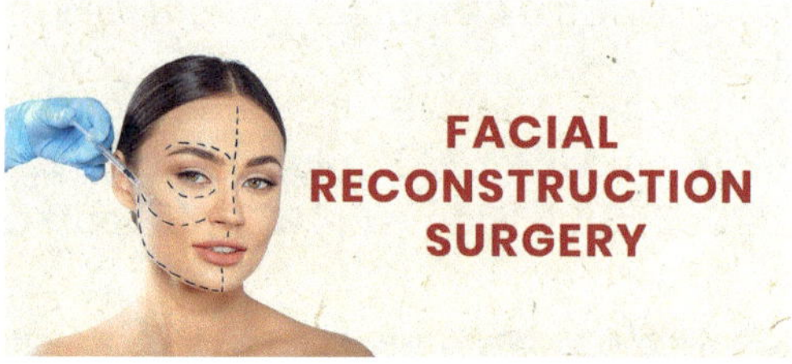

Figure 14.7. Role of reconstruction in facial cosmetic surgery.

Source: https://external-content.duckduckgo.com/iu/?u=https%3A%2F%2Famandeephospital.org%2Fwp-content%2Fuploads%2F2023%2F06%2FFacial-Reconstruction-Surgery.webp&f=1&nofb=1&ipt=83c386ff65aa8d01d146479063b17799f93538f2fa757da65fc6d0229d1e24f4.

Thus, the role of reconstruction in facial cosmetic surgery is more than corporeal, and it is an integral part of comprehensive cancer care intended to enhance quality of life as well as psychosocial well-being for survivors as they step into the bewildering realm of life after treatment (Figure 14.7).

14.2.1. Definition and Purpose of Reconstructive Surgery

Reconstructive surgery is a fundamental component of clinical treatment that entails the reconstruction of form and function following trauma, disease, or surgery. The term "reconstructive surgery" extends beyond the exclusive esthetic correction and comprises the rehabilitation of not only physical integrity but also psychological health of those patients who have experienced significant loss, particularly following oncological surgery. It frequently entails the rebuilding of complicated areas of anatomy in which malignancies have required massive excisions, for example, facial tumors. Reconstructive surgery, beyond cosmetic repair, is meant to allow for necessary physiological processes such as mastication, communication, and respiration, which can be impaired as a result of tumor resections or cancer therapy deformities. In particular, in the oncologic and post-tumoral reconstructive fields, the reconstructive surgery methodology is focused on enhancing the survivor's level of quality of life. The procedures may involve the use of a large variety of state-of-the-art methodologies, including flap techniques, which utilize the patient's own tissue to restore volume, shape, and function. The applicability of such procedures is best illustrated through breast reconstruction following lumpectomy, whereby incorporation of pedicled perforator flaps restores breast loveliness following cancerous tissue excision. The effectiveness of such procedures has been demonstrated in research to produce positive outcomes in functional as well as psychological reconstruction, substantiating the importance of reconstructive surgery in cancer management in its entirety (Cillino et al., 2010). Furthermore, improvements in surgical techniques, such as the development of ultrasonic osteotomes, illustrate the ongoing evolution of reconstructive surgery. These innovations have portrayed a noticeable improvement in the precision and outcomes of surgical interventions, minimizing destruction of adjacent tissues and refining recovery times. Understanding micromorphology and surface roughness of osteotomized bone surfaces has been beneficial, particularly in craniofacial reconstruction, where delicate facial bones require close attention. As reconstructive surgery advances and utilizes newer technologies, its purpose remains constant in rehabilitating function and form for the victims of cancer as well as the psychological impact of disfigurement and trauma (Anesi et al., 2014) (Figure 14.8).

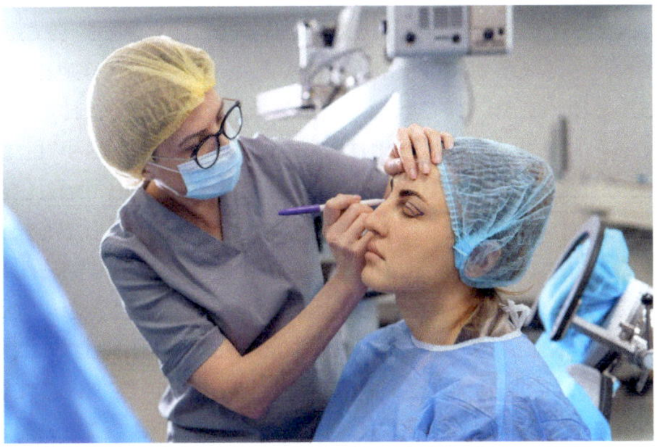

Figure 14.8. Purpose of reconstructive surgery.

Source: https://external-content.duckduckgo.com/iu/?u=https%3A%2F%2Fcachevalleyent.com%2Fstorage%2F2023%2F10%2FReconstructive-Surgery-by-Cache-Valley-ENT-in-Logan-UT-scaled.jpeg&f=1&nofb=1&ipt=2799cefeb77b86f258a57cf0c898ab54ff23c34f1626cfd74cfbd729e77d35d8.

14.2.2. Techniques Used in Facial Reconstruction

There are various surgical techniques used to attain facial function and aesthetics in oncologic and post-tumor reconstruction. Soft tissue reconstruction is generally performed through the usage of local flaps, such as the rotation or advancement flaps, which transfer tissue within the vicinity for the aim of covering defects with minimal disfigurement. Free tissue transfer techniques involving microvascular anastomosis have also become increasingly popular, with the possibility of transferring tissue from more distant sites. This technique not only facilitates the reconstruction of large defects but also facilitates the restoration of function, which is paramount to the overall quality of life in the patient. The nature of the technique varies significantly based on the size and location of the defect, the general well-being of the patient, and their desired aesthetic result; thus customized treatment planning is essential in achieving the most desirable outcome. Another significant feature of facial reconstruction is the management of facial paralysis of the facial nerve, a not uncommon complication of head and neck cancer surgery. The procedures employed to address this condition need to be tailored for each patient based on individual anatomy and functional requirements. For instance, reinnervation methods, where remaining segments of nerves are utilized to stimulate facial musculature, are able to offer more natural motion compared with static reconstructive methods. However, the intricacy of facial innervation often defies complete restoration, and surgeons find it necessary to combine neurotization with other surgeries, such as muscle transfers, to provide better function and cosmetic result. The subtle dance of anatomy and surgical potential demands close understanding of the pathway of the facial nerves and the patient's functional deficit (Anderson et al., 2012). Lastly, the incorporation of advanced technologies has transformed facial reconstruction methods in the recent past. Computational models and 3D printing have become useful resources when it comes to planning and performing intricate reconstructive procedures. Surgeons are able to design accurate patient-specific models for simulating the surgical procedure before it, enabling greater accuracy throughout the actual procedure. Moreover, evolution in biomaterials used for tissue engineering and grafting has the potential for enormous opportunities for designing individually tailored solutions for unique defects. This convergence of technology and surgery not only optimizes healing but also optimizes aesthetic and functional outcomes for patients undergoing tumor resection (de Bree et al., 2017). As science continues to evolve, future research will likely provide increasingly advanced methods for addressing facial reconstruction challenges (Figure 14.9).

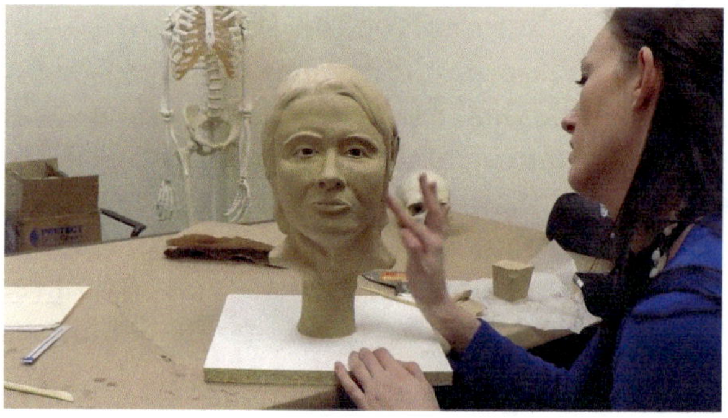

Figure 14.9. Techniques used in facial reconstruction.

Source: https://i.ytimg.com/vi/tQ95nVPJvEE/maxresdefault.jpg.

14.2.3. Psychological Impact of Facial Reconstruction on Patients

The psychological effect of facial reconstruction on oncologic patients is intense and complex. Patients with facial disfigurement from tumors typically experience deep emotional distress, which impacts their self-esteem and social conduct. Appearance of the face automatically equates with individual identity and social acceptance, and reconstructive surgery can be a catalyst for recovery of appearance and psychological well-being. Anticipation of surgical outcome, especially restoration of facial appearance, can influence patients' psychological state because the majority anticipate that improved appearances will be followed by reintegration with society and enhanced quality of life. Noted, facial dynamics restoration is not merely cosmetic rehabilitation but was deeply entangled with mental health, wherein successful reconstruction could restore a sense of normalcy and confidence among facial trauma victims. And the success of reconstructive surgeries also largely lies in the surgical techniques themselves, which can vary in their effectiveness depending on circumstances. The communication among the patient, oncologist, and surgeon is most important in achieving maximum outcome through potential pre-prosthetic surgical preparation that influences global satisfaction with the reconstruction. According to clinical reports, when integrated treatment with comprehensive pre-surgical planning is provided to the patient, the resultant improvement in function and form can greatly reduce anxiety and optimize post-procedure satisfaction. Proper communication throughout the process enables patients to understand their options, get their concerns addressed, and participate actively in their own healing. Not only does this interaction improve surgical results, but also has long-term impacts on patients' psychological health, affirming again the importance of shared medical care in the process of recovery. Moreover, following reconstruction, ongoing care by healthcare providers is essential in developing psychological resilience in paticnts. Thc majority of individuals face an intricate process of adjustment as they strive to deal with their new identity after undergoing surgery, grappling with both physical changes and the emotional consequences that result from them. The process of coping with societal attitudes and self-concept issues can lead them to become anxious or depressed, particularly where outcomes are less expected. Therefore, psychological counseling following surgery becomes essential in solving such issues, assisting patients in coping and enhancing their self-concept. Positive outcomes in facial reconstruction ultimately result in increased social interaction and readaptation, as patients slowly begin viewing their reconstructed faces as symbols of resilience rather than reminders of their past, validating the role of psychological support after facial cosmetic surgery (Anderson et al., 2012; Fattah et al., 2012) (Figure 14.10).

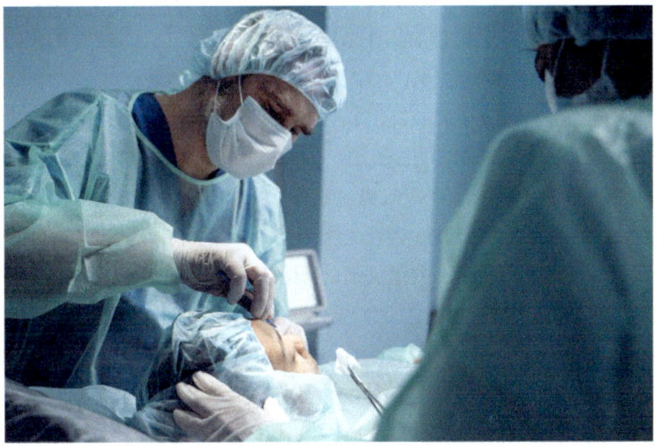

Figure 14.10. Psychological impact of facial reconstruction on patients.

Source: https://nevadaoms.com/wp-content/uploads/2024/04/2149352203.jpg.

Test Your Knowledge

1. Why is reconstructive surgery important after tumor removal in facial cosmetic surgery?
2. How does reconstructive surgery improve both the appearance and functional abilities of patients after oncologic surgery?

14.3. Preoperative Considerations

Learning Outcome

1. Patient Assessment and Evaluation
2. Importance of Multidisciplinary Teams
3. Planning for Aesthetic Outcomes

Preoperative considerations are the limelight in oncologic and post-tumor reconstruction in facial cosmetic surgery for the best operating outcomes. High on the list is multidisciplinary coordination among oncologists, surgeons, and prosthodontists. Preoperative planning secures that surgical technique is tailored to the patient's specific needs, particularly after procedures such as maxillectomy. The research highlights the importance of pre-prosthetic surgical preparation that can significantly enhance the prognosis of oral cancer patients by preserving key structures, i.e., alveolar bone or adjacent teeth, which are vital for successful prosthetic management. Preoperative planning with such attention to detail enables not just the rehabilitation of functional capacity but also the aesthetic form, thereby enhancing the quality of life in patients post-surgery (Fattah et al., 2012). Another highly significant consideration is assessment of the patient's psychological status pre-surgery. Patients undergoing oncologic interventions can be discovered to be extremely anxious and emotionally upset, both on account of the diagnosis per se and on account of the alterations they expect in their appearance. Addressing these psychological factors is paramount in ensuring compliance and satisfaction by the patient post-surgery. Preoperative counseling can help patients establish realistic expectations of the reconstructive outcome and adopt coping strategies to nurture their mental and emotional well-being during recovery. Involving the patients in decision-making also confers on them a sense of autonomy and control that can significantly improve the global satisfaction with the surgical outcome (Cortese et al., 2021). In addition, the incorporation of contemporary technology and methods of preoperative planning has revolutionized facial cosmetic surgery following tumor removal. Preoperative imaging and 3D modeling can facilitate visualization by surgeons of the particular anatomical hurdles presented by defects from tumor removal. This sophisticated preparation enables more accurate surgical interventions and assists in the success of postoperative cosmetic and functional restorations. Furthermore, technologies such as the use of hyaluronic acid fillers are now valuable adjuvants in treating surgical sequelae, presenting a minimally invasive technique that contributes to aesthetic results after reconstruction. Surgical teams can decrease disability and enhance cosmetic outcome with these new methods, which is finally the greatest aim of rehabilitating patients' social relationships and self-confidence (Cortese et al., 2021) (Figure 14.11).

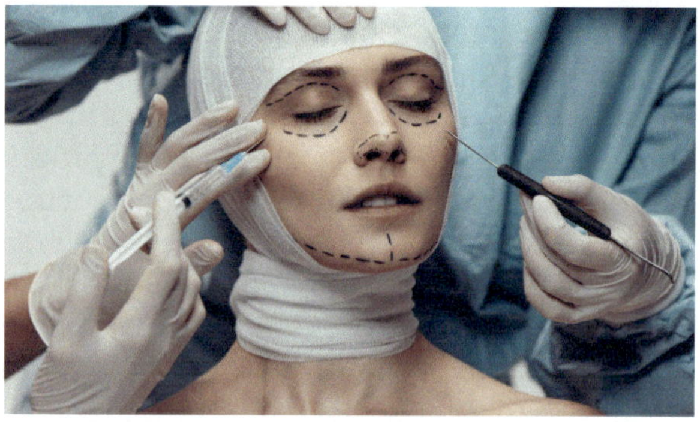

Figure 14.11. Oncologic and post-tumor reconstruction in facial cosmetic surgery.

Source: https://www.vaidam.com/sites/default/files/tests-before-cosmetic-surgery-intro-image-09-23.png.

14.3.1. Patient Assessment and Evaluation

Successful oncologic and post-tumor reconstruction in facial cosmetic surgery is founded on good patient assessment and evaluation. This comprehensive process begins with meticulous clinical history that includes not just the patient's cancer diagnosis and treatment but their psychosocial status and functional issues as well. Considerations such as tumor invasion extent and aesthetic impact are carefully weighed. By incorporating multidisciplinary consultation involving oncologists, surgeons, and counseling support staff, the entire holistic picture is considered so that all elements of patient health and welfare are taken into account in order to plan individualized reconstructive measures. The purpose of this thorough examination is to establish an individualized plan of treatment for the physical as well as psychological stresses of cancer therapy, ultimately resulting in improved patient outcomes and satisfaction. Physical examination is another salient feature of patient examination, with a focus on the specific anatomical region being reconstructed. Careful evaluations of facial balance, vascularization, and tissue integrity are significant as they direct the choice of surgical interventions and prosthetic appliances. For instance, after surgeries such as maxillectomy, the evaluation needs to take into account how defects resulting from such surgeries will impact functions such as speech and mastication. Coordination of reconstructive specialists and oncologic surgeons is required here in order to ensure that pre-prosthetic preparations, such as the preservation of overlying structures, support the patient's potential for successful rehabilitation. This caution is imperative in optimizing not just functional results of the surgery but also cosmetic results that significantly affect the patients quality of life, and which underscores the importance of a careful process of assessment. In addition, psychological testing is a part of patient assessment in oncologic and post-tumor reconstruction cases. Psycho-emotional impact from cancer and its treatments is usually debilitating in nature and results in body image disturbance, anxiety, and depression. These psycho-emotional factors should be evaluated as part of the overall plan of treatment since they play an important role in recuperation as well as in the patient's willingness to undertake reconstructive surgeries. Understanding the emotional and mental state of a patient allows health care professionals to give individualized care and support that may be needed in effective rehabilitation. In organizing reconstructive treatment, as suggested by literature, consideration of possible psychosocial impacts can improve not only aesthetic results but also allow for more satisfactory and holistic recovery, as reported by studies evaluating the significance of pre-prosthetic surgical interventions and their effect on patient rehabilitation (Fattah et al., 2012) (Figure 14.12).

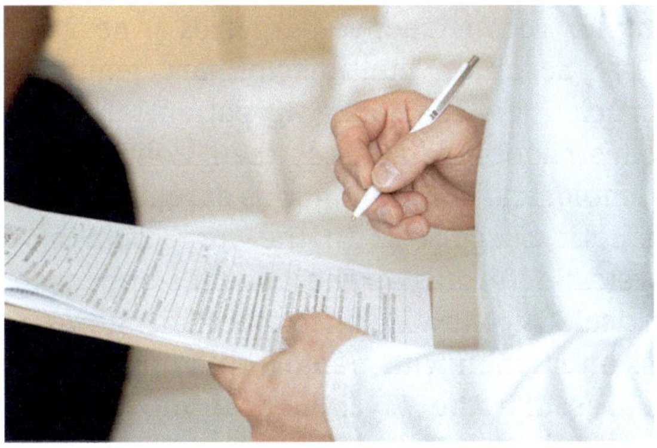

Figure 14.12. Patient assessment and evaluation.

Source: https://external-content.duckduckgo.com/iu/?u=https%3A%2F%2Fi0.wp.com%2Fstudent-nurse-life.com%2Fwp-content%2Fuploads%2F2023%2F03%2Fintroduction-to-assessing-and-implementing-care.jpg%3Ffit%3D1024%252C683&f=1&nofb=1&ipt=4c5422de406e21ec18239f6d1b9328f3d5f0c91e4892276b1ff60eb14ddd4645.

14.3.2. Importance of Multidisciplinary Teams

The complexity of oncologic and post-tumor reconstruction of facial cosmetic surgery demands the formation of multidisciplinary teams, with a balance of various expertise and specializations. This collaboration brings together oncologists, plastic surgeons, dermatologists, radiologists, and even mental health professionals, all with their unique expertise and skills. This cooperative approach is at the core of designing complete treatment plans based on specific patient needs. For instance, integration of oncological knowledge into surgical decisions ensures full understanding of the tumors behavior and associated risks of recurrence. One article emphasized how the use of advanced technology like Piezosurgery has the capacity to enhance surgical precision to a very significant degree while preserving valuable surrounding tissues, thus ensuring that collaboration between team members is necessary to ensure maximum results in complex reconstructive surgeries (Anesi et al., 2014). Secondly, multidisciplinary teams play a crucial role in managing patients following reconstruction to address their holistic needs. Psychological counseling is as essential in facial cosmetic surgery as in the correction of the physical deformity in the patient's appearance, particularly following oncological disfigurement. This interaction with mental health professionals ensures that the psychological and emotional effects of cancer treatment and reconstruction are optimally addressed, thus enhancing the overall recovery of patients. The successful reconstruction of scalp defects, as exemplified in recent case series using autologous grafts and dermal matrices, shows how interdisciplinary collaboration within specialties yields improved operating results and greater patient satisfaction (Gonzaga et al., 2019). The same support system in various aspects is needed in dealing with the intricate process of healing and reintegrating into society after surgery. The advantages of multidisciplinary practice extend beyond clinical effectiveness; they also promote a culture of cross-learning and innovation among medical practitioners. Collaboration of various expertise pushes practitioners to remain updated with the latest developments in methodologies and technology, which is a must in an increasingly evolving specialty like facial cosmetic surgery. By sharing knowledge and experiences, team members can identify best practices and refine protocols, leading to continuous improvement in patient care. Furthermore, such collaboration cultivates a strong professional network that can facilitate research and development initiatives, ultimately pushing boundaries in oncologic reconstruction methodologies. In summary, interaction among various specialties not only benefits but is essential for advancing oncologic and post-tumor reconstruction in facial aesthetic surgery (Figure 14.13).

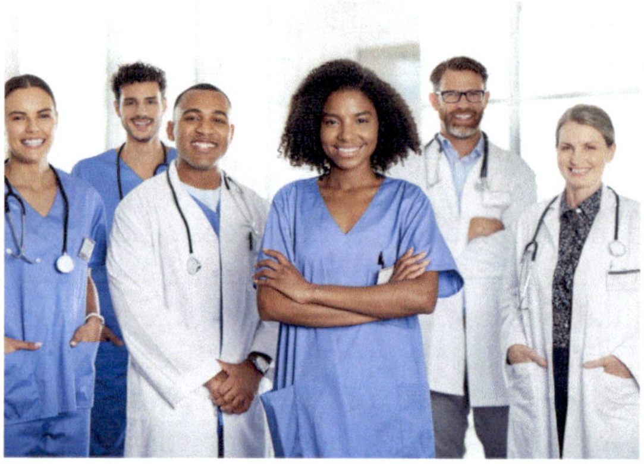

Figure 14.13. Importance of multidisciplinary teams.

Source: https://external-content.duckduckgo.com/iu/?u=https%3A%2F%2Fgettraumainformed.com%2Fwp-content%2Fuploads%2F2022%2F03%2FUntitled-design-e1647928342547-1024x744.png&f=1&nofb=1&ipt=3df54e0f9ebf6af805c237b956853e701afcc53c33a0bf64ae44ebc6fa469596.

14.3.3. Planning for Aesthetic Outcomes

Planning for aesthetic results in oncologic and post-tumor reconstruction of the facial structures is directly associated with the interdisciplinary interaction between oncologists and reconstructive surgeons. This collaboration is particularly crucial in procedures such as maxillectomy, whose size and site of resection significantly influence the possibility of an aesthetically pleasing result. The combination of measures directed at the preservation of adjacent structures, such as premaxilla or alveolar bone, holds the potential to enhance functional and cosmetic results for patients undergoing prosthetic rehabilitation. Pre-prosthetic surgical preps like these allow for an ideal platform for prostheses to be secured on, which further results in successful aesthetic rehabilitation. Efficient communication and planning can therefore not only enhance the prosthetic outcome but also the patient's psychosocial rehabilitation following surgery, underlining the importance of aesthetic components in the overall treatment plan (Fattah et al., 2012).

In oncologic breast reconstruction, careful consideration of aesthetic outcomes has a groundbreaking effect on patient recovery and the quality of life. Use of techniques such as pedicled perforator flaps allows for an accurately recreated breast shape and size with minimal scarring visible. The success of such reconstructive techniques depends on their application in preoperative treatment planning, thereby obliterating symmetry and aesthetic issues prior to proceeding. With the achievement of acceptable restoration of size and shape, reconstructive surgeons can mitigate loss and disfigurement feelings normally experienced by patients after mastectomy. Also, since donor site scars are well-placed, they remain concealed, hence contributing to the ultimate aesthetic result.

Such planning in totality accentuates reconstruction as more than a functional necessity; it is reconstructing identity and womanhood after cancer treatment (Cillino et al., 2010). Furthermore, patient education regarding expectations and the cosmetic nature of reconstructive surgery is important for achieving desired results. The presentation of patients with an in-depth discussion of potential outcomes and the limitations of reconstruction has the ability to empower them and synchronize their expectations with reasonable ones.

These are informed consent, where patients learn about the techniques used and the effects on appearance as a result. Facial symmetry and normal contour correction should be highlighted as features, which will enable the patients to see the end result of their treatment. Support systems psychological should also be incorporated into preoperative care to deal with physical alteration anxieties after surgery. Lastly, concern being shown towards aesthetic outcomes in oncologic reconstruction not only increases physical results but also emotional recovery and patient satisfaction with their recovery process (Figure 14.14).

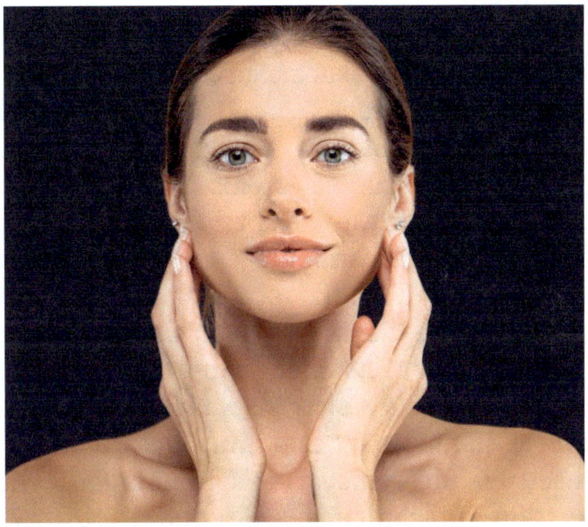

Figure 14.14. Planning for aesthetic outcomes.

Source: https://external-content.duckduckgo.com/iu/?u=https%3A%2F%2Fempireondemand.com%2Fcdn%2Fshop%2Ffiles%2FUnlockingAdvancedAestheticOutcomesCombinationTherapywiththeV-SeriesPlatform-horizontal.webp%3Fv%3D1726258974&f=1&nofb=1&ipt=fdb2fc76441eba71facef7b5c1255a48aa6642fb8088cfb1976a7222eb921bb8.

Test Your Knowledge

1. What factors must surgeons evaluate before performing facial reconstructive surgery?
2. Why is patient assessment and surgical planning essential for successful reconstructive outcomes?

14.4. Surgical Techniques in Reconstruction

Learning Outcome

1. Flap Techniques and Their Applications
2. Grafting Methods in Facial Reconstruction
3. Innovations in Surgical Technology

Surgical methods in reconstruction following oncologic surgery are heavily responsible for the restoration of function and aesthetics of the facial region. The complexity of reconstructive processes is highlighted by the need to overcome unique issues caused by the removal of cancerous tissues, particularly in areas with intricate anatomical structures such as nerves and vascular systems. Surgeons must skillfully assess the extent of tissue damage and formulate treatments that allow optimal healing with minimal scarring and loss of function. Free tissue transfer and local flap procedures, for instance, allow repositioning of adjacent tissues or transplantation of tissue from a distant part and thus bridge defects caused by the removal of a tumor. This wise selection of techniques is essential in restoring the patients to as much of their preoperative form and function, and therefore the quality of life. Paralysis of the face due to oncologic surgery complicates the reconstructive process further. Surgical techniques need to be adapted not only to restore the physical deformity, but also to restore facial symmetry and expression. Therapies may be directed toward grafting or repair of nerves, local muscle transfer, and static or dynamic sling placement for support of injured facial structures. When reinnervation is feasible, reconnections within the current musculature lead to more natural and functional outcomes. Nonetheless, the intricate facial nerve anatomy typically poses problems for complete rehabilitation. Thus, the synergy of newer surgical methods and a sound understanding of facial dynamics is needed to address the dual requirements of aesthetics and function following tumor removal (Anderson et al., 2012).

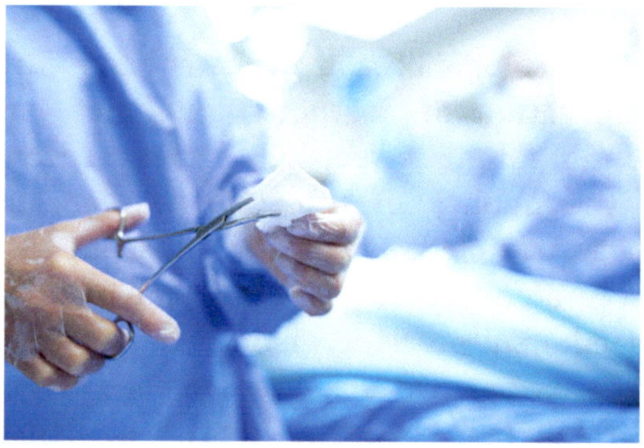

Figure 14.15. Surgical techniques in reconstruction.

Source: https://external-content.duckduckgo.com/iu/?u=https%3A%2F%2Fi0.wp.com%2Ffabknowledge.com%2Fwp-content%2Fuploads%2F2020%2F05%2F2240-scaled.jpg%3Fzoom%3D3%26resize%3D700%252C480%26ssl%3D1&f=1&nofb=1&ipt=31b72e76c89b7ee7a404dc3398fb372cb5323310735c2e77fb4472613fdee480.

Reconstruction after oncologic surgery is not only concerned with achieving the short-term aesthetic outcome, but also with considering the long-term factors influencing the patient's psychosocial status. An understanding of the interplay between physical appearance and self-image is essential for reconstruction success. The employment of modern adaptations of established surgical methods may offer optimal results in restoring facial appearance with maintenance of functional integrity. Knowledge of basic surgical principles is relevant, as the reconstructive techniques must be adapted to meet the individual patient's needs, particularly with large tumor resections (Garey et al., 2018). By including these factors in the reconstructive plan, surgeons can optimize overall success of oncologic and tumor-post reconstruction in removing both the physical and psychological scars of surgery (Figure 14.15).

14.4.1. Flap Techniques and Their Applications

Flap techniques are the most important technique in oncologic and post-tumor reconstruction, in the restoration of tissue function, aesthetics, and integrity. Flap techniques are used for the transfer of skin, muscle, and fat from one body area to another and the creation of a flap that is nourished by its own blood supply. Flap procedures are particularly relevant in the context of tumor resection for facial cosmetic surgery, where loss of tissue is highly impactful upon both shape and functional capacity, such as speech and swallowing. Recent studies have demonstrated the usefulness of the pedicled perforator flap application in successful volume and envelope skin restoration, particularly in partial breast reconstruction following tumor excision, thereby indicating the versatility of flap procedures in other facial and breast reconstructive operations (Cillino et al., 2010). One additional interesting aspect of flap techniques is the manner in which these procedures can be adapted to confront other reconstructive problems presented by oncologic surgery, most notably in the head and neck. Facial anatomy presents too much complexity to allow proper selection of the applicable flap type based on defect size and location. A systematic review has outlined several locoregional flaps, i.e., the infrahyoid, nasolabial, and submental flaps, which have been successfully employed for oral cavity reconstruction after tumor removal. Not only does this approach correct the immediate anatomical deficits, but it also enhances aesthetically better outcomes, so that the patients have not only functional rehabilitation but also the return to a more normal appearance. Complications of flap procedures are generally low and in reports of flap necrosis in a minimal percentage of procedures, further confirming the reliability of the technique (Accoronna et al., 2024). Moreover, studies using flap techniques in the follow-up of tumor resection have increased over time with advancements in surgical procedures and patient care. Surgeons now make use of cutting-edge imaging technologies and innovative surgical planning to optimize flap design and improve operative results. This patient-specific system allows for more precise reconstructions that meet the special demands of each patient, thereby increasing the satisfaction with both the aesthetic and functional results. Although flap techniques continue to expand in scope of popularity in oncologic and post-tumor reconstruction, clinical trials and research will certainly aid in further evolving these techniques, expediting recovery times, and minimizing complications wherever possible, overall enhancing patient outcomes in the domain of facial cosmetic surgery.

14.4.2. Grafting Methods in Facial Reconstruction

The grafting technique of methods of facial reconstruction is key to successful facial aesthetics and function restoration following oncologic surgery. Skin grafting, normally applied for facial defect resulting from the removal of a tumor, can be classified into various types including split-thickness and full-thickness grafts. Split-thickness grafts, which include the epidermis and part of the dermis, are most often employed for larger defects since they are convenient and cause less donor site morbidity. Both layers of the skin, full-thickness grafts, however, give better cosmetic results and should be utilized on small, more visible sites like the mouth and nose. The literature reports that appropriate grafting technique choice significantly influences healing time and surgical outcome, particularly requiring surgeons to customize their technique to the specific patient needs and individual presentations of the tumor. In the event of major loss of face tissue from oncologic resections, the reconstructive alternatives extend beyond merely skin grafts to more complex techniques that include local flaps and free tissue transfer. Local flaps are useful in that they utilize adjacent tissues to fill in the defects without disrupting vascular supply and typically yield better functional results. For instance, the modified crescentic flap procedure has been successful in correcting defects in the area around the nose to facilitate both functional reconstruction and cosmetic enhancement through adequately camouflaging scars within natural contours. Research has established that such regional methods prefer faster recovery and less postoperative complications, emphasizing their importance in oncologic reconstruction (Arginelli et al., 2016). With accurate planning of these procedures, surgeons can develop the best aesthetic results with fewer psychological disturbances to patients recovered from facial anomalies caused by cancer. Apart from the cosmetic nature, the functional implications of facial grafting methods in tumor post-reconstruction cannot be overstated. Paralysis of the facial nerve is a common complication of head and neck surgery, and individualized rehabilitation programs are needed to establish innervation and musculature for an optimal functional outcome. Grafting techniques involving a combination of nerve repair and tissue reconstruction can provide patients with significant improvement in mobility and expression for a more natural appearance and enhanced quality of life. Secondly, the selection of the method of grafting needs to consider not only aesthetic, but functional outcomes, as some methods will be more accommodating to achieving both objectives. Lastly, the use of grafting in facial reconstruction is critical, as both the physical and psychological dimensions of healing from oncologic surgery are being attended to (Anderson et al., 2012).

14.4.3. Innovations in Surgical Technology

The cosmetic surgery world, particularly in the areas of oncologic and post-tumor reconstruction, is being significantly revolutionized by advances in surgical technology. Contemporary practices are revolutionizing how surgeons approach complex defects, primarily by facilitating enhanced functional and aesthetic outcomes. Much of this paradigmatic change can be attributed to advancements in flap surgery and regenerative medicine, which offer alternative avenues for reconstructive issues. For instance, perforator flap techniques have also achieved an astonishing 96.5% success rate, which has been significantly improved in relation to functional restoration over traditional pedicled flaps. Given that aesthetic satisfaction is highest in facial surgery, these developments are of great promise to enhance patient recovery with reduced complications, further showing the importance of iterative technological developments in surgical techniques (Bernal et al., 2024). An essential component of these advancements is the application of virtual surgical planning (VSP) and computer-aided design/manufacturing (CAD/CAM) systems. These technologies aid in precise anatomical reconstructions, especially important in complex situations such as maxillectomy, where critical defects require meticulous restoration of form and function. Evidence proves that the addition of VSP may streamline operational efficiency, reducing the duration of surgeries while improving the precision of osseous reconstructions. As a result, patient outcomes are greatly enhanced, both aesthetically and in terms of rehabilitation. Furthermore, the aforementioned technologies minimize the risk of complications associated with traditional techniques, presenting a compelling case for the adoption of sophisticated technology in facial reconstructive surgery (Datarkar et al., 2024). Surgical procedures using regenerative medicine are transforming healing processes and realizing optimal recovery results in oncologic patients. Techniques such as the use of platelet-rich plasma (PRP) and bioengineered scaffolds are now viable adjuncts, facilitating wound healing at a rapid rate and drastically lowering the rates of infection. Experiments have also proven that application of these regenerative methods can improve graft survival to up to 90%, a significant improvement over conventional methods. Also, the combination of advanced flap methods with regenerative therapy greatly minimizes complications while providing robust functional and cosmetic results. These developments underscore the necessity for ongoing research and development in surgical technology, with emphasis on their role in the future of oncologic and post-tumor reconstruction in facial cosmetic surgery (Bernal et al., 2024).

Test Your Knowledge

1. What are the common surgical techniques used in facial reconstruction after oncologic surgery?
2. How do grafts and flap techniques help restore facial form and function?

14.5. Postoperative Care and Recovery

Learning Outcome

1. Importance of Follow-up Care
2. Managing Complications and Risks
3. Rehabilitation And Support For Patients

The postoperative recovery following oncologic and post-tumor reconstruction in facial cosmetic surgery is paramount, as it plays a vital role both in the immediate recovery and long-term outcomes. Appropriate care at this stage can avoid complications, minimize discomfort, and improve rehabilitation. Appropriate pain control is a cornerstone of postoperative care, generally dealt with by a combination of pharmacological and non-pharmacological interventions. Individualized management of pain requires frequent assessment of the surgical field and general condition, so patients can carry out necessary activities such as eating and speaking with minimal distress. Closely monitoring for infection, dehiscence, or complications is crucial since these variables can disrupt healing and negatively affect cosmetic results. Postoperative care includes supportive management that facilitates recovery. In maxillary reconstructive surgery, for instance, the employment of a multimodality team of oncologists, plastic surgeons, prosthodontists, and rehabilitation specialists ensures patients receive comprehensive care tailored to their specific surgical experiences. Pre-prosthetic surgical alterations have the potential to enhance prosthetic fit conditions, which subsequently influence functionality and aesthetics after maxillectomy. There is evidence that suggests that there is a significant role contributed by surgeon-prosthodontist interaction toward post-surgical rehabilitation success, for example, research emphasizing the role of preoperative planning and collaborative action in ensuring a satisfactory outcome (Fattah et al., 2012). Such an approach of a team ensures not only current medical needs but also continuity of care along the course of recovery. Modalities and timing of rehabilitation are most crucial in setting the postoperative course of recovery. Newer methods, such as the use of ultrasonic osteotomes, have emerged as useful options for craniofacial surgery and have advantages in bone healing due to accuracy and less injury to surrounding tissues (Anesi et al., 2014). The ability of such equipment to cut smoothly supports better maintenance of important structures, which supports better surgical outcomes and, possibly, better aesthetics. Along with postoperative care, this technique underscores the necessity for the adoption of modern surgical practices that allow for faster recovery and enhanced cosmetic outcomes. Through an emphasis on innovative practice and whole patient care, healthcare professionals can help patients who have had oncologic and facial reconstruction surgery regain function and confidence as they continue down their path to recovery.

14.5.1. Importance of Follow-up Care

For oncologic and post-tumor reconstruction in facial cosmetic surgery, follow-up care cannot be overstated. Post-op management is important to monitor possible complications and ensure optimal recovery. For reconstructive surgery, patients are faced with numerous issues, including handling pain, surgical site infections, and the psychological impact of their appearance. Regular follow-up allows medical specialists to timely address and resolve such issues, which can significantly affect the quality of life of a patient and overall contentment with the outcome of the surgery. Periodic visits provide an opportunity for patients to share their doubts, receive support, and become capable of accessing necessary help, thereby making the rehabilitation process easier after tumor resection and reconstruction. Moreover, follow-up care is necessary to ensure maximum success of prosthetic rehabilitation following maxillectomy or similar surgery. As seen through research, pre-prosthetic surgical preparation substantially optimizes the success of prosthetic treatment among patients of maxillary reconstruction. Interdisciplinary collaboration between oncologists and maxillofacial surgeons during preparatory procedures can optimize sites for prosthetic placement, as described in Fattah et al. (2012). When follow-up care is integrated into this system, it establishes the foundation for adjustments that respond to evolving patient needs, ensuring that what is delivered as prosthetic restoration satisfies functional requirements as well as visual and aesthetic satisfaction. Regular inspections present a chance to make timely adjustments and refinements, which are key to maintaining patient confidence and social adjustment. In addition, the follow-up care function also entails monitoring the physiological impact of the surgical intervention on tissue viability and bone regeneration. The use of advanced technology, such as Piezosurgery, has been observed to have the capability of minimizing trauma to surrounding structures, thereby affecting post-operative recovery. Evaluating the outcome of different osteotomy techniques, as reported in Anesi et al. (2014), is important in deciding the most effective method to facilitate proper recovery and healing after facial reconstructive operations. Postoperative follow-up sessions provide significant insights about healing patterns of bone and soft tissues so that surgeons can analyze whether chosen techniques provide the best results in terms of recovery rate and quality. This unified assessment can have a profound impact on long-term cosmetic results and functional rehabilitation, verifying the position of follow-up management as an integral component of oncologic facial reconstructive practice.

14.5.2. Managing Complications and Risks

Effective management of complications and risks is necessary in oncologic and post-tumor reconstruction in facial cosmetic surgery. The treating surgeons should anticipate potential problems such as infection, wound dehiscence, and necrosis to enhance patient results. Technological innovation, particularly ultrasonic osteotomes, has been found to assist in minimizing bone trauma during surgical procedures. Comparisons of various osteotomy devices discovered that ultrasound-guided equipment, such as Piezosurgery®, produces surfaces with advantageous micromorphologies that can promote bone healing and reossification. These technologies not only address the physical aspect of reconstruction but also minimize risks associated with traditional methods, including rotating or sawing instruments, that lead to increased complications (Anesi et al., 2014). Through their integration, surgeons can optimize the safety and efficacy of facial cosmetic procedures, leading to an overall improvement in the quality of life among cancer survivors. Post-operative complications can potentially change the course of recovery for patients following oncologic reconstruction. Age, pre-existing health conditions, and the size of the original tumor are risk factors that should be evaluated in an attempt to plan surgical procedures accordingly. Certain patients may be at greater risk for complications if they have extensive tissue loss or require high reconstructive procedures, for instance. Surgery teams are stimulated to utilize comprehensive preoperative assessment to determine subjects with high risk and therefore, utilize personalized protocols to minimize post-surgical complications. Furthermore, ongoing education on the latest surgical techniques and materials can improve the capacity of health professionals to manage probable complications confidently. Such practices are instrumental in building a safer operating room and boosting recovery rates among patients undergoing facial reconstruction after tumor resection (Ndongo et al., 2010). Post-operative care and complication management are also important, as early detection encourages timely intervention to improve outcomes from the operation. Postoperative checkups and follow-up make the detection of signs of complications early on possible, allowing them to be treated in due time. Patient education regarding potential signs of infection or other side effects also empowers them to actively seek medical care. Adoption of a standard follow-up schedule, coupled with a patient-centered care approach, is crucial in ensuring the effective management of complications without compromising the overall well-being and satisfaction of the patient and the reconstructive result. With facial cosmetic surgery continuing to advance, emphasis on balanced risk management approaches is pivotal in achieving optimal results in patients who are undergoing oncologic surgery (Anesi et al., 2014).

14.5.3. Rehabilitation And Support For Patients

The rehabilitation and support of oncologic and post-tumor reconstruction patients are multifaceted and include both functional and psychological concerns. The patient, following facial surgery for tumor removal or reconstruction, will often have an extreme change in appearance and function. Such changes are distressing psychologically and potentially impacting self-esteem and quality of life. Therefore, an effective rehabilitation program will include psychological support services so that patients can cope with their new realities. Counseling or support groups, for instance, can offer a forum in which patients can share experiences and strategies, accelerate emotional healing as well as physical recovery. It is significant to note the psychological components of recovery since this can significantly enhance compliance with rehabilitation routines, lead to optimal outcomes, and build resilience during recovery. For patients with facial paralysis secondary to cancer therapies, individualized rehabilitation protocols help ensure maximum recovery of function. Facilitation of the recovery process is most often impeded by the complexity of facial innervation; individualized evaluation takes precedence. As varied as therapy to restore the function of the muscles or surgery for nerve repair and reinnervation, treatment is outlined in Anderson et al. (2012). These approaches not only address cosmetic concerns but also focus on improving functional abilities such as speech, swallowing, and facial expression. Additionally, the integration of new technologies, such as biofeedback systems or electrical stimulation units, can offer alternative avenues for treatment, hence boosting patient motivation and involvement in their rehabilitation. By prioritizing functional recovery as the first step in overall patient care, healthcare practitioners are able to put patients on the path to greater independence and improved quality of life. Pre-prosthetic surgical preparation as a component for realizing best rehabilitation outcomes cannot be overstated. Following operations like maxillectomy, the resulting defects need successful prosthetic replacement to facilitate restoration of function and aesthetics, and this is crucial for the reintegration of patients into social settings. Such success hinges on collaborative efforts between oncologists and maxillofacial surgeons to help ensure effective preservation of the remaining anatomy during primary surgery, as emphasized in Fattah et al. (2012). Such collaboration aids in formulating a pre-prosthetic plan that may include the preservation of significant anatomical structures to maximize function of the prosthetic devices as a whole. An in-depth knowledge of prosthetic and surgical principles can enhance patient outcomes, addressing key areas like speech intelligibility and social interaction after reconstruction. An integrated rehabilitation and support program, thus, is essential in order to optimize physical and psychosocial aspects of rehabilitation for patients undergoing facial cosmetic surgery due to cancer therapy.

Test Your Knowledge

1. What are the key components of postoperative care following facial reconstructive surgery?
2. How does proper postoperative care influence healing and long-term surgical results?

14.6. Ethical Considerations in Oncologic and Reconstructive Surgery

Learning Outcome

1. Informed Consent and Patient Autonomy
2. Balancing Aesthetics with Medical Necessity
3. Addressing Disparities in Access to Care

In the practice of oncologic and reconstructive surgery, moral principles should come first in surgeons' decision-making. The confrontation between the demand for life-saving procedures and the intention to preserve beauty is embedded in complex dilemmas. Doctors must navigate the ethical landscape between the urgency of patients' health and the accommodation of the psychosocial impacts of disfiguration by tumors. The process generally entices a high level of subtlety in obtaining informed consent for high-pressure treatments that may sacrifice on appearance and balancing realistic patient expectations regarding the end result of reconstructive surgeries. This is compounded when resource availability, patient-informed consent, and the potential for unequal access to high-technology reconstructive modalities are considered, ultimately confronting surgeons with their ethical responsibilities beyond the solution of the immediate clinical challenges of oncologic disease. Furthermore, ethics in reconstructive and oncologic surgery extend to postoperative rehabilitation and aesthetic requirements. The use of new techniques, such as the use of HA fillers as adjuvants in reconstructive surgery, illustrates an even greater ethical concern when it comes to patient satisfaction and quality of life. These methods, previously used for cosmetic reasons, can bring about significant functional and aesthetic gains following surgery, thus improving patient confidence. Still, their introduction challenges the issue of potential over-treatment and the commodification of surgical outcomes, where the outcome becomes more focused on aesthetics than on clinical necessity. The surgeons will need to consider the implications of using such methods, particularly in sensitive cases where a patient's psychological and emotional healing is interwoven with his or her physical appearance. The ethical responsibility is to make these processes work responsibly, weighing patient safety and satisfaction without compromising the limits of professional medical practice (Cortese et al., 2021). In addition, the social and cultural components of patient decision-making in reconstructive and oncologic surgery call for an ethical approach that is more nuanced. Personal convictions, cultural norms of beauty, and how accessible the reconstructive procedures are, all come into play in a patient's thought processes regarding what they wish to have done. The multi-faceted scenario necessitates surgeons to confront their own prejudices and be attuned to body image and personal identity cultural subtleties. Open dialogue with patients regarding what they desire, expect, and fear becomes important in developing an open way of doing things concerning treatment planning. Ethically, surgeons have a responsibility to equip patients with a complete set of information to allow them to make appropriate decisions regarding their treatment in alignment with their own values and conception of healing. These discussions become essential in bridging the gap between surgical technicality and the very personalized process of healing after oncologic operations (Accorona et al., 2024).

14.6.1. Informed Consent and Patient Autonomy

The importance of informed consent in the situation of oncologic and post-tumor reconstruction of facial cosmetic surgery cannot be overstressed. Informed consent is a fundamental principle that allows patients to make autonomous decisions regarding their medical treatment. This practice raises the patient from the status of a passive recipient of medical attention to that of an active participant in their own medical attention. In reconstructive facial procedures, particularly following oncologic surgery, patients are faced with complex decisions that are usually charged with emotional, psychological, and physical implications. Ethical practice necessitates health professionals to communicate risks, benefits, and potential outcomes of accessible surgical options in depth, not only upholding medical practice ethical standards but also respecting the autonomy and personal beliefs of the patient. The formation of informed consent is in harmony with the overall principles of patient autonomy, which becomes particularly important in the field of cancer following reconstructive surgery. Autonomy is an individuals' capacity to exercise control over their decision-making, based on values and wants, particularly in an exceedingly personal and life-changing circumstance such as facial cosmetic surgery. Surgeons should make sure that patients know about the different procedures that can be undertaken, their implications, and what recovery paths to expect. By allowing patients to comprehend the subtleties of their surgical choices, surgeons give them the power to fully participate in the decision-making process.

This becomes important to facilitating their emotional recovery and constructive self-concept upon treatment, because patient autonomy can positively enhance overall satisfaction with surgical outcomes, thereby solidifying the importance of informed consent in facilitating patient-centered care. Healthcare providers' responsibility for facilitating informed consent is not merely to convey information but also to create a supportive therapeutic relationship. As a dynamic blend of humanism and science, clinical practice demands practitioners not just to transmit technical information but also to talk to the emotional domain of patient care (Kalaskar et al., 2016). Building trust between the health care team and the patient is crucial in getting patients to relax and open up about their concerns and reconstruction preferences. These relationships also play a significant role in managing the complex terrains of cosmetic surgery decision-making, since patients may seek to balance their individual choices with broader social expectations. In the end, a holistic approach to informed consent prioritizing patient autonomy, emotional support, and honest communication guarantees that the health care process is holistic, dignified, and consonant with the values and projected outcomes of the patients.

14.6.2. Balancing Aesthetics with Medical Necessity

In the context of oncologic and post-tumor reconstruction, the intersection between aesthetics and medical necessity becomes a critical factor for consideration among both surgeons and patients. The physical and psychological impact of facial disfigurement necessitates consideration of both functional recovery and aesthetic restoration. In the majority of patients, particularly those recovering from procedures like mastectomy or radical tumor resections, a natural appearance is a significant part of their psychological well-being and readjustment to society. Reconstructive surgery therefore, must focus not only on restoring anatomical continuity but also on maximizing the aesthetic outcome, as reflected in the many strategies used by reconstructive surgeons. The prevalence of psychological distress following facial surgery renders this balance essential to patient satisfaction and thereby substantiates the intuition that reconstructive activity transcends medical necessity alone to encompass aesthetic desire. The conflicts of balancing aesthetic desires against clinical realities predominantly arise in preoperative consultations, wherein communication between healthcare providers and patients is of paramount importance. Identification of determinants influencing decision-making is of critical concern, particularly in patients undergoing significant reconstruction of their facial appearance. Evidence has shown that breast cancer patients tend to look at cosmetic considerations when deciding on reconstructive operations, similar to the behaviors of facial reconstructive surgery patients (Ndongo et al., 2010). Surgeons must navigate this ground with sensitivity, acknowledging the differing emotional responses of patients to disfigurement while presenting the medical justification for some operations. This serves to emphasize the need for an individualized approach, acknowledging that patients' notions of success of reconstruction can be extremely individualized and intertwining their body shape with their self-concept. With continually evolving surgical techniques and technology, the possibilities for innovative solutions in the marriage of form and functional necessity only expand. Surgeons are driven to integrate new technologies, such as 3D modeling and bioprinting, into practice, allowing increased degrees of customization of reconstruction and increased ability to address aesthetic issues without compromising medical success. This crossing alludes to an avant-garde trend in the field, whereby technologies facilitate the creation of naturally occurring-looking results that promote healing as well as contentment. These advancements bring with them, however, ethics related to access and equity of care, meaning that surgeons must be sensitive to disparities in patient access to reconstructive options (Ndongo et al., 2010). Hence, the balance between aesthetic and medical needs is not just a clinical objective but is also a reflection of the evolution of patient treatment in oncology and aesthetic surgery.

14.6.3. Addressing Disparities in Access to Care

Gaps in access to care have an important influence on the outcomes of oncologic and post-tumor reconstruction facial cosmetic surgery patients. Social determinants of health, such as socioeconomic status, location, and insurance coverage, usually determine patients' capacity to receive timely and appropriate care. For instance, patients in economically backward communities will have issues pertaining to transportation, which leads to delayed consultations and treatments. Delaying the process not only lowers the success rate of initial oncologic procedures but also complicates further reconstructive procedures. Addressing these disparities is crucial to ensuring equal access to care, which ultimately improves prognosis and quality of life for the suffering patients. Overall, policies aimed at addressing awareness and access to medical care are necessary in bridging the gap in healthcare availability, particularly for disadvantaged communities disproportionately affected by facial tumors and the resultant reconstruction needs. Besides these disparities in care and accessibility, biases among healthcare practitioners can similarly hinder equal access to oncologic and reconstructive care. Studies have demonstrated that racial and ethnic minorities are most likely to receive levels of care consistent with presumed abilities to tolerate pain or compliance with treatment recommendations. These biases may lead to suboptimal control of pain, decreased referrals for reconstructive surgery, and ultimately, poorer cosmetic results. The addition of cultural competency education to medical school curricula may be the bridge to crossing these biases. Through the provision of a healthcare environment that respects and honors various backgrounds, practitioners can enhance communication, build trust, and promote better care for all patients regardless of demographics. Meticulous training and sensitization can enable practitioners to break through their presuppositions, ultimately enhancing the provision of oncologic and post-tumor reconstructive surgeries for the underrepresented populations. In addition, community outreach programs play a key role in addressing disproportionate access to care in the areas of oncologic and post-tumor reconstruction. Through their direct engagement with communities, medical centers can better identify common hurdles in obtaining care. Educational programs can demystify reconstructive procedures and position them at the forefront of the cancer care process. Secondarily, partnerships with local organizations can promote advocacy for underinsured patient coverage and reimbursement for reconstructive treatment. Outcomes reveal that outreach programs will similarly encourage awareness and utilization of surgical therapy. In anticipation of the growing tumor-related deformity burden, active community outreach is necessary. Investment in such outreach is not only altruistic; it is required to create a more equitable model of healthcare that provides all patients with the ability to access reconstructive care that they need and deserve (Ndongo et al., 2010; Kalaskar et al., 2016).

Test Your Knowledge

1. What ethical responsibilities do surgeons have when performing oncologic and reconstructive facial surgery?
2. Why is informed consent important in oncologic and reconstructive surgical procedures?

SUMMARY

In oncologic and post-tumor reconstruction in facial cosmetic surgery, the key is to integrate high-tech surgical expertise and personalized patient care. As demonstrated in this essay, effective outcomes for facial reconstruction following oncological surgery rely on a combined vision of both aesthetic and functional needs. Facial anatomy's inherent complexities render the process more individualized, particularly in the case of addressing issues such as facial nerve paralysis due to cancer treatment. Careful assessment of residual nerve segments and musculature can lead to successful reinnervation methods, ultimately restoring patients closer to their original form and higher mobility. This complementarity of oncologic control and reconstructive surgery emphasizes the necessity of a multidisciplinary treatment, involving surgeons, oncologists, and rehabilitation specialists (Anderson et al., 2012). Furthermore, the pursuit of aesthetic reconstruction after oncological intervention presents unique challenges and opportunities for innovation in surgical techniques. The pedicled perforator flap is now considered a choice for breast reconstruction following tumor removal and is a suitable metaphor for facial reconstruction. Just as in breast reconstruction, the addition of tissue can reconstructively restore contour and volume, so too can these concepts be used in facial reconstruction, restoring both function and appearance following surgery. The early outcomes present promising results, with complete flap survival and satisfactory restoration of size and form, toward the possibility of improving patient satisfaction and global quality of life in this region (Cillino et al., 2010). In the end, the conclusion reached by this discussion of oncologic and post-tumor reconstruction in facial cosmetic surgery is that the future lies in continued refinement of the technique and the fostering of an empathic appreciation of patient experience. The gains achieved in terms of function and appearance can have a very powerful impact on the psychological and emotional well-being of patients subsequently. Thus, embracing a patient-centered approach that guarantees personalized treatment protocols will not only advance surgical outcomes but also the quality of care provided to oncologic surgery and subsequent reconstruction candidates. Engaging patients in their reconstructive process guarantees long-term satisfaction and improved quality of life after oncological complications.

The oncologic principles applied to facial cosmetic surgery signify the significance of addressing the aesthetic as well as functional issues of post-tumor reconstruction. Advances in technology and surgery have significantly enhanced the outcomes of patients with facial reconstruction after oncologic treatment. A key factor is selecting proper osteotomes, which have been altered with the development of ultrasonic tools such as Piezosurgery® and the newer models. These instruments have shown improved micromorphology and reduced osteotomized bone surface roughness compared to the standard rotating and sawing instruments. The implications of these findings are enormous; not just do they highlight the importance of precision in surgical procedures, but they also reflect improved bone healing and reossification, thereby maximizing the reconstructive process in cranio-facial surgery (Anesi et al., 2014). In addition to the reconstructive aspects, the application of fat grafting has emerged as a significant field of interest for enhancing aesthetic results following tumor removal. Autologous adipose tissue serves various purposes, including restoration of contour and volumetric support. However, challenges such as variability in long-term volume retention necessitate optimal knowledge of the factors controlling fat graft survival. Research on adipose tissue-derived stem cells (ASCs) has led to new techniques to improve outcomes. Enrichment of lipoaspirate with ASCs has been reported by studies to increase angiogenesis and viability of adipocytes, addressing the universal issue of graft resorption. With regard to these techniques, in addition to issues of oncological safety, a complex setting in which fat grafting can improve or complicate reconstruction (Vyas, 2016) is raised. It is important to address the subtleties of oncologic and cosmetic surgery simultaneously in order to provide the optimal patient outcome. Aesthetic enhancement versus oncologic safety is a compromise that must be made a priority, as evidenced by research and regulatory interest in the significance of ASCs for fat grafting. An integrated understanding of the interactions between cancer biology, surgical techniques, and tissue engineering techniques will guarantee future improvements in facial cosmetic surgery after a tumor. Therefore, the new paradigms in the specialty emphasize multidisciplinary approaches, integrating surgical innovation and oncologic precision to enhance quality of life in patients undergoing reconstructive surgery (Vyas, 2016).

KEY TERMS FROM THIS CHAPTER

- Tumor Resection
- Mohs Surgery
- Basal Cell Carcinoma
- Melanoma
- Local Flap
- Free Flap
- Skin Grafting
- Bone Reconstruction
- Margins of Excision
- Cutaneous Malignancy
- Squamous Cell Carcinoma
- Defect Reconstruction
- Regional Flap
- Microvascular Anastomosis
- Soft Tissue Reconstruction
- Functional Restoration

CRITICAL THINKING QUESTIONS

1. **The most common malignant tumor of the facial skin is:**
   a. Melanoma
   b. Basal cell carcinoma
   c. Squamous cell carcinoma
   d. Merkel cell carcinoma
2. **What is the most important consideration in reconstruction of nasal ala defects?**
   a. Skin color match
   b. Structural support restoration
   c. Scar position
   d. Donor site morbidity
3. **Which technique is considered the gold standard for margin control in facial skin cancer?**
   a. Wide excision
   b. Cryotherapy
   c. Mohs micrographic surgery
   d. Laser excision
4. **The primary goal of oncologic facial reconstruction is:**
   a. Aesthetic enhancement
   b. Functional restoration and cosmesis
   c. Immediate scar reduction
   d. Symmetry correction only
5. **A full-thickness defect of the lower eyelid is best reconstructed using:**
   a. Advancement flap
   b. Mustardé flap
   c. Hughes tarsoconjunctival flap
   d. Skin graft

Short Answer Questions

1. What are the primary goals of oncologic reconstruction in facial surgery?
2. Why is achieving clear surgical margins essential in facial tumor excision?
3. What makes Mohs micrographic surgery particularly suitable for facial skin cancers?
4. How does the location of a tumor influence the choice of reconstruction technique?
5. What factors determine whether a skin graft or a local flap is used after tumor removal?
6. What is the role of sentinel lymph node biopsy in the management of facial melanoma?
7. How does defect size affect reconstruction planning following tumor excision?

Answers to Critical Thinking Questions

1. (b) 2. (b) 3. (c) 4. (b) 5. (c)

REFERENCES

1. Accorona, R., Achena, A., Awny, S., Cremasco, et al. (2024). *Oral reconstruction with locoregional flaps after cancer ablation: A systematic review of the literature.* https://core.ac.uk/download/638813116.pdf (accessed on 14th July 2025).
2. Adams, N. J., Adrián, T. M., Allen, L. R., Arcelus, et al. (2022). *Standards of care for the health of transgender and gender diverse people, Version 8.* http://diposit.ub.edu/dspace/bitstream/2445/189561/1/Standards%20of%20Care%20for%20the%20Health%20of%20Transgender%20and%20Gender%20Diverse%20People%20Version%208.pdf (accessed on 14th July 2025).
3. Anderson, Asaoka, Berghaus, Booth, Coulson, Cross, Croxson, et al. (2012). *Re-animation and rehabilitation of the paralyzed face in head and neck cancer patients.* https://deepblue.lib.umich.edu/bitstream/2027.42/89486/1/21286_ftp.pdf (accessed on 14th July 2025).
4. Anesi, A., Cavani, F., Chiarini, L., Ferretti, et al. (2014). *Preliminary findings of a potenziated piezosurgical device at the rabbit skull.* https://core.ac.uk/download/80171725.pdf (accessed on 14th July 2025).
5. Arginelli, F., Bellini, P., Ferrari, B., Losi, et al. (2016). *Crescentic flap for the reconstruction of the nose after skin cancer resection.* https://core.ac.uk/download/84495439.pdf (accessed on 14th July 2025).
6. Bernal, J. G. T., Galindo, A. S., García, M. F. R., Javier, et al. (2024). *Advances in flap surgical techniques and regenerative approaches for reconstruction of extensive defects in cutaneous squamous cell carcinoma: A systematic review of functional and aesthetic outcomes.* https://core.ac.uk/download/635338710.pdf (accessed on 14th July 2025).
7. Cillino, M., Cordova, A., D'Arpa, S., Liuzza, et al. (2010). *Algorithm of partial breast reconstruction with pedicled perforator flaps.*2nd ITALIAN MEETING ON PERFORATOR FLAPS – Bologna, 26th-27th November 2010. ASTRACT BOOK Cured by: Dott.ssa Rossella Sgarzani Dott. Luca Negosanti brought to you by COREView metadata, citation and similar papers at core.ac.ukprovided by Archivio istituzionale della ricerca - Università di Palermo https://core.ac.uk/download/53293997.pdf (accessed on 14th July 2025).
8. Cortese, A., Chirico, F., Tartaro, G., Audino, G., Colella, G., Rugge, L., Sgaramella, N., et al. (2021). *Non-surgical touch-up with hyaluronic acid fillers following facial reconstructive surgery.* https://core.ac.uk/download/599516555.pdf (accessed on 14th July 2025).
9. Datarkar, A., Daware, S., & Khruomo, A. (2024). *Methods for functional and aesthetic rehabilitation of maxillectomy defect: A systematic review.* https://core.ac.uk/download/620836611.pdf (accessed on 14th July 2025).
10. de Bree, R., Ferlito, A., Olsen, K. D., Quer, et al. (2017). *Deep Lobe Parotidectomy—Why, When, and How?* https://core.ac.uk/download/604637332.pdf (accessed on 14th July 2025).
11. Garey, L., & Maillard, G. F. (2018). *Plastic Surgery After Ablative Cancer Surgery.* https://core.ac.uk/download/159156664.pdf (accessed on 14th July 2025).
12. Goldhirsch, A., Curigliano, G., Petit, J. Y., Rietjens, M., & Lohsiriwat, V. (2011). *Autologous fat transplantation in patients with breast cancer: Silencing or fueling cancer recurrence.* https://core.ac.uk/download/572847921.pdf (accessed on 14th July 2025).

13. Gonzaga, C. B., Glória Filho, E., Miqueloti, M. B., Freire, R. A. V., & Ribeiro, V. da S. A. (2019). *Scalp reconstruction after wide resection of an angiosarcoma*. https://core.ac.uk/download/587685526.pdf (accessed on 14th July 2025).
14. Lankage, D. L. M. (2023). *Factors influencing patient choice in type of breast reconstruction: A qualitative study*. https://core.ac.uk/download/571214680.pdf (accessed on 14th July 2025).
15. Deepak M. Kalaskar, Peter E. Butler, Shadi Ghali. (2016). *Textbook of Plastic and Reconstructive Surgery*. ISBN: 978-1-910634-37-0 (Hbk.) https://core.ac.uk/download/79526588.pdf
16. (accessed on 14th July 2025).
17. Ndongo, B. N., Mballa, G. A. E., Hyder, A. A., Juillard, et al. (2010). *Patterns of injury and violence in Yaoundé Cameroon: An analysis of hospital data*. https://core.ac.uk/download/323075033.pdf (accessed on 14th July 2025).
18. Vyas, K. S. (2016). *The role of fat grafting and adipose-derived stem cells in breast reconstruction*. https://core.ac.uk/download/232574356.pdf (accessed on 14th July 2025).

ADVANCES, TECHNOLOGIES, AND PRACTICE MANAGEMENT IN FACIAL COSMETIC

15

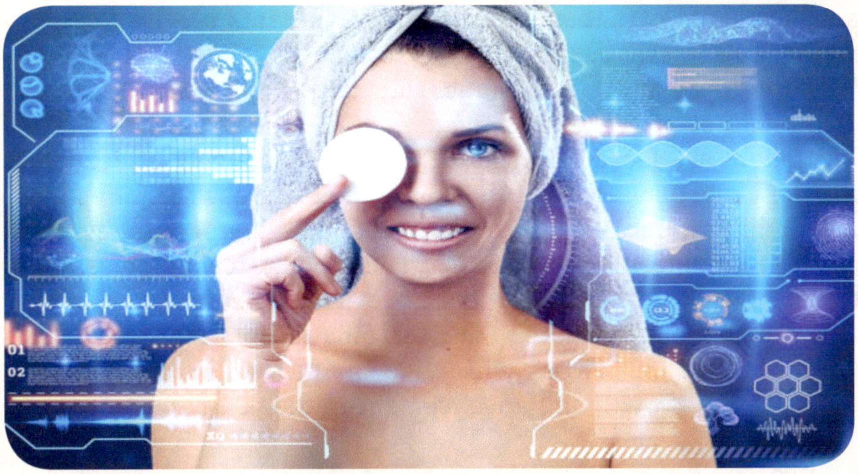

LEARNING OBJECTIVES

After studying this chapter, you will be able to:

1. Describe the historical perspective of facial cosmetics;
2. Highlight the latest technologies in facial cosmetics;
3. Define the non-surgical cosmetic treatments;
4. Discuss the surgical technological advances in facial cosmetics;
5. Comprehend practice management in cosmetic clinics;
6. Be familiar with regulatory and ethical considerations.

Introduction

Over the past decade, facial cosmetics have witnessed revolutionary advances fueled by the wave of technology innovation as well as changing consumer expectations. The use of cutting-edge technologies is transforming many facets of cosmetic procedures, from the formulation and application to overall effectiveness. From advanced imaging systems to nanotechnology, clinicians now have available to them technology that not only enhances the application process but also results in more targeted and effective outcomes. An important tendency in this area is the greater application of nanomaterials, which have emerged as the most important tools to prepare cosmetics and skincare products with improved penetration into the skin and with improved therapeutic effects. With the industry increasingly embracing such advancements, a certain understanding of their implications on practice management remains the utmost priority, so that practitioners can utilize such technologies effectively to meet the needs of their clients according to safety and efficacy parameters (Joseph et al., 2023). Furthermore, with the continuous advancements in facial cosmetics, practitioners are compelled to reconsider their management strategies in order to best capitalize on these developments. Effective practice management in today's world is necessitated by a comprehension of the technology landscape as well as consumer patterns. While minimally invasive facial treatments and personalized skincare regimes are on the rise, practitioners are presented with a complex landscape where exposure to newer technologies, including machine learning and artificial intelligence, becomes increasingly vital. These technologies facilitate evidence-based decision-making, allowing practitioners to tailor treatments to individual patients in a relevant manner. However, the implementation of such advanced technologies also calls for ongoing training and education for practitioners to ensure there is a dynamic and sensitized workforce that is capable of optimizing practice outcomes. With increasingly complex cosmetic treatments, practice management work in facilitating the integration of such advancements is fundamental to ensure patients receive the optimal quality of care (de Vries & Schallig, 2022). The destiny of facial cosmetics is also shaped by technological progress, as well as the importance of ethical practice and care for patients. With more access to aesthetic treatments, concerns over safety, effectiveness, and ethical marketing practices come into the limelight. Practitioners are faced with the dilemma of balancing ethical standards when promoting effective technology that benefits patients. This kind of approach requires constant dialogue among stakeholders, including researchers, practitioners, and regulatory bodies, to govern the changing landscape of cosmetic enhancement judiciously. Focusing on technological advancement and ethics, the application of facial cosmetics can continue in such a manner as to attain greater patient confidence and satisfaction. Ultimately, the combination of technology, practice management, and regulation in an ethical framework will guide the pace of innovation in this rapidly evolving domain towards sustained growth and advancement in the years to come.

Definition of Facial Cosmetics

Facial cosmetics form a broad range of cosmetic products and treatments intended to enhance or modify the appearance of an individual, primarily in the cosmetic definition of the face. This category includes items such as foundations, concealers, blush, eyeshadow, lipstick, and highlighters, which are applied to create a more enhanced natural appearance or totally transform one's look. The history of facial cosmetics dates back thousands of years, indicating a rich timeline reflecting cultural, social, and economic influences throughout the years. Thus, these products are not only tools of beautification but also symbols of identity and methods of self-expression, entrenched deeply in societal norms and expectations. In current practice, advances in formulation technology have enabled the production of lighter, longer-lasting, and more functional products that cater to diverse skin types and personal desires. The significance of face makeup extends far beyond simple enhancement; it plays a crucial role in one's self-esteem and social interactions. The psychological impact of cosmetics has long been established, linking the use of such products to enhanced confidence and self-image. Such is an indication of the intersection of individual identity and cultural norms of beauty standards. In an era where mass media and instantaneous visual information dominate the public sphere, the need for creative solutions in facial cosmetics has skyrocketed. Practitioners finding themselves in this environment need to comprehend the multiple layers of customer motivation to develop effective practice management techniques in the area of facial cosmetics. The responsiveness of the industry to customers' needs fuels constant innovation in product lines and educational initiatives, emphasizing the need for a balanced approach towards satisfaction and loyalty in customers. Advances in the IoT space have also witnessed the infusion of technology in the domain of facial cosmetics, making it not just easier to develop products but also providing for bespoke experiences for customers. Technologies such as augmented reality applications allow consumers to experiment with products virtually prior to purchase, thus transforming the shopping experience. Moreover, the sustainability and clean beauty trend has compelled cosmetic businesses to rethink ingredients and production, emphasizing safe, eco-friendly products that cater to enlightened consumers (Boyen et al., 2025). With a changing market, professionals must be adaptable and aware of these trends to maintain competitiveness. Through exposure to scientific research and consumer feedback, professionals will not only be enriching their product knowledge but will also become contributory forces for shaping the future of facial cosmetics and creating a more embracing and innovative industry landscape (Kivnick et al., 2014) (Figure 15.1).

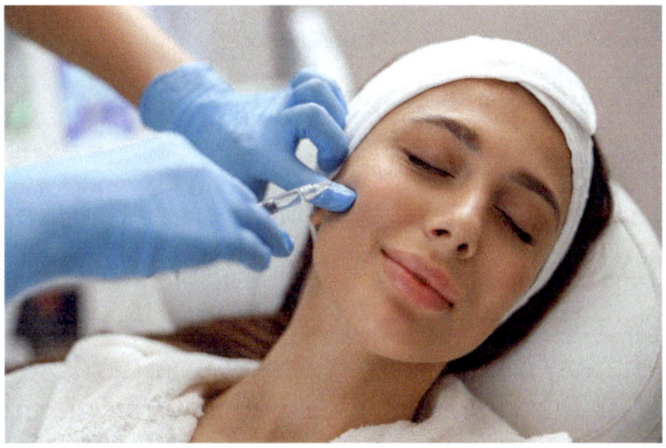

Figure 15.1. Woman getting injection in her face at plastic surgery.

Source: https://virginiaoralsurgeryspecialists.com/wp-content/uploads/2022/07/woman-getting-injection-in-her-face-at-plastic-sur-2022-04-05-15-41-43-utc-scaled.jpg.

Importance of Advances in Technology

The rapid speed of technology has a determining role in reshaping the facial cosmetic scene, both by making treatment more efficient and the information more accessible to the consumer. Advances in non-surgical cosmetic treatments, such as laser therapy and injectable fillers, are an incredible shift towards safer, more effective alternatives to traditional surgery. The integration of advanced technologies has decreased recovery times and lowered risks, appealing to increasingly educated patient groups that value efficacy and safety. Further, patients utilizing extensive information resources on cosmetic procedures have a greater satisfaction rate and increased self-confidence following treatment, emphasizing the value of educated decision-making within this evolving environment (Reisenwitz & Fowler, 2021). This access fuels not only consumer trust but also a competitive marketplace, placing technological advancement as a central component among practice management strategies for cosmetic practitioners. Technological advancements also provide invaluable tools for marketing and patient engagement in the facial cosmetics marketplace. Creating platforms for social media marketing and virtual consultations enables an instant line of contact between practitioners and potential clients, promoting new procedures and in-the-moment results. This shift toward web engagement is reflective of changing consumer sentiment, particularly among newer generations that are inherently predisposed toward online information and visual content. Notably, patients who embrace the full continuum of accessible cosmetic information have proven to possess a reduced cognitive age and greater response to targeted marketing efforts, further highlighting the importance of technology strategy implementation (Reisenwitz & Fowler., 2021). The combined use of technology and aesthetics brings to life a colorful marketing world, where offices are in a position to effectively establish brand loyalty and have a steady stream of clients. Moreover, the interplay of developments in artificial intelligence (AI) and the visualization of aesthetic treatments has become a revolutionary aspect of office management. Immersive systems utilizing AI-generated images produce tailor-made experiences for prospective patients, allowing decision-making to be streamlined from a previously uncertain process. Considering AI-generated images portrays how these technologies can reaffirm or complicate gender stereotypes and norms in the beauty industry. This advanced sensitivity to the visual representation is in harmony with broader social trends and facilitates the practitioner's role in promoting varied and inclusive concepts of beauty. As technology further improves, its impact on practice management in facial cosmetics will increasingly become more profound, allowing more individualized and efficient care while adapting to the more diverse source base of client populations (Figure 15.2).

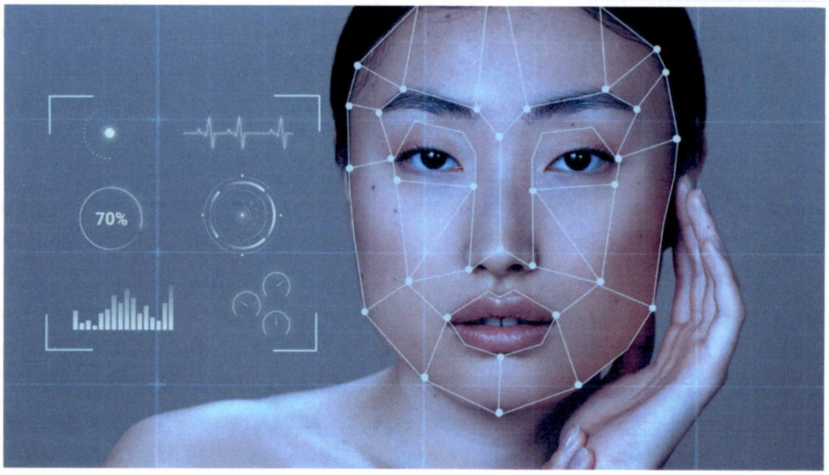

Figure 15.2. Evolution of technology in reshaping the landscape of facial cosmetics.

Source: https://sprivil.com/wp-content/uploads/2025/01/2150038888-1.webp.

Overview of Practice Management in the Industry

Successful practice management in the facial cosmetics sector is more necessary than ever with technology and innovation development altering consumer needs and industry standards. The integration of management strategies within practices in the cosmetic field is closely connected to the enhanced quality of services provided. With the competition that now exists in clinics, the implementation of holistic systems of practice management that include scheduling appointments, patient communication, and data management has become unavoidable. By streamlining operations as well as adopting patient-centered approaches, practitioners can enhance client relationships, hence achieving maximum patient satisfaction and loyalty. On foundations established within other sectors, for instance, marine research as defined by the Marine Board, the cosmetic sector can borrow such common ground to identify best practices that eventually enhance both clinical efficacy and business acumen (Boyen et al., 2025). Furthermore, evolving perspectives of aesthetic treatments compel practitioners to adapt to technological advancements to ensure effective management. Technologies such as telemedicine, emerging imaging technology, and online marketing technology make up invaluable devices to enhance cosmetic practice operational capability. With the application of these technologies, practitioners are in a position to offer bespoke solutions that meet unique client needs, establishing a new platform for client engagement and retention. But the test comes in reconciling potential ethical challenges concerning consumer perceptions and commercialization, most importantly, that of reconciling best practices with the way brand identity is represented. This is all within broader corporate branding concerns where corporations must considerably connect their practices to community norms and expectations without compromising ethical standards (Avery et al., 2007). Lastly, facial cosmetic practice management is an intricate ballet of clinical excellence, technology integration, and moral practice. On one hand, practitioners hone their technique through comments received from consumers and industry norms, yet they must also stay abreast of the swift rate of aesthetic advancement by virtue of continuous education and workforce development. Their success is not just dependent on clinical skill but also on the synergistic application of management theory that builds a positive work environment and enhances the patient experience. As we examine the intersection of technology innovation with successful practice management, it is certain that the future of the business will be shaped by those who prioritize a balanced and ethical strategy for the provision of cosmetic care.

15.1. Historical Context of Facial Cosmetics

Learning Outcome

1. Evolution of Cosmetic Practices
2. Key Milestones in Cosmetic Technology
3. Focus on Cultural Influences on Cosmetic Use

The history of facial cosmetics starts way back in ancient times, when the use of paraphernalia was not merely for beauty but also took on cultural and social functions. In Ancient Egypt, for instance, cosmetics were applied by both men and women as a protection against the intense sun, as well as for ritual purposes. Khol and face paints were common, symbolizing status and a deity figure. As societies progressed towards the Greco-Roman era, cosmetic applications rose because of the influence of class divisions. The elite would depict elaborate face makeup, whereas societal opinions started blending beauty with morality. Thus, the history of cosmetics reflects the positive tension between utilitarian functionality and cultural values and results in modern practices of facial cosmetics that are prompted by aesthetic necessity and deep societal consequences. The Renaissance was a turning point in beauty's understanding with the development of art and philosophy, defining the finer points of cosmetic use. It was also during this time that the beautified image of womanhood arose, and with it, facial cosmetics multiplied within the affluent classes. Ingredients like lead powders and vivid pigments came to symbolize beauty, though at a cost to health. This was a time of opulent depictions of beauty within works of art, and it strengthened the view that cosmetics were used to express social standing and identity. These historical changes highlight the inherent richness of cosmetic practices and herald an evolution that continued through into the Enlightenment, eventually providing the foundations for the commodified beauty industry that exists today. As the modern period progressed, advances in industry created major changes in the production and availability of cosmetics. The late 19th and early 20th centuries saw the emergence of brands that capitalized on the beauty revolution, transitioning cosmetics from homemade concoctions to mass-produced goods. Innovations in marketing, inclusive of widely circulated advertisements, began linking cosmetics to notions of modernity and empowerment, thus reshaping societal standards. Furthermore, movements advocating for women's rights intertwined with beauty norms, revealing a unique relationship between empowerment and appearance. The rich negotiation of such themes, coupled with the commercialization of beauty, directs consideration toward how long-standing facial cosmetics history continues to be underpinned by changing historical context, reflecting complex social narratives and shaping practice management in the field today (Avery et al., 2007; Garrisi et al., 2018) (Figure 15.3).

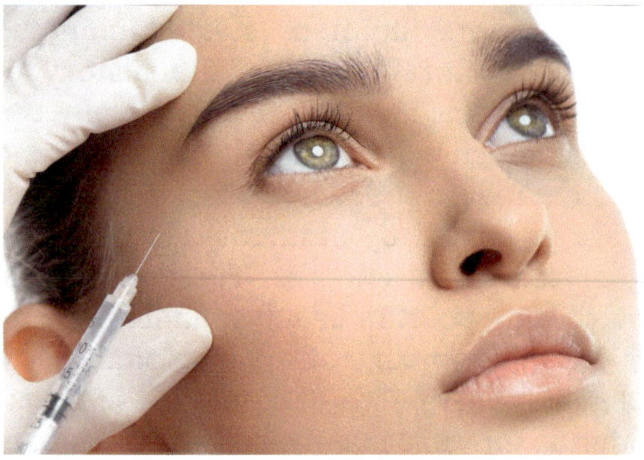

Figure 15.3. Historical evolution of facial cosmetics.

Source: https://hedoxclinic.co.uk/wp-content/uploads/2021/02/botox-1024x680.jpg.

15.1.1. Evolution of Cosmetic Practices

The evolutionary history of cosmetic practices has witnessed substantial changes, particularly since the advent of advanced technologies and techniques. Conventional cosmetics comprised mostly natural substances, such as minerals and plant extracts, applied for beautification and social communication. With the progress of societies, so evolved the cosmetic techniques and ingredients, culminating in synthetic products. This shift was driven by a demand for range, affordability, and durability, allowing cosmetic corporations to sell to a broader segment. The introduction of chemical technologies during the latter 20th century, as well as the worldwide homogenization of beauty standards, triggered the increase in product complexity and diversity that eventually reshaped assumptions regarding efficacy and safety. This continuous development is a reflection not just of progress in technology but also of greater convergence between culture and personal identity in shaping cosmetics, marking a distinct watershed in the art of facial aesthetics. Practice of cosmetic procedures has expanded dramatically in recent years with impetus coming from advances in non-surgical aesthetics (NSA). The growing popularity of minimally invasive procedures, such as dermal fillers and Botox, is symptomatic of a consumer preference for subtle enhancement over mainstream surgery. All of these developments allow for tailored alterations with less downtime, and prioritize above all safety and convenience. But the rapid growth of NSA procedures has raised training and standardization concerns across the industry. As described in research dedicated to the necessity for a well-structured postgraduate program in NSA, there is a strong need for complex education and training systems to equip practitioners with skills and knowledge to deliver these techniques correctly. The growth of such educational platforms is a reflection of the dynamic nature of cosmetic procedures and the importance of evidence-based education in delivering quality patient outcomes amidst this dynamism (Kumar, 2021). Along with procedural development, technology infusion in cosmetic procedures also encompasses marketing and patient management. Social media has transformed consumer engagement, with individuals being able to influence trends and make products popular. This shift demands that cosmetic professionals embrace electronic tools not only for marketing but also to educate patients and manage post-treatment. Additionally, using data analytics in practice management simplifies clinical operations, leading to better patient outcomes through individualized treatment protocols. With the rising need for cosmetic treatments, it is important that one addresses cosmetic practice management with a strategic plan encompassing clinical competency and effective communication skills. With such an interdisciplinary approach , practitioners are well-positioned to address the challenges in the current cosmetic age, rendering patient satisfaction and safety as the utmost concern of practice (Boyen et al., 2025) (Figure 15.4).

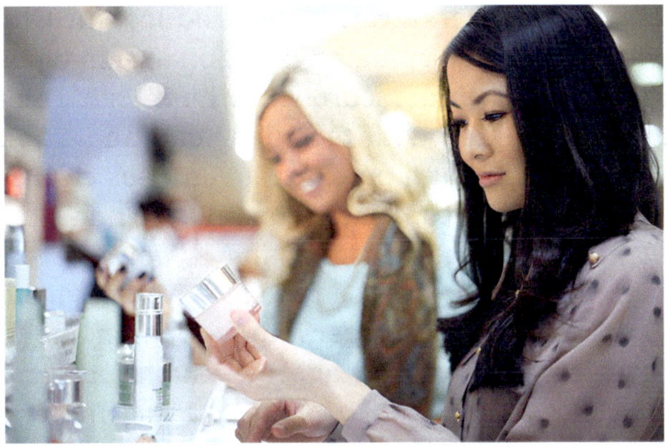

Figure 15.4. Cosmetic practices.

Source: https://mscosmeticslab.com/wp-content/uploads/2024/07/gettyimages-171278045-170667a-1-2.jpg.

15.1.2. Key Milestones in Cosmetic Technology

Evolution in cosmetic technology has been marked by some significant milestones that have had an overwhelming influence on facial cosmetics. One of the most significant has been the coming of minimally invasive treatment, which promoted a shift in public perception towards aesthetic treatments. This has been particularly realized in the popularity of injectable treatments like Botox and dermal fillers. Not only do these treatments provide instant gratification, but they also offer faster recovery times, making cosmetic treatments more affordable to more individuals. Further, advances in the formulation and delivery of cosmetic active ingredients enabled a better understanding of how the product would interact with skin appearance and health. These advancements have hastened consumer buying of products that provide transformational effects while, at the same time, enhancing overall skin health, thus merging beauty and health in new ways. Another trend in the cosmetic industry is the formulation of non-surgical aesthetic (NSA) treatments, which mark a dramatic shift away from traditional surgical alternatives towards less intrusive solutions. The increasing popularity of NSA treatments has required the development of official training and education programs tailored specifically to these technologies. While the integration of NSA training within postgraduate clinical education has been challenging, efforts to develop an evidence-based curriculum have been robust. This move toward formal education is a sign of the mounting appreciation for NSAs role within the cosmetic industry.

Programs that focus on standardized assessment techniques, such as the objective structured practical examination (OSPE) and the objective structured clinical examination (OSCE), have been effective in improving practitioners' training. Such models of learning provide necessary skills and knowledge that are relevant in a dynamically changing industry, ensuring safe and effective practices for patients. The use of digital technologies in cosmetic practice is a sea change that shifts the manner in which practitioners engage with patients and provide their services. The arrival of virtual and augmented reality in the cosmetic consultation field allows patients to preview how they might appear post-treatment, leading to better-informed choices. Simulations of procedures in real time reduce fear and enhance satisfaction with the chosen treatment. Furthermore, advancements in data analysis contribute to the robustness of practice management, enabling clinics to learn better about treatment effectiveness, patient needs, and market trends. Through this method of analysis, customized treatment plans are achieved, with services being adjusted to suit patients' needs and maximize success rates. As thus cosmetic technology continues to evolve, the inclusion of new treatments and efficient practice management becomes increasingly important in adapting to changes in the industry (Figure 15.5).

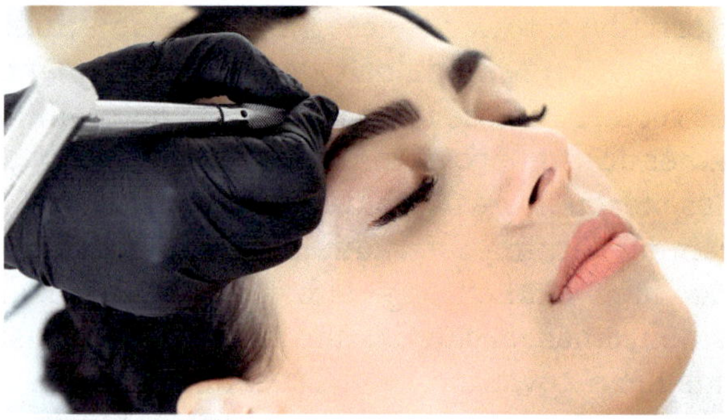

Figure 15.5. Cosmetic technology.

Source: https://soulskinclinic.com/wp-content/uploads/2022/11/Micro-Blading-2.webp.

15.1.3. Cultural Influences on Cosmetic Use

Cultural influences significantly affect the use and perception of cosmetic products, and they become an integral part of societal norms and identity. Beauty standards in other societies are typically dictated by economics, history, and society. For instance, in the majority of Western nations, youthfulness is the preferred norm, and due to this, there has been an increase in the demand for anti-aging treatments and products. Contrastingly, there have been Asian cultures where the desire for light skin has continued the use of whitening creams and sunblock. These are not shallow beauty standards; they affect individuals' self-esteem and can drive their choice concerning the use of cosmetics. Knowing the cultural dimensions is of utmost importance to facial cosmetic practitioners because it forms the basis of effective marketing and the development of suitable products for target consumer groups. The cosmetic industry has come to further realize the importance of cultural narratives, and this has witnessed an explosion of products that cater to diverse beauty standards. Such an adaptation stems from a recognition of diverse cultural worldviews regarding aesthetics, which can drive purchasing habits strongly. For example, increased campaigns for inclusive beauty have led to the diversification of product lines by brands to reflect a greater variation in skin types and colors. It underscores how appreciation of culture, coupled with technological innovation in formulation and production, enables clearer alignment with consumer demands. In addition, with digital platforms making it possible for beauty trends to diffuse quickly—ranging from social media influencers to virtual makeup products in the metaverse—such cultural influences continue to change. Practitioners, have to remain vigilant to such changes to be able to manage product innovation and marketing strategies capable of communicating effectively with current consumer emotions (Damar, 2022).

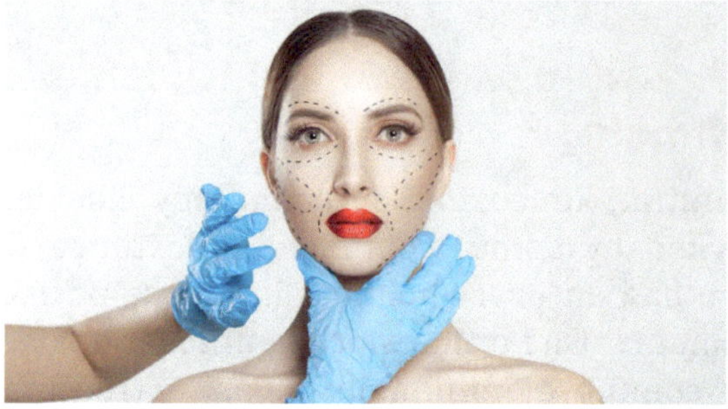

Figure 15.6. Cultural influences on cosmetic use.

Source: https://external-content.duckduckgo.com/iu/?u=https%3A%2F%2Fbioscops.com%2Fwp-content%2Fuploads%2F2024%2F10%2FCultural-Influences-on-Modern-Cosmetic-Surgery-Trends.webp&f=1&nofb=1&ipt=c8b9075f2a2ae00c402d04bda3a937826a94438754ae11d0b151aa79c8293922.

The intersection of such cultural influences with modern technology also offers new possibilities for the cosmetic industry. Artificial intelligence advancements, for example, enable the offering of tailored experiences in cosmetic use, tailoring products to individual preferences based on culture. AI can identify consumer trends and tastes across various populations and thereby inform product innovation and niche marketing. Coupling augmented reality capability enables consumers to try cosmetic products virtually, enhancing their shopping experience and inducing trial over cultural divides. These technologies are particularly relevant when it comes to globalization, where cultural exchanges introduce new standards and practices of beauty. Cosmetic practitioners, therefore, must engage with such technologies in mind while being sensitive to culture, so that the products and services they offer resonate closely with their multicultural clientele (Kazimierczak et al., 2024) (Figure 15.6).

Test Your Knowledge

1. What are some key milestones in the evolution of cosmetic technology throughout history?
2. How have cultural and societal influences shaped the use of facial cosmetics in different regions?
3. Describe the major historical developments that contributed to modern facial cosmetic practices.

15.2. Current Technologies in Facial Cosmetics

Learning Outcome

1. Understand Innovations in Cosmetic Formulations
2. Focus on Advances in Application Techniques
3. Discuss the Role of Digital Technology in Cosmetic Design

The development of current technologies in facial makeup has allowed a transformation of the way consumers perceive and consume these products. Through the integration of artificial intelligence and machine learning, companies in the beauty industry are now able to personalize their suggestions based on the individual's skin tone, skin type, and personal preferences. Such a customized approach not only enhances the level of user satisfaction but also promotes a self-interactive consumption. Such technologies encompass augmented reality (AR) technology, whereby customers are able to try out products virtually prior to buying them, bridging the gap between physical and web stores. Uptake of such leading-edge tools is part of a broader trend among the cosmetic industry toward personalization to meet the range of needs consumers have, so the products resonate on a deeper level, resulting in increased sales and brand loyalty. Moreover, nanotechnology application in skin cosmetics has provided new avenues of product performance and safety. Nanoparticles are used in products more frequently to enable increased penetration and absorption that lead to more effective delivery of active ingredients to the skin. It allows the development of light, fast-absorbing products that provide amazing results without interfering with the health of the skin. However, as paramount in recent studies, the use of nanoparticles also necessitates a thorough understanding of their possible toxicity and environmental impact, thus sparking ongoing research in their long-term effects on human health and the environment (Joseph et al., 2023). As the industry progresses, the prudent balancing of innovation and safety will be crucial in guaranteeing consumer trust and sustainable growth. Furthermore, with the development of biotechnological advancements, the formulation of cosmetic products has also evolved, with much focus on ethicality and sustainability. The majority of brands today utilize bioengineered ingredients that are able to mimic the performance of traditional cosmetics while reducing reliance on non-renewable sources. This not only responds to the consumer's demand for green products but also demonstrates the growing concern regarding the ecological impact of the cosmetics sector. Advances such as gene editing and cellular agriculture are unveiling possibilities for sustainable manufacturing, aligning with global sustainability goals. With continuous innovation in the sector, such technological advancements have the potential to reorient standards and shift norms within the realm of cosmetic formulation (de Vries & Schallig, 2022) (Figure 15.7).

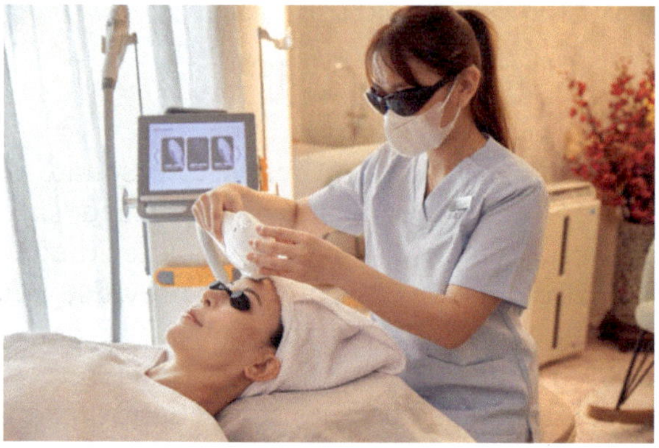

Figure 15.7. Current technologies in facial cosmetics.

Source: https://kellyoriental.com/wp-content/uploads/2022/05/Facial-600x400.jpg.

15.2.1. Innovations in Cosmetic Formulations

The cosmetic formulation history has been strongly impacted by the introduction of nonsurgical facial rejuvenation treatments. Increased public demand for these noninvasive procedures has led to revolutionary breakthroughs in product development and technological advancement. In the past decade, there has been an increase in treatment modalities for cosmetic professionals, in large part due to the inception of botulinum toxin and a variety of dermal fillers. As referenced in Bowler et al. (2009), the facial rejuvenation market has altered with increased physicians providing these treatments to address rising demand. This evolution has also impacted the behavior of consumers and compelled the medical community to embrace and advance their methods of cosmetic improvement, with the ultimate result being an enhanced understanding of the subtleties in facial appearance. Among the cosmetic innovations, the most prevalent and successful method for managing facial aging has been hyaluronic acid (HA) dermal fillers. Time impacts the aging process by inducing various cellular and anatomical changes that lead to a reduction in soft tissue volume, as elaborated in Brandt et al. (2008).

HA filler development has revolutionized the treatment of these aging changes among medical professionals, shifting the way they craft facial contouring. Hyaluronic acid's unique properties, including its amazing water-binding ability, make it an amazing treatment for plumping and shaping the face. These types of fillers are a safe, temporary solution that allows clients to achieve their desired aesthetic outcome without the downtime and hassles of surgery. To this, the use of HA fillers has been majorly fueled by demographics, namely the baby-boomer generation. This group has a desperate desire to appear "young" and yet still live an active life; thus, safe and effective cosmetic products are more desirable than ever. Eight HA dermal fillers are now approved by the Food and Drug Administration for sale in the United States, and this represents growing acceptance and use of these new products in facial aesthetics. As noted by Brandt et al. (2008), HA product futures look promising, and research on further improving their performance and expanding their applications for facial rejuvenation continues. Practice management and client expectations, therefore, will be affected by advances in cosmetic formulations in the ever-evolving realm of facial cosmetics (Figure 15.8).

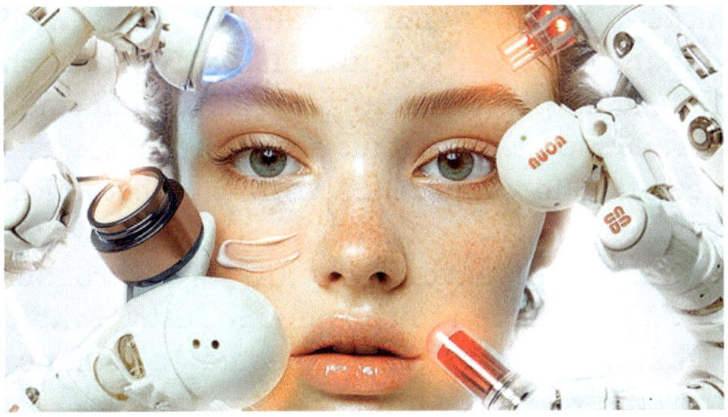

Figure 15.8. Cosmetic formulations.

Source: https://img.gcimagazine.com/files/base/allured/all/image/2025/01/Head_Banner_Pic.677c19bd73e8d.png?auto=format%2Ccompress&q=70&w=700.

15.2.2. Advances in Application Techniques

The evolution of application techniques in facial cosmetics has revolutionarily transformed the industry, enhancing product functionality and presentation. Previously, application techniques were rudimentary, resulting in uneven results or a weird look. Nowadays, advanced developments have initiated a variety of new tools and techniques that not only enhance user experience but also support a variety of skin types and preferences. For instance, technological improvements in airbrushes now allow for a smooth finish that simulates natural skin texture and also buildable coverage. Furthermore, application methods such as baking and strobing are now popular, allowing individuals to achieve radiant skin or long-lasting makeup, respectively. Such innovations encourage an independent approach to beauty, allowing individuals to embrace their unique features while at the same time enhancing their overall look. Moreover, where cosmetics have converged with technology, a new age of application methods has arisen in the form of online platforms. Augmented reality (AR) technology and Android apps allow consumers to test products virtually prior to purchasing, making product selection efficient without causing dissatisfaction. Not only does this technological advance revolutionize the buying process of consumers but also provides brands with more efficient means of engaging with consumers. By providing detailed lessons and instant feedback, these apps foster a culture of self-enablement and makeup application skill development. Moreover, business houses have started using data analytics to refine their offerings and fine-tune marketing to make them more targeted, ensuring they are aligned with shifting consumer preferences and tastes.

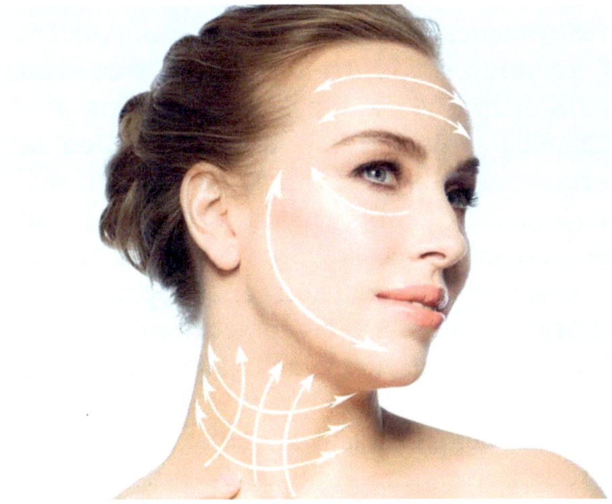

Figure 15.9. Application techniques in facial cosmetics.

Source: https://iicad.org/wp-content/uploads/2024/06/IICAD-Mumbai-1-1200x600.png.

More sustainable practice in the business has also influenced application trends, compelling brands to become innovative for the eco-conscious consumer. Waste-reducing methods—reusable applicators and refillable containers—are on the rise. This not only addresses the environmental concern, but it also encourages a more mindful approach to beauty treatments. While companies are striving to decrease their impact, eco-friendly application methods take center stage, creating a sense of responsibility among consumers, now better informed about the impact of their actions. In addition, the use of educational content on sustainable use in product advertising raises responsible consumption significance, therefore brand loyalty and consumer accountability. With these new ways, the facial cosmetic industry is technical as well as ethical in orientation, with a thorough change in practice management (Figure 15.9).

15.2.3. Role of Digital Technology in Cosmetic Design

In the practice of cosmetic design, the application of technology is transforming traditional methods into vibrant, precise ones. One of the technologies that has empowered cosmetic artists to create very detailed and personalized designs to a high degree of precision is computer-aided design (CAD). This allows for a smooth synthesis of creative imagination and technological innovation, elevating the practice within facial cosmetics. Furthermore, augmented reality (AR) technologies enable clients to visualize possible outcomes before actually undergoing procedures. Through the simulation of various cosmetic procedures in a virtual environment, clients are more confident in their choices, resulting in a generally improved experience. The use of digital technologies not only streamlines the design process but also allows practitioners to refine their skills, offering customized solutions that respond to the diverse needs of their patients, a reflection of the evolving world of facial cosmetic treatments. The use of developments in artificial intelligence (AI) also plays an important role in shaping cosmetic design. Using machine learning algorithms and deep learning models, AI can learn from large sets of facial images and derive personalized traits and suggest best cosmetic treatments. In oral and maxillofacial (OMF) cosmetic surgery, specifically, AI assists in preoperative planning and prediction of outcomes, optimizing the surgeon's ability and minimizing risks with human analysis. The increasing reliance on AI readies practitioners for making informed therapeutic decisions, thus ensuring the aesthetic ideals are in congruence with the anatomical features of each patient. This shift towards digital intelligence is typical of a broader paradigm within the cosmetic industry, where technology is not only expected to enhance procedural efficacy but also has a primary role to play in issues of ethical importance about patient information and treatment transparency, such as in emerging technologies applied in medical practice (Rokhshad et al., 2023). Of greater significance is that the development of the metaverse represents an epoch-changing platform for the integration of digital technology and cosmetic design.

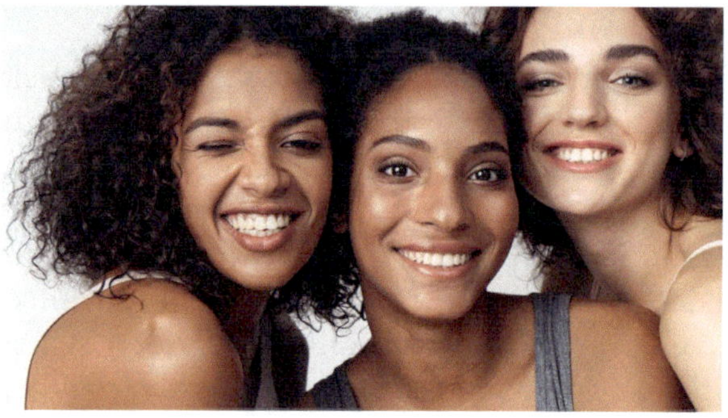

Figure 15.10. Role of digital technology in cosmetic design.

Source: https://www.thequeenzone.com/wp-content/uploads/2024/11/gorgeous-woman.-Dean-Drobot-via-Shutterstock.jpg.

With the application of virtual reality (VR) and augmented reality (AR), the metaverse offers unprecedented opportunities for immersive client consultations and interactive learning opportunities for professionals. With clients engaging with avatars that display their potential cosmetic outcomes within an imaginary space, they are able to explore many design options in real time, thus helping them make more informed decisions on their cosmetic journey.

This innovation extends beyond client consultation, with metaverse platforms being used by health practitioners to simulate training, refining their techniques in a risk-free environment. With recent technological advances, incorporating metaverse elements into the cosmetic design process represents a significant shift in practice management, with increased client satisfaction and improved surgical outcomes on the horizon (Damar, 2022) (Figure 15.10).

Test Your Knowledge

1. What recent innovations in cosmetic formulations have improved efficacy and safety in facial cosmetics?
2. How have advances in application techniques enhanced precision and outcomes in cosmetic procedures?
3. What role does digital technology play in modern cosmetic design and treatment planning?

15.3. Non-Surgical Cosmetic Procedures

Learning Outcome

1. Overview of Popular Non-Surgical Treatments
2. Focus on Safety and Efficacy of Non-Surgical Options
3. Explain Patient Satisfaction and Outcomes

The rising popularity of non-surgical cosmetic treatments is an overall trend toward beautification with minimal recovery time and risk. Treatments such as dermal fillers, Botox injections, and chemical peels are now routine, as individuals desire subtle but noticeable changes. The treatments have many benefits, including immediate results, less risk than surgical procedures, and relatively low costs. Consequently, practitioners in the main are faced with more demand from patients starved for rejuvenation but not with the burden of traditional surgical interventions. Besides, faster developments in formulations of products, methods of application, and delivery systems have entrenched non-surgical options firmly as viable alternatives, thereby altering the landscape of facial aesthetics entirely. Increased availability and popularity of such treatments reflect their pivotal role in the beauty standards today, in support of the contention that patients are able to achieve desired outcomes more easily than ever before. In addition to their functional uses, technological improvements have spawned enormous innovation in the field of non-surgical cosmetic therapy. Non-invasive treatments like laser treatment and ultrasound treatments use innovative mechanisms to enhance the quality of skin, reduce the perceptibility of wrinkles, and stimulate collagen production. These techniques take advantage of innovations like nanotechnology to target drugs at the intended locations and maximize therapeutic impacts, thereby enhancing the effectiveness of interventions (Joseph et al., 2023). Furthermore, the incorporation of 3D printing technologies has already begun transforming practice management through the capability for printing patient-specific models for pre-procedure simulation and planning. This incorporation enhances efficiency and outcome while showing remarkable synergy between technology and non-surgical care. With professionals embracing such advances, patients benefit from enhanced procedural tailoring, which equates to improved satisfaction as well as superior aesthetic results. Despite the rapid expansion and demand for non-surgical cosmetic treatments, there are still a few issues within the practice management space. Some of the practitioners hurrying to be in the business might be unaware of regulating and ethics requirements, which are indispensable to ensure patient safety and satisfaction as well. Additional training in the existing technologies, techniques, and materials required to maintain high-quality care is the success factor. As new emerging solutions and technologies arise, healthcare practitioners will be required to catch up with trends that might affect the outcome of procedures, such as the expansion of personalized treatments, driven by advancements in 3D printing and enhanced imaging (Meyer-Szary et al., 2022). Developing an ethic of continuous learning and adaptation is therefore necessary for practitioners who will be capable of effectively handling the complexities in non-surgical cosmetic practice. This focused approach will not only improve the safety and satisfaction of patients but will also maintain the professionalism and credibility of the aesthetics field (Figure 15.11).

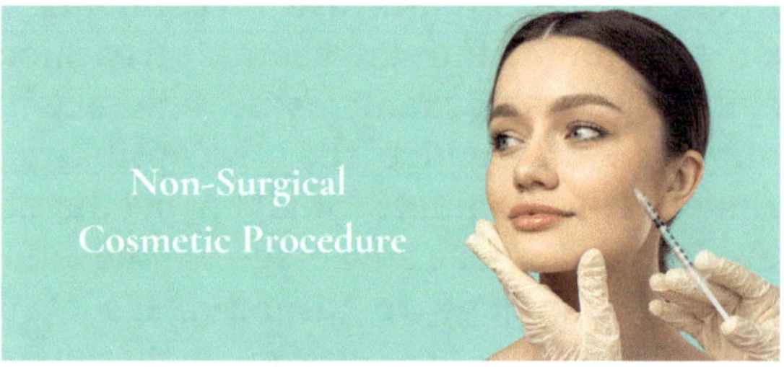

Figure 15.11. Non-surgical cosmetic procedures.

Source: https://drlouisedelange.com/wp-content/uploads/2025/03/BLOG-DE-LANGE-1.png.

15.3.1. Overview of Popular Non-Surgical Treatments

In the practice of facial cosmetics, non-surgical treatments have become extremely popular, allowing patients to avail themselves of techniques to enhance their appearance without going through invasive surgeries. Among the most popular treatments are injectable applications, such as botulinum toxin and dermal fillers. Minimal and brief in application, these procedures take little to no downtime, thereby making them highly desirable for a broad population. Botulinum toxin relaxes facial muscles to the point of reducing the appearance of dynamic wrinkles, while dermal fillers replace contour and volume in areas that have been changed by age. These treatments not only treat beauty but also fit into an expanding societal emphasis on self-improvement and maintenance, validating the role of non-surgical interventions in contemporary cosmetic care. Another novel non-surgical facial rejuvenation method is photodynamic therapy (PDT), which takes advantage of the interaction between light and photosensitizers to treat a range of skin disorders. PDT is increasingly known for its utility in the treatment of precancerous cells, sun-damaged skin, and even acne, demonstrating its versatility. With its ability to facilitate targeted cell destruction while modulating the immune response, PDT has become a holistic therapeutic avenue in dermatology. As the ease of delivery of treatment increases, so too can the dermatologist easily offer PDT as an option, thereby facilitating the patient experience by means of non-invasive treatment. This greater acceptance of PDT by the cosmetic industry is reflective of a shift towards the introduction of advanced applications of technology to face treatments, emphasizing the demand for non-surgical methods of present-day care. In addition, LED-red light therapy is also attracting interest for its ability to modulate cellular activity in skin fibrosis, a source of concern for most patients who receive facial cosmetic procedures. The efficacy of LED-RL has already been depicted in preliminary clinical trials of minimizing post-surgical scarring, which indicates its promise as an adjuvant treatment in cosmetic care. Harnessing specific wavelengths of light to control fibroblast activity and collagen production, LED-RL provides a new, non-invasive therapeutic modality for enhancing the quality of postoperative outcomes. Beyond cosmetics, its potential is to improve skin quality in general as well as the healing process. As is confirmed in studies, integration of LED-RL into cosmetic treatment regimens can potentially pave the way for setting the trend for elevated standards of facial appearance, affirming the paradigm shift towards non-surgical, safer procedures while focusing on both outcome and patient well-being (Heilman et al., 2019; Lin et al., 2014) (Figure 15.12).

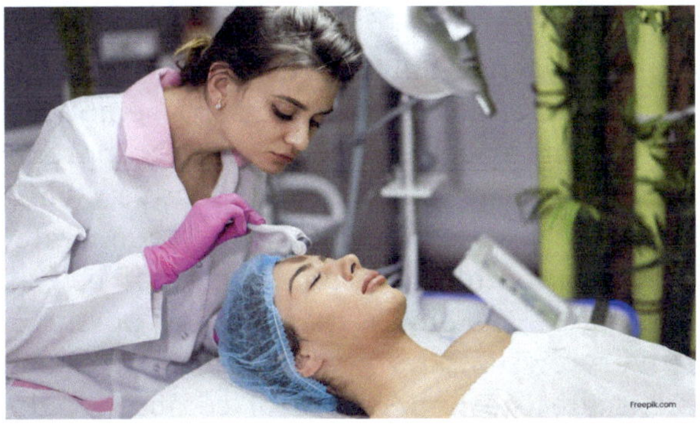

Figure 15.12. Popular non-surgical treatments.

Source: https://www.osvidermatology.com/wp-content/uploads/2023/11/advance-treatment.jpg.

15.3.2. Safety and Efficacy of Non-Surgical Options

The revelation of non-surgical modalities in facial cosmetics has gained popularity on a wide scale due to their safety and efficiency in enhancing quality without the dangers associated with surgery. Techniques such as dermal fillers, neurotoxin injections, and platelet-rich plasma (PRP) therapy are now highly demanded alternatives that promise rejuvenation with less downtime.

The efficacy of treatments like these is pointed out by their ability to create focused results, such as wrinkle relaxation and volume increase, while reducing recovery times traditionally required by surgical interventions. As observed in recent studies, non-surgical interventions have been shown to have a significant impact on patient satisfaction and aesthetic results, thus being valid choices in modern-day facial cosmetic treatment, where client safety and natural results remain priorities. Particularly, PRP therapy is gaining popularity for its diverse applications in cosmetic dermatology. With the application of the body's own inherent healing process, PRP enhances the skin texture, promotes hair growth, and accelerates the wound healing process.

Because PRP employs the patient's own plasma, it is less likely to cause any harmful reactions, thus possessing a good safety profile. Current literature points to its application not just in improving the appearance of the skin but also in treating chronic wounds and reversing aging skin. With an understanding of the mechanism of PRP being augmented, its utilization in aesthetics has continued to rise, underlining the importance of evidence-based practices in ensuring safety and efficacy in non-surgical aesthetic interventions (Patel et al., 2023). Although generally there is less danger of complications linked with non-surgical treatments than with surgery, it is nonetheless required to answer to the regulatory and technological frameworks that govern their administration.

The Food and Drug Administration (FDA) has established stringent standards for medical treatments and devices, developing a whole process for the regulation and approval of non-surgical cosmetic therapies. This rule seeks to guarantee that the devices used in such therapies are effective and safe. In addition, with emerging technology, innovations such as artificial intelligence and Internet of Things (IoT) are revolutionizing practice management by allowing practitioners to use data-driven intelligence to advance patient care (Tettey et al., 2023). By keeping an eye on the regulatory framework and adopting innovation, practitioners can significantly enhance the safety and efficacy of non-surgical procedures in facial cosmetology (Figure 15.13).

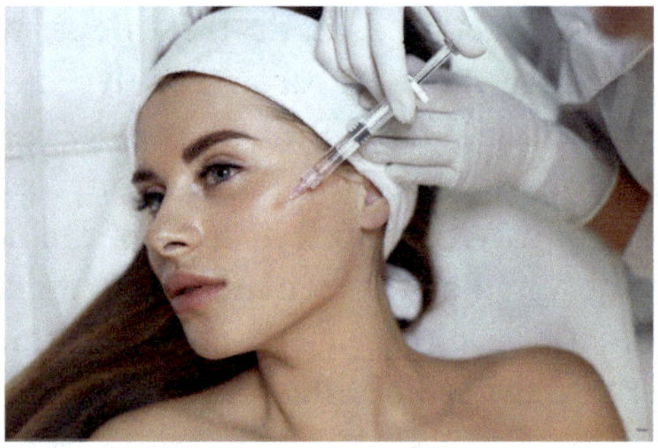

Figure 15.13. Safety and efficacy of non-surgical options.

Source: https://cdn.jasonbdiamond.com/wp-content/uploads/2023/12/14155942/Shutterstock_1724712010.jpg.

15.3.3. Patient Satisfaction and Outcomes

Given the extremely competitive facial cosmetics market in today's world, patient satisfaction is a key indicator of success for both the practitioner and the quality of procedure carried out. Recent advances in technology and methodology in aesthetic medicine have transformed the industry to a great extent, making treatments more personalized. Patients today expect customized approaches to treating their particular concerns, which is key to providing favorable outcomes. Emerging studies have emphasized the pivotal relationship between appropriately created training for non-surgical aesthetic (NSA) treatments and improved patient experiences. These procedures, many of which are carried out in private clinics, call for an elaborate model of training to guarantee practitioners possess the technical ability as well as people skills required to optimize patient interactions and, in the process, create more satisfaction (Kumar, 2021). The integration of feedback from patients into practice management has been increasingly important in guaranteeing facial cosmetic treatments yield positive results. Growing literature supports the assertion that patient-reported outcomes are essential indicators in assessing the success of aesthetic interventions. Practitioners are urged to adopt evidence-based models that not only track clinical outcomes but also carefully monitor patients' emotional and psychological states. A holistic approach focuses on the client's perspective, which significantly adds to overall satisfaction rates. As the somatology profession evolves, the blending of systematic training, as portrayed in overviews of the practice area, works to accentuate the importance of comprehending the technical and emotional aspects of caring for patients (Vosloo, 2025). Consequently, education and skill acquisition cannot be overstressed in facial cosmetic practice. Continuing professional education via a robust curriculum is the impetus for enhanced patient outcomes and satisfaction rates. There is evidence to show that organized courses of education, such as those built via the Delphi method, can foster critical thinking and practical skills needed within this very complex area of practice. Also, developing effective rapport between somatologists and patients raises the prospects of compliance by patients with post-treatment instructions and follow-ups, eventually leading to better aesthetic results. The practitioners must thus be responsive to both technological advancements and educational needs to ensure that they are adequately equipped to counter evolving patient expectations while promoting long-term satisfaction (Kumar, 2021; Vosloo, 2025).

Test Your Knowledge

1. How is the safety and efficacy of non-surgical cosmetic procedures evaluated?
2. What factors influence patient satisfaction and outcomes following non-surgical cosmetic treatments?

15.4. Surgical Advances in Facial Cosmetics

Learning Outcome

1. Discuss Latest Techniques in Facial Surgery
2. Focus on Minimally Invasive Surgical Options
3. Explain the Ethical Considerations in Surgical Practices

Recent surgical advancements in facial cosmetics have revolutionized procedures that plastic surgeons and other specialists employ. Previously, procedures were considered invasive and complex. However, due to technological improvements, there has been apparent procedural simplification. For instance, the application of minimally invasive techniques such as endoscopic brow lifts and transconjunctival blepharoplasty has minimized downtime while enhancing aesthetic outcomes. Surgeons can now utilize procedures that minimize scarring and bruising, thus making aesthetic surgery less intimidating for patients. Additionally, the new technology of 3D imaging systems offers precise pre-surgical assessments, optimizing surgical planning and allowing more accurate post-surgical result predictions, thus enhancing patient satisfaction.

As cosmetic surgery advances, patient-centric and accuracy-focused approaches are likely to impact further development within the specialty so that surgery remains at the center of enhancing facial attractiveness as per the patient's wish. Another improvement in surgical technology is the increasing use of fat grafting as a means of facial rejuvenation. This technique has volumetric augmentation with natural results through the utilization of the patient's adipose tissue and has superior results compared to traditional filler injections. The recent innovations have improved the procedure, such as the development of advanced harvesting and purifying techniques, which enhance the survival of the graft and reduce complications. Physicians now have sophisticated liposuction techniques through which they can harvest good-quality grafts that yield esthetically pleasing facial contour refinement. In addition, the suggested surge in minimally invasive procedures can also be interpreted in terms of the trend towards preserving the natural appearance of the face. Therefore, not only does the procedure indicate a tendency towards natural outcomes, but also a broader trend for cosmetic procedures that is concerned with safety and long-term satisfaction for patients who receive facial enhancement.

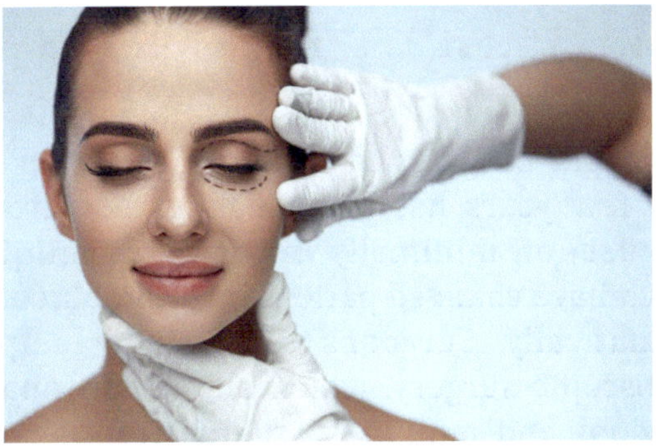

Figure 15.14. Surgical advances in facial cosmetics.

Source: https://external-content.duckduckgo.com/iu/?u=https%3A%2F%2Fpoppcosmeticsurgery.com%2Fwp-content%2Fuploads%2F2021%2F12%2FCosmetic-Surgery.jpg&f=1&nofb=1&ipt=3ebf983c95a023a892981ea711f48b483996e3cb7c8408433e597b1067838bca.

The addition of interdisciplinary collaboration has also taken center stage as one of the most important trends in surgical facial cosmetics. With further developed comprehension of the intricacy of facial anatomy, practitioners from all fields, such as dermatology, maxillofacial surgery, and oculoplastic surgery, are coming together to offer whole-brained care to patients. This collaborative practice is also observed by joint procedures, wherein surgeons address multiple cosmetic concerns simultaneously, resulting in effective treatment schedules and higher overall patient satisfaction. Moreover, the adoption of new standards of direction, as realized within the cosmetic practice, enhances the significance of an integrated approach to handling facial cosmetic treatment, enabling experts to share information and enhance the quality of patient treatment. Finally, the cosmetic surgical future lies at the nexus of collaboration and innovation, leading to more streamlined treatment paradigms and happier patients in the field of cosmetics (Figure 15.14).

15.4.1. Latest Techniques in Facial Surgery

The rapid progress in facial surgery over the past few years has been highlighted through the use of minimally invasive techniques, which have changed patient care and outcomes dramatically. Surgeons increasingly employ endoscopic surgery, which allows for smaller incisions and minimal tissue destruction, and thus rapid recoveries and reduced scarring. This method has proven particularly valuable in operations such as brow lifts and facelifts, which once generated a lot of downtime. Growing expertise with these operations is part of a broader movement toward patient satisfaction and safety, in which individuals can achieve their cosmetic objectives with less physical and psychological cost. Such innovation not only enhances the surgery process but also demonstrates the capability of the medical sector to react and adapt to the increasing demand for effective but minimally invasive facial cosmetic surgeries. Moreover, the role of technology in facial surgery has seen spectacular advancement, particularly through the use of 3D imaging and virtual simulation. Surgeons can create very accurate anatomical replicas of patients' faces that enable easier preoperative planning and better visualization of expected outcomes. It enhances the precision of surgery and offers more tailored approaches based on each patient's unique anatomy. Increased dependence on such cutting-edge equipment fosters greater communication between surgeons and patients as the visual aids assist in creating proper patient expectations. Besides, the advancement of surgical procedures through improved imaging assists in continuous learning and professional development in the profession to enable practitioners to maintain efficiency in carrying out contemporary approaches. With these advancements in technology, they too can continue to revolutionize facial surgery procedures in the field of cosmetics.

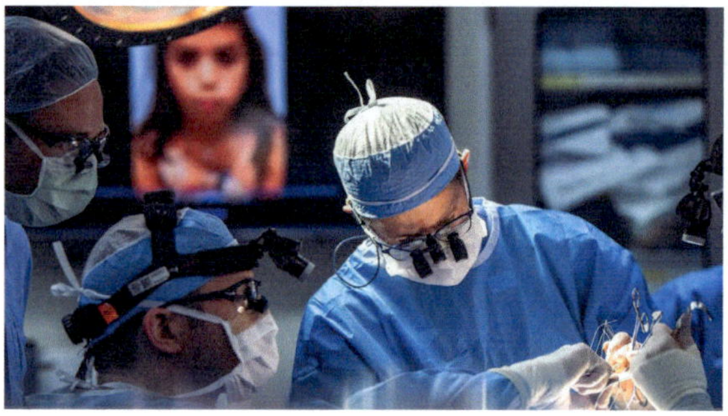

Figure 15.15. Advances in facial surgery.

Source: https://assets.clevelandclinic.org/transform/LargeFeatureImage/69603611-5eca-4061-9dde-ecb8b5c86bfc/CCC_2191938_06-08-21_349_AMO.

The record-breaking need for facial cosmetic procedures has also been driven by the call for holistic education and training in non-surgical aesthetics. In order to fill the knowledge gap, evidence-based postgraduate programs are being designed, emphasizing the newest non-surgical techniques like fillers and botulinum toxin therapy. Development of formal training systems is important to ensure that the standards of care are upheld, as there are increased professionals entering the field by virtue of public interest in the noninvasive treatments (Bowler, 2009). This educational focus is paramount, given that an educated practitioner can significantly influence patient satisfaction and safety. Furthermore, the incorporation of approaches such as objective structured clinical examinations (OSCE) allows for testing of fundamental competencies in aesthetic practice (Kumar, 2021). As facial cosmetics evolve with newer techniques and technology, the movement towards structured education paths is vital for long-term growth in the industry (Figure 15.15).

15.4.2. Minimally Invasive Surgical Options

Minimally invasive surgical options have significantly transformed the face of facial cosmetic procedures, giving patients efficient options over traditional surgeries. These innovative techniques are characterized by small incisions, less trauma to the surrounding tissues, and shorter recovery times, and as such, more patients are turning to them to attain their desired aesthetic enhancements. Given facial aging's complex interaction of intrinsic and extrinsic forces, the combination of surgical and non-invasive methods provides a holistic approach to treatment. Therapies such as Ultherapy and fat grafting exemplify the trend as they achieve remarkable outcomes in rejuvenation without long recoveries typical of more invasive treatments. This shift towards refinement in surgical intervention is a growing recognition of taste in aesthetics and a desire for naturally appearing outcomes, and hence minimally invasive treatments form a major part in practice management strategies (Portilla et al., 2024). In addition to lifts and tightening, the growing popularity of neurotoxin injections and fillers has transformed the landscape of minimally invasive cosmetics. All of these non-surgical therapies ease the anxieties of risk and cost that otherwise accompany traditional surgical procedures. With therapies like Botox and dermal fillers, doctors can create significant facial enhancements with minimal downtime, corresponding to the expanding need for convenient and effective cosmetic treatments. These therapies, in turn, provide a lower-risk profile, with complications being rare and generally temporary. According to existing evidence, the rates of patient satisfaction with such minimally invasive techniques are remarkably high, further validating their efficacy and widespread use in contemporary practice. This dual technique, applying both minimally invasive surgical and non-surgical treatments, allows practitioners to provide a diverse array of interventions tailored to every patient's interests and requirements (Timraz et al., 2025).

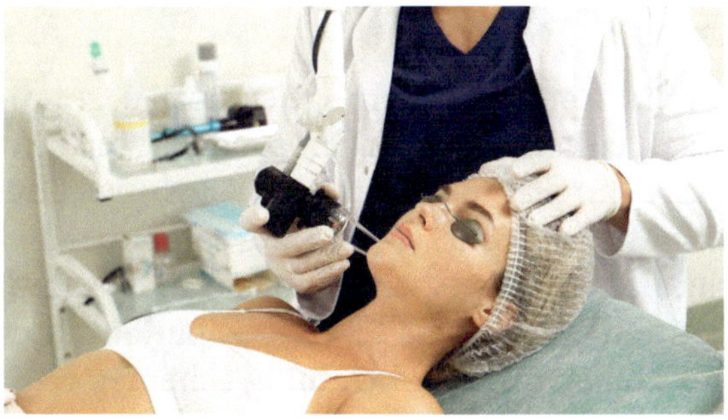

Figure 15.16. Minimally invasive surgical options.

Source: https://symbiosishospital.com/wp-content/uploads/2022/03/Symbiosis-Invasive-Surgeries.jpg.

The use of newer technology in minimally invasive surgery has raised procedural precision and patient outcomes, a great advancement of facial cosmetic surgery. Procedures such as thread lifts, where polydioxanone (PDO) and polylactic acid (PLA) materials are used, are great examples of how this branch has evolved to provide effective lifting and contouring with minimal downtime. These treatments stimulate collagen generation, giving patients not just immediate aesthetic gains but also long-term rejuvenating effects in the future. Moreover, technologies like high-intensity focused ultrasound (HIFU) and radiofrequency procedures have further expanded the scope of non-invasive treatments, enabling practitioners to tailor treatments based on individual patient needs. With the help of these technological developments, practitioners are able to increase their service, enhance patient satisfaction, and manage the practice efficiently in a competitive market. Synergistic application of minimally invasive approaches and new technologies emphasizes the evolving dynamics in facial cosmetic surgery (Portilla et al., 2024) (Figure 15.16).

15.4.3. Ethical Considerations in Surgical Practices

With the rapidly evolving age of facial cosmetics, ethical considerations in surgical practices acquire further significance. With procedure availability being ever more enabled by technology, the specter of inapt training among practitioners can lead to serious patient injury. The absence of formal training schemes within non-surgical aesthetics has highlighted the imperative for an evidence-based curriculum, as evidenced recently in a study that identified current knowledge gaps in the specialty (Kumar, 2021). This points to the ethical obligation of medical staff to not just take up continuous learning but also engage in comprehensive learning programs that ensure proficiency with new technologies. The necessity of maintaining patient safety and joy still remains topmost, since any lapse in ethics would result in bodily and psychological harm to patients undergoing cosmetic enhancement. Another pressing ethical concern of surgical practice is that of the process of informed consent, which underlies patient autonomy. Surgeons and practitioners have a duty to ensure that patients understand risks, benefits, and achievable outcomes of cosmetic procedures, particularly because social media and advertising have a tendency to shape expectations in misleading ways (Fedorchenko, 2024). This poses a threat of misalignment between patient expectations and surgical reality. Ethical practice demands that physicians not only provide full disclosure but also sympathetic counseling that accepts patients' motivations for such treatments. Failure to uphold these ethical standards creates a climate of misinformation and exploitation, which ultimately undermines the trust so essential to the doctor-patient relationship. Last, the social implications of aesthetic enhancement deserve ethical scrutiny, particularly the perpetuation of unrealistic beauty ideals. The increasing volume of cosmetic surgeries can promote a culture with a higher value of physical appeal than other attributes, further increasing body dysmorphic disorder and low self-worth in vulnerable groups. As trends currently indicate, the increase in procedures is often accompanied by social pressures, thus making the ethical climate for practitioners even more difficult (Fedorchenko, 2024). It is incumbent upon practicing professionals not only to be responsive to these pressures but also to labor on behalf of patient-centered care that supports healthy body image and psychological well-being. Knowledge of the broader social context in which these ethical concerns operate is essential in traversing the sensitive terrain of surgical practice in facial aesthetics.

<u>Test Your Knowledge</u>

Test Your Knowledge

1. What are the latest techniques in facial cosmetic surgery that have improved surgical outcomes?
2. How have minimally invasive surgical options changed the approach to facial cosmetic procedures?
3. What ethical considerations must surgeons keep in mind when performing facial cosmetic surgeries?

15.5. Practice Management in Cosmetic Clinics

Learning Outcome

1. Importance of Effective Management Strategies
2. Staff Training and Development
3. Patient Relationship Management

Practice management in aesthetic clinics has also become more complex as the changes brought about by advancing technology reshape the landscape of cosmetic medicine. Modern practices are confronted not only with traditional business protocol but also with the procedures of integrating new procedures that address the client's demand for outcome-based treatments. As the cosmetic surgery market continues to grow, professionals are tasked with adopting multidimensional management processes including patient education, operational efficiency, and financial prudence. The inclusion of new methods, such as dorsal augmentation (DA) rhinoplasty, calls for advanced training and ongoing professional development to remain up-to-date with this competitive market. By implementing effective practice management systems, clinics are able to enhance patient satisfaction, provide superior treatment results, and ultimately develop a sustainable practice that answers changing consumer demands and the rapid rate of technological advances (Nikparto et al., 2024). In addition to safeguarding patient safety and quality of care, which are foremost concerns in the field of cosmetic procedures, effective practice management becomes imperative. The incorporation of regenerative medicine techniques, such as the use of platelet-rich plasma (PRP) for wound healing, underscores the need to have stringent procedure protocols instituted by cosmetic clinics. Management strategies that prioritize safety can reduce the possibility of new technology pitfalls, thus creating a culture of trust among consumers. Monitoring clinical practice and vigilant observation of patient outcomes over time can form the foundation of quality improvement initiatives. Having adequate guidelines and staff training adds an overall enhancement in patient experience through an informed and compassionate setting that favors the long-term operation of the clinic in the highly regulated setting of cosmetic services (Patel et al., 2023). Finally, the financial sustainability of cosmetic clinics is reliant on a good practice management plan that considers operational costs as well as generating revenues.

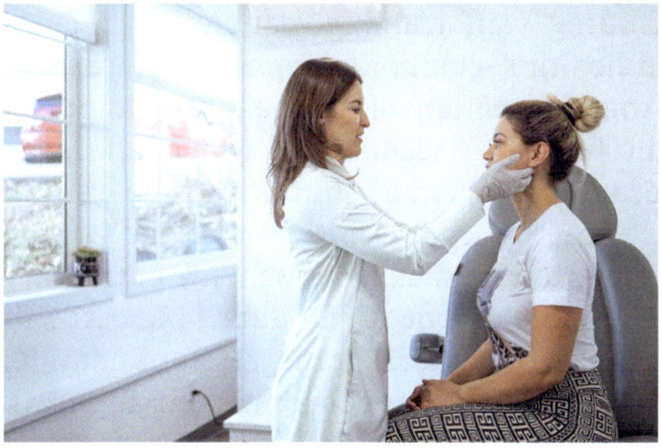

Figure 15.17. Practice management in cosmetic clinics.

Source: https://medizinonline.com/wp-content/uploads/2018/09/iStock-1359714290.jpg.

With the increasing popularity of beauty treatments, clinics must develop a strong grasp of consumer behavior and market trends in order to devise appropriate pricing mechanisms based on the value of service. Leveraging the most up-to-date technology in marketing campaigns, such as social media interaction and online consultation, can enhance client acquisition and retention activities. In addition, effective financial planning steps like cost-benefit analysis and resource allocation allow clinics to be competitive without sacrificing sustainable development. Through a mix of the latest advances in cosmetic treatments and effective management of practice, clinics can position themselves in an increasingly dynamic and evolving business sector in facial aesthetics (Figure 15.17).

15.5.1. Importance of Effective Management Strategies

Effective management of facial cosmetic treatment advancements is essential in ensuring patient safety and satisfaction. With technologies evolving constantly, practitioners must develop effective management strategies in order to handle the changes. The strategies involve an extensive array of business practices, including staff training, patient engagement, and health regulation compliance. An example is the application of light-emitting diode-red light (LED-RL) technology, which offers new therapeutic avenues, but its usage requires best-practice comprehension of the protocol in order to gain maximum benefits of treatment and avoid side effects. Evidence indicates that excessive procedural transgressions may lead to suboptimal consequences in their application for the management of skin fibrosis, which highlights the mutualistic relationship between technology, practice management, and clinical results (Heilman et al., 2019). Considering these facts, the importance of strategic management in practice cannot be exaggerated, as it has a direct impact on enhanced patient outcomes and service quality. Apart from operational management, effective marketing and education also play a significant role in disseminating new technology in facial cosmetics. Building patient awareness of new treatments such as LED-RL therapy requires not just a marketing approach, but also gaining an understanding of patient fears and perceptions. A good management approach can allow for informational campaigns that address these topics, thereby establishing patient confidence and enhancing treatment uptake rates. Equally important is staff education to ensure all staff deliver uniform, credible information on procedures and outcomes. Since education and marketing have priority in effective sound management strategies, practice can excel in a competitive marketplace, resulting in increased patient engagement and loyalty (Nova Southeastern University, 2014). The intersection of education and management, thus, offers windows of opportunity for effective integration of state-of-the-art technologies in practice. Lastly, the impact of flawed management strategies directly affects clinical success and patient health in the rapidly changing field of facial cosmetics. Incompetent management may not only risk the efficacy of treatment but also cause patient dissatisfaction and safety risks. For example, incompetent standardized practices when applying LED-RL can produce inaccurate results and potential complications. Therefore, developing management guidelines that maintain the guidelines for treatment and safety standards is necessary. This includes regular checks on procedure and results to enable consistent improvement. Emphasizing management's adoption of technology is crucial in order to promote patient safety, enhance treatment outcomes, and maintain practice in cosmetic practice. While forward steps continue to redefine the arena, good management practice will remain crucial in bridging challenges and maximizing gains in facial cosmetics (Heilman et al., 2019).

15.5.2. Staff Training and Development

Staff training and development in the field of facial cosmetics cannot be overstated, particularly in a company that keeps changing with new technologies and evolving customer preferences. Continuous education courses, as pointed out by recent studies, are required to equip employees with the information and skills necessary to cope with the complexities of cosmetic products and treatments. As observed in a cosmetic and dermatologic sciences continuing medical education (CME) initiative launched in 2008, the training significantly enhanced practitioners' understanding of cosmetic formulations, dermatologic sciences, and legal requirements. This knowledge gap, as typically experienced by practitioners and consumers, may generate misperceptions on product efficacy and safety, which ultimately impacts client confidence and satisfaction (Huo et al., 2023). Hence, expert training programs are necessary to equip employees not just with theoretical expertise but also with real-world expertise that enhances professional abilities. Furthermore, the integration of advanced technology within training programs will further strengthen the learning experience of the staff in the face cosmetic industry. For example, the utilization of digital platforms for the delivery of training videos, virtual simulations, and interactive sessions can facilitate staff in comprehending complex ideas more effectively. These methodologies not only bridge the gap between traditional education and modern learning patterns but also address different styles of employees to learn. By unveiling the positive comments from the CME program trainees, the incorporation of practical sessions and recent developments in cosmetic science assists in enhancing their knowledge and enthusiasm for their work. This strategy not only acquaints the workers with the delivery of maximum service to customers but also gives them the confidence to deal with the evolving problems in an intensely competitive marketplace (Huo et al., 2023). Ultimately, well-framed training modules can lead to improved employee performance and customer satisfaction with facial cosmetics. Besides, creating a corporate culture of highest regard for employee training and development is consistent with general industry goals of maintaining public trust and skin well-being. Subject to pressure from community standards and consumer demands, businesses are compelled to tread carefully on branding and employee conduct to avoid conflicts over workplace discrimination and harassment, as most labor and legal studies have noted. By ensuring employees are effectively trained to understand and implement ethical branding practices, companies can assist in avoiding risks for deceptive advertising and enhance their reputations. Training should not only include cosmetic science but also customer interaction facets and corporate social responsibility so employees can advocate accurate information and client well-being. By doing so, ongoing training reinforces the innate correlation between staff development and overall company success within the ever-changing universe of facial cosmetics.

15.5.3. Patient Relationship Management

With the rapidly changing universe of facial cosmetics, effective patient relationship management (PRM) has become an intrinsic part of practice management. The nature of cosmetic procedures demands not just technical competence but also a mature understanding of patient expectations and emotional needs. Developing a robust PRM strategy ensures effective communication and enhancing confidence, which is vital in addressing patients' complaints regarding treatment outcomes. As practitioners adopt advanced equipment to enhance the delivery of services, integrating such gadgets within a formalized PRM system ensures constant engagement with the patients, thus allowing them to make informed decisions. The emphasis on building relationships in such an environment is of top priority, since patient satisfaction depends largely on trust, with follow-up visits and recommendations that are key to business growth. The setup of evidence-based training has also transformed the dynamics of patient care in non-surgical aesthetics (NSA), putting further focus on the work of PRM in a niche sector. Modern training programs, findings of current studies now indicate, emphasize the practitioner's requirement to not only be technical experts but also to possess interpersonal skills that will allow them to practice PRM effectively. By fostering a curriculum grounded in extensive literature reviews and global needs analysis, educational institutions can better prepare their aesthetic practitioners to appropriately engage with their patients. This approach is with the growing realization that high-quality patient experience increasingly hinges on personalized interactions that are susceptible to being augmented by media that enable continuous interaction and feedback between the practitioner and patient and are hence in line with the core tenets of patient relationship management (Kumar, 2021). Corporate branding and patient experience cross-linking makes the landscape of PRM in facial cosmetics even more complex. As practices develop marketing strategies that are sensitive to community values, they must guard against the use of branding that would subtly reinforce stereotypes or be harmful to patient interactions. The challenge is finding a balance between aesthetics and professional norms so that marketing does not detract from the quality of services provided. The practitioners must institute a PRM approach that not only highlights their skills but also addresses any body image and personal identity issues that are present in the community, as these are directly tied to patient loyalty and satisfaction. Effective PRM in branding can enhance the overall patient experience, ultimately locking in the practitioner's reputation in a competitive market (Avery et al., 2007).

Test Your Knowledge

1. Why are effective management strategies important for the success of a cosmetic clinic?
2. How does staff training and development contribute to quality patient care in cosmetic practices?
3. What are key approaches to building and maintaining strong patient relationships in cosmetic clinics?

15.6. Regulatory and Ethical Considerations

Learning Outcome

1. Focus on Importance of Effective Management Strategies
2. Explain the Staff Training and Development
3. Discuss the Patient Relationship Management

The world is more regulated and guided by ethical factors that are pivotal in ensuring consumer safety, as well as industry integrity. With technological advances breeding novel cosmetic treatments and products, regulatory authorities must lay out detailed guidelines. The regulations must ensure not only product safety and efficacy but also the ethical aspects of this marketing practice that can deceive consumers. For instance, cosmetic misuse as a result of misinformation may result in ill effects, necessitating a regulatory mechanism that bridges the existing gap in knowledge among users and cosmetic practitioners, as facilitated by the evidence of ongoing continuing medical education (CME) programs tailored for cosmetic practitioners (Huo et al., 2023). Such a convergence of education and regulation builds good practice and promotes public trust in cosmetic sciences. Besides regulatory stipulations, ethical considerations are the basis for practice management for the facial cosmetics business. Practitioners must adhere to ethical principles such as beneficence, where clients' well-being is the principal concern. An ethical informed consent and avoidance of deceptive advertising claims are highly critical factors that clinicians should not forget during their encounters with patients. Industry players' focus on professionalism is supplemented by education efforts; training courses in cosmetic and dermatologic sciences have demonstrated a remarkable increase in clinicians' understanding of the scientific as well as ethical aspects of practice (Huo et al., 2023). This unification of ethical principles into everyday practice not only enhances the quality of care that is being delivered but also works to enhance the image of the cosmetic industry as a whole, thereby creating a climate where consumers have confidence in their choices. In addition, the interdisciplinary discussion facilitated by regulatory bodies can go a long way to enhance the overall ethical discussion within the cosmetic industry. By facilitating discourse among researchers, clinicians, and policy makers, organizations can work towards having more responsive and coherent policies that encompass the high pace of technological developments. Marine science organizations' efforts, as noted in the Marine Board-ESF work, highlight that efforts should be made to foster an interdisciplinary platform to address complex scientific as well as ethical issues. A similar approach in the cosmetic field would have regulators and practitioners joining together to develop regulations protecting consumers and professional standards alike. Thus, embracing an all-encompassing approach incorporating regulatory oversight, continued education, and ethical practice is crucial in regulating the emerging face of facial cosmetics.

15.6.1. Overview of Regulations Governing Cosmetic Practices

The regulation governing cosmetic practice is also multifaceted, encompassing numerous considerations from efficacy and safety to marketing and distribution. In the USA, the Food and Drug Administration (FDA) is the primary regulator of the cosmetics industry. Unlike pharmaceuticals, which are subjected to rigorous pre-market approval, cosmetic products in themselves are not subject to such a high degree of assessment before being placed on the market. This regulatory climate is a potential danger to the consumer because the products may contain poisonous substances or lack the advertised benefits. With the technology of cosmetics evolving through new processes and technologies, the need for updated rules that take into consideration current innovations is more pressing. A comprehensive organization covering the educational and operating skills of the practitioners and consumer protection is essential in managing the challenges and advancements of facial cosmetics. Increased popularity for non-surgical aesthetic treatments has raised demands for improved training and regulation within the cosmetic industry. Although non-surgical aesthetic (NSA) procedures are becoming increasingly popular, their dominance within private clinics, as opposed to academic medical centers, has resulted in a void of vigilance and education. To close this gap, the establishment of evidence-based postgraduate curricula for NSA has emerged as a necessary requirement for guaranteeing that practitioners not only meet ethical standards but also clinical competencies. Evidence has been discovered regarding how literature systematic reviews and Delphi studies can inform curriculum development, thereby forming a solid basis that integrates critical thinking and enquiry-based learning in NSA training (Kumar, 2021). This systematic method can enhance the level of care given in facial cosmetic treatment by professionalizing education. The intersection of race and gender in cosmetic control has an additional complexity that needs to be thoroughly interrogated. The control of skin-lightening cosmetics provides a useful case study, with the extensive racial and gender assumptions included in cosmetic law. Women of color, who are disproportionately targeted by these products through hostile marketing and toxic chemicals, are in grave danger of health complications due to the absence of regulatory intervention. The legacy exclusion of women from trials has contributed to such issues, rendering an intersectional framework for analysis indispensable in guiding policy reforms (Campbell et al., 2024). Such an analytic focus not only assists in understanding the unique health impacts felt by minority groups but also emphasizes the necessity of inclusive regulatory frameworks, placing emphasis on the well-being and protection of all as consumers. The construction of cosmetic regulation must therefore be attentive to plural experiences to create equitable standards regarding health and safety.

15.6.2. Ethical Dilemmas in Cosmetic Procedures

More cosmetic surgery over the last few years has garnered serious ethical issues, particularly with the fast pace of technology that has enabled such procedures to become more accessible. The main issue is the risk of the medical profession indulging in cosmetic desires over genuine healthcare requirements. This shift of focus raises serious issues regarding informed consent since the patients are not going to be given proper insight into what the implications of such elective procedures will be. Dermatosurgery is now walking the thin line between medical and cosmetic intentions, befuddling physicians' ethical requirements. The task of harmonizing patient satisfaction and medical ethics has increased as social norms of beauty evolve (Ekomwereren et al., 2023). As the demand for cosmetic surgery increases, practitioners must carefully work on these ethical issues to ensure patients' safety and well-being and preserve standards of care. Furthermore, the commercialization of cosmetic surgery presents added ethical challenges. The market dynamics of the cosmetic industry foster aggressive marketing practices tending to deceive about the nature of these surgical procedures. Patients can be under pressure to achieve unrealistic beauty ideals, which worsens the ethical challenge that is encountered by practitioners. Profit may be achieved at the expense of clinical judgment, and this can result in over-treatment or ignoring the patient's mental health. Mental wellness is particularly important to address, as people are getting cosmetic treatments to correct underlying psychological issues instead of for aesthetic needs that are genuine. As is observed by Ekomwereren et al. (2023), open communication between medical professionals and patients is important in averting such risks. It is the role of health practitioners to uphold professional ethics while meeting the growing demand for cosmetic surgery within a society that only continues to place more emphasis on looks. As a result of technological advancement, ethical questions are also complicated by the integration of artificial intelligence (AI) within the management and execution of procedures. As AI becomes more engagement by AI in forming patient experience and outcomes, there are pressing issues about data privacy and security. Misuse of personal information is a concerning issue around consent and transparency. Incorporation of AI into cosmetic practice must be undertaken with vigilance to ensure that patient rights are not violated. The performance of AI in translating patient desires over medical needs continues to evolve. As theorized in, human-AI cooperation may revolutionize ethical frameworks in healthcare, with careful observation being needed to prevent exploitation or harm. It will be essential to strike a delicate balance between ethics and innovation in creating a system that ensures patient autonomy without stifling accountable practice in an evolving environment.

15.6.3. Impact of Regulations on Practice Management

The impact of regulation on practice management in the facial cosmetics industry has come more sharply into focus as the industry continues to evolve. As technology and methods of treatment evolve, practices are forced to deal with a highly regulated climate that monitors their actions. Regulation systems intended to ensure patient safety and practitioner responsibility can also pose significant challenges for practice management. For instance, compliance with certification requirements and health standards necessitates ongoing training and investment. Hence, practitioners are compelled to make investments in terms of keeping abreast with these regulations, detracting from time and investment that otherwise could be spent on enhancing services and being creative within practice. Lastly, the interplay between regulatory standards and corporate branding makes it problematic to strategize practice management in facial cosmetics. Businesses typically seek to establish a specific brand image so that they can compete better, but this must go hand in hand with legal compliance. Marketing procedures and the advertisement of plastic surgery are subject to laws that demand a balancing act between effective branding and adherence to ethical standards. As mentioned, in environments where sexualized branding does not align with what is accepted by society, laws may intervene and ban practices leading to unwanted working environments. This dynamic also shows the importance of having an understanding of local community norms, the ethical implications of branding in the regulated space, and thereby influencing practice decision-making processes. Finally, the influence of regulations on practice management also reaches into establishing certain professional standards and guidelines that must be followed by practitioners. Regulating authorities provide useful frameworks that can enhance practice quality through structured guidelines and recommendations. However, simultaneously, these regulations can suppress innovation when they are overly restrictive. Clarity and flexibility of regulations are crucial so that there is an appropriate setting for embracing technological advances in clinical practices. Facial cosmetic professionals struggle to maintain the vagueness of adhering to regulations and the need to deal with new practices that take care of patients' needs and expectations. Lastly, the intersection of practice management and regulation is an ideal area for continued study, as how successfully one can accommodate these forces will influence the future course of the facial cosmetics industry.

Test Your Knowledge

1. How does staff training and development ensure compliance with ethical and legal standards?
2. What ethical principles should guide patient relationship management in cosmetic clinics?

SUMMARY

It should be evident that the advancement of this career is highly influenced by scientific discovery and technological integration. Within the past few decades, practitioners have witnessed a drastic shift in patient expectations as well as treatment methods. With the development of new technologies and materials, they have transformed the landscape of aesthetic treatments so that practitioners are able to offer more effective and safer treatments that can treat a large population of patients. Utilization of advanced technologies such as nanotechnology and biocompatible fillers not only enhanced results but also promoted more interest in the study of aesthetic medicine underway. This trend underscores the necessity of continuous professional education and a responsive nature in practitioners to offset the dynamic nature of the practice. The facial cosmetics revolution is also underscored by heightened emphasis on individually tailored treatment protocols, driven by a viewpoint of unique anatomy and aesthetic goals. With diagnostic methods and materials still being developed, practitioners are now in a position to individualize treatment more effectively according to patient requirements, thus raising satisfaction and efficacy. In the recent past, minimally invasive treatments have also made facial cosmetic treatments more and more accessible, more so in an attractive and viable way for a wider populace. This democratization of cosmetic care is a cultural revolution, in which beauty and self-care are not only material aspirations, but essential components of healthful living. Such demographic advancement mandates that there be ongoing discussion regarding ethical practice, best practices, and patient education, so that the expansion of access is accompanied by commitment to safety and efficacy. Lastly, the conclusion drawn via evaluation of facial cosmetics innovation is that an integrated approach that merges technology, patient care, and severe management practices is required. As the industry innovates, practitioners need to remain informed about emerging technologies and their applications, such as innovations of Joseph et al. (2023), which stated the significance of nanotechnology in advancing medical treatments. Moreover, with specialties such as cutaneous conditions being addressed in the domain of cosmetics, marrying aesthetic practice with knowledge from other medical specialties, as envisioned in de Vries & Schallig (2022), paves the way for future innovations. The future demands adherence to the ethics of practice, lifelong learning, and adherence to standards of care for the achievement of both aesthetic and patient safety.

The facial cosmetic environment is undergoing a dramatic change due to the advancement of technology, enhancing patient experience and practitioner capabilities. Central to this change is the integration of the latest modalities, which not only maximize aesthetic enhancement but also patient safety and satisfaction. Intelligent devices have transformed practice management, allowing practitioners to become more bespoke in their engagements with clients. For instance, the application of artificial intelligence in cosmetic treatments for the face assists with predictive analysis to ensure treatment plans are optimized to meet individual needs. Such a paradigm shift is a representation of embracing innovative technologies that are in agreement with ethical standards and professional practices, leading to better patient outcomes as well as enhanced industry relations. The role of social media and forums in facial cosmetic treatment has become increasingly influential, shaping public perception and patient demand. Particularly, the beauty blogging phenomenon enables individuals with facial disfigurement to narrate their experiences and rebuild their identity. These self-narrative accounts, as opposed to normalized journalistic accounts, bear witness to the complexity with respect to disability and beauty. By examining the narrative exchanged between beauty bloggers and traditional journalism, it becomes evident that these platforms can coexist to enrich societal understanding of disfigurement and challenge conventional representations. As practitioners keenly observe these communications, they are better equipped to engage with diverse patient narratives, fostering an inclusive approach to cosmetic enhancement that respects individual stories and experiences (Garrisi et al., 2018). Moreover, progress in artificial intelligence and smart technologies brings forth prospects and issues for the cosmetics industry. Personalized experiences have increasingly become popular, necessitating the development of convergence platforms that will be capable of fulfilling varied consumer demands in addition to guaranteeing accessibility. Innovations such as the Internet-of-Mirrors (IoM), encompassing networked smart mirrors, register this prospect as it offers interactive and tailored consultations for beauty and health routines. Nonetheless, gaping holes in the existing portfolios still remain, especially in relation to their mass adoption and uptake into day-to-day practice. To be able to maximize these developments, the sector has to place greater importance on research and development activities designed to bridge these loopholes as well as further improve the functionality of autonomous solutions. In this way, practitioners are able to improve service provision, better bringing it in line with modern-day consumer expectations (Fatima et al., 2023).

KEY TERMS FROM THIS CHAPTER

- 3D Imaging
- Virtual Surgical Simulation
- Intraoperative Navigation
- Laser Technology
- Ultrasound-Guided Procedures
- Injectable Therapies
- Electronic Medical Records (EMR)
- Quality Assurance
- Computer-Aided Surgical Planning
- CAD/CAM Technology
- Endoscopic Techniques
- Radiofrequency Devices
- Robotic-Assisted Surgery
- Patient Workflow Optimization
- Teleconsultation
- Regulatory Compliance

CRITICAL THINKING QUESTIONS

1. **Which technology has greatly improved preoperative planning in facial cosmetic surgery?**
   a. Laser Doppler
   b. 3D imaging and simulation
   c. Ultrasound
   d. Traditional photography
2. **Computer-assisted surgical guides are primarily used for:**
   a. Minimizing anesthesia
   b. Accurate implant placement and bone reconstruction
   c. Skin resurfacing
   d. Hair transplantation
3. **Which energy-based device is commonly used for non-invasive skin tightening?**
   a. Radiofrequency
   b. Scalpel
   c. Cryotherapy
   d. Electrocautery
4. **What is a major advantage of minimally invasive facial cosmetic procedures?**
   a. Permanent results
   b. Reduced downtime and faster recovery
   c. No anesthesia needed
   d. No follow-up required
5. **Fractional lasers are primarily used for:**
   a. Hair removal only
   b. Skin resurfacing and rejuvenation
   c. Deep bone contouring
   d. Fat reduction

Short Answer Questions

1. How has 3D imaging and simulation improved preoperative planning in facial aesthetics?
2. What role do computer-assisted surgical guides play in facial reconstruction and implant placement?
3. Describe the advantages of using laser and energy-based devices in modern facial rejuvenation.
4. How has the development of minimally invasive techniques changed patient recovery and outcomes?
5. What are the key considerations in maintaining patient safety while adopting new cosmetic technologies?
6. Explain the importance of digital documentation and patient record management in facial cosmetic practice.

Answers to Critical Thinking Questions

1. (b) 2. (b) 3. (a) 4. (b) 5. (b)

REFERENCES

1. Timraz, J. H., Bakour, H. A., Samman, R. R., Alawi, K. M., Bava, F. S. M., Alkhdaidi, F. A., AlGhorab, M. A., Alabbassi, M. A., Thalib, H. I., Khan, S., Makki, F., & Alsolamy, A. (2025). Advancements in Non-Invasive Plastic Surgery Techniques: Evaluating Efficacy, Safety, Patient Outcomes and Potential Complications. *South Eastern European Journal of Public Health*, 4078–4099. https://doi.org/10.70135/seejph.vi.5983(accessed on 14th July 2025).

2. Araya, D., & Marber, P. (2023). *Augmented Education in the Global Age*. Routledge eBooks. https://doi.org/10.4324/9781003230762.

3. Avery, D., & Crain, M. (2007). *Branded: Corporate image, sexual stereotyping, and the new face of capitalism*. https://core.ac.uk/download/62548098.pdf (accessed on 14th July 2025).

4. Bowler P. J. (2009). Impact on facial rejuvenation with dermatological preparations. *Clinical interventions in aging*, *4*, 81–89. https://doi.org/10.2147/cia.s3524(accessed on 14th July 2025).

5. Boyen, C., Børresen, T., Dobson, A., Höfle, et al. (2025). *Marine biotechnology: A new vision and strategy for Europe*. https://core.ac.uk/download/pdf/29241634.pdf (accessed on 14th July 2025).

6. Brandt, F. S., & Cazzaniga, A. (2008). *Hyaluronic acid gel fillers in the management of facial aging*. https://core.ac.uk/download/pdf/8185430.pdf (accessed on 14th July 2025).

7. Campbell, C. (2024). *Intersectionality Matters in Food and Drug Law*. https://core.ac.uk/download/647851141.pdf (accessed on 14th July 2025).

8. Portilla, A. S. P., Portilla, C. S. P., Palacios, G. S. G., Rodríguez, B. S. P., Castillo, S. G. A., Espin, N. E. P., & Pita, G. P. M. (2024). The integration of surgical and dermatological techniques in the treatment of cutaneous aging: multidisciplinary approaches and clinical outcomes - a comprehensive systematic review of current literature. *International Journal of Research in Medical Sciences*, *12*(5), 1659–1667. https://doi.org/10.18203/2320-6012.ijrms20240943(accessed on 14th July 2025).

9. Damar, M. (2022). What the literature on medicine, nursing, public health, midwifery, and dentistry reveals: An overview of the rapidly approaching metaverse. *Journal of Metaverse*, *2*, 62–70. https://doi.org/10.57019/jmv.1132962.

10. de Vries, H. J. C., & Schallig, H. D. F. H. (2022). Cutaneous leishmaniasis: A 2022 updated narrative review into diagnosis and management developments. *American Journal of Clinical Dermatology*, *23*, 823–840. https://doi.org/10.1007/s40257-022-00726-8.

11. Edmonds, A. (2014). *Surgery-for-life: Aging, sexual fitness and self-management in Brazil*. Anthropology & Aging Quarterly 2014: 34 (4) https://core.ac.uk/download/28979727.pdf (accessed on 14th July 2025).

12. Ekomwereren, O., Shehryar, A., Yahya, N. A., Rehman, A., Affaf, M., Chilla, S. P., Kumar, U., et al. (2023). Mastering the art of dermatosurgery: Aesthetic alchemy in medical excellence. *Cureus*. https://doi.org/10.7759/cureus.49659.

13. Fatima, H., Imran, M. A., Mohjazi, L., Taha, et al. (2023). *Internet of mirrors for connected healthcare and beauty: A prospective vision*. http://arxiv.org/abs/2311.14734 (accessed on 14th July 2025).

14. Fedorchenko, Y. (2024). ANTI-AGING COSMETIC PROCEDURES: BENEFITS AND RISKS. *Anti-Aging Eastern Europe, 3*(3), 135-140. https://doi.org/10.56543/aaeeu.2024.3.3.04(accessed on 14th July 2025).

15. Reisenwitz, Timothy and Fowler, Jie G. (2021) "An Analysis on Engaging "Beauty Work"," Atlantic Marketing Journal: Vol. 10 : No. 2 , Article 6. Available at: https://digitalcommons.kennesaw.edu/amj/vol10/iss2/6 (accessed on 14th July 2025).

16. Garrisi, D., Johanssen, J., Johanssen, et al. (2018). *Competing narratives in framing disability in the UK media: A comparative analysis of journalistic representations of facial disfigurement versus practices of self-representations online.* https://core.ac.uk/download/161104198.pdf (accessed on 14th July 2025).

17. Heilman, E., Isseroff, R. R., Jagdeo, J. R., Jakus, et al. (2019). *A dose-ranging, parallel group, split-face, single-blind phase II study of light emitting diode-red light (LED-RL) for skin scarring prevention: Study protocol for a randomized controlled trial.* https://core.ac.uk/download/323070347.pdf (accessed on 14th July 2025).

18. Huo, W., Wang, X., Wang, X., Wang, X., Shu, X., & Li, Y. (2023). *Promoting public skin health through a national continuing medical education project on cosmetic and dermatologic sciences: A 15-year experience.* https://core.ac.uk/download/593349901.pdf (accessed on 14th July 2025).

19. Joseph, T. M., Mahapatra, D. K., Esmaeili, A., Piszczyk, Ł., Hasanin, M. S., Kattali, M., Haponiuk, J. T., et al. (2023). Nanoparticles: Taking a unique position in medicine. *Nanomaterials, 13*, 574–574. https://doi.org/10.3390/nano13030574.

20. Kazimierczak, N., Kazimierczak, W., Serafin, Z., Nowicki, P., Nożewski, J., & Janiszewska-Olszowska, J. (2024). AI in orthodontics: Revolutionizing diagnostics and treatment planning—A comprehensive review. *Journal of Clinical Medicine, 13*, 344–344. https://doi.org/10.3390/jcm13020344.

21. Kivnick, H. Q., Twigg, J., & Martin, W. (2014). *The Challenge of Cultural Gerontology.* https://core.ac.uk/download/30339730.pdf (accessed on 14th July 2025).

22. Kumar, Narendra; (2021) Design, Development and Implementation Framework for a Postgraduate Non-Surgical Aesthetics Curriculum. Doctoral thesis (Ph.D), UCL (University College London).(accessed on 14th July 2025).

23. Lin, J. Y., & Wan, M. T. (2014). *Current evidence and applications of photodynamic therapy in dermatology.* https://core.ac.uk/download/28949556.pdf (accessed on 14th July 2025).

24. Meyer-Szary, J., Luis, M. S., Mikulski, S., Patel, A., Schulz, F., Tretiakow, D., Fercho, J., et al. (2022). The role of 3D printing in planning complex medical procedures and training of medical professionals—Cross-sectional multispecialty review. *International Journal of Environmental Research and Public Health, 19*, 3331–3331. https://doi.org/10.3390/ijerph19063331.

25. Mubashir, M. (2024). *The gendered dress of DALL-E 2: Exploring profession-based images in the Indian context.* https://core.ac.uk/download/616689178.pdf (accessed on 14th July 2025).

26. Naik, M. (2015). Donate eyes, not patients!. *Indian Journal of Ophthalmology, 63*, 564, 565. https://www.semanticscholar.org/paper/725523a9575cbdbb3e3af205ca0a8d83e9856093.

27. Nikparto, N., Yari, A., Mehraban, S. H., Bigdelou, M., Asadi, A., Darehdor, A. A., Nezaminia, S., et al. (2024). The current techniques in dorsal augmentation rhinoplasty: A comprehensive

review. *Maxillofacial Plastic and Reconstructive Surgery, 46*. https://doi.org/10.1186/s40902-024-00418-9.

28. Nova Southeastern University. (2014). *Academic Impressions, 2014*. https://core.ac.uk/download/51073269.pdf (accessed on 14th July 2025).
29. Patel, H., Pundkar, A., Shrivastava, S., Chandanwale, R., & Jaiswal, A. M. (2023). A comprehensive review on platelet-rich plasma activation: A key player in accelerating skin wound healing. *Cureus*. https://doi.org/10.7759/cureus.48943.
30. Rokhshad, R., Keyhan, S. O., & Yousefi, P. (2023). *Artificial intelligence applications and ethical challenges in oral and maxillo-facial cosmetic surgery: A narrative review. Maxillofacial Plastic and Reconstructive Surgery, 45*. https://doi.org/10.1186/s40902-023-00382-w.
31. Tettey, F., Parupelli, S. K., & Desai, S. (2023). A review of biomedical devices: Classification, regulatory guidelines, human factors, software as a medical device, and cybersecurity. *Deleted Journal, 2*, 316–341. https://doi.org/10.1007/s44174-023-00113-9.
32. Vosloo, M. (2025). *A framework to position the somatology profession in South Africa*. https://core.ac.uk/download/222966444.pdf (accessed on 14th July 2025).

INDEX

A

Abnormalities 370, 371, 372, 373, 380, 381, 382, 385, 386, 389, 394
Acoustic Neuroma 147
Acoustic Reflex Testing 178
Acute Otitis Media 117
Adenoid Cystic Carcinoma 271
Adenoid Hypertrophy 253, 271
Adenoiditis 271
Adenoids 28
Adenotonsillitis 331
Adhesive Otitis Media 117
Adipose-derived stem cells (ASCs) 402
Adjunctive treatments 339
Aesthetic 3, 5, 12, 15, 22, 27
Aesthetic beauty 369
Aesthetic treatments 434, 435, 436, 439, 457, 460
Afflicted body 402
Air Conduction Testing 178
Allergies 101, 103, 293, 295, 296
Anatomical Abnormalities 101, 104
Anatomy 1, 4, 5, 6, 35, 39, 43, 47, 95, 149, 153, 156, 157, 185, 187, 188, 195, 196, 211, 214, 243, 247, 275, 277, 278, 282, 303, 305, 308, 309
Anosmia 216
anti-aging treatments 440
Antibiotic Resistance 22, 23
Artificial intelligence (AI) 435, 444, 458
Arytenoid Cartilages 301
Assessment 402, 414, 415, 421, 422, 423, 428
Asymmetry 340
Atresia 87
Audiogram 178
Audiological Assessments 16, 19, 109, 111, 165, 168
Audiology 28
Audiometric Testing 134, 136
Auditory Brainstem Response (ABR) 178
Auditory Canal 39, 40
Auditory Information 51, 54
Auditory Nerve 47, 50, 62
Augmented reality (AR) 441, 444
Aural Polyp 117
Auricle 60
Autologous bone 337, 344, 348, 358, 362
Avulsion Injuries 363

B

Bacterial infection 67, 71, 73
Bacterial pathogens 115
Balance crucial 402
Barotrauma 117
Basal Cell Carcinoma 429
Basal cell carcinoma (BCC) 406
Benign Paroxysmal Positional Vertigo (BPPV) 126, 129, 135, 143, 147
Bilateral vestibulopathy (BVP) 124

Bioactive materials 338
Biological 369
Bone Conduction Testing 178
Bone Grafting 363
Bone morphogenetic proteins (BMPs) 338
Bone Reconstruction 429
Bony Labyrinth 60
Brain 30, 55, 57
Brand identity 437

C

CAD/CAM Technology 461
Canal Stenosis 87
Cancer microenvironments 402
Cauliflower Ear 87
Cellulitis 87
Cerumen Impaction 87
Chemotherapy 22, 23, 31
Choanal Atresia 271
Cholesteatoma 94, 97, 99, 109, 117, 121
Chronic Otitis Media 117
Chronic Pharyngiti 331
Chronic suppurative otitis media (CSOM) 23
Chronic Tonsilliti 331
Circumstance 338
Circumstances 413
Cleft Lip 373, 396
Cleft Palate 396
Client engagement 436
Clinical competency 438
Clinical efficacy 436
Clinical operation 438
Clinical skill 437
Cochlea 28, 47, 48, 60
Cochlear Duct 60
Cognitive development 371
Common Diseases 67, 68
Common Disorders 55, 203, 246, 251, 293, 296
Communication 409, 411, 413, 417, 426, 427
Complex deformities 370
Complex structure 185
Comprehension 338
Comprehensive treatment protocols 370
Computer-Aided Surgical Planning 461
Concha Bullosa 237
Configurations 36
Congenital malformation 370, 380
Consistency 338
Consumer engagement 438
Consumer patterns 434
Contusion Management 363
Corniculate Cartilages 301
Cosmetic design 444, 445
Cosmetic industry 439, 440, 441, 444, 446, 455, 457, 458
Cosmetic practices 437, 438, 441, 456
Cosmetic professionals 406
Cosmetic technology 439, 441
Cosmetic therapy 445
Craniofacial Anomalies 396
Craniofacial reconstruction 339, 358, 411
Craniosynostosis 374, 375, 396, 397
Cribriform Plate 212
Cricoid Cartilage 301
Cricothyroid Membrane 301
Cultural influences 440
Cuneiform Cartilages 301
Cutaneous integrity 402
Cutaneous Malignancy 429
Cutting-edge technologies 433

D

Deep learning 444
Defect Reconstruction 429
Dermatitis 68, 87
Deviated Nasal Septum (DNS 237
Diagnosis 11, 16, 17, 30, 70, 71, 72, 74, 75, 91, 93, 107, 108, 109, 110, 120, 123, 124, 127, 128, 134, 165, 167, 180, 181, 222, 224, 227, 240, 241, 246, 254, 257, 312, 314, 320, 322
Diagnostic Audiometry 178
Diagnostic Tools 16, 165
Digital technologies 439, 444
Disease 403, 406, 411, 425
Disfigurement 402, 405, 411, 412, 416, 417, 426
Diversity 35, 53

Dizziness 130, 131, 134
Dysfunction 44, 55, 64, 97, 99, 119, 132, 200, 239, 247, 264
Dysmorphisms 372

E

Ear Care Practices 82, 83
Ear Diseases 79, 80
Ear Disorders 9, 93, 94, 95, 97, 101, 105, 109, 113, 126, 134
Ear Health 66, 79, 80, 82, 84
Ear Pain 105, 107
Earwax Impaction 68, 70
Economy 95
Eczema 87
Effective communication skills 438
Effective management 436, 454, 456
Efficacy 403, 405, 423
Effusion 117
Electronic Medical Records (EMR) 461
Emotional impact 369, 372
Endolymph 60
Endolymphatic Hydrops 147, 151
Endoscopic Procedures 12, 13, 162
Endoscopic Techniques 461
Endoscopy 13, 16, 18, 165, 167, 207, 224, 226, 257, 319
Enlarged vestibular aqueduct (EVA) 94, 104
Environmental exposure 370, 382
Environmental Factors 79, 80, 101, 103
Epidermis 406, 420
Epiglottis 28, 301
Epipharyngeal Catarrh 271
Epistaxis 237
Equilibrium 55, 56
Eustachian Tube 28, 43, 45, 64, 97, 99, 120
Eustachian Tube Dysfunction 271
Exclusive esthetic 411
External Ear Diseases 72, 73, 76
External Nose 212
External Structures 189

F

Facial artery perforator (FAP) 338
Facial bony skeleton 338
Facial cosmetics 433, 434, 435, 436, 437, 438, 439, 441, 442, 443, 444, 445, 446, 447, 448, 449, 451, 452, 454, 455, 456, 457, 458, 459, 460
Facial deformities 369, 370, 371, 376, 378, 379, 380, 381, 382, 383, 384, 386, 387, 388, 389, 390, 393, 394, 397
Facial Fractures 363
Facial injuries 339, 340, 341, 342, 345, 352
Facial Symmetry Restoration 363
Facial trauma 337, 338, 340, 341, 342, 343, 344, 345, 346, 349, 351, 352, 353, 355, 356, 357, 358, 362, 363, 364
Flexibility 36, 44, 45, 46
Fluid Drainage 105, 108
Fluorouracil 22
Free Field Testing 178
Free Flap 429
Frontal Sinus 212
Functional Impairment 396
Functional Rehabilitation 363
Functional Restoration 429
Function restoration 340
Furunculosis 87, 237

G

Genetic defects 370, 380
Genetic Predispositions 79, 81
Global sustainability 442
Glottis 301
Glue Ear 117

H

Hair Cells 51, 53
Hallucinations 94, 97, 113
Hard Palate 212
Healthcare Professionals 72, 74
Health professionals 370, 379, 384, 390
Hearing Assessment 153
Hearing Threshold 178

Hematoma Auris 87
Hemifacial Microsomia 375, 396, 398
Hemotympanum 117
Heterogeneity 22, 23, 373, 375, 379
Holistic approach 401, 426
Home Remedies 76, 78, 228, 231, 232, 323, 325
Human papillomavirus (HPV) 406
Humidity 185, 199
Hyaluronic acid (HA) 442
Hyoid Bone 301
Hypersecretion 66

I

Impacted Cerumen 87
Impedance Audiometry 178
Incus 43, 44, 60
Infection 94, 95, 96, 97, 98, 99, 100, 101, 102, 103, 106, 107, 108, 109, 113, 114, 115
Infections 30, 71, 101, 102, 221, 222, 262, 265, 266, 269, 334
Inferior Turbinate 212
Inflammation 101, 102, 197, 240, 297
Injectable Therapies 461
Inner Ear 47, 55, 57, 89, 123, 124, 126, 134
Innovation 433, 434, 436, 437, 440, 441, 442, 444, 445, 447, 450, 458, 459, 460
Innovations 12, 15, 16, 173
Intraoperative Navigation 461
Invasive Surgery 12, 15
Isolation 142, 143

K

Keratosis Obturans 87

L

Laryngeal Structures 157
Laryngology 28
Laryngopharynx 301
Larynx 158, 161, 250, 275, 276, 282, 284, 289, 296, 298, 301
Laser Technology 461
Lipotransfer techniques 405
Local Flap 429
Locally advanced squamous cell carcinoma (LA SCCHN) 22
Ludwig's Angina 331
Lumpectomy 411
Lymphoid Hyperplasia 271

M

Machine learning algorithms 444
Macrognathia 396
Magnitude 405
Malleus 43, 44, 60
Mandibular Fracture Fixation 363
Margins of Excision 429
Market trends 439, 453
Mastoiditis 117
Maxillary Sinus 212
Maxillectomy 403, 407, 410, 414, 415, 417, 420, 421, 422, 424, 431
Maxillofacial Trauma 363
Meatus 212
Mechanotransduction 51, 53
Medical management 113, 114, 115
Medical Management 113, 258, 259
Medical professionals 3, 19, 20, 23
Medical technology 340
Medical Treatments 76
Medications 138, 139, 228, 229, 232
Melanoma 406, 429, 430
Membranous Labyrinth 60
Methodology 411
Micrognathia 396
Micromorphology 405, 410, 411, 428
Microtia 370, 375, 377
Microvascular Anastomosis 429
Middle Turbinate 212
Midface Hypoplasia 396
Mixed Reality (MR) 408
Mohs Surgery 429
Moisture accumulation 67
Molar-Incisor Hypomineralization (MIH) 373
Monitor ear health 115
Morphological aspect 369

Morphology 35, 48
Motion Sickness 147
Multidisciplinary Approach 20, 22, 90, 119, 149, 169, 171
Multidisciplinary Management 396
Muscle transfers 402, 412
Muscular function 402
Musical Ear Syndrome 94, 97, 113, 121

N

Nanotechnology 433, 441, 445, 460
Nasal Cavity 4, 6, 156, 188, 190, 195, 198, 212
Nasal Obstruction 9, 11
Nasal Polyps 219, 237
Nasal Septum 28, 191, 212
Nasal Valve 212
Nasal Vestibulitis 237
Nasopharyngeal Carcinoma 252, 271
Nasopharyngeal Stenosis 271
Nasopharyngitis 271
Nasopharynx 96, 101, 301
Nausea 130, 133
Neck Conditions 12, 14
Neck disease 2, 14, 23, 24
Neck Structures 7
Neck surgery 153, 154, 155, 156, 162, 165, 166, 173, 174
Neck Surgery 1, 3, 4, 11, 12, 19, 20, 27, 30, 120, 150, 154, 155, 156, 162, 165, 173, 184
Nerve Injury Assessment 363
Nervous system 370, 396, 400
Neural Processing 51, 54
Neurotization 407, 412
Noise-Induced Hearing Loss 147
Non-steroidal anti-inflammatory drugs (NSAIDs) 66
Non-surgical aesthetics (NSA) 438, 455

O

Objective structured clinical examination (OSCE) 439
Objective structured practical examination (OSPE) 439
Obstructive sleep apnea syndrome (OSAS) 1
Ocular Protection 363
Olfactory Bulb 212
Olfactory Epithelium 212
Oncologic 401, 402, 403, 404, 405, 406, 407, 408, 409, 410, 411, 412, 414, 415, 416, 417, 418, 419, 420, 421, 422, 423, 424, 425, 426, 427, 428, 429, 430
Oncologic surgery 401, 402, 403, 405, 406, 408, 409, 410, 418, 419, 420, 423, 425, 428
Online marketing technology 436
Open Reduction and Internal Fixation (ORIF) 363
Operational capability 436
Oral and maxillofacial (OMF) 444
Oral squamous cell carcinoma (OSCC) 406
Orbital Floor Repair 363
Oropharynx 301
Orthognathic surgery 369, 380, 387, 388, 393, 394, 400
Ossicles 28, 43, 44
Ossicular Chain 60
Ossicular Discontinuity 117
Otitis externa 67, 68, 69, 86
Otitis Externa 68, 69, 87, 91
Otitis Media 9, 89, 97, 98, 119, 158, 159, 273, 274
Otitis Media with Effusion 271
Otoacoustic Emissions (OAE) 178
Otology 28
Otomycosis 87
Otorhinolaryngology 186, 196, 199, 201, 207, 208, 209
Otosclerosis 94, 117
Ototoxicity 147
Outer Ear 39

P

Paranasal Sinuses 28, 156, 185, 186, 195, 196, 199, 200, 214
Parapharyngeal Abscess 331
Patient management 1, 20, 438
Patient Management 20, 22, 169, 171
Patient Workflow Optimization 461
Perichondritis 68, 71, 87
Perilymph Fistula 147

Peritonsillar Abscess 315, 331, 334
Pharyngitis 317, 318, 331, 333
Pharyngology 28
Pharynx 279, 301
Physical aspect 338
Physical deformity 338
Physical Examination 109, 110, 134, 135, 207, 208, 320
Physical trauma 65
Physiology 35, 51, 52, 55, 62, 185, 187, 192, 199, 214, 247, 275, 277, 285, 289, 303
Postgraduate program 438
Postnasal Drip 271
Postoperative Care 20, 21, 169, 171
Practice management 433, 434, 435, 436, 437, 438, 439, 444, 445, 447, 448, 451, 453, 454, 455, 456, 458, 459, 460
Practitioners 434, 440, 448, 456
Preoperative Assessment 20, 169, 170
Presbycusis 147
Pre-surgical planning 413
Prevention Strategies 82, 232, 326
Preventive Measures 76, 78, 113, 115, 266
Primary operation 401
Production 434, 435, 437, 440, 445, 446
Propensity 404
Psychological 401, 402, 403, 404, 405, 406, 408, 410, 411, 412, 413, 414, 415, 416, 417, 419, 420, 422, 423, 425, 426, 428
Psychological issues 338
Psychological recovery 339, 340, 344
Psychosocial adaptation 371, 376
Psychosocial sequelae 402
Psychosocial well-being 373
Pure Tone Audiometry 178

Q

Quadrantectomy 408
Quality Assurance 461
Quinsy 331

R

Radiofrequency Devices 461
Reconstructive surgeon 402
Recovery 20, 21, 169, 171
Recruitment 178
Recurrent Laryngeal Nerve 301
Regional Flap 429
Regulatory Compliance 461
Rehabilitation 50, 116, 138, 140, 151, 153, 154, 162, 164, 169, 182, 184
Respiratory Epithelium 212
Responsibility 444, 455, 458
Retraction Pocket 117
Retropharyngeal Abscess 271, 331
Rhinitis 218, 233, 237, 239, 241
Rhinology 28
Rhinosinusitis 23, 30, 237, 241
Rigid Fixation 363
Robotic-Assisted Surgery 461
Round Window 60

S

Salivary gland tumors 406
Scar Revision 363
Screening Audiometry 178
Semicircular Canals 28, 60
Septal Hematoma 237
Signal Transmission 47, 50
Sinusitis 9, 11, 158, 160, 200, 203, 205, 214, 221, 222, 223, 237, 240
Skin cells 94, 99, 112
Skin Grafting 429
Social Implications 142, 143
Social interaction 403, 408, 413, 424
Societal consequences 437
Societal opinions 437
Soft Palate 212
Soft Tissue Laceration Repair 363
Soft Tissue Reconstruction 363, 429
Sound Amplification 43, 46
Speech Audiometry 178
Squamous Cell Carcinoma 429
Squamous cell carcinoma (SCC) 406
Strategic planning 407
Subglottis 301

Surgical Interventions 76, 77, 113, 114, 138, 140, 228, 230, 232, 258, 260, 323, 325
Surgical outcome 445, 452
Surgical techniques 369, 375, 376, 388, 389, 391, 392, 396
Surgical Techniques 12, 14, 162, 163
Sustainable growth 441
Swimmer's Ear 69, 87
Symmetry 371, 372, 375, 376, 377, 378, 389, 391, 395
Symptoms 65, 68, 72, 73, 93, 105, 106, 119, 123, 128, 130, 144, 149, 203, 205, 215, 224, 225, 243, 252, 254, 255, 258, 260, 296, 297, 312, 313, 316, 318
Syndromic congenital 372
Syndromic Deformities 396
Systemic lupus erythematosus (SLE) 93, 105

T

Technology infusion 438
Teleconsultation 461
Tendency 433, 449, 452
Therapy 89, 138, 140, 273
Thornwaldt's Cyst 271
Throat 2, 4, 7, 9, 11, 153, 155, 157, 275, 276, 278, 281, 285, 293, 295, 326, 329, 333
Thyroid Cartilage 301
Titanium Plates and Screws 363
Tonsillar Hypertrophy 331
Tonsillitis 313, 314, 331
Tornwaldt's Disease 271
Toxicity 441
Transferring tissue 412
Trauma reconstruction 337, 338, 339, 340, 341, 342, 344, 345, 346, 347, 348, 349, 350, 353, 354, 355, 356, 357, 358, 359, 360, 361, 362, 363, 364, 366
Traumatic injuries 338, 341
Tubal Tonsil Hypertrophy 271
Tube Dysfunction 117
Tumor Removal 162, 163
Tumor Resection 429
Turbinate Hypertrophy 237
Turbinates 28, 212
Tympanic Membrane 28, 39, 42, 60, 120
Tympanic Membrane Perforation 117
Tympanometry 178
Tympanosclerosis 117

U

Ultrasound-Guided Procedures 461
ultraviolet (UV) 406

V

Vehicular accident 338
Vertigo 126, 129, 130, 131, 135, 143, 147
Vestibular 9, 36, 47, 49, 50, 55, 56, 64, 119, 120, 121, 123, 124, 125, 126, 127, 128, 130, 131, 138, 140, 142, 143, 147, 149, 150, 151, 152
Vestibular Disorders 64, 120, 123, 125, 130, 142, 143, 152
Vestibular Folds 301
Vestibular Migraine 147
Vestibular System 28, 47, 49, 55, 56, 124
Vestibule 212
Vestibulo-ocular reflex (VOR) 124
Virtual Surgical Simulation 461
Vocal Cord Nodules 158, 161, 296, 298
Vocal Cords 283, 301

W

Wave Transmission 51, 53

Z

Zygomaticomaxillary Complex (ZMC) 363